Drugs and the
Developing Brain

ADVANCES IN BEHAVIORAL BIOLOGY

Drugs and the Developing Brain

Edited by

Antonia Vernadakis

Associate Professor
Departments of Psychiatry and Pharmacology

and

Norman Weiner

Professor and Chairman
Department of Pharmacology

University of Colorado
School of Medicine
Denver, Colorado

PLENUM PRESS • NEW YORK - LONDON

Library of Congress Cataloging in Publication Data

Main entry under title:

Drugs and the developing brain.

(Advances in behavioral biology, v. 8)
Sponsored by Pfizer Pharmaceuticals.
Includes bibliographies.
1. Neuro-psychopharmacology. 2. Developmental neurology. I. Vernadakis,
Antonia, 1930- ed. II. Weiner, Norman, 1928- ed. III. Pfizer Pharmaceuticals.
[DNLM: 1. Brain—Drug effects—Congresses. 2. Brain—Embryology—Congresses.
3. Brain Chemistry—Drug effects—Congresses. W3 AD215 v. 8 1972/WL300
S89d 1972]
RM315.D83   615'.78   74-640
ISBN-13: 978-1-4684-3065-3   e-ISBN-13: 978-1-4684-3063-9
DOI: 10.1007/978-1-4684-3063-9

Proceedings of the symposium on "Drugs and the Developing Brain," held at
the University of Colorado, School of Medicine, Denver, Colorado,
December 18-20, 1972

© 1974 Plenum Press, New York
Softcover reprint of the hardcover 1st edition 1974

A Division of Plenum Publishing Corporation
227 West 17th Street, New York, N.Y. 10011

United Kingdom edition published by Plenum Press, London
A Division of Plenum Publishing Company, Ltd.
Davis House (4th Floor), 8 Scrubs Lane, Harlesden, London, NW10 6SE, England

ACKNOWLEDGMENTS

This symposium was sponsored by PFIZER PHARMACEUTICALS 235 East 42nd Street, New York, N.Y.

The editors are grateful to Miss Marilyn Robbins for her assistance throughout the organization of the symposium and the preparation of the proceedings.

PREFACE

The thalidomide tragedy which occurred slightly more than a
decade ago made public officials and the general public acutely
aware of the teratogenic potential of drugs. Although specialists
in pharmacology and developmental biology had been studying this
problem many years before, this catastrophic episode triggered
the passage of legislation which required that information about
the teratogenicity of drugs be produced before the drugs could be
available to the general public. Gross deformities in man produced
by drugs are frequently difficult to reproduce in experimental
animals and the changes which are produced in other animals are
frequently not translatable to humans. The problem of evaluating
the potential that drugs have to produce gross malformations is
small, however, compared to the evaluation of subtle but permanent
behavioral effects which drugs may exert upon the developing
organism. Nevertheless, many experimental studies in recent
years indicate that subtle biochemical changes produced by drugs
on brain tissue during critical periods of fetal or early postnatal maturation may become manifest subsequently as behavioral
deviations in early childhood or adolescence. Hyperkinetic
disorders, epilepsies and other developmental disabilities may
have a subtle biochemical imbalance, perhaps drug induced, as an
underlying factor.

This symposium was organized with the intent of bringing together prominent investigators who are working in different aspects
of brain development and who are interested in the effects of drugs
on the developing brain in order to discuss their findings, pro-
pose new theories, and open new avenues for future research. It
is only by discussing and exploring the enormous complexities of
brain development, the critical periods during which the developing brain is most vulnerable to exogenous agents, and the molecular
basis for brain vulnerability, that we will begin to understand
the nature and the significance of the actions of drugs on the
developing brain.

This symposium focuses on brain development, both at the cellular and organismic levels and covers such physiological aspects as electrical activity, myelinogenesis, neurotransmission, the blood-brain-barrier, the metabolism of the brain and the influence of drugs, hormones and environment (e.g., high altitude) thereon. An attempt has been made to relate molecular neurobiology to developmental disabilities such as epilepsy and the hyperkinetic syndrome. Evaluation of the therapy of these disorders also is discussed.

Although not all aspects of brain development have been covered in this symposium, we hope that these proceedings offer basic information and present experimental models which can be used to obtain information useful for clinical application. Finally, we hope that these proceedings will stimulate further research in the vitally important and growing field of Developmental Neuropharmacology.

Antonia Vernadakis and Norman Weiner

CONTENTS

CNS DRUGS: FUNCTIONAL DEVELOPMENT
Dominick P. Purpura, Chairman

DEVELOPMENT OF SYNAPTIC SUBSTRATES FOR DRUG ACTIONS

IN IMMATURE BRAIN

Dominick P. Purpura

Department of Anatomy and the Rose F. Kennedy Center

for Research in Mental Retardation and Human

Development, Albert Einstein College of Medicine,

Yeshiva University, Bronx, New York

INTRODUCTION AND DEFINITION OF PROBLEMS

Studies of the effects of drugs and hormones on the immature brain must of necessity proceed from an understanding of the nature of the neural and synaptic substrate that constitutes the primary target of action of the pharmacological agent under investigation. Unfortunately this has rarely been possible for the obvious reason that there is a paucity of data available on the organization and properties of different subsystems during the development of the central nervous system in different species. Development implies change, and this cardinal feature of maturation introduces variables in the assessment of drug action in immature animals which may be major determinants of overt effects. An instructive example of the manner in which the developmental processes may influence drug actions is illustrated in Fig. 1 which summarizes data obtained over a decade ago in studies of the effects of topically applied aliphatic ω-amino acids on the immature brain (Purpura, 1961a). In these studies local responses elicited by cortical surface stimulation were utilized to determine the responsiveness of axodendritic synaptic pathways (Purpura, 1961b) to ε-amino caproic acid, a six-carbon aliphatic ω-amino acid which in adult animals produces rapid potentiation of superficial negative responses and subsequent convulsant activity (Purpura et al., 1959). In contrast to this effect observed in adult animals, topically applied ε-amino caproic acid produced only minimal depression of the superficial negative response of cortex in

3

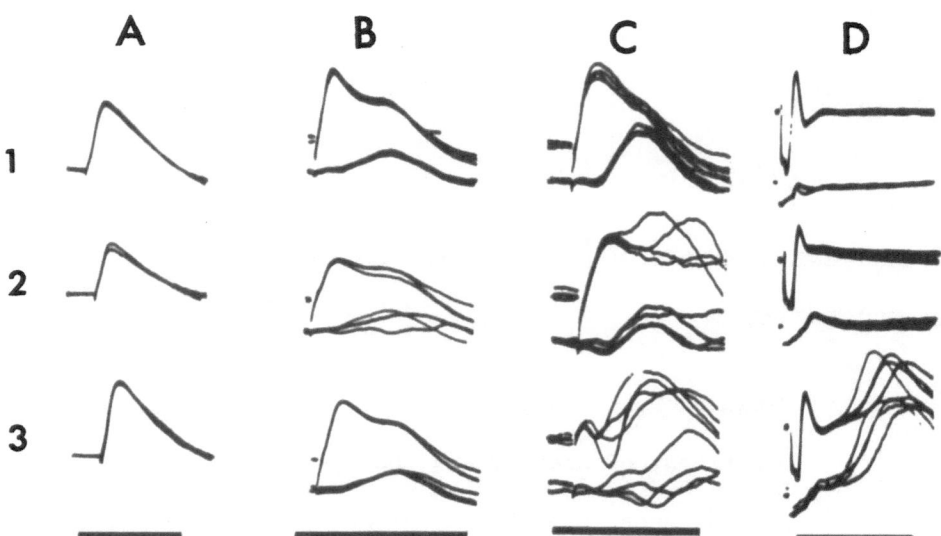

Fig. 1. A-C: Changing responsiveness of superficial neocortical axodendritic synaptic pathways to topically applied ε-amino caproic acid (C_6). A, newborn kitten; b, 7-day-old kitten; c, 15-day-old kitten. In these studies superficial negative responses were elicited by local cortical stimulation and recorded monopolarly close to the site of stimulation in A and upper channels in B and C. Lower channel responses in B and C were recorded at 5 and 6 mm, respectively from the site of stimulation. 1, control responses; 2, effect of topically applied C_6; 3, responses observed after removal of C_6. Note in C onset of seizure activity. D: Responses recorded at two sites along the ventricular surface of the exposed hippocampus in a 2-day-old kitten. Upper channel, response to fimbrial stimulation recorded at the fimbrial-hippocampal junction. Lower channel, responses several millimeters away. 1, control; 2, few seconds after C_6 application to hippocampal surface; 3, development of convulsant activity due to C_6. Time bar: 1 sec throughout. A-C, modified from Purpura, 1961a; D, unpublished observations.

newborn kittens (Fig. 1A). Similar effects were observed even as late as the end of the first postnatal week (Fig. 1B). Indeed this agent did not produce convulsant effects typically observed in adult animals until the second postnatal week (Fig. 1C). At this time much of the development of axodendritic and axosomatic synaptic systems in kitten neocortex has been completed (Noback and Purpura, 1961; Purpura et al., 1964; Voeller, Pappas and Purpura, 1963). By way of contrast it should be noted that whereas ε-amino caproic acid was relatively inert when applied to the neocortex of the very young kitten such was not the case when the amino acid was applied to the exposed ventricular surface of the hippocampus in neonatal animals. Responses elicited from the hippocampus by fimbria or fornix stimulation were found to be potentiated by the drug (Fig. 1D).

Despite several years of additional morphophysiological studies on the immature feline brain it is still not possible to provide a completely satisfactory explanation for the changing responsiveness of cortical synaptic systems to convulsant ω-amino acid drugs during postnatal development. Brief discussion of Fig. 1 may serve to underscore the nature of the problem at hand.

Consider the question of the differential responsiveness of hippocampal as opposed to neocortical neuronal organizations to the amino acid in the neonatal animal. One obvious explanation of this difference in drug responsiveness may be sought in the relative maturational status of synaptic systems in these fundamentally different types of cortical structure. Unlike the situation encountered in the neocortex, pyramidal neurons of the hippocampus in the neonatal kitten exhibit a precocious development of their dendritic systems (Purpura, 1964; Purpura and Pappas, 1968). Additionally, electron microscope observations indicate a relatively mature appearing neuropil containing many axodendritic and axo-spinodendritic synapses in the neonatal kitten hippocampus (Schwartz, Pappas and Purpura, 1968). However, as in the case of the neocortex (Voeller, Pappas and Purpura, 1963) axosomatic synapses on pyramidal neurons are rarely encountered in the neonatal period (Schwartz, Pappas and Purpura, 1968). Thus whatever differences in synaptic substrate may account for the increased responsiveness of hippocampal neuronal organizations to ε-amino caproic acid in the neonatal period must be referable solely to the accelerated maturation of axodendritic synaptic systems in the hippocampus as compared to neocortex. This raises the question of what differences if any are detectable in the functional activity of synapses in the two cortical structures in the neonatal period and during postnatal development. Answers to this question require data that can only be obtained by intracellular recording from immature neurons. Before considering the synaptic events observed in studies of immature neocortical and hippocampal neurons an additional point may be made in respect to the findings summarized in Fig. 1. At the time these studies were published (Purpura, 1961a) it seemed reasonable to assume that the lack of responsiveness of immature neocortical neurons to the convulsant amino acid could be explained by the delayed development of axodendritic inhibitory synapses whose blockade by the amino acid was postulated to be the basis for the convulsant action observed in adult animals (Purpura et al., 1959). Suffice it to say that this proposed interpretation exposed the hazards of what Gasser referred to as "trying to define a process from a potential". Fortunately, the notion that inhibitory synaptic pathways in immature cortex are

poorly developed in the neonatal period could be put to the test of
intracellular recording, which failed to substantiate this hypothesis, as will be shown below. However, the lesson learned from
attempts to define drug actions from studies of gross evoked
potentials merits consideration particularly since this method is
likely to be preferred in ontogenetic studies because of the
technical difficulties of applying microphysiological approaches to
studies of the immature brain. In a word gross evoked potential
studies alone can never provide sufficient information on the
nature of the synaptic organization of neurons participating in the
generation of the evoked potential. While there may be significant
and predictable correlations between different components of evoked
potentials and extracellularly recorded single unit or multiunit
discharges of neurons (Purpura, 1959) only by combining extracellular field potential analysis with intracellular recording can
the complexity of the synaptic events which underlie the production
of evoked potentials be appreciated (Purpura, 1972a). This is not
to say that studies of changes in evoked potentials during postnatal development, when correlated with morphological analyses
(Purpura et al., 1964; Laemle, Benhamida, and Purpura, 1972) can
not provide important clues concerning changes in underlying
synaptic organization. But due to the complexity of the alterations in neuronal connectivity patterns during brain maturation
the simultaneous application of several neurophysiological strate-
gies is required in studies of drug actions on the immature brain.

INTRACELLULARLY RECORDED SYNAPTIC EVENTS
IN IMMATURE CORTICAL NEURONS

Intracellular studies of immature neocortical (Purpura,
Shofer and Scarff, 1965) and hippocampal neurons (Purpura, 1969;
Purpura, Prelevic and Santini, 1968) have disclosed several
features of the electrophysiological properties of these elements
and their synaptic relations which can be expected to significantly
influence the effects of a wide range of drugs, putative transmitters or hormones on the immature brain. First, it is evident
that immature neurons do not exhibit the range of spontaneous or
evoked discharge frequencies that are characteristically observed
in mature cortical neurons (Purpura, 1972a). Indeed although
relatively large amplitude EPSPs may be elicited in immature
cortical neurons in very young kittens, these rarely evoke more
than one or two spike potentials (Fig. 2A). This low level
repetitive responsiveness is undoubtedly related to spike potential
recovery processes although the kinetics underlying these events
in immature neurons remain obscure. (Detailed quantitative studies
of membrane properties of immature cortical neurons have not as yet
been successful due to technical difficulties of maintaining satisfactory recording conditions during bridge stimulation.)

A feature of the PSPs recorded from immature cortical neurons is their relatively long duration when compared with PSPs elicited by similar modes of stimulation in mature animals (Purpura, 1972a; Purpura et al., 1965) (Fig. 2). This applies to both EPSPs and IPSPs although the latter are by far the most prominent in both neocortical (Fig. 2D,E) and hippocampal neurons (Fig. 2F,G). The fact that prolonges IPSPs similar to those observed in mature hippocampal neurons can be observed in hippocampal neurons of neonatal animals following fimbria or fornix stimulation is of special interest from the standpoint of the mode of initiation of such inhibitory activities. In adult animals emphasis has been placed on the role of inhibitory basket cell-axosomatic synapses onto pyramidal neurons in the production of those IPSPs (Andersen, Eccles and Løyning, 1964a, 1964b). However, electron microscopic observations indicate that in the neonatal period axosomatic synapses of the type postulated to mediate the IPSPs of mature pyramidal neurons are rarely encountered in the stratum pyramidale (Schwartz, Pappas and Purpura, 1968). Consequently it must be inferred that the IPSPs observed in hippocampal pyramidal neurons of very young kittens are generated by axodendritic synaptic inputs and only later in the postnatal period are axosomatic inhibitory synapses acquired by pyramidal neurons (Purpura, 1969). It should be noted that recent morphological studies of the comparative development of synaptic pathways related to dendritic systems of hippocampal neurons as opposed to the cell bodies of these elements (basket cell plexus of the stratum pyramidale) have confirmed the relatively delayed maturation of axosomatic systems in the human hippocampus (Purpura, 1973).

The observations pointing to a dramatic change in the organization of inhibitory synaptic inputs to cortical neurons during postnatal development clearly require close attention in assessment of the mechanisms of drug actions on cortical structures at different developmental stages. This is especially pertinent to studies of pharmacological agents which may exert their effects largely at inhibitory synapses. As yet there is no evidence that axosomatic inhibitory synapses on a particular class of neurons are pharmacologically different from axodendritic inhibitory synapses. But this possibility has not been excluded and remains an intriguing problem for future investigators in developmental neuropharmacology.

Immature cortical neurons differ from neurons encountered in adult animals in respect to the frequency with which they exhibit partial responses and propagating spike potentials in dendrites (Purpura, 1967; Purpura, Shofer and Scarff, 1965; Purpura, Prelevic and Santini, 1968). Examples of these dendritic partial responses and spikes are illustrated in Fig. 2C and 2H, respectively. The capacity of dendrites of immature cortical neurons to show spike initiation and propagation may be viewed as a mechanism for

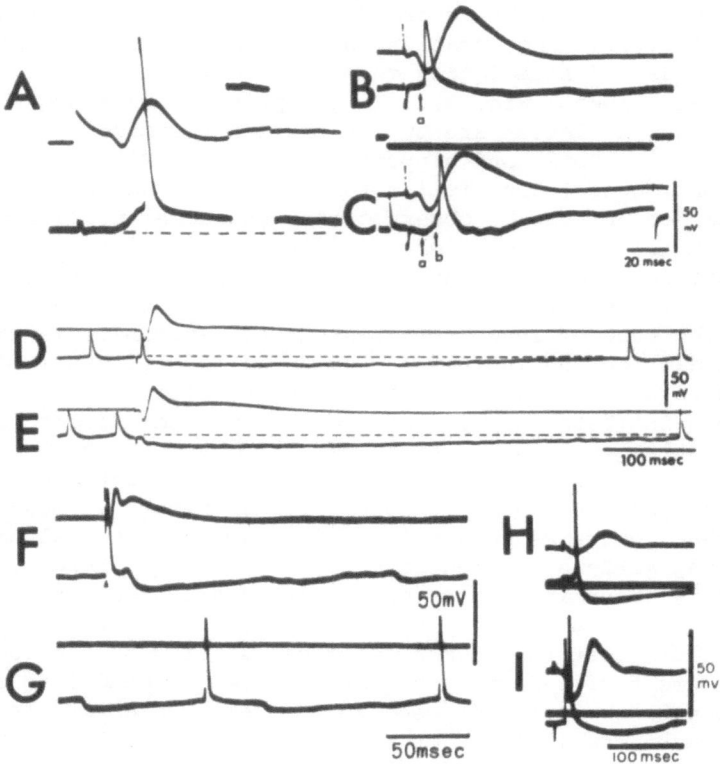

Fig. 2.   Examples of spike potentials and synaptic activities intracellularly recorded from neocortical and hippocampal neurons in the
neonatal and young kitten.   A: Prolonged EPSP (80 to 100 msec)
evoked by ventrolateral thalamic stimulation in a sensorimotor cortex neuron from a 6-day-old kitten.   In this and other dual-channel
recordings, the upper channel records indicate cortical surface
activity, negativity upwards.   Weak stimulation elicits and 18- to
20 msec latency EPSP with a slow rise time and prolonged declining
phase.   Calibration: 50 mV, 20 msec.   B and C: Appearance of
partial response during induced soma hyperpolarization in a neuron
from a 24-day-old kitten.   B: Ventrolateral thalamic stimulation
elicits a 5 msec latency small EPSP (at arrow, A) and a cell discharge.   C: During soma hyperpolarization (indicated by first
trace), the EPSP is augmented and a second component is revealed,
b, which is succeeded by a spike potential.   The response revealed
at b, is presumably due to a dendritic partial spike.   D and E:
Prolonged IPSPs recorded from a sensorimotor cortex neuron in a
24-day-old kitten.   Examples are shown of two responses to single-
shock stimulation of the ventrolateral thalamus.   Broken horizontal lines are drawn through base lines to facilitate estimation of
IPSP duration, which may attain a value of 600 msec.   F and G:
Spontaneous and evoked IPSPs in a hippocampal pyramidal neuron from
a 3-day-old kitten.   Upper trace, hippocampal surface evoked response

enhancing the effectiveness of sparsely distributed excitatory
synapses at early developmental stages (Purpura, 1969). This
property is generally "suppressed" in normal adult neocortical
neurons and only partially "suppressed" in mature hippocampal
neurons (Purpura, 1967, 1972a). Nothing can be said at this time
as to how the property of dendritic spike electrogenesis may influence the responsiveness of immature cortical neurons to convulsant pharmacological agents. Examination of the effects of
topically applied penicillin to kitten neocortex has as yet provided no evidence that the paroxysmal activity recorded in
immature neurons is referable to spike generation and propagation
in dendrites (Prince and Gutnick, 1971).

FACTORS INFLUENCING PROPAGATION OF EVOKED ACTIVITY
IN IMMATURE CORTEX

Two factors determine the ease with which topically applied
convulsant agents may initiate seizure activity which propagates
from the area of drug application. The first is related to the
responsiveness of elements at the site of seizure initiation; the
second depends upon the degree of synaptic coupling between locally
involved neurons and distant neuronal organizations. In the case
of immature cortex local responsiveness, as indicated above, may
be determined by the developmental states of the synaptic substrate
for the drug action, the excitability of activated neurons and the
degree to which relatively well developed local inhibitory circuits
are simultaneously activated along with excitatory synaptic pathways. Given the situation in which a "critical mass" of immature
cortex becomes involved in paroxysmal activity the capacity for
spread of this activity to distant cortical sites will be determined
by the extent to which short and long intracortical synaptic pathways have attained structural and functional maturation.

Fig. 2 (cont'd). to fimbrial stimulation. H and I. Examples of
changing characteristics of spike potentials recorded in a sensorimotor cortex neuron from a 3-week-old kitten during single shock
(H), and during 5/sec ventrolateral thalamic stimulation (I) which
elicited cortical surface augmenting responses. In H, the thalamic
stimulus evokes a typical spike potential which arises from an EPSP.
During summation of IPSPs, thalamic stimulation elicits spikes
without depolarizing prepotentials which arise from a level of increased membrane polarization. Such spikes are generated in dendrites and propagate in an all-or-none fashion into the soma.
A-E, H and I, modified from Purpura et al., 1965; F and G from
Purpura et al., 1968.

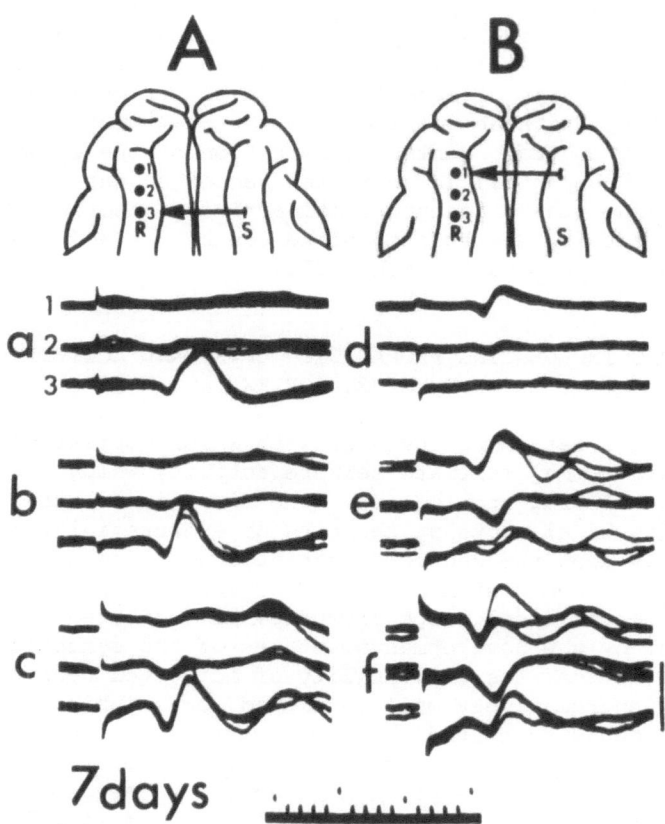

Fig. 3. Spread of transcallosally evoked responses in AMSG of a 7-day-old kitten. Diagrams illustrate stimulating conditions for each column of records in A and B. A, Stimulation of the homotopic-R_3 site. (a) Weak stimulation (twice threshold, 2T) at 0.5/sec elicits a prominent homotopic-R_3 response. (b) Increase in strength of stimulation (3T) increases the surface-positive component of the homotopic-R_3 TCR and produces a small response at the nonhomotopic-R_2 site. (c) Supramaximal stimulation produces little change in the homotopic-R_3 TCR but elicits small responses at R_2 and R_1. B, (d-f) Stimulus intensities as in a, b and c, respectively. Note that supramaximal stimulation (f) elicits prominent responses of different configuration at nonhomotopic R_2 and R_3 sites. The data indicate a preferential spread of TCRs in the rostral-to-caudal direction. Calibrations 100 cycle/sec, 200 µV.
From: Shofer and Purpura, 1972.

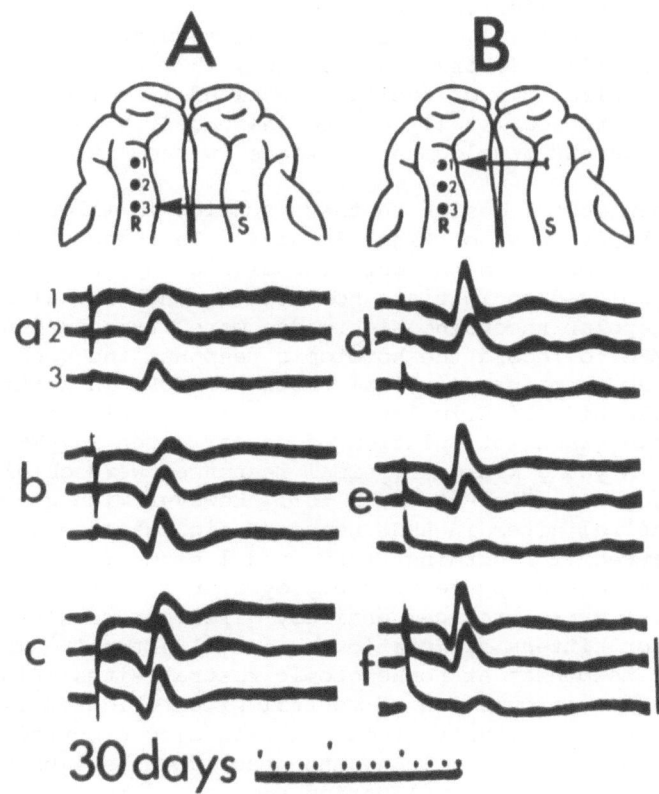

Fig. 4. Spread of transcallosally evoked responses in AMSG of a
30-day-old kitten. Diagrams illustrate stimulating conditions for
each column of records in A and B. A, Stimulation of the homo-
topic-R_3 site. (a) Weak stimulation (0.5/sec) elicits TCRs which
are detectable at all recording sites. (b and c) Progressive increase in stimulus strength enhances all TCRs. B, (d-f) Stimulus
intensities in a, b and c, respectively. Supramaximal stimulation
(f) elicits prominent responses at the R_1 and R_2 site but only a
very small long-latency response is detectable at the nonhomo-
topic-R_3 site. The data indicate a preferential spread of TCRs in
the caudal-to-rostral direction (compare with Fig. 3). Calibrations 100 cycle/sec, 300 μV. From: Shofer and Purpura, 1972.

It has not been recognized until recently that spread of evoked activity in cortex initiated by direct (Brown and Pinsky, 1971) or synaptic activation (Shofer and Purpura, 1972) may occur in a nonuniform fashion but exhibit preferential directionality. What is more the preferred direction of spread of evoked activity may change as a function of the postnatal maturation of intra-cortical connections (Shofer and Purpura, 1972). Figs. 3 and 4 serve to summarize some of the data obtained in recent studies of the spread of transcallosally evoked responses in association cortex at different developmental stages in the kitten.

The experimental design in these studies is illustrated with respect to the diagrams of Figs. 3 and 4. In these studies local stimulation of cortex in the anterior middle suprasylvian gyrus (AMSG) was employed to initiate homotopic transcallosal responses (TCRs). Monopolar recording electrodes were arranged linearly along the AMSG to record the homotopic response and nonhomotopic TCRs resulting from intracortical spread of TCRs in cortex contra-lateral to the side of stimulation (S). The results of Fig. 3 show that when graded stimulation of caudal sites in AMSG was carried out in young kittens minimal responses were observed at nonhomotopic sites (Fig. 3A, a, b, c). However with graded stimu-lation of rostral sites in AMSG nonhomotopic responses were readily observed in recordings from caudal sites (Fig. 3B, d, e, f). The same experimental procedures employed in studies of kittens older than 3-4 weeks produced entirely different results (Fig. 4). In these older kittens stimulation of caudal sites in AMSG resulted in prominent responses at nonhomotopic rostral sites (Fig. 4A, a, b, c) whereas stimulation at rostral sites elicited little or no significant evoked activity at caudal recording electrode place-ments (Fig. 4B, d, e, f). These and other data have been taken to indicate that in the neonatal period and up to about the second postnatal week transcallosally evoked activity spreads preferential-ly in a rostral-to-caudal direction. At a later developmental stage this preferred direction of spread reverses so that caudal-to-rostral spread predominates (Shofer and Purpura, 1972).

The significance of the foregoing observations cannot be assessed apart from suggesting the obvious, i.e., that this develop-mental change in the preferred direction of propagation of trans-callosally evoked activity may be related to the functional de-velopment of interhemispheric transactions in association cortex. The reversal of preferred cortical spread of transcallosally evoked activity during late postnatal development represents a maturational change in the functional organization of cortex that could not have been predicted from previous morphophysiological studies on the immature brain.

For present purposes the manner in which the studies of TCR spread in immature association cortex may be utilized in evaluating

pharmacological actions of agents such as dibutyryl cyclic adenosine monophosphate (Purpura and Shofer, 1972) is shown in Figs. 5
and 6. Dibutyryl cyclic AMP when topically applied to recording
sites in AMSG in very young kittens in Ringer's solution containing 0.2 mM of the nucleotide, results in rapid potentiation of
homotopic TCRs (Fig. 5E). In these early stages of enhanced
excitability convulsant activity is generally confined to homotopic
sites of maximal TCR input. Of particular interest are observations indicating that dibutyryl cyclic AMP may enhance the development of nonhomotopic TCRs, presumably by facilitation of intracortical synaptic pathways (Fig. 5H). After continued application
of the cyclic nucleotide to all sites of registration convulsant
activity may appear at all sites (Fig. 5J). However a singular
feature of this activity is its independent nature at different
sites of registration which is indicative of the relatively poor
synaptic coupling between adjacent areas of immature cortex in the
early postnatal period (cf. also Fig. 6).

The excitatory effects of dibutyryl cyclic AMP on immature
cortical neuronal organizations demonstrate a remarkable <u>potential</u>
functional capacity of immature neuronal and synaptic subsystems
when these have been appropriately activated. However, again it
must be emphasized that the overt convulsant action of dibutyryl
cyclic AMP on immature cortex as reflected in changes in transcallosally evoked responses or spontaneous seizures provides no
information on the synaptic or neural substrate that is predominantly affected by the cyclic nucleotide. What is clear is that
the previously reported inhibitory effects of dibutyryl cyclic AMP
on Purkinje cells of the cerebellum (Siggins <u>et al.</u>, 1971) cannot
be generalized to other synaptic systems unless one postulates that
the convulsant effects observed in immature cortex are a consequence
of selective inhibition of an inhibitory system that limits the
excitability of a considerable number of cortical neurons. In view
of preliminary studies indicating that IPSPs are prominently displayed in transcallosally evoked intracellular synaptic events in
immature cortex (Fig. 7) it must be left for future work to determine the action of dibutyryl cyclic AMP and other cyclic nucleotides
on these inhibitory activities.

DEVELOPMENT OF INTRATHALAMIC SYNAPTIC ORGANIZATIONS

The ready accessibility of cortical structures for evoked potential and extra- and intracellular studies has undoubtedly contributed to the relatively large number of investigations in which
immature cerebral and cerebellar cortex have been emphasized to the
virtual exclusion of subcortical neuronal subsystems. Still it
must be recognized that the cerebral cortex does not carry out its
complex functions in isolation but in conjunction with thalamic
nuclear organizations that give rise to the major afferent projection

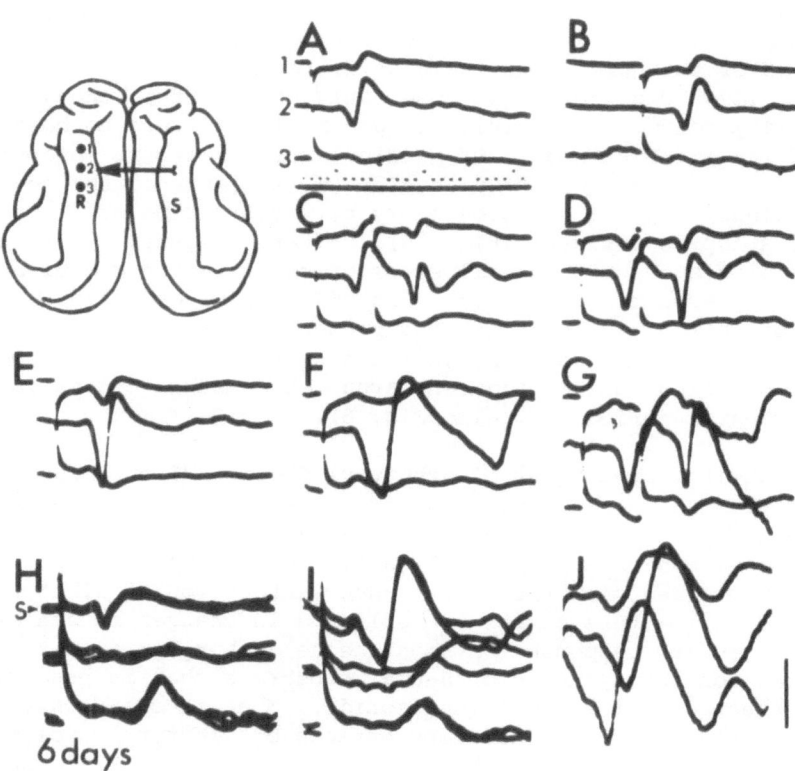

Fig. 5. Effects of topically applied dibutyryl cyclic AMP on transcallosal evoked responses (TCR) and spontaneous activity of immature
feline cerebral cortex (6-day-old kitten). Inset shows arrangement
of three monopolar recording electrodes on left suprasylvian gyrus
(indifferent electrode on temporal muscle). Separation of 2 mm
between adjacent pairs of recording electrodes. The homotopic site
opposite the R_2 recording electrode was stimulated to evoke the
responses shown in A-G. A and B, Conditioning and testing responses,
respectively (negativity upwards). C, Paired responses. D, 10 min
following application of 0.2 mM dibutyryl cyclic AMP to all recording sites. E, 5 min after D. F and G, 10 min after additional dibutyryl cyclic AMP. Convulsant activity is evident. In H and I
stimulation was homotopic to R_1. Note the appearance of a prominent
surface negative response at R_3. J, Seizure activity recorded with
different temporal and electrographic characteristics at the three
recording sites. Time calibration, 10 msec intervals. Amplitude
0.2 mV. From: Purpura and Shofer, 1972.

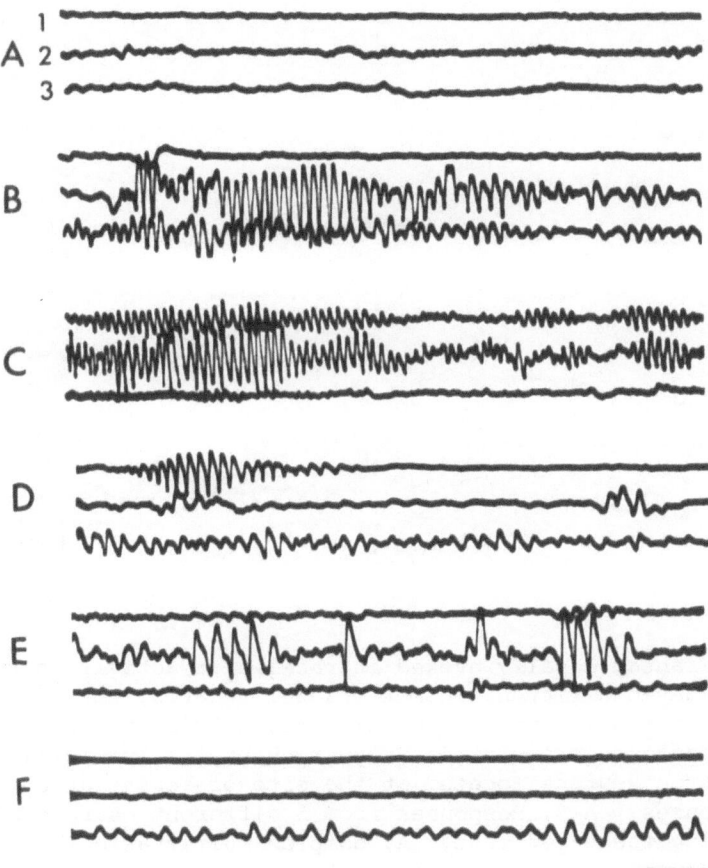

Fig. 6. Convulsant action of topically applied dibutyryl cyclic
AMP in a 6-day-old kitten. 1, 2, 3: Activity recorded monopolarly
from a linear array of electrodes located on the middle suprasylvian
gyrus, each electrode separated by 2 mm. A: Interictal activity.
B-F: Various stages during the action of the dibutyryl cyclic AMP.
Note that convulsant activity may be limited to sites 2 and 3 (B),
1 and 2 (C), 2 (E), or 3 (F). This independence of convulsant
activity is indicative of loose synaptic coupling between areas of
registration. From: Purpura, 1972b.

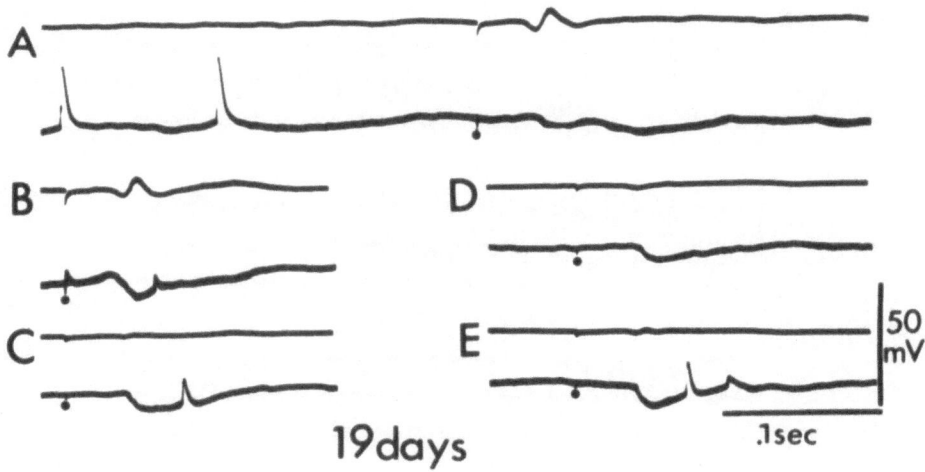

Fig. 7. Transcallosally evoked intracellular activities recorded
from a 19-day-old kitten. Upper channel records, cortical surface
responses evoked in anterior middle suprasylvian gyrus by contra-
lateral homotopic stimulation. Lower channel: Intracellular recordings from neurons located at the site of registration of surface responses. A-E, Responses from 5 different neurons at varying
times during the experiment. A, complex multiphasic IPSPs are
elicited in association with the TCR. In B, the IPSP is preceded
by a small EPSP. C, D and E, Long latency IPSPs are detected in
cortical neurons despite the absence of significant surface evoked
potential activity. Partial responses are observed on falling
phases of IPSPs in B, C and E as a consequence of partial restoration of membrane potential by IPSPs in damaged neurons.
From: Shofer and Purpura, unpublished observations.

systems to cortex. Thus without an adequate appreciation of the
maturational status of intrathalamic synaptic pathways involved in
the regulation of cortical activity analyses of cortical neuronal
organizations alone must be considered incomplete, at best. For
this reason recent studies from our laboratory (Thatcher and Purpura,
1972) have focused on attempts to define the functional characteristics of intrathalamic synaptic pathways which in adult animals play
a major role in the production of EEG-synchronization and EEG-
desynchronization.

As background for these studies it should be recalled that in
adult animals low-frequency (6-12 per sec) stimulation of medial
and intralaminar "nonspecific" thalamic nuclei typically elicits
recruiting responses in widespread areas of cortex as a consequence
of the production of prolonged EPSP-IPSP sequences in thalamic
neurons, many of which have projections to cortex (Purpura and
Cohen, 1962; Purpura and Shofer, 1963). The discovery of these
EPSP-IPSP sequences has provided the basis for an understanding of
how intrathalamic, internuclear synaptic pathways operate to produce synchronized discharges in many organizations of thalamic
neurons (Purpura, 1970, 1972a). It has been shown that the most
significant synaptic event in the intrathalamic synchronization
process is the prolonged 100-200 msec IPSP observed during low-
frequency medial thalamus (MTh) stimulation in a large proportion
of thalamic neurons. Such IPSPs are also observed in adult animals
during spontaneous and evoked spindle-waves in thalamus and cortex
(Purpura, 1972a). Characteristic of the transition from EEG-
synchronization to EEG-desynchronization elicited by high-frequency
stimulation of medial thalamic nuclei is the rapid inhibition of
synchronizing-IPSPs and the production of powerful excitatory synaptic drives in thalamic neurons (Purpura and Shofer, 1963).

It has long been known that in very young kittens low-frequency
stimulation of thalamic and brain stem reticular regions does not
result in typical recruiting responses (Purpura, 1961b). Studies
of the ontogenesis of sleep-wakefulness activities in a variety of
mammals have revealed a paucity of slow-wave or spindle bursts and
a predominance of low-voltage activity during sleep stages
(cf. Clemente, Purpura and Mayer, 1972). Indeed it seems likely
that the maturation of sleep patterns in altricial mammals involves
largely the development of slow wave or "quite" sleep which comes
to dominate a larger proportion of the total sleep time with advancing postnatal age.

Since the development of thalamic synaptic processes underlying
the maturation of thalamocortical synchronization can be expected to
be of considerable importance in studies of drug effects on sleep
mechanisms in immature animals it is appropriate to briefly summarize preliminary findings on this subject (Thatcher and Purpura,
1972).

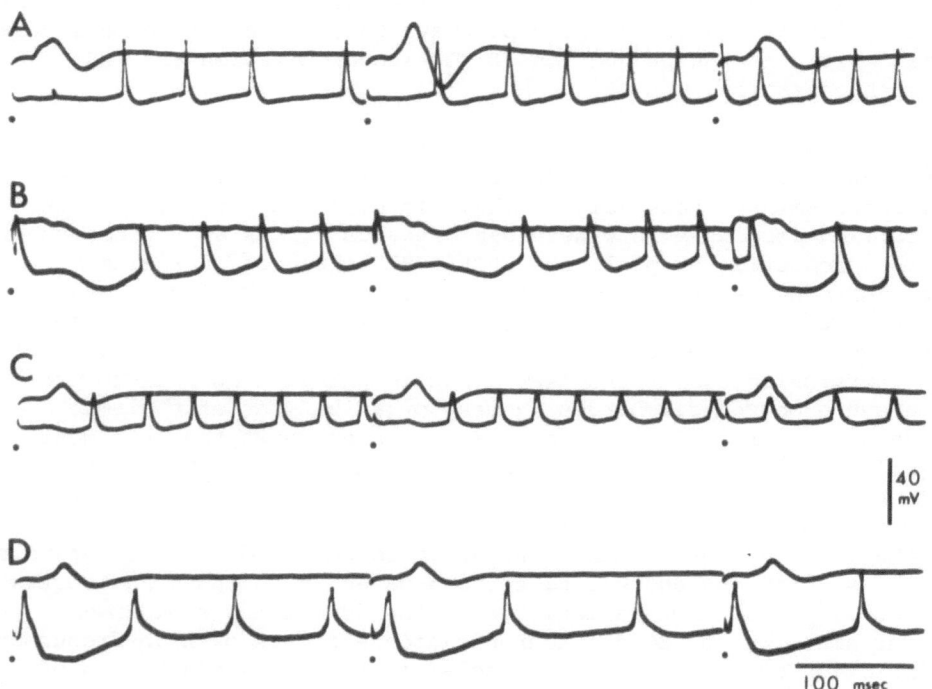

Fig. 8. Examples of intracellularly recorded responses in 4 different thalamic neurons during low-frequency (3/sec) medial thalamic
(MTh) stimulation. A, C and D, from the same 3-day-old kitten.
B, from a 2-day-old kitten. Upper channel records (negativity
upwards) show responses evoked from sensorimotor cortex during continued MTh-stimulus. A, MTh-stimulation does not elicit a detectable IPSP but there is slowing of discharge rate during period
corresponding to evoked IPSPs in other cells from the same preparation (C and D). Note multiple spike components in D. Such
spike potential discontinuities are often seen in immature neurons
partially damaged by impalement (Purpura, Shofer and Scarff, 1965).
 Several of the IPSPs in B and C exhibit small superimposed EPSPs
which are curtailed by late phases of the IPSP.
From: Thatcher and Purpura, 1972.

Intracellular recordings from thalamic neurons have revealed that unlike the responses observed in mature animals during low-frequency medial thalamic (MTh) stimulation, such stimulation in neonatal and young kittens does not result in prolonged EPSP-IPSP sequences. Although IPSPs have been detected in a large proportion of thalamic neurons during very low frequency (3 per sec) MTh stimulation such IPSPs lack the prolonged duration observed in older kittens and adult animals (Fig. 8). Another difference between young and older kittens is to be seen in the relatively few and weak MTh-evoked EPSPs observed in the neonatal and young kittens. Thus the failure to produce typical recruiting responses in very young kittens must be ascribed to the functional immaturity of intrathalamic internuclear synaptic pathways involved in the thalamocortical synchronizing process. Specifically in the absence of prolonged IPSPs (in excess of 100 msec) and prior EPSPs there is little or no effective widespread synchronization of thalamic neuronal discharges.

The relative weakness of excitatory synaptic activity evoked in thalamic neurons of very young kittens by low-frequency MTh-stimulation undoubtedly contributes to the failure of high-frequency MTh-stimulation to produce sustained depolarizations in immature thalamic neurons as is the case in adult animals (Purpura and Shofer, 1963). Instead of a rapid and sustained depolarization which is typical of adult animals high-frequency MTh-stimulation in very young kittens results in sustained membrane hyperpolarization of thalamic neurons (Fig. 9).

Results obtained to date indicate that it is only after the second postnatal week that prolonged synchronizing IPSPs of the type observed in adult animals are detectable in intracellular recordings of immature thalamic neurons during low-frequency MTh-stimulation (Thatcher and Purpura, 1972) (Fig. 10). At the same time high-frequency MTh-stimulation becomes effective in producing sustained summation of EPSPs, a process that characterizes thalamically in-duced reticulocortical activation (Purpura and Shofer, 1963). Blockade of prolonged IPSPs with high-frequency MTh-stimulation also becomes prominent at this developmental stage as does the period of post-activation suppression of synchronizing-IPSPs as observed in mature cats (Fig. 10).

Summarizing the findings illustrated in Figs. 8-10, it can be concluded that whereas prolonged IPSPs are commonly observed in neocortical neurons of very young kittens such prolonged IPSPs are not observed in thalamic neurons. Rather as a consequence of the relatively short duration of MTh-evoked IPSPs (and the absence of well-developed EPSPs) widespread synchronization of thalamic neuronal discharge does not occur. Hence the lack of 8-12 per sec evoked synchronization or spindle bursts in neocortex in very young kittens is largely a consequence of the functional immaturity of interneuronal

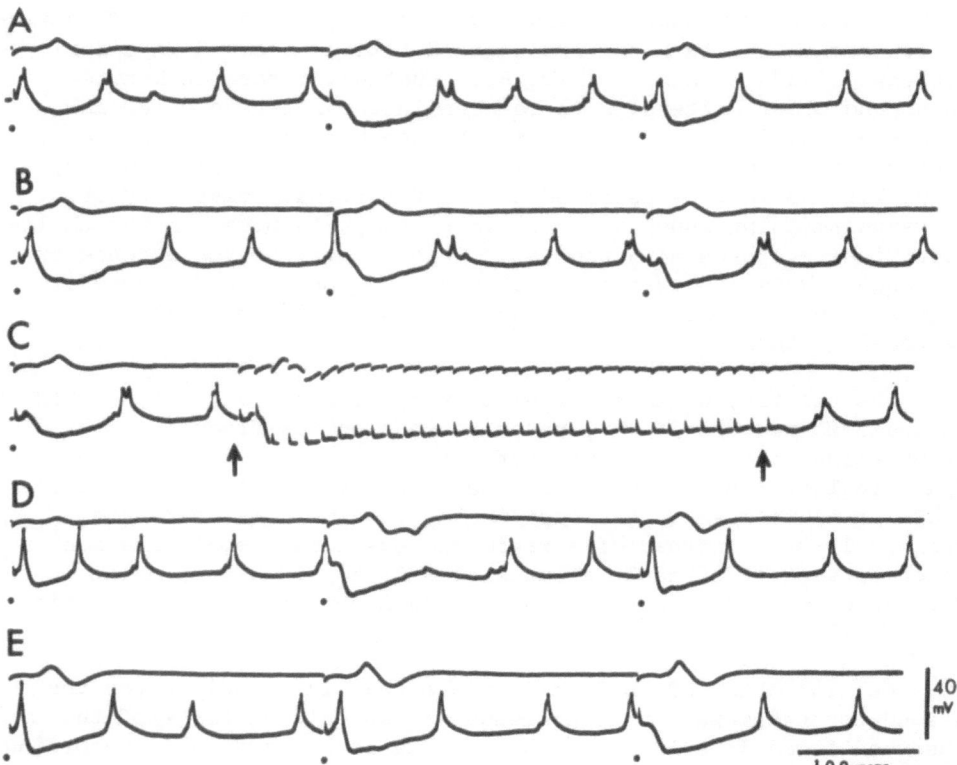

Fig. 9. Comparison of the postsynaptic effects of low (3/sec) and
high (80/sec) frequency MTh-stimulation observed in a thalamic
neuron in a 3-day-old kitten. A-E, continuous recording. A and B,
3/sec MTh-stimulation (dots) elicits prominent IPSPs. In C, between arrows, a period of high-frequency MTh-stimulation is introduced. Note summation of IPSPs and the attenuation of the IPSP
elicited by the last stimulus of the repetitive train. D, resumption of low-frequency stimulation (first dot) results in a markedly
attenuated IPSP. Subsequent IPSPs are simular to IPSPs elicited
prior to high-frequency MTh-stimulation.
From: Thatcher and Purpura, 1972.

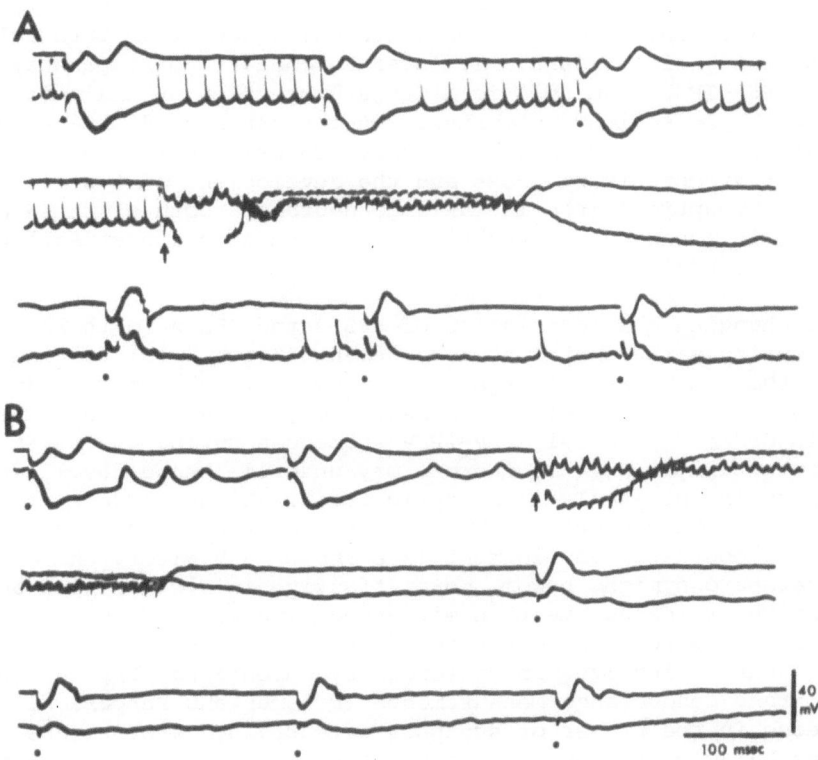

Fig. 10. Comparison of the postsynaptic effects of low (3/sec) and
high (80/sec) frequency MTh-stimulation observed in a thalamic neuron
in a 14-day-old kitten. A and B, recordings from two different
neurons. A, low frequency stimulation (dots) elicits prominent and
prolonged IPSPs which effectively suppress injury discharges. In
the second row high-frequency stimulation is initiated (at arrow).
The initial IPSP is followed by a sustained depolarization which
decreases slowly after termination of the stimulus. Resumption of
low-frequency stimulation (third row) now results in EPSPs which
initiate spike discharges but IPSPs remain blocked or attenuated.
B, same as in A but high-frequency stimulation is initiated towards
the end of the first row of records. Note the post-activation
facilitation of EPSPs and persisting attenuation of IPSPs. The
results of high-frequency MTh-stimulation in the 2-week-old animal
contrast sharply with the results shown in Fig. 9 from the 3-day-
old kitten. From: Thatcher and Purpura, unpublished observations.

synaptic organizations linked to nonspecific thalamic nuclei. This
implies that the maturation of sleep behavior which is largely reflected in the development of slow-wave or "quiet" sleep depends
upon the development of powerful synchronizing activities in thalamic neuronal organizations. Such synchronization is in turn related
to the capacity of intrathalamic interneuronal synaptic pathways to
generate EPSP-IPSP sequences in a large proportion of thalamic
neurons with projections to cortex. On the other hand EEG-desynchronization produced by high-frequency MTh-stimulation requires
blockade of synchronizing IPSPs and the development of powerful
excitatory synaptic drives in thalamic neurons. Both of these processes attain functional maturation after the second postnatal week
in the feline brain.

     The changing characteristics of EPSPs and IPSPs in thalamic
neurons during early postnatal development (Figs. 8-10) provide
evidence that intrathalamic synaptic pathways which are already
functional in the neonatal period become more effective in generating prolonged and powerful EPSP-IPSP sequences during the first two
weeks postnatally. Several factors may underlie these developmental
alterations in intrathalamic synaptic organizations. Since it is
known that immature neurons exhibit a greater repetitive responsiveness during postnatal development (see above) inhibitory and excitatory interneurons might become more effective in synthesizing and
releasing their respective transmitters during repetitive activity.
Indeed there are reasons to suspect continued transmitter action on
thalamic neurons involved in prolonged synchronizing IPSPs as judged
from membrane conductance measurements (Feldman and Purpura, 1970).
An increase in the number of synapses effected by interneurons in
the intrathalamic internuclear pathways may further contribute to
the functional maturation of EPSP-IPSP sequences.

     Electron microscope studies of the fine structural alterations
in thalamic synaptic organizations during the early postnatal period
suggest that there is indeed an increase in the number of axodendritic synapses observed during this developmental phase. However,
axosomatic synapses, which are infrequently encountered on thalamic
neurons in adult animals (Pappas, Cohen and Purpura, 1966) are rarely
observed in neonatal and even in 2-3 week old kittens. In searching
for difference in thalamic synaptic organization in neonatal and
older kittens one of the most intriguing findings has been noted in
respect to the development of complex synapses in glomerular arrange-
ments (Pappas and Purpura, in preparation). This can be appreciated
by comparison of the electron micrographs shown in Figs. 11 and 12
from 3-days old and 17-days old kittens, respectively. Although
axodendritic synapses are readily identified at both stages these
are diffusely distributed on trunks and spines of dendrites in the
neonatal period (Fig. 11). Characteristically in older kittens
some axodendritic synapses are surrounded by glial processes which
tend to segregate complex synapses into clusters that resemble the

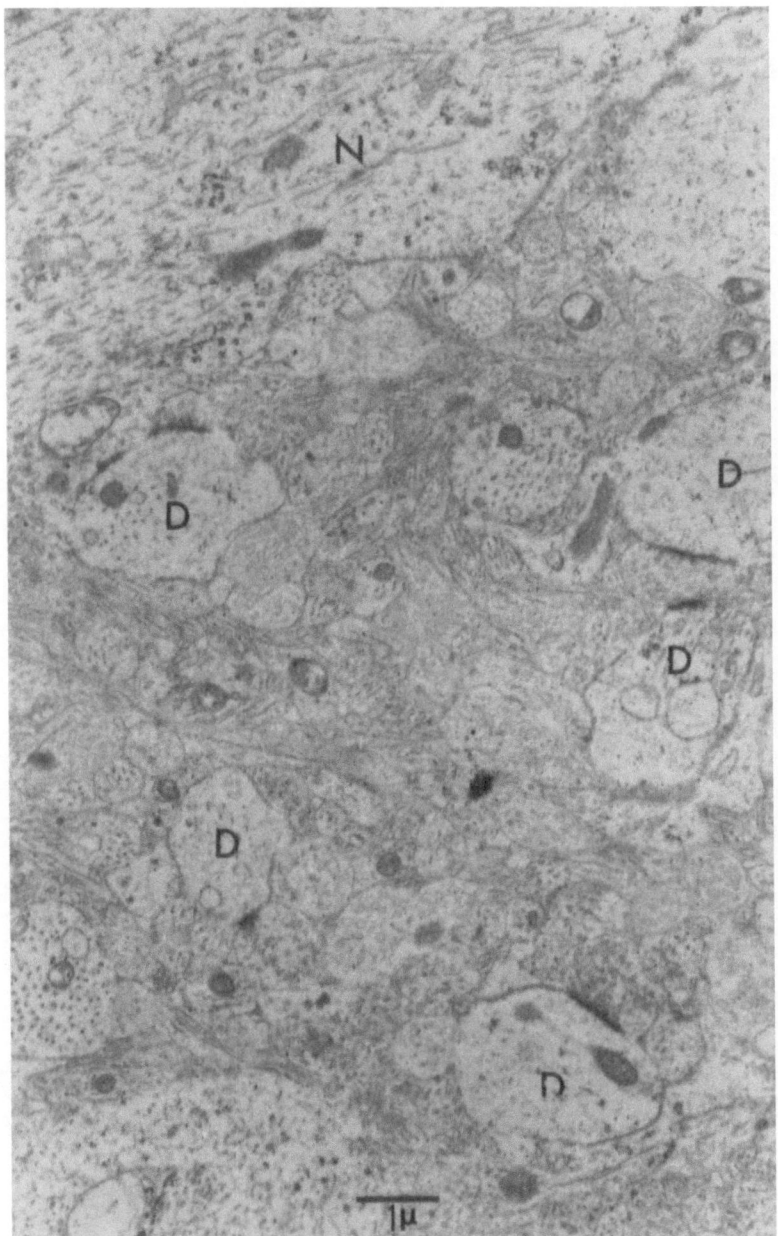

Fig. 11. Electron micrograph of a portion of the neuropil of the ventrolateral thalamus of a 3-day-old kitten. Typically no axosomatic synapses are present at this age. In the neuropil profiles of large dendritic processes can be seen as well as axodendritic synapses. N=neuron cell body; D=dendrites. Bar, 1 μm (X 12,000).
From: Pappas and Purpura, in preparation.

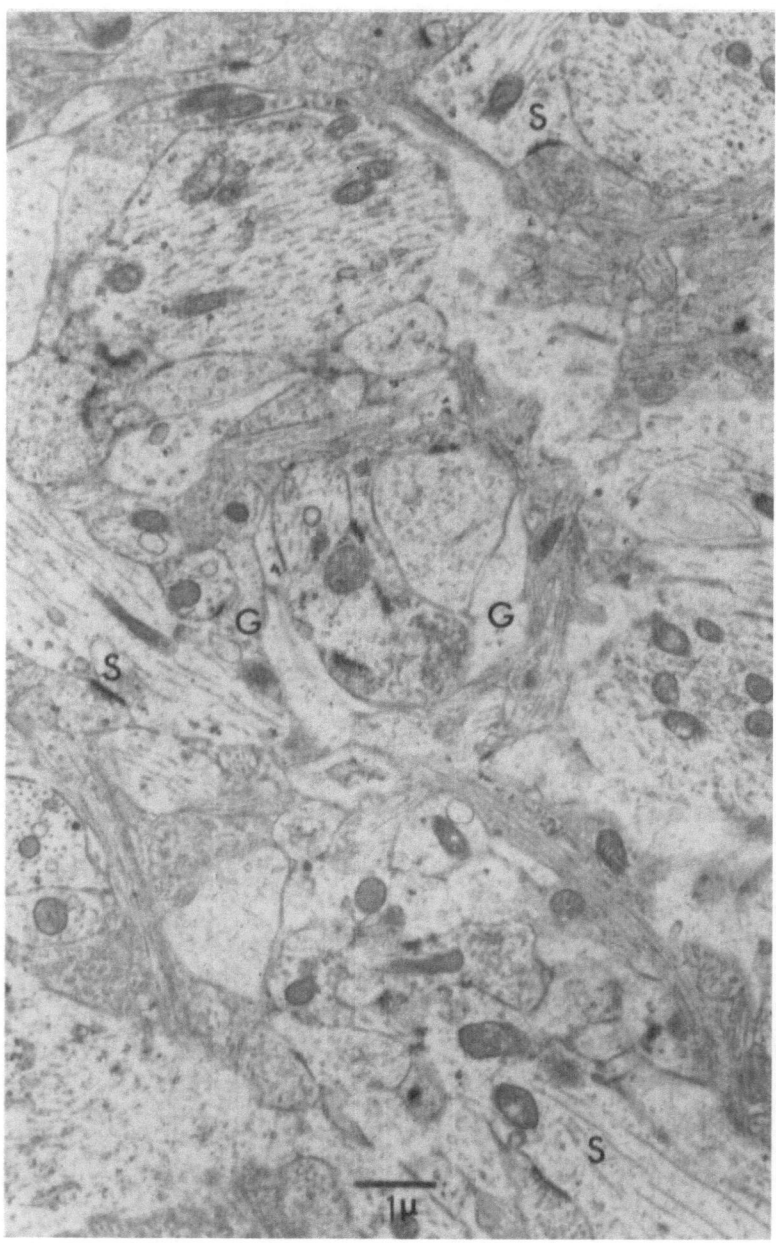

Fig. 12. Electron micrograph of a portion of the ventrolateral thalamus of a 17-day-old kitten. At this age small clusters of synapses are surrounded by glial processes (G), in glomerular arrangement. Isolated axodendritic synapses (S) are also detectable in the neuropil. Bar, 1 μm (X 12,000). From: Pappas and Purpura, in preparation.

glomerular structures of adult animals (Fig. 12). The question as
to whether this morphological development plays any role in pro-
longing the effectiveness of released transmitter at such synapses
remains unanswered. But it would be surprising indeed if these
morphological changes had no relation to the changing functional
operation of interneuronal synaptic pathways in thalamic neuronal
organizations during postnatal development.

It would be fatuous to maintain that the morphophysiological
alterations in intrathalamic synaptic pathways observed in the first
few weeks postnatally in the kitten are the sole determinants of the
maturation of the neural substrate underlying sleep-wakefulness behavior in this species. Evidence has accumulated in recent years
to the effect that a variety of complex basal forebrain and brain
stem subsystems rich in indole and catechol amines are implicated
in the development of sleep-wakefulness behaviors (Clemente, Purpura
and Mayer, 1972). How such serotonergic, dopaminergic and noradrenergic systems interact with cholinergic and other (GABA, glutamate,
taurine, glycine, etc.) transmitter operated systems remains a major
problem of general neurobiology. In the final analysis the functional development of these subsystems must be defined in terms of the
properties of neurons, synapses and probably glia at different
neuraxial sites. However technically difficult it may be to provide
rigorous neurophysiological and neuropharmacological data on these
subsystems in the immature brain, it is unreasonable to hope for the
emergence of a coherent body of information concerning 'developmental neuropsychopharmacology' without making an effort equal to the task.

SUMMARY

Several approaches to the analysis of synaptic substrate development are discussed in respect to the problem of defining the actions
of pharmacological agents on the immature brain. Studies of evoked
potentials and intracellularly recorded synaptic events in immature
cortical and thalamic neurons provide evidence that the time-course
of development of excitatory and inhibitory synaptic inputs to these
elements as well as the effectiveness of such inputs follows temporal
patterns which vary in different neuronal organizations. These
factors are emphasized in studies of the development of thalamic
organizations contributing to the production of evoked electrocortical synchronization and desynchronization. They serve to illustrate
the kind of data that must be forthcoming for the emergence of
developmental neuropsychopharmacology as a productive enterprise
in which drug actions can be specified in relation to the maturation
of identifiable synaptic subsystems.

ACKNOWLEDGMENTS

The work described in this paper has been supported in part by a grant from the Alfred P. Sloan Foundation and the National Institute of Neurological Diseases and Stroke (NS-07512).

REFERENCES

Andersen, P., Eccles, J.C., and Løyning, Y., 1964a, Location of postsynaptic inhibitory synapses on hippocampal pyramids, J. Neurophysiol. 27: 592.

Andersen, P., Eccles, J.C., and Løyning, Y., 1964b, Pathway of postsynaptic inhibition in the hippocampus, J. Neurophysiol. 27: 608.

Brown, J.D., and Pinsky, C., 1971, Nonuniform transmission and directional preference in the spread of surface positive burst responses in cerebral cortex: Evidence for ordered groups of neurons in the cerebral cortex, Exp. Neurol. 30: 251.

Clemente, C.D., Purpura, D.P., and Mayer, F.E., 1972, "Sleep and the Maturing Nervous System", Academic Press, New York.

Feldman, M.H., and Purpura, D.P., 1970, Prolonged conductance increase in thalamic neurons during synchronizing inhibition, Brain Res. 24: 329.

Laemle, L., Benhamida, C., and Purpura, D.P., 1972, Laminar distribution of geniculo-cortical afferents in visual cortex of the postnatal kitten, Brain Res. 41: 25.

Noback, C.R., and Purpura, D.P., 1961, Postnatal ontogenesis of cat neocortex, J. Comp. Neurol. 117: 291.

Pappas, G.D., Cohen, E.B., and Purpura, D.P., 1966, Fine structure of synaptic and nonsynaptic neuronal relations in the thalamus of the cat, in "The Thalamus", (D.P. Purpura and M.D. Yahr, eds.), pp. 47-71, Columbia Univ. Press, New York.

Prince, D.A., and Gutnick, M.J., 1971, Cellular activities in epileptogenic foci of immature cortex, Trans. Amer. Neurol. Assoc. 96: 88.

Purpura, D.P., 1959, Nature of electrocortical potentials and synaptic organizations in cerebral and cerebellar cortex, Int. Rev. Neurobiol. 1: 47.

Purpura, D.P., 1961a, Ontogenetic analysis of some evoked synaptic activities in superficial neocortical neuropil, in "Nervous Inhibition", (E. Florey, ed.), pp. 495-514, Pergamon Press, New York.

Purpura, D.P., 1961b, Analysis of axodendritic synaptic organizations in immature cerebral cortex, Annals N.Y. Acad. Sci. 94: 604.

Purpura, D.P., 1964, Relationship of seizure susceptibility to morphologic and physiologic properties of normal and abnormal immature cortex, in "Neurological and Electroencephalographic Correlative Studies in Infancy", (P. Kellaway and I. Petersen, eds.), pp. 117-154, Grune and Stratton, New York.

Purpura, D.P., 1967, Comparative physiology of dendrites, in "The Neurosciences: A Study Program", (G.C. Quarton, T. Melnechuck and F.O. Schmitt, eds.), pp. 372-393, Rockefeller Univ. Press, New York.

Purpura, D.P., 1969, Stability and seizure susceptibility of immature brain, in "Basic Mechanisms of the Epilepsies", (H.H. Jasper, A.A. Ward and A. Pope, eds.), pp. 481-505, Little, Brown and Co., Boston.

Purpura, D.P., 1970, Operations and processes in thalamic and synaptically related neural subsystems, in "The Neurosciences, Second Study Program", (G.C. Quarton, T. Melnechuck and G. Adelman, eds.), pp. 458-470, Rockefeller University Press, New York.

Purpura, D.P., 1972a, Intracellular studies of synaptic organizations in the mammalian brain, in "Structure and Function of Synapses", (G.D. Pappas and D.P. Purpura, eds.), pp. 257-302, Raven Press, New York.

Purpura, D.P., 1972b, Ontogenetic models in studies of cortical seizure activities, in "Experimental Models of Epilepsy - A Manual for the Laboratory Worker", pp. 531-556, Raven Press, New York.

Purpura, D.P., 1973, Normal and aberrant development of synaptic pathways in human hippocampus, Trans. Amer. Neurol. Assoc. 98: (in press).

Purpura, D.P., and Cohen, B., 1962, Intracellular recording from thalamic neurons during recruiting responses, J. Neurophysiol. 25: 621.

Purpura, D.P., Girado, M., Smith, T.G., Callan, D., and Grundfest, H., 1959, Structure-activity determinants of pharmacological effects of amino acids and related compounds on cortical synapses, J. Neurochem. 3: 238.

Purpura, D.P., and Pappas, G.D., 1968, Structural characteristics of neurons in the feline hippocampus during postnatal ontogenesis, Exp. Neurol. 27: 379.

Purpura, D.P., Prelevic, S., and Santini, M., 1968, Postsynaptic potentials and spike variations in the feline hippocampus during postnatal ontogenesis, Exp. Neurol. 22: 408.

Purpura, D.P., and Shofer, R.J., 1963, Intracellular recording from thalamic neurons during reticulo-cortical activation, J. Neurophysiol. 26: 494.

Purpura, D.P., and Shofer, R.J., 1972, Excitatory action of dibutyryl cyclic adenosine monophosphate on immature cerebral cortex, Brain Res. 38: 179.

Purpura, D.P., Shofer, R.J., Housepian, E.M., and Noback, C.R., 1964, Comparative ontogenesis of structure-function relations in cerebral and cerebellar cortex, in "Growth and Maturation of the Brain", (D.P. Purpura and J.P. Schade, eds.), Prog. in Brain Res., pp. 187-221, Elsevier, Amsterdam.

Purpura, D.P., Shofer, R.J., and Scarff, T., 1965, Properties of synaptic activities and spike potentials of neurons in immature neocortex, J. Neurophysiol. 28: 925.

Schwartz, I.R., Pappas, G.D., and Purpura, D.P., 1968, Fine structure of neurons and synapses in the feline hippocampus during postnatal ontogenesis, Exp. Neurol. 22: 394.

Shofer, R.J. and Purpura, D.P., 1972, Spread of transcallosally evoked responses in immature association cortex, Exp. Neurol. 37:431.

Siggins, G.R., Oliver, A.P., Hoffer, B.J., and Bloom, F.E., 1971, Cyclic adenosine monophosphate and norepinephrine: effects on transmembrane properties of Purkinje cells, Science 171: 192.

Thatcher, R.W., and Purpura, D.P., 1972, Maturational status of inhibitory and excitatory synaptic activities of thalamic neurons in neonatal kitten, Brain Res. 44: 661.

Voeller, K., Pappas, G.D., and Purpura, D.P., 1963, Electron microscope study of development of cat superficial neocortex, Exp. Neurol. 7: 107.

SELECTIVE DEPRESSION OF ORGANOTYPIC BIOELECTRIC ACTIVITIES OF CNS TISSUE CULTURES BY PHARMACOLOGIC AND METABOLIC AGENTS

Stanley M. Crain

Department of Physiology and Rose F. Kennedy Center for

Research in Mental Retardation and Human Development,

Albert Einstein College of Medicine,

Yeshiva University, Bronx, New York

INTRODUCTION

Electrophysiologic studies of fetal rodent cerebral cortex and spinal cord explants have demonstrated that small fragments (ca. 1 cu mm) of these tissues can generate progressively more complex organotypic bioelectric activities as they mature in culture (e.g. Fig. 1; Crain, 1966, 1969; Crain and Bornstein, 1964; Crain and Peterson, 1964, 1967). The present studies emphasize the pharmacologic properties of these CNS explants, and they illustrate the value of this model system to supplement analyses of factors which regulate excitability of the central nervous system in situ, especially during development. Attention will be focused primarily on two groups of chemical agents: a) those which depress all types of Ca^{++}-dependent, synaptically mediated activities by decreasing availability of Ca^{++} to the neural tissue; and b) those which depress synaptic network discharges by selective effects at inhibitory receptor sites, e.g., hyperpolarization or increased membrane conductance, in mimicry of inhibitory transmitters.

DEPRESSION OF COMPLEX ACTIVITY BY ACUTE Ca^{++}-DEPRIVATION AND RESTORATIVE EFFECTS OF CYCLIC AMP AND CAFFEINE

Introduction of procaine (4×10^{-4}M) or xylocaine (ca. 10^{-4}M) into CNS cultures produces selective depression of complex discharges mediated by polysynaptic circuits without blocking simple

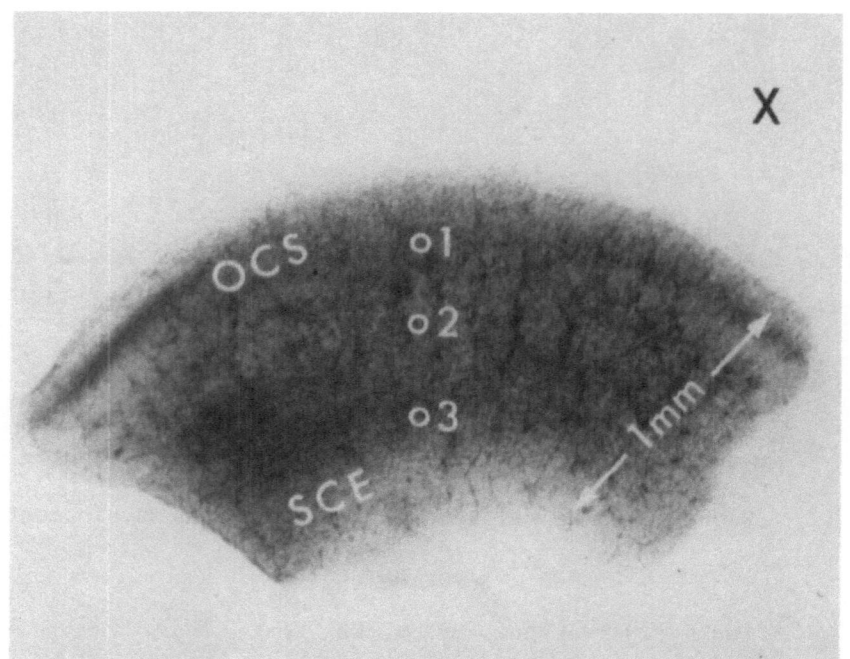

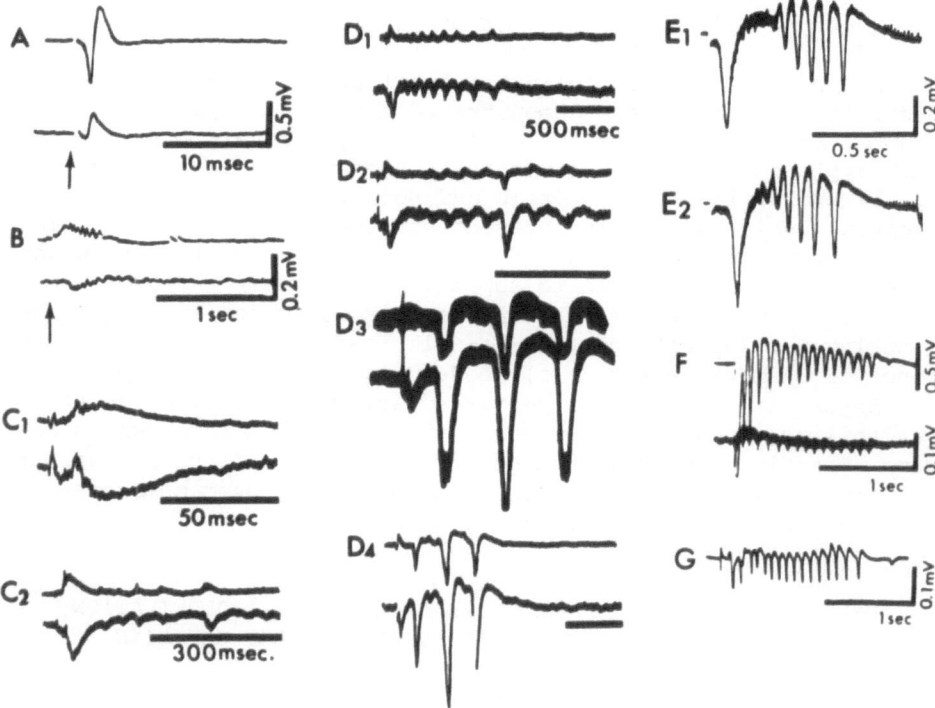

Fig. 1. Transition from simple to complex evoked responses in explants of newborn mouse cerebral cortex tissue during first 2 weeks
in vitro. (X): Photomicrograph of freshly prepared explant of neonatal mouse cerebral cortex (about 0.5 mm thick). OCS: original
cortical surface; SCE: subcortical edge. (A): Simultaneous records
showing simple spikes evoked in 3-day culture, at "cortical depths"
of 200 μ (site 1 in X, upper sweep) and 400 μ (site 2) by stimulus
applied near subcortical edge of explant (site 3). (B): Early signs
of complex response patterns recorded, at much slower sweep rate, at
same loci as in (A). Long-duration negativity appears with long
latency after early superficial spike (upper sweep), and long-duration positivity develops with still longer latency after early deep
spike. Arrow indicates onset of dual stimuli (50 msec apart).
Note that the second pair of stimuli, applied 1 sec after first
pair, is ineffective. (C_1): Simultaneous records of characteristic
evoked potentials in 10-day culture at cortical depths of 250 μ
(upper sweep) and 650 μ following stimulus applied at deeper site.
Note 60 msec negative evoked response in superficial region and deep
positive response of longer duration and greater latency. (C_2): At
slower sweep rate, small amplitude repetitive potentials (10-20 per
sec) are seen to follow primary responses at both sites and are also
of opposite polarities. (D_1): After introduction of d-tubocurarine
$(10^{-4}M)$, repetitive afterdischarge becomes more pronounced. (D_2):
Sudden increase in amplitude of one of the positive potentials in
deep response (lower sweep) and reversal of polarity of corresponding potential in superficial response. (D_3): Large increase in amplitude of all positive potentials in superficial response. Note
marked decrease in frequency of repetitive discharge. (D_4): Subsequent decrease in amplitude of the large paroxysmal waves. (E): Repetitive oscillatory afterdischarge evoked in cerebral explant after
3 weeks in vitro by single stimulus applied several hundred μ from
recording site. Note variation in latency of onset of oscillatory
discharge following initial, positive evoked potential (in two
successive responses at same stimulus strength.) (F): Similar longer-
lasting oscillatory (ca. 10 per sec) afterdischarges occurring syn-
chronously at 2 sites in another cerebral explant. (G): Characteristic repetitive afterdischarge sequence evoked in cerebral cortical
slab in 5-day-old kitten, 3 days after neuronal isolation, in situ.
Note similarity between this response pattern and those obtained from
the cerebral explants in vitro. (X,A-E: Crain, 1964; F: Purpura and
Housepian, 1961.) In this and all subsequent figures, time and amplitude calibrations apply to all succeeding records, until otherwise
noted. Upward deflection indicates negativity at active recording
electrode, and onset of stimuli is indicated by arrow, or by initial
sharp pulse or brief gap, near beginning of each sweep. All records
made in BSS (see Fig. 3) or modified culture medium, at 33-35°C and
pH of 7.2-7.4, using Ag-AgCl electrodes with saline-filled pipettes
(tip diameters for recording: 3-5 μ and for stimulating: 8-10 μ).
Stimuli were square pulses of 0.2-0.5 msec in duration and up to
100 μamp in strength (Crain, 1972a, 1973a).

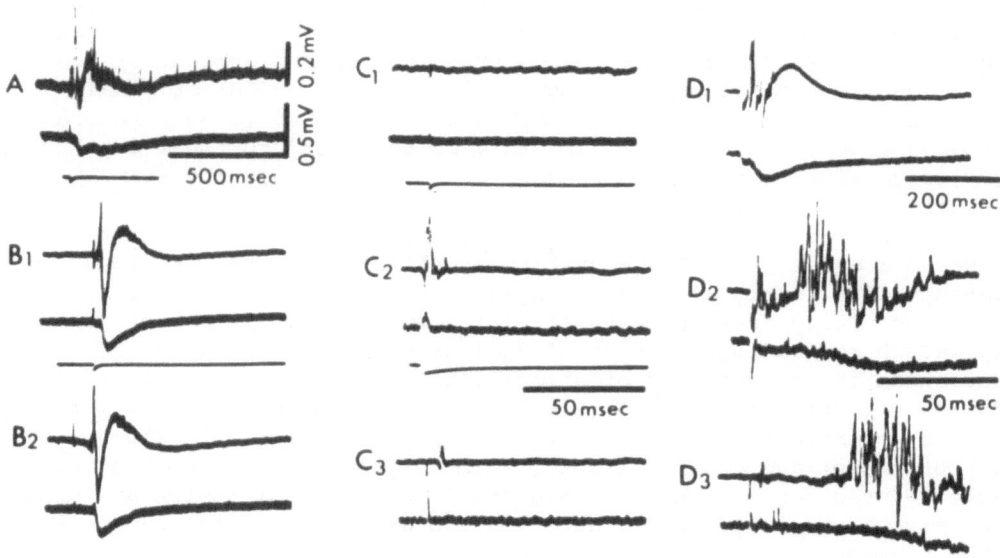

Fig. 2. Characteristic evoked responses in cerebral explant after
2 months in vitro, and selective block with procaine. (A): Simultaneous records at cortical "depths" of 50 μ (upper sweep) and 250 μ
showing long-lasting responses following a single superficial stimulus applied about 500 μ away from the first recording electrode.
Note complex, triphasic, predominantly negative potential at superficial site (upper sweep) and simpler positivity of similar duration,
recorded at deeper site. Also note large negative spikes superimposed on slow waves in superficial response. (B1): After procaine
(4x10^-5M) superimposed spikes are no longer seen. (Increased amplitude of positive potentials appeared earlier following preliminary
application of d-tubocurarine.) (B2): Same recording conditions as
in B1, but stimulus applied to subcortical region at "depth" of about
1 mm. Note large increase in response latency to about 60 msec.
(C1): Several minutes after increasing procaine concentration to
4x10^-4M. Note complete block of evoked long-duration responses
(cf. B1). (C2): Faster sweep rate reveals that early-latency spike
potentials are still evoked (cf. C1). (C3): After stimulus to subcortical region only small spike appears, with 5 msec latency, at
superficial site (cf. B2). (D1): Within 5 min after restoration of
control medium. Note almost complete reappearance of characteristic
evoked responses, in both superficial and deep records, following a
superficial stimulus (cf. A and B1). (D2): Faster sweep rate shows
details of spike barrages which occur prior to slow-waves (cf. C2).
(D3): After a subcortical stimulus, a 35-msec silent period occurs
between appearance of the first spike potential (cf. C3) and the
spike barrage preceding the slow waves (cf. B2). (From Crain and
Bornstein, 1964.)

propagated spike potentials (Fig. 2; Crain et al., 1968a). Similar
effects can be produced by increasing the Mg^{++} concentration of the
culture medium from 1 to 5-10 mM (Figs. 3A, 4B$_2$), by removal of Ca^{++}
from the medium (Fig. 5F), or by addition of the chelating agent,
EGTA (10^{-3}M). The latter three procedures decrease the availability
of Ca^{++} to the CNS tissue and xylocaine may act similarly (Blaustein
and Goldman, 1966; Kuperman et al., 1968; Dettbarn, 1971). Addition
of strychnine (10^{-6}-10^{-7}M) in normal balanced salt solution (BSS)
(see legend, Fig. 3) generally leads to rapid enhancement of
synaptically-mediated discharges and often initiates spontaneous
convulsive activity (Crain, 1966, 1969, 1972a). Although introduction of strychnine along with these blocking agents does not
effectively prevent these Ca^{++}-deficit depressions, caffeine (10^{-3}M)
produces, within a few minutes, a transient (up to 15 min) restoration of the original complex bioelectric discharges, after complete
blockade in high Mg^{++} (Fig. 3B; Crain and Pollack, 1973). Previous
experiments had shown that caffeine (10^{-3}M) elicited convulsive discharges in cerebral cortex explants (Crain, 1966), resembling
characteristic hyperexcitability produced by caffeine in the CNS
in situ (Ritchie, 1970). Since this methylxanthine inhibits cerebral
cyclic AMP-phosphodiesterase (Butcher and Sutherland, 1962; Cheung,
1970), the possibility arose that the excitatory effects in cultured
cerebral tissues could be due to an increased level of endogenous
cyclic AMP following interference with its normal rate of hydrolysis
by this enzyme. Introduction of low concentrations (ca. 10^{-6}M) of
cyclic AMP (or its dibutyryl derivative) to Ca^{++}-deprived spinal
cord and cerebral cortex explants does, indeed, produce similar restorative effects as 10^{-3}M caffeine, not only after high Mg^{++}, but
also after Ca^{++}-free and xylocaine blockades (Figs. 4 and 5; Table 1;
Crain and Pollack, 1973). These dramatic effects have been obtained
with 14- to 18-day fetal rodent spinal cord and cerebral cortex explants after 1 to 4 weeks in vitro (comparable in development to CNS
tissues in situ during the first 2-3 weeks after birth). Similar
restorative effects during high Mg^{++}-blockades have also been produced with a much lower concentration (ca. 10^{-6}M) of another phosphodiesterase inhibitor, SQ 66,442 (Table 1; this agent is about
100-fold more potent than caffeine as an inhibitor of cerebral PDE--
M. Chasin, personal communication; Chasin et al., 1972). Furthermore,
addition of 5' AMP (10^{-6}M) or ATP (10^{-6}M) to Mg^{++}-blocked cultures
did not restore complex bioelectric activity (Fig. 4C), whereas
subsequent introduction of dibutyryl cyclic AMP in the same cord
explants did, indeed, restore activity (Fig. 4F). These experiments
provide support for specificity of action by cyclic AMP in relation
to its precursor (ATP) and primary breakdown product (AMP).

In some CNS explants monitored over periods of several hours in
regular BSS, introduction of cyclic AMP or dibutyryl cyclic AMP at
low concentrations (ca. 10^{-6}M) often produced convulsive bioelectric
effects, but the degree of excitation was quite variable, both in
regard to enhancement and prolongation of complex responses as well

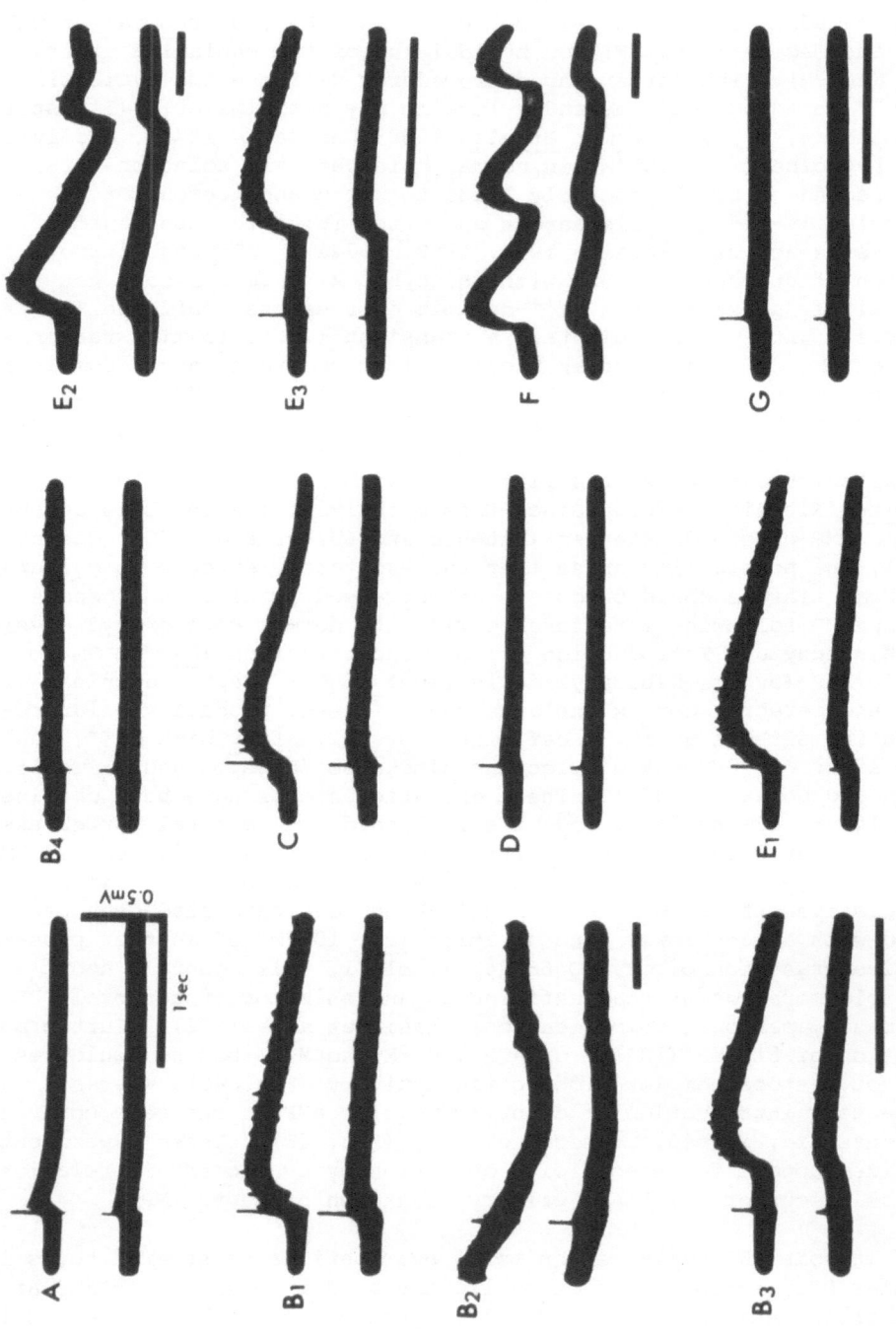

as spontaneous discharges (Crain and Pollack, 1973). Long-lasting
cyclic sequences of complex spike-barrages and slow-waves occurred
in several of the 2- to 3-week-old cord explants during 1-2 hrs of
exposure to dibutyryl cyclic AMP, but these convulsive effects were
milder or absent in most of the younger or older explants tested.
The excitatory effects of cyclic AMP where similar to those of dibutyryl cyclic AMP, but the latter generally resulted in a greater
degree of complex activity and persisted for a longer time.

    There did not appear to be any obvious relationship between
the age of an explant in vitro and its responsiveness to cyclic
AMP-restoration of a blockade, though there did seem to be an
optimal period during which direct excitatory effects of cyclic AMP
on bioelectric activity in regular BSS were observed (as noted above).
Furthermore, in many of the explants were no clearcut convulsive
activity could be detected during exposure to cyclic AMP in normal
media, restorative effects of cyclic AMP after acute Ca^{++}-deprivation
were, nevertheless, demonstrable.

Fig. 3. Restorative effects of caffeine on complex discharges in
fetal mouse spinal cord explant after acute depression in high-Mg^{++}/
BSS (13 days in vitro). (A): Almost complete depression of characteristic complex discharges of cord explant (in response to single
cord stimuli) several min after increasing Mg^{++} concentration from
1 to 5 mM (10^{-6}M strychnine present during entire experiment: A-G).
(B): Long-lasting negative slow-wave and spike-barrage responses
are restored (B_1) about 1 min after adding 10^{-3}M caffeine to the
5 mM Mg^{++}/BSS. (Note: The balanced salt solution (BSS) used in these
experiments (Figs. 3-7) contained the following salt concentrations
(mM): NaCl (137), KCl (2.7), $CaCl_2$ (1.0), $MgCl_2$ (1.0), Na_2HPO_4 (1.36),
NaH_2PO_4 (0.15), $NaHCO_3$ (6.0), and glucose (5.5) in glass-distilled
water.) Similar large amplitude discharges also begin to occur
spontaneously (B_2) and continue for about 5 min. By 7 min, latency
of evoked responses increases markedly to about 300 msec (B_3), and
complete depression ensues about 1 min later (B_4). (C): Complex
discharges are restored after return to regular BSS. (D): Sustained
block occurs within 1 min after increasing Mg^{++} level again to 5 mM.
(E): Within 2 min after adding 10^{-3}M caffeine to the 5 mM Mg^{++}/BSS
responses are even larger than those in regular BSS (cf. $E_{1,2}$ vs. C).
By 7 min, however, response latencies again become very long (500
msec in E_3) and complete blockade develops soon afterwards (as in
$B_{3,4}$). (F): Convulsive series of discharges occur shortly after
return to regular BSS. (G): Nevertheless, increasing Mg^{++} level to
5 mM still results in rapid and complete depression. (From Crain
and Pollack, 1973.)

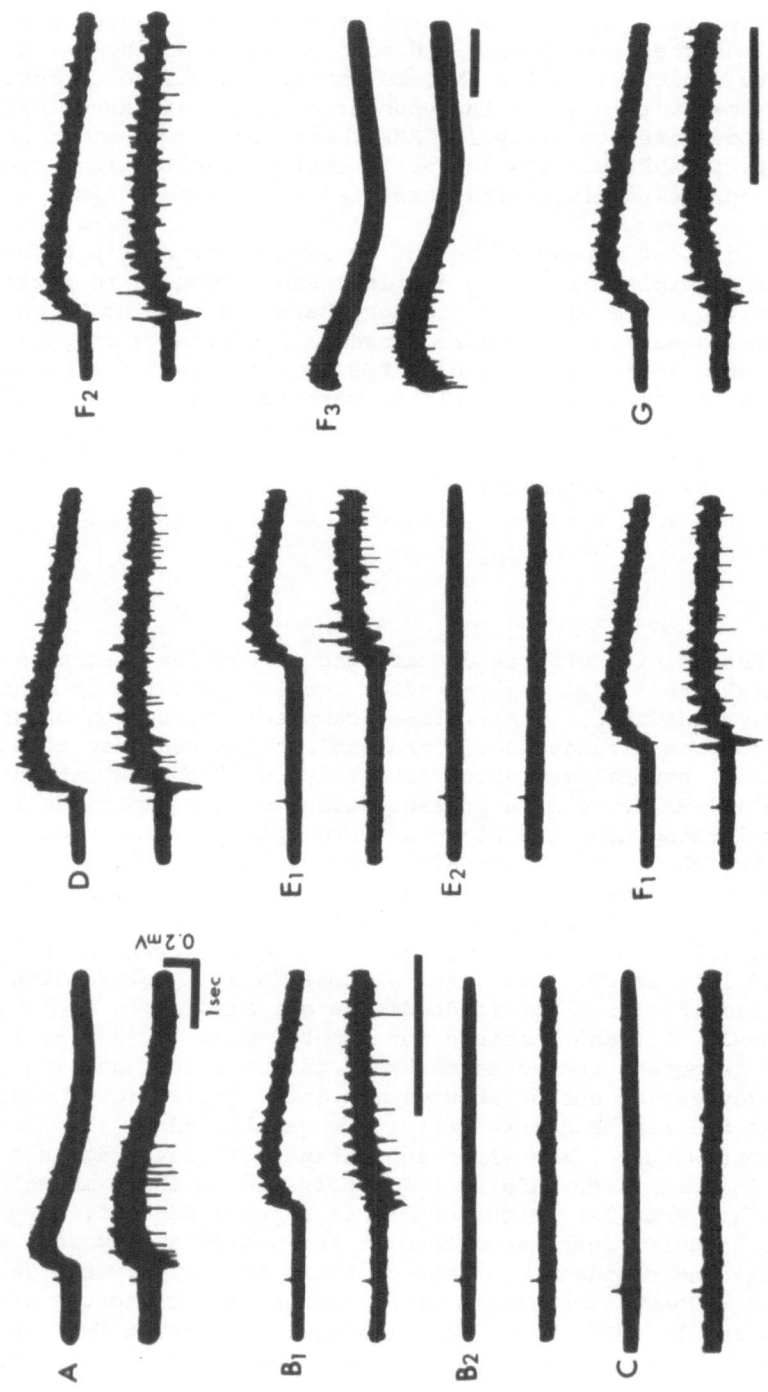

    In preliminary developmental studies of 18-day fetal mouse
cerebral neocortex hippocampus explants (Crain and Bornstein, in
preparation), introduction of caffeine (10^{-3}M) at stages shortly
before the usual appearance of complex synaptically-mediated discharges (3-4 days in vitro) led to precocious generation of long-
lasting repetitive spike-barrage and slow-wave responses to electric
stimuli instead of simple spike potentials. Similar precocious,
synaptically-mediated bioelectric discharges have also been evoked
under caffeine (10^{-3}M) in 14-day fetal mouse spinal cord explants
after 3-4 days in vitro (Crain and Peterson, in preparation). In
both types of CNS explants these caffeine effects could be produced
at stages prior to the characteristic onset of strychnine sensitivity.
These preliminary data suggest that low Ca^{++} or low cyclic AMP levels
may be a significant factor underlying the high thresholds and extreme lability of synaptically-mediated discharges shortly after
synaptogenesis in the CNS, and that strychnine-sensitive inhibitory
circuits (Crain, 1969, 1973b; Crain and Peterson, 1967) may become
functional after an additional brief period of maturation.

Fig. 4. Restorative effects of dibutyryl cyclic AMP on complex
discharge activity of fetal spinal cord explant after acute depression in high-Mg^{++} BSS (13 days in vitro). (A): Organotypic
slow-wave and spike-barrage responses evoked in 2 regions of cord
explant by single stimulus to another cord site, during exposure
to low concentration of strychnine (10^{-6}M) in BSS. (Strychnine
concentration maintained at 10^{-6}M during entire experiment: A-G.)
(B_1): Responses at both sites occur with much longer latency
(ca. 400 msec) when similar or larger stimulus is applied following
increase of Mg^{++} level from 1 to 5 mM. (B_2): About 2 min later,
complex cord discharges can no longer be evoked even with very large
cord stimuli (only an early-latency spike potential can be detected
at faster sweep). (C): Block of complex activity continues after
addition of 5'-AMP (10^{-6}M) to the 5 mM Mg^{++}/BSS. (D): Restoration
of characteristic discharges after return to regular BSS. (E):
Similar partial (E_1) and complete (E_2) depression of complex responses within 1-2 min after increasing Mg^{++} again to 5 mM. Note
unusually long (1 sec) latencies in E_1. (F): Within 1 min after
addition of dibutyryl cyclic AMP ($2x10^{-6}$M) to the 5 mM Mg^{++}/BSS,
organotypic cord discharges can again be evoked with a single cord
stimulus (F_1; cf. B_1 and E_1). Soon afterwards, these complex responses occur with shorter latency (F_2; cf. D), and similar discharges begin to appear spontaneously at both cord sites (F_2; cf. A),
occurring sporadically during the next 10 min, and then followed by
complete depression as in B_2 and E_2. (G): Restoration of original
responses after return to regular BSS. (From Crain and Pollack, 1973.)

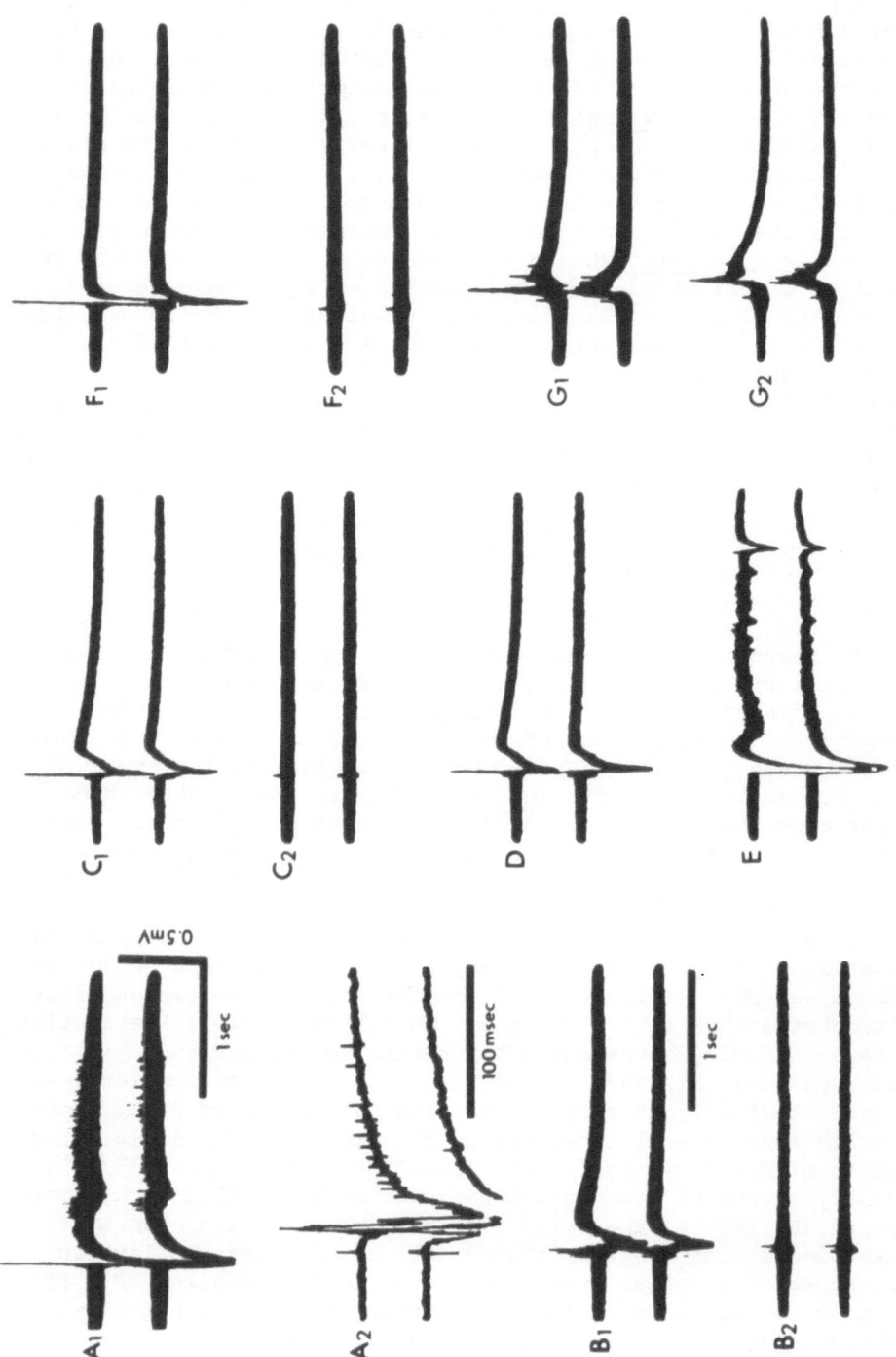

MECHANISMS OF RESTORATIVE ACTION OF CYCLIC AMP

The low level of cyclic AMP (10^{-6}M) which produced direct
functional effects in these experiments is of particular significance,
since it appears to be the first demonstration of excitatory effects
on vertebrate CNS tissue at concentrations which approach the physiological range (Hardman et al., 1971). In other CNS preparations
where significant excitatory phenomena have been observed with exogenous cyclic AMP, concentrations of 10^{-4} to 10^{-3}M have generally
been required (Gessa et al., 1970; Purpura and Shofer, 1972;
Auerbach and Purpura, 1972, and personal communication) presumably
because of greater diffusion barriers in situ (see also Chagas
et al., 1972; Forn et al., 1972).

The effects of cyclic AMP on rat neuromuscular junctions provide a useful model for analysis of mechanisms underlying the mode
of action of this agent at CNS synapses (Goldberg and Singer, 1969;
Singer and Goldberg, 1970). Partial blockade of neuromuscular transmission was produced by appropriate concentrations of Mg^{++} (22 mM)
or d-tubocurarine. Addition of dibutyryl cyclic AMP (4×10^{-3}M)
clearly enhanced the amplitude of the endplate potentials at these

------

Fig. 5. Restorative effects of dibutyryl cyclic AMP on evoked
potentials in mouse cerebral cortex explant after acute depression
in high-Mg^{++} or Ca^{++}-free BSS (18-day fetus; 3 weeks in vitro).
(A): Complex long-lasting discharges (A_1) evoked in 2 regions of
cerebral explant by single stimulus at third site (in BSS). Initial
phases of these elaborate slow-wave and spike-barrage responses are
seen more clearly at faster sweep (A_2). (B): Partial depression of
these complex responses several min after increasing Mg^{++} concentration from 1 to 10 mM (B_1), and complete block (except for small,
early-latency spike) within 5 min (B_2). (C): After addition of
2×10^{-6}M dibutyryl cyclic AMP to the 10 mM Mg^{++}/BSS, the primary
phases of the original complex evoked discharges are restored (C_1)
(cf. A_1, B_1). Within 5 min, however, complete depression develops
again (C_2). (D): Second restoration of complex evoked responses in
2×10^{-6}M dibutyryl cyclic AMP + 10 mM Mg^{++}, after interim return to
regular BSS and subsequent blockade in 10 mM Mg^{++} for 10 min. Responses could again be elicited for about 5 min. (E): Restoration
of original long-lasting discharges after return to regular BSS
(cf. A). (F): Partial depression of evoked discharges within 2 min
after introduction of Ca^{++}-free BSS (F_1) and complete block shortly
thereafter (F_2). (G): Prominent negative slow-wave discharges can
be elicited within 30 sec after addition of 2×10^{-6}M dibutyryl cyclic
AMP to the Ca^{++}-free BSS. Latency of these responses increases within
1 min (G_2) and complete block soon occurred (reversible after return
to regular BSS, as in E). (From Crain and Pollack, 1973.)

TABLE 1

RESTORATIVE EFFECTS OF CYCLIC AMP AND PDE INHIBITORS
ON CNS ACTIVITY

Medium Producing Sustained Depression of Complex Bio-Electric Discharges of Spinal Cord Explant[a]	Agent Added to Blocking Medium Which Restored Original Activity for 1-20 Minutes[b]
high Mg^{++} ($5-10 \times 10^{-3}$M)-BSS	cyclic AMP (3×10^{-6}M)[c]
"	dibutyryl cyclic AMP (2×10^{-6}M)[d]
"	caffeine (10^{-3}M)
"	SQ-65,442 (3×10^{-6}M)[e]
Ca^{++}-free BSS	dibutyryl cyclic AMP (2×10^{-6}M)[d]
EGTA (10^{-3}M)-BSS	"
Xylocaine (10^{-4}M)-BSS	"

[a]In some cases, strychnine (10^{-7}M) was added during entire experiment to enhance contrast between excited and depressed states.

[b]Restorative agent was generally added shortly after blockade developed.

[c]ATP and 5'-AMP were ineffective when tested at same concentration on these explants.

[d]Same effect also obtained on explant of mouse cerebral cortex in high Mg^{++} and Ca^{++}-free media.

[e]Synthetic phosphodiesterase inhibitor (Squibb; see text).

depressed junctions. The cyclic AMP effects were interpreted as a facilitation of the release of acetylcholine from the presynaptic neuron since intracellular recordings showed an increase in frequency of miniature endplate potentials (MEPPs) without an increase in their average amplitude (see also Breckenridge and Bray, 1970), resembling epinephrine-enhancement of neuromuscular transmission (Krnjevic and Miledi, 1958; Jenkinson et al., 1968). Furthermore, the same enhancement in frequency of MEPPs was obtained at these depressed junctions after addition of the methylxanthine PDE-inhibitors, theophylline and caffeine ($0.2-2 \times 10^{-3}$M), in agreement with similar observations by Elmqvist and Feldman (1965) after

application of caffeine ($5x10^{-3}$M) to neuromuscular preparations
blocked in calcium-free solutions. In both studies it was suggested
that caffeine may act in the nerve terminal by mobilizing bound
calcium stores, but the more recent data obtained by Singer and
Goldberg (1970) permitted additional speculation that the methylxanthine effects might be mediated by enhanced levels of endogenous
cyclic AMP following PDE-inhibition.

The present experiments extend these neuromuscular studies to
CNS tissues in vitro, and they may provide significant clues to
mechanisms underlying cyclic AMP effects on synaptic transmission
in the CNS in situ. Following blockade of complex, synaptically-
mediated bioelectric activity in CNS explants by 4 different modes
of acute Ca^{++}-deprivation (low Ca^{++}, high Mg^{++}, EGTA and xylocaine),
a low concentration of exogenous cyclic AMP is capable of promoting
a temporary restoration of that activity. In view of the well-
established effects of cyclic AMP in mobilizing membrane-bound
calcium in a variety of gland cells so that Ca^{++}-dependent
secretion can be restored in Ca^{++}-free media (Rasmussen, 1970;
Farese, 1971; Prince et al., 1972), it is tempting to speculate
that this may also be the mechanism of action of exogenous cyclic
AMP in restoring Ca^{++}-dependent, synaptically-mediated bioelectric
activity in CNS explants following depression by Ca^{++}-deprivation
(see also Singer and Goldberg, 1970; Breckenridge and Bray, 1970;
Torda, 1972). The similar restorative effects obtained with PDE
inhibitors (caffeine and SQ-65,442) in the cultures might then be
interpreted as due to the resulting increase in endogenous levels
of cyclic AMP, leading to mobilization of membrane-bound calcium
in presynaptic terminals and thereby facilitating neurotransmitter
release.

Ample supplies of bound calcium for translocation to synaptic
vesicles are probably present in membranes of axonal endoplasmic
reticulum (Henkert, 1972) and mitochondria (e.g., Baker et al.,
1971; Llinás et al., 1972; Rasmussen, 1970) in presynaptic terminals
of CNS neurons (Birks, 1966; Korneliussen, 1972; Teichberg and
Holtzman, 1973). Furthermore, cyclic AMP, adenyl cyclase, and PDE
activity have been demonstrated to be present in synaptic vesicle
fractions from presynaptic nerve endings of mammalian brain
(Cheung and Salganicoff, 1967; Johnson et al., 1972), as well as
in postsynaptic membranes (Florendo et al., 1971). The remarkably
long stimulus-response latencies (1-2 sec) of the synaptic network
discharges in CNS explants which occur during development of Ca^{++}-
deprivation blockades (e.g., Figs. $3B_3$, E_3; $4B_1$, E_1), and the rapid
restoration of normal latencies after addition of cyclic AMP, add
further support to a mechanism involving facilitation of stimulus-
secretion coupling through mobilization of calcium. It is unlikely
that decreased conduction velocity of nerve impulses in the CNS
explants could account for much of this increased latency, since
the lengths of the conductile neurites in the networks are quite

short (ca. 1 mm) and propagation normally occurs at rates of the order of 0.1-1 m/sec in these small diameter (ca. 1 μ) fibers (Crain and Bornstein, 1964; Crain and Peterson, 1964, 1967; Hild and Tasaki, 1962). Conduction velocities would have to be drastically decreased to the order of 1 mm/sec to account for the long stimulus-response latencies in Ca^{++}-deprived media. It is more probable that these increased latencies are related to the effects of Ca^{++}-deficits on complex multi-synaptic circuits, since characteristic synaptic delays in situ appear to involve primarily the mechanism by which Ca^{++} triggers release of synaptic transmitter in axon terminals (Katz, 1969; Katz and Miledi, 1965a, 1965b, 1968). Similar long stimulus-response latencies have also been observed in immature CNS explants in normal medium, as well as in older ones when small, barely threshold stimuli are applied (Crain and Peterson, 1964; Crain and Bornstein, 1964; Crain et al., 1968b; see also Figs. 1B, E; $2B_2$, D_3). Finally, the transient nature of these restorative periods (1-20 min) indicates that cyclic AMP is not simply substituting for Ca^{++} (since this should lead to more permanent restoration); it may, indeed, reflect limits to the releasable membrane-bound "calcium stores" in the terminals.

The electrophysiologic properties of these CNS explants, are, however, quite complex and extracellular recordings are relatively indirect indicators of the synaptic activities involved. It is, therefore, quite possible that the observed restorative effects of cyclic AMP may also involve direct transmitter-like depolarizing actions which enhance the sensitivity of postsynaptic or other neuronal membranes, independent of intracellular calcium mobilization [analogous to the hyperpolarizing effects of cyclic AMP on cerebellar Purkinje cells (Siggins et al., 1971a, 1971b) and sympathetic ganglion cells (McAfee and Greengard, 1972)]. It should be noted, however, that even high concentrations of cyclic AMP ($4x10^{-3}$M) did not produce direct depolarizing effects in muscle (Singer and Goldberg, 1970) nor in superior cervical ganglion cells (McAfee and Greengard, 1972). Iontophoretic application of cyclic AMP to cerebellar Purkinje cells produced only hyperpolarization (Siggins et al., 1971a, 1971b) even when tested in neonatal rats before the onset of synaptogenesis (Hoffer, 1971). It is also of interest that caffeine ($2x10^{-3}$M) does not alter the resting potential of muscle fibers (Axelsson and Thesleff, 1958; Marco and Nastuk, 1968).

If cyclic AMP does, in fact, facilitate synaptic transmission by mobilization of membrane-bound calcium in presynaptic terminals, it should enhance both inhibitory as well as excitatory synapses. Some of the variability in the observed excitatory effects of cyclic AMP on CNS explants in normal media may thus be attributable to predominance of inhibitory circuits in certain explants. In the latter case, strychnine or picrotoxin could evoke marked excitatory effects by selective blocking of inhibitory receptor sites, whereas cyclic AMP might appear to be ineffective when monitored for overt activity

with extracellular electrodes. Furthermore, after depressing the
complex bioelectric activity of spinal cord explants by increasing
the concentration of the postulated inhibitory synaptic transmitter,
glycine (Curtis et al., 1968; Curtis et al., 1971; Werman et al.,
1968), to 10^{-3}M, preliminary experiments indicate that cyclic AMP
and caffeine do not overcome this type of blockade, whereas low concentrations of strychnine (10^{-7}M) can readily neutralize it (Fig. 6;
see also Part 4). The considerations led to the use of strychnine
as a means of enhancing the restorative effects of cyclic AMP during
the high-Mg^{++} and other Ca^{++}-deficit blockades (vide supra), even
though strychnine alone was ineffective against these generalized
synaptic depressions.

DEVELOPMENTAL ASPECTS OF CYCLIC AMP EFFECTS

The potent effect of caffeine in facilitating precocious
synaptically-mediated repetitive-spike and slow-wave responses to
electric stimuli during the earliest stages of synaptogenesis in CNS
explants suggests that endogenous cyclic AMP levels may already be
an important factor in regulation of synaptic transmission at the
onset of synaptic function in the CNS in situ. These data are consonant with studies of convulsive activity produced by topical application of dibutyryl cyclic AMP to 6-day-old kitten cerebral neocortex
(Purpura and Shofer, 1972), indicating that elaborate excitatory
synaptic networks are already well-organized but not normally active
at this neonatal stage (see Purpura, this volume). Long-lasting
sequences of repetitive discharges elicited by exogenous cyclic AMP
in 14-day fetal cord explants after 2 to 3 weeks in vitro are in good
agreement with these observations in situ. The absence of marked
convulsive effects during the first week after synaptogenesis in
cord explants may be related to a predominance of inhibitory components in the synaptic networks during this developmental stage
(Crain and Peterson, 1967; Crain, 1973b). It may also be due, in
part, to immaturity of cellular components associated with cyclic
AMP functions, e.g., calcium-binding sites on endoplasmic reticulum
and mitochondria in presynaptic terminals; protein kinases and adenyl
cyclase at synapses. The protein kinase system in rat brain, for
example, is not fully developed until 10 days after birth (Gaballah
et al., 1971). On the other hand, the variability and frequently
weak excitatory effects of cyclic AMP on older cord explants (after
4 weeks in vitro) in regular media may be partly attributable to
poor penetration through sheaths that tend to form over the tissues
during long-term culture (Guillery et al., 1968), and also to a return
to increased dominance of inhibitory synaptic circuits in these older
cultures after an interim period of hyperexcitability (Crain, 1969,
1973b).

The sensitivity of organotypic bioelectric activities of fetal
spinal cord and cerebral explants to cyclic AMP and PDE inhibitors

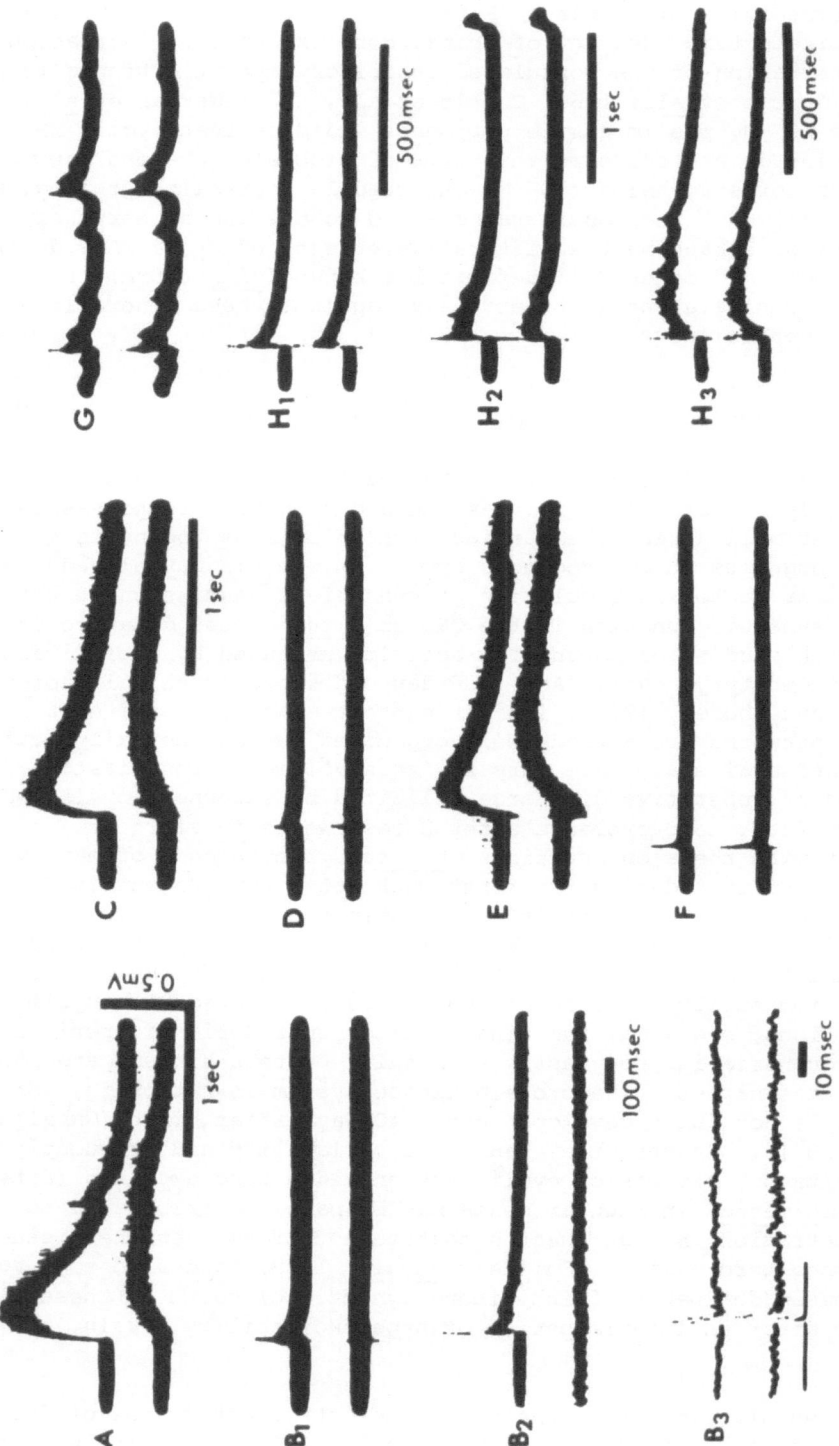

indicates that organized CNS tissue cultures can be utilized as a
model system to investigate mechanisms underlying the complex effects
of cyclic nucleotides on brain function in the adult, as well as
during critical developmental stages. Furthermore, the restorative
effects of cyclic AMP on synaptic activity during acute Ca^{++}-depri-
vation of cultured neural tissues may provide a valuable experimental
paradigm for studies related to CNS plasticity, e.g., synaptic
facilitation and post-tetanic potentiation (Breckenridge and Bray,
1970; Greengard and Kuo, 1970; Miledi and Thies, 1967), as well as
to pathologic conditions involving Ca^{++}-deficits in presynaptic
nerve terminals (e.g., Lambert and Elmqvist, 1971; Takamori, 1972).

DEPRESSION OF NETWORK DISCHARGES BY AMINO ACIDS
WHICH MIMIC INHIBITORY TRANSMITTERS

In contrast to the blocking effects of agents which decrease
availability of Ca^{++} to the neural tissue, several amino acids
produce a rather different type of depression of synaptic network
discharges of CNS explants. Introduction of 10^{-3}M glycine, for
example, leads to rapid depression of most of the complex discharges
of spinal cord explants, and only brief spike-bursts or simple mono-
phasic slow-wave responses can be evoked (Fig. 6B,D,F). Whereas
strychnine is ineffective against high-Mg^{++} or low Ca^{++} blockades,

---

Fig. 6. Selective depression of major components of complex synaptic
network discharges of fetal spinal cord explants in high-glycine/BSS
and complete recovery after addition of strychnine. (A): Complex
slow-wave and spike-barrage responses evoked in 2 regions of cord
explant in BSS, by single stimulus to another cord site (1 month
in vitro). (Many of the individual spike potentials are obscured
or only faintly visible in the records at slow sweep rates.) $(B_{1,2})$:
Rapid disappearance of most components of complex afterdischarge
following introduction of 10^{-3}M glycine. After several min almost
complete block occurs (B_3). (C): Original complex responses are
rapidly restored after return to BSS. (D): Sustained depression
occurs again after return to 10^{-3}M glycine. (E): About 1 min after
introduction of 10^{-6}M strychnine + 10^{-3}M glycine almost complete
restoration of complex discharges occurs (and is maintained in this
solution as well as after return to BSS). Note spontaneous spikes
occurring prior to onset of stimulus, as well as long-lasting spike
barrage during slow-wave responses. (F): Similar block with 10^{-3}M
glycine in another cord explant (2 weeks in vitro). (G): Restoration
of long-lasting rhythmic afterdischarge in BSS. (H_1): Partial
depression after return to 10^{-3}M glycine + 10^{-7}M strychnine. Within
2 min, however, complex afterdischarge pattern began to reappear
(H_2) and became still more prominent after another min (H_3).

as noted above, the glycine depression can be prevented by concomitant addition of a low concentration of strychnine (10^{-7} to 10^{-6}M; Fig. 6E,H). Introduction of 10^{-7}M strychnine into the culture medium is probably comparable to the 0.1 mg/kg dosage used intravenously in the adult cat to produce selective reduction of synaptic inhibition in spinal neurons (Bradley et al., 1953; Curtis et al., 1971). On the other hand, whereas caffeine and cyclic AMP are quite effective in overcoming Ca^{++}-deficit blockades, no restorative action has been detected after glycine depression of cord explants. These data suggest that strychnine-enhancement of bioelectric discharges of CNS explants may be due to selective interference with glycine-sensitive receptors, possibly related to inhibitory synaptic membranes, as occurs in situ (e.g., Curtis et al., 1971).* Caffeine and cyclic AMP, on the other hand, appear to produce a general enhancement of transmission at both excitatory as well as inhibitory synapses (see Part 3). Therefore, whereas sustained hyperpolarization or increased membrane conductance effects on neurons in a high glycine medium could be efficiently reduced by strychnine they might actually be augmented by caffeine. The depressant effects of glycine perfusion on synaptically-mediated discharges of spinal cord explants are consonant with the demonstration by Hösli et al. (1971) that electrophoretic application of glycine produces hyperpolarization and increased membrane conductance of neurons in similar rat spinal cord explants (as occurs in situ - Curtis et al., 1968; Werman et al., 1968).

The specificity of glycine depression of spinal cord explant discharges is further supported by the following evidence: 1) in cultures of cord-innervated skeletal muscle (Crain et al., 1970), coordinated muscle contractions can still be evoked by ventral cord (or root) stimuli during this glycine blockade of internuncial CNS activity; 2) explants of cerebral neocortex show little or no depression in 10^{-3}M glycine, whereas 10^{-4}M γ-aminobutyric acid (GABA) may produce marked cerebral blocking effects; 3) 10^{-3}M GABA also produces serious depression of spinal cord discharges (Fig. 7B,D), but 10^{-7}M strychnine is ineffective in preventing this blockade - even 10^{-6}M strychnine produces only intermittent recovery (Fig. 7C); 4) picrotoxin and penicillin, on the other hand, which appear to antagonize GABA-receptor sites in situ (Curtis et al., 1971, 1972; Davidoff, 1972), can produce sustained recovery from GABA blockades of cord explants at concentrations which are ineffective against glycine-depressions; 5) a series of peptides including glycyl-γ-aminobutyric acid, glycyl-tryptophan and glycyl-glycyl-glycine show no depressing effects at 10^{-3}M concentrations, and some may even

---

*The dramatic enhancement of complex oscillatory afterdischarges which often occurs in CNS explants after introduction of d-tubocurarine (e.g., Fig. 1D) may also be due to selective blockade of inhibitory receptor sites - in this case, cholinergic (see Bhargava and Meldrum, 1969, 1971; Phyllis and York, 1968a, 1968b).

produce excitatory effects, on cord and cerebral explants. The
latter data are in agreement with earlier observations of Purpura
(1960) indicating that topical application of γ-aminobutyryl-γ-amino-
butyric acid on adult cat cerebral cortex in situ markedly augmented
surface-negative cortical evoked responses, in contrast to the powerful depressant effects of GABA. The absence of depression and the
possible excitatory effects of these peptides provides further
support for specificity of action of the component amino acids, and
it also suggests that enzymatic control of the formation and breakdown of simple peptides may be a significant mechanism for regulation
of CNS excitability. It will be of interest to determine whether
some of these peptides may produce excitatory effects by acting as
competitive antagonists of their component inhibitory amino acids.

Although high concentrations (10^{-3}M) of glycine and GABA were
used in the bathing fluid to produce these profound depressions of
synaptically-mediated discharges in CNS explants, the controls noted
above suggest that the effects may nevertheless be of physiological
significance. Normal glycine levels in cerebrospinal fluid are of
the order of 10^{-5}M (Dickinson and Hamilton, 1966), but local concentrations in the vicinity of CNS neurons may reach much higher
values. Using intraventricular or intrathecal injections of glycine
in adult cats (3-4 kg), 2.5-5 mg was required to produce marked
selective inhibition of flexor and crossed extension reflexes and
5-15 mg to abolish the facilitation of these reflexes produced by
10 μg of strychnine (Dhawan et al., 1972). The concentrations of
glycine and strychnine which developed in the cerebrospinal fluid
following these injections may well be comparable to the levels used
to bathe the CNS explants. Furthermore, the requirement of 1,000-
fold higher concentration of glycine to neutralize strychnine effects
in the cat is quite similar to the glycine/strychnine ratios used in
the CNS cultures. Also, chronic exposure of cord-muscle explants to
10^{-3}M glycine for several weeks did not produce any detectable cyto-
logic damage to the cells. Neuromuscular transmission was not blocked
during this period of sustained depression of internuncial cord activity, and complex organotypic cord discharges could be evoked after
return to normal medium (Crain and Peterson, in preparation).*

DEVELOPMENTAL ASPECTS OF AMINO ACID DEPRESSANTS

Glycine produces characteristic depressant effects on fetal
spinal cord explants within a few days after synaptogenesis in vitro,
and strychnine is concomitantly effective in augmenting complex discharges (Crain and Peterson, 1967; see also Parts 1 and 3). Similarly, GABA shows potent depressant effects on explants of fetal cerebral

---

*It is of interest in this regard that some of the standard
synthetic tissue culture media, e.g., Puck's medium N-16 (Puck et al.,
1958), include glycine concentrations of 10^{-3}M!

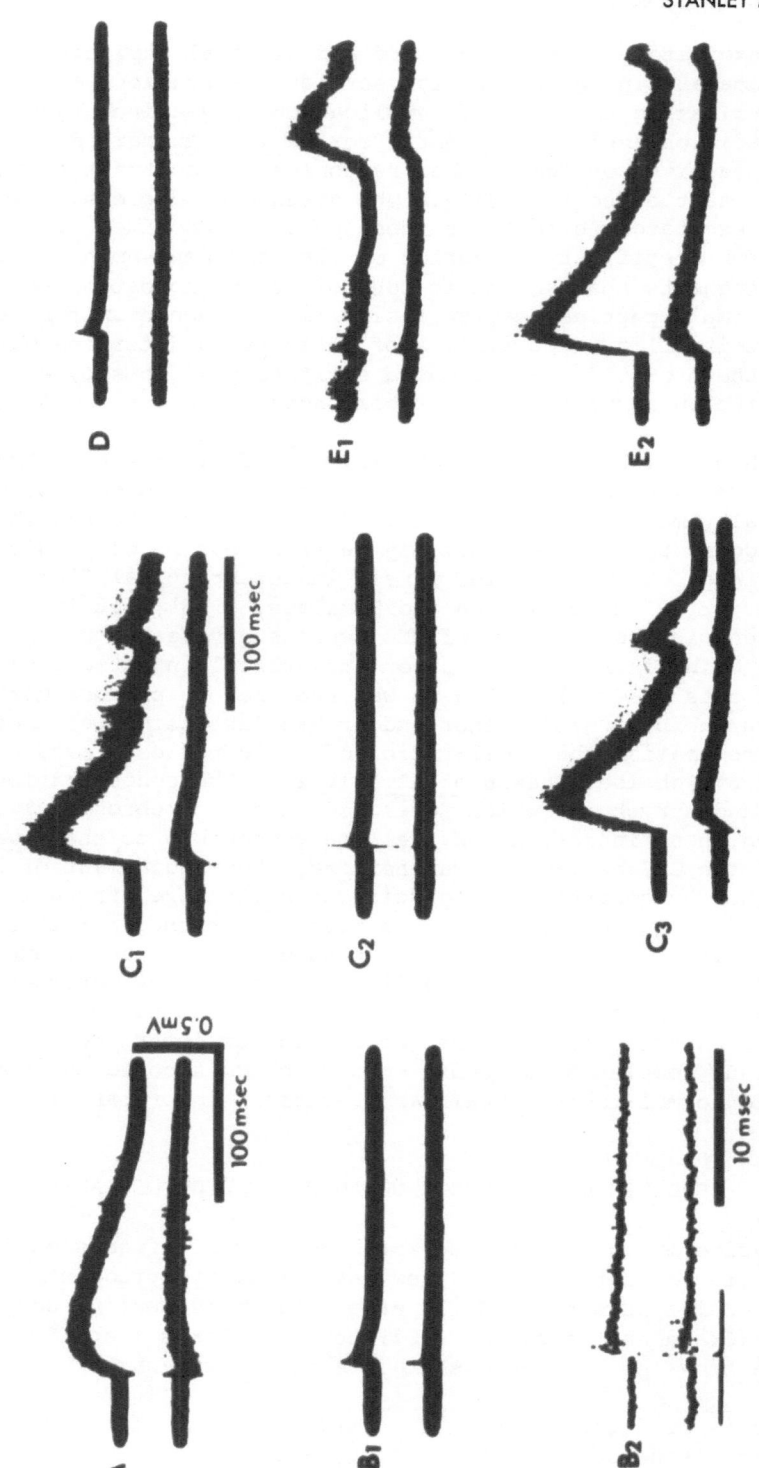

neocortex and hippocampus shortly after synaptogenesis _in vitro_ and penicillin (as well as strychnine) produces marked enhancement of discharges in these immature cerebral tissues (Crain and Bornstein, in preparation). These data suggest that inhibitory synapses are already functional during early stages of formation of CNS synaptic networks (Crain, 1966, 1969, 1973b; Pollack and Crain, 1972; Purpura, this volume). Further work is needed to clarify whether the amino acid depressants act as specific transmitters at inhibitory synapses or as more generalized regulators of neuronal excitability by action on diffusely-distributed receptor sites. Intracellular recordings from CNS explants during maturation _in vitro_ should provide valuable data on the mechanisms underlying these pharmacologic effects (e.g., Zipser _et al._, 1973). Similar studies of dissociated CNS neurons reaggregating in culture (Crain and Bornstein, 1972; Fischbach, 1972; Peacock _et al._, 1973) may permit still more critical analyses, expecially in conjunction with microelectrophoretic application of chemical agents to specific CNS cells under direct microscopic ob-servation (e.g., Hösli, 1971). Correlation of these bioelectric studies with direct analyses in CNS cultures of stimulus-dependent release of radio-isotope-labeled glycine, GABA, and other possible transmitter agents, will also be of great interest (e.g., Roberts and Mitchell, 1972).

ACKNOWLEDGMENTS

     The author wishes to express his appreciation to Murray B. Bornstein and Edith R. Peterson, Department of Neurology, for pro-viding the CNS cultures used in these studies. The nerve tissue culture laboratory at the Rose F. Kennedy Center is supported in part by grants NS-06735 and NS-08770 from NINDS, and MS-433 from the National Multiple Sclerosis Society. The work described in this paper has been supported by research grants NS-06545 from NINDS, grant MS 760-A from the National Multiple Sclerosis Society, and a grant from the Alfred P. Sloan Foundation. Dr. Crain has been supported by a Kennedy Scholar Award.

Fig. 7. Selective depression of synaptic network discharge of fetal cord explant in high-GABA/BSS and partial recovery after addition of strychnine. (A): Complex slow-wave and repetitive spike-barrage re-sponses evoked in 2 regions of cord explant, in BSS, by single sti-mulus to another cord site (1 month _in vitro_). ($B_{1,2}$): Rapid block in 10^{-3}M GABA. (C_1): Transient recovery and enhancement of discharges after addition of 10^{-6}M strychnine + 10^{-3}M GABA, but complete de-pression resumed about 1 min later (C_2). Within another min original complex responses resumed, but block continued to occur intermittently (in contrast to maintained protection by strychnine against glycine depression, e.g. Fig. 6E). (10^{-7}M strychnine did not antagonize this GABA blockade; cf. Fig. 6H.) (D): Return to 10^{-3}M GABA/BSS produced sustained depression again. (E): Rapid recovery of spontaneous (E_1) and evoked (E_2) discharges in BSS.

REFERENCES

Auerbach, A.A., and Purpura, D.P., 1972, Effects of dibutyryl cyclic AMP at giant fiber synapses in the hatchetfish, Fed. Proc. 31: 403.

Axelsson, J., and Thesleff, S., 1958, Activation of the contractile mechanism in striated muscle, Acta Physiol. Scand. 44: 55.

Baker, P.F., Hodgkin, A.L., and Ridgway, E.B., 1971, Depolarization and calcium entry in squid giant axon, J. Physiol. 218: 709.

Bhargava, V.K., and Meldrum, B.S., 1969, The strychnine-like action of curare and related compounds on the somatosensory evoked response of the rat cortex, Brit. J. Pharmacol. 37: 112.

Bhargava, V.K., and Meldrum, B.S., 1971, Blockade by eserine of the cerebral cortical effects of strychnine and curare, Nature 230: 152.

Birks, R.I., 1966, The fine structure of motor nerve endings at frog myoneural junction, Ann. N.Y. Acad. Sci. 135: 8.

Blaustein, M.P., and Goldman, D.E., 1966, Action of anionic and cationic nerve-blocking agents: Experiment and interpretation, Science 153: 429.

Bradley, K., Easton, D.M., and Eccles, J.C., 1953, An investigation of primary or direct inhibition, J. Physiol. 122: 474.

Breckenridge, B. McL., and Bray, J.J., 1970, Cyclic AMP and nerve function, in "Role of Cyclic AMP in Cell Function," (P. Greengard and E. Costa, eds.), pp. 325-333, Raven Press, New York.

Butcher, R.W., and Sutherland, E.W., 1962, Adenosine 3',5'-phosphate in biological materials. I. Purification and properties of cyclic 3',5'-nucleotide phosphodiesterase and use of this enzyme to characterize adenosine 3',5'-phosphate in human urine, J. Biol. Chem. 237: 1244.

Chagas, M.C., Esquibel, M.A., and Milhaud, M.G., 1972, Action d'inhibiteurs de la phosphodiesterase sur la décharge électrique de l'électroplaque isolée de l'Electrophorus electricus (L.), Comptes Rendus Acad. Sc. Paris 274: 1341.

Chasin, M., Harris, D.N., Phillips, M.B., and Hess, S.M., 1972, 1-Ethyl-4-(isopropylidenehydrazino)-1-H-pyrazolo (3,4-b)-pyridine-5-carboxylic acid, ethyl ester, hydrochloride (SQ 20009) A potent new inhibitor of cyclic 3',5'-nucleotide phosphodiesterases, Biochem. Pharmacol. 21: 2443.

Cheung, W.Y., 1970, Cyclic nucleotide phosphodiesterase, in "Role of Cyclic AMP in Cell Function," (P. Greengard and E. Costa, eds.), pp. 51-65, Raven Press, New York.

Cheung, W.Y., and Salganicoff, L., 1967, Cyclic 3',5'-nucleotide phosphodiesterase: localization and latent activity in rat brain, Nature 214: 90.

Crain, S.M., 1964, Development of bioelectric activity during growth of neonatal mouse cerebral cortex in tissue culture, in "Symposium: Neurological and Electroencephalographic Correlative Studies in Infancy," (P. Kellaway and I. Petersén, eds.), pp. 12-26, Grune and Stratton, New York.

Crain, S.M., 1966, Development of "organotypic" bioelectric activities in central nervous tissues during maturation in culture, Internat. Rev. Neurobiol. 9: 1.

Crain, S.M., 1969, Electrical activity of brain tissue developing in culture, in "Basic Mechanisms of the Epilepsies," (H.H. Jasper, A.A. Ward and A. Pope, eds.), pp. 506-516, Little, Brown, Boston.

Crain, S.M., 1972a, Tissue culture models of epileptiform activity, in "Experimental Models of Epilepsy," (D.P. Purpura, J.K. Penry, T. Tower, D.M. Woodbury and R. Walter, eds.), pp. 291-316, Raven Press, New York.

Crain, S.M., 1972b, Depression of complex bioelectric activity of mouse spinal cord explants by glycine and γ-aminobutyric acid, In Vitro 7: 249.

Crain, S.M., 1972c, Selective depression of organotypic bioelectric discharges of CNS explants by glycine and γ-aminobutyric acid. Soc. Neuroscience, 2nd Ann. Mtg, Houston, Abstr. p. 131.

Crain, S.M., 1973a, Microelectrode recording in brain tissue cultures, in "Methods in Physiological Psychology," Vol. 1, "Bioelectric Recording Techniques: Cellular Processes and Brain Potentials," (R.F. Thompson and M.M. Patterson, eds.), Academic Press, New York, pp. 39-75.

Crain, S.M., 1973b, Tissue culture models of developing brain
    functions, in "Developmental Studies of Behavior and the Nervous
    System," Vol. 2, "Aspects of Neurogenesis," (G. Gottlieb, ed.),
    Academic Press, pp. 69-114.

Crain, S.M., and Bornstein, M.B., 1964, Bioelectric activity of neo-
    natal mouse cerebral cortex during growth and differentiation
    in tissue culture, Exper. Neurol. 10: 425.

Crain, S.M., and Bornstein, M.B., 1972, Organotypic bioelectric
    activity in cultured reaggregates of dissociated rodent brain
    cells, Science 176: 182.

Crain, S.M., and Peterson, 1964, Complex bioelectric activity in
    organized tissue cultures of spinal cord (human, rat and chick),
    J. Cell. Comp. Physiol. 64: 1.

Crain, S.M., and Peterson, E.R., 1967, Onset and development of
    functional interneuronal connections in explants of rat spinal
    cord-ganglia during maturation in culture, Brain Res. 6: 750.

Crain, S.M., and Pollack, E.D., 1973, Restorative effects of cyclic
    AMP on complex bioelectric activities of cultured fetal rodent
    CNS tissues after acute Ca^{++}-deprivation, J. Neurobiol.,
    4: 321.

Crain, S.M., Bornstein, M.B., and Peterson, E.R., 1968a, Maturation
    of cultured embryonic CNS tissues during chronic exposure to
    agents which prevent bioelectric activity, Brain Res. 8: 363.

Crain, S.M., Peterson, E.R., and Bornstein, M.B., 1968b, Formation
    of functional interneuronal connections between explants of
    various mammalian central nervous tissues during development
    in vitro, in "Ciba Found. Symposium, Growth of the Nervous
    System," (G.E.W. Wolstenholme and M. O'Connor, eds.), pp. 13-31,
    Churchill, London.

Crain, S.M., Alfei, L., and Peterson, E.R., 1970, Neuromuscular
    transmission in cultures of adult human and rodent skeletal
    muscle after innervation in vitro by fetal rodent spinal
    cord, J. Neurobiol. 1: 471.

Curtis, D.R., Hösli, L., Johnston, G.A.R., and Johnston, I.H., 1968,
    The hyperpolarization of spinal motoneurones by glycine and
    related amino acids, Exper. Brain Res. 5: 235.

Curtis, D.R., Duggan, A.W., and Johnston, G.A.R., 1971, The specificity of strychnine as a glycine antagonist in the mammalian spinal cord, Exper. Brain Res. 12: 547.

Curtis, D.R., Game, C.J.A., Johnston, G.A.R., McCulloch, R.M., and Maclachlan, R.M., 1972, Convulsive action of penicillin, Brain Res. 43: 242.

Davidoff, R.A., 1972, Penicillin and presynaptic inhibition in the amphibian spinal cord, Brain Res. 36: 218.

Dettbarn, W.D., 1971, Local anesthetics, in "Handbook of Neurochemistry," Vol. 6, (A. Lajtha, ed.), pp. 423-439, Plenum Press, New York.

Dhawan, B.N., Sharma, J.N., and Srimal, R.C., 1972, Selective inhibition by glycine of some somatic reflexes in the cat, Brit. J. Pharmacol. 44: 404.

Dickinson, J.C., and Hamilton, P.B., 1966, The free amino acids of human spinal fluid determined by ion exchange chromatography, J. Neurochem. 13: 1179.

Elmqvist, D., and Feldman, D.S., 1965, Calcium dependence of spontaneous acetylcholine release at mammalian motor nerve terminals, J. Physiol. 181: 487.

Farese, R.V., 1971, Calcium as a mediator of adrenocorticotrophic hormone action on adrenal protein synthesis, Science 173: 447.

Fischbach, G.D., 1972, Synapse formation between dissociated nerve and muscle cells in low density cell cultures, Develop. Biol. 28: 407.

Florendo, N.T., Barrnett, R.J., and Greengard, P., 1971, Cyclic 3',5'-nucleotide phosphodiesterase: Cytochemical localization in cerebral cortex, Science 173: 745.

Forn, J., Tagliamonte, A., Tagliamonte, P., and Gessa, G.L., 1972, Stimulation by dibutyryl cyclic AMP of serotonin synthesis and tryptophan transport in brain slices, Nature (New Biology) 237: 245.

Gaballah, S., Popoff, C., and Sooknandan, G., 1971, Changes in cyclic 3',5'-adenosine monophosphate-dependent protein kinase levels in brain development, Brain Res. 31: 229.

Gessa, G.L., Krishna, G., Forn, J., Tagliamonte, A., and Brodie, B.B., 1970, Behavioral and vegetative effects produced by dibutyryl cyclic AMP injected into different areas of the brain, in "Role of Cyclic AMP in Cell Function," (P. Greengard and E. Costa, eds.), pp. 371-381, Raven Press, New York.

Goldberg, A.L., and Singer, J.J., 1969, Evidence for a role of cyclic AMP in neuromuscular transmission, Proc. Natl. Acad. Sci. 64: 134.

Greengard, P., and Kuo, J.F., 1970, On the mechanism of action of cyclic AMP, in "Role of Cyclic AMP in Cell Function," (P. Greengard and E. Costa, eds.), pp. 287-306, Raven Press, New York.

Guillery, R.W., Sobkowicz, H.M., and Scott, G.L., 1968, Light and electron microscopical observations of the ventral horn and ventral root in long term cultures of the spinal cord of the fetal mouse, J. Comp. Neurol. 134: 433.

Hardman, J.G., Robison, G.A., and Sutherland, E.W., 1971, Cyclic nucleotides, Ann. Rev. Physiol. 33: 311.

Henkart, M., 1972, Structure and function of the endoplasmic reticulum in the squid giant axon, Soc. Neuroscience, 2nd Ann. Mtg., Houston, Abstr. p. 103.

Hild, W., and Tasaki, I., 1962, Morphological and physiological properties of neurons and glial cells in tissue culture, J. Neurophysiol. 25: 277.

Hoffer, B.J., 1971, Discussion in: Symp. on Cyclic AMP Cell Function, Ann. N.Y. Acad. Sci. 185: 555.

Hösli, L., Andres, P.F., and Hösli, E., 1971, Effects of glycine on spinal neurones grown in tissue culture, Brain Res. 34: 399.

Jenkinson, D.H., Stamenovi, B.A., and Whitaker, B.D.L., 1968, The effect of noradrenaline on the end-plate potential in twitch fibers of the frog, J. Physiol. 195: 743.

Johnson, G.A., Boukama, S.J., Lahti, R.A., and Mathews, J., 1972, Cyclic AMP and cyclic nucleotide phosphodiesterase activity in synaptic vesicles, Fed. Proc. 31: 513.

Katz, B., 1969, "The Release of Neural Transmitter Substances," C.C. Thomas, Illinois.

Katz, B., and Miledi, R., 1965a, The measurement of synaptic delay, and the time course of acetylcholine release at the neuromuscular junction, Proc. Roy. Soc. London, Series B, 161: 483.

Katz, B., and Miledi, R., 1965b, The effect of calcium on acetyl-
    choline release from motor nerve terminals, Proc. Roy. Soc.
    London, Series B, 161: 496.

Katz, B., and Miledi, R., 1968, The role of calcium in neuromuscular
    facilitation, J. Physiol. 195: 481.

Korneliussen, H., 1972, Ultrastructure of normal and stimulated motor
    endplates, Z. Zellforsch. 130: 28.

Krnjevic, K., and Miledi, R., 1958, Some effects produced by adren-
    aline upon neuromuscular propagation in rats, J. Physiol.
    141: 291.

Kuperman, A.S., Altura, B.T., and Chezar, J.A., 1968, Action of
    procaine on calcium efflux from frog nerve and muscle, Nature
    217: 673.

Lambert, E.H., and Elmqvist, D., 1971, Quantal components of end-
    plate potentials in the myasthenic syndrome, Ann. N.Y. Acad.
    Sci. 183: 183.

Llinás, R., Blinks, J.R., and Nicholson, C., 1972, Calcium transient
    in presynaptic terminal of squid giant synapse: Detection with
    aequorin, Science 176: 1127.

Marco, L.A., and Nastuk, W.L., 1968, Sarcomeric oscillations in frog
    skeletal muscle fibers, Science 161: 1357.

McAfee, D.A., and Greengard, P., 1972, Adenosine 3',5'-monophosphate:
    Electrophysiological evidence for a role in synaptic transmission,
    Science 178: 310.

Miledi, R., and Thies, R.E., 1967, Post-tetanic increase in frequency
    of miniature end-plate potentials in calcium-free solutions,
    J. Physiol. 192: 54.

Peach, M.J., 1972, Stimulation of release of adrenal catecholamine
    by adenosine 3':5' cyclic monophosphate and theophylline in the
    absence of extracellular Ca^{2+}, Proc. Natl. Acad. Sci. 69: 834.

Peacock, J.H., Nelson, P.G., and Goldstone, M.W., 1973, Electro-
    physiologic study of cultured neurons dissociated from spinal
    cord and dorsal root ganglia of fetal mice, Devel. Biol.,
    30: 137.

Phillis, J.W., and York, D.H., 1968a, An intracortical cholinergic
    inhibitory synapse, Life Sciences 7: 65.

Phillis, J.W., and York, D.H., 1968b, Pharmacological studies on a cholinergic inhibition in the cerebral cortex, Brain Res. 10: 297.

Pollack, E.D., and Crain, S.M., 1972, Development of motility in fish embryos in relation to release from early CNS inhibition, J. Neurobiol. 3: 381.

Prince, W.T., Berridge, M.J., and Rasmussen, H., 1972, Role of calcium and adenosine-3':5'-cyclic monophosphate in controlling fly salivary gland secretion, Proc. Nat. Acad. Sci. 69: 553.

Puck, T.T., Cieciura, S.J., and Robinson, A., 1958, Genetics of somatic mammalian cells. III. Long-term cultivation of euploid cells from human and animal subjects, J. Exp. Med. 108: 945.

Purpura, D.P., 1960, Pharmacological actions of ω-amino acid drugs on different cortical synaptic organizations, in "Inhibition in the Nervous System and Gamma-Aminobutyric Acid," (E. Roberts, C.F. Baxter, A. Van Harreveld, C.A.G. Wiersma, W.R. Adey and K.F. Killam, eds.), pp. 495-514, Pergamon Press, New York.

Purpura, D.P., and Housepian, E.M., 1961, Morphological and physiological properties of chronically isolated immature neocortex, Exper. Neurol. 4: 377.

Purpura, D.P., and Shofer, R.J., 1972, Excitatory action of dibutyryl cyclic adenosine monophosphate on immature cerebral cortex, Brain Res. 38: 179.

Rasmussen, H., 1970, Cell communication, calcium ion, and cyclic adenosine monophosphate, Science 170: 404.

Ritchie, J.M., 1970, Central nervous stimulants. II. The xanthines, in "The Pharmacological Basis of Therapeutics," (L.S. Goodman and A. Gilman, eds.), pp. 358-370, Macmillan, New York.

Roberts, P.J., and Mitchell, J.F., 1972, The release of amino acids from the hemisected spinal cord during stimulation, J. Neurochem. 19: 2473.

Siggins, G.R., Hoffer, B.J., and Bloom, F.E., 1971a, Response to Godfraind, J.M. and R. Pumain, Cyclic adenosine monophosphate and norepinephrine: effect on Purkinje cells in rat cerebellar cortex, Science 174: 1257.

Siggins, G.R., Oliver, A.P., Hoffer, B.J., and Bloom, F.E., 1971b, Cyclic adenosine monophosphate and norepinephrine: effects on transmembrane properties of cerebellar Purkinje cells, Science 171: 192.

Singer, J.J., and Goldberg, A.L., 1970, Cyclic AMP and transmission
    at the neuromuscular junction, in "Role of Cyclic AMP in Cell
    Function," (P. Greengard and E. Costa, eds.), pp. 335-348, Raven
    Press, New York.

Takamori, M., 1972, Caffeine, calcium and Eaton-Lambert syndrome,
    Arch. Neurol. 27: 285.

Teichberg, S., and Holtzman, E., 1973, Axonal agranular reticulum
    and synaptic vesicles in cultured embryonic chick sympathetic
    neurons, J. Cell Biol., 57: 88.

Torda, C., 1972, Effect of cyclic adenosine 3',5'-monophosphate
    (c-AMP) on synaptic spike generation, in "Advances in Cyclic
    Nucleotide Research," Vol. 1, "Physiology and Pharmacology of
    Cyclic AMP," (P. Greengard, R. Paoletti and G.A. Robison, eds.),
    p. 589, Raven Press, New York.

Werman, R., Davidoff, R.A., and Aprison, M.H., 1968, Inhibitory
    action of glycine on spinal neurons in the cat, J. Neurophysiol.
    31: 81.

Zipser, B., Crain, S.M., and Bornstein, M.B., 1973, Intracellular
    recordings of complex synaptically mediated discharges in
    explants of fetal hippocampal cortex during maturation in
    culture, Fed. Proc., 32: 420.

Zipser, B., Crain, S.M. and Bornstein, M.B., 1973, Directly evoked
    "paroxysmal" depolarizations of mouse hippocampal neurons in
    synaptically organized explants in longterm culture, Brain Res.,
    in press.

CNS DRUGS: BEHAVIORAL DEVELOPMENT
C.O. Rutledge, Chairman

FACTORS INFLUENCING THE EFFECTS OF DRUGS ADMINISTERED DURING

DEVELOPMENT ON ADULT BEHAVIOR

C.O. Rutledge

Department of Pharmacology, University of Colorado

School of Medicine, Denver, Colorado

Studies on the effects of drugs administered during development on the subsequent behavior of the adult animal were given new direction about 10 years ago with a series of investigations by Werboff and his colleagues (Werboff et al., 1961; Werboff and Dembicki, 1962; Werboff and Havlena, 1962; Werboff and Kesner, 1963). In one of these studies (Werboff and Havlena, 1962) pregnant rats were treated chronically with either reserpine, meprobamate or chlorpromazine. After the offspring had matured, their behavior was compared to the behavior of offspring of untreated rats. It was found that there was motor impairment in the offspring of treated rats: their ability to move up an inclined plane was impaired. It was also observed that motor activity, as measured in an open field test, was reduced in offspring of treated animals. Although these studies have been criticized for inadequate control of postnatal rearing effects (see Joffe, 1969), they serve to illustrate the numerous variables which must be controlled before one can interpret the effects of a drug given during development on the subsequent behavior of the adult. These variables have been described in detail by Joffe (1969) and Kornetsky (1970).

Some of these variables are illustrated in Fig. 1. The initial factor in determining the behavior of an adult animal is the genotype of the animal (1 in Fig. 1). The fact that one can have strains of mice and rats with markedly different behavioral characteristics illustrated the importance of the genotype in influencing behavior. In a well controlled study of the role of genetic factors in determining behavior, Joffe (1969) mated two strains of rats which differed in their open field motor activity and in their conditioned avoidance behavior. He observed the effect of stress to the mother on the behavior of the offspring. Although the results were complex

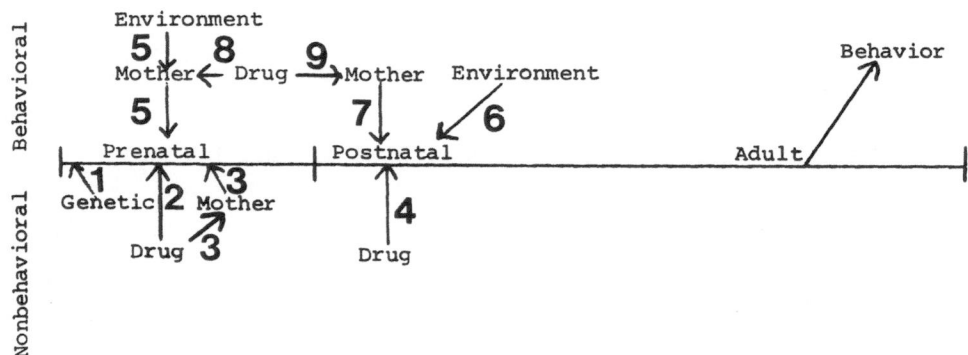

Fig. 1. Pre- and postnatal determinants of behavior. The horizontal line represents the prenatal, postnatal and adult life span of an animal. The nonbehavioral (below the line) and the behavioral (above the line) determinants of a behavioral response of the adult animal are illustrated. The numbers adjacent to each determinant are explained in the text.

---

due to the large number of necessary controls, he suggested that maternal genotype determines the extent of the effects of prenatal stress on offspring behavior and that the offspring genotype determines the direction of the changes in behavior when bidirectional effects occur.

Most of the pharmacological studies on the development of behavior have been on the effect of a drug, given either prenatally or postnatally, on the developing central nervous system (2 and 4 in Fig. 1). Two examples of this type of interaction are presented in this symposium. Dr. Whalen describes the effects of sex hormones given to rats during development on their subsequent sexual behavior and Dr. Sparber describes the effects of drugs which alter the biochemistry of neurotransmitters on subsequent conditioned and unconditioned behavior in the rat.

In addition to acting directly on the developing neurons, drugs also alter the developing central nervous system indirectly through the mother (3 in Fig. 1). By altering the nutritional state (Cowley and Griesel, 1962) oxygen supply (Vierck et al., 1966), blood epinephrine levels (Thompson and Goldenberg, 1962) or blood corticos-

teroid levels (Joffe, 1969) of the pregnant female, the behavior of
the offspring can be changed. This is presumably due, at least in
part, to a physiological impairment of the development of the fetus.
A drug may also alter behavior by changing the development of other
systems which are important in specific behaviors (2 and 4 in Fig. 1).
For example, changing the development of the penis has been shown to
be important in sexual behavior (Whalen, 1968; Beach et al., 1969).
The administration of testosterone at birth to castrated male rats
altered differentiation of the penis so that changes in sexual behavior in the adult were due, at least in part, to changes in phallic
development.

     Perhaps the variables which most confound interpretation of the
effects of drugs on the development of behavior are the behavioral
determinants of subsequent behavior. There are numerous studies
which indicate that the behavioral experience of the mother as well
as the offspring have marked effects on the subsequent behavior of
the offspring. These effects can occur either before or after birth.
Prenatal behavioral effects on subsequent behavior of the offspring
(5 in Fig. 1) have been studied by Joffe (1969). He subjected rats
to stress during pregnancy and observed the behavior of the offspring.
There were differences between the offspring of stressed and nonstressed mothers on both open field motor activity and conditioned
avoidance responses. These experiments were controlled by cross-
fostering the offspring to nonstressed rats.

     Most behavioral influences on the developing organism are post-
natal effects. Denenberg and Whimbey (1963) demonstrated that the
manipulation of the environment (6 in Fig. 1) of rats during infancy
not only can have detectable effects on their behavior but on the
behavior of their offspring as well. Infant rats were handled daily
by simply removing the pups from their nest and putting them into a
can of shavings for 3 minutes a day and then replacing them in their
home cage. This treatment alters the behavior of the infant rats.
When the rats were adult the females were mated randomly with un-
handled males from the colony. Litters born to some of these females
were left with their natural mothers, litters born to others were
fostered to mothers which had not received the handling treatment.
It was found that the type of mother which reared the litter affected
the behavior of the pups: pups reared by mothers which had been handled in infancy had different open field activity scores than pups
raised by mothers which had not been handled in infancy. Defecation
scores were used as an index of reaction to stress and were significantly higher in animals reared by mothers which had been handled in
infancy than in animals reared by nonhandled mothers. Thus, handling
the mothers in their infancy in some way altered the behavior of the
mothers so that behavior of their pups was changed, presumably by a
behavioral interaction (7 in Fig. 1).

The interaction of the mother with pups may be influenced by prenatal drug administration. Ordy et al. (1966) in a well controlled study has shown that chlorpromazine administered to pregnant rats altered conditioned avoidance behavior and motor activity of the offspring. Through fostering procedures they were able to demonstrate that the drug had both prenatal effects (8 in Fig. 1) on the offspring as well as postnatal fostering effects (9 in Fig. 1). It was obvious that the treatment of the mothers during pregnancy altered the interaction of the mother with the offspring after the pups were born.

It is clear that drugs act on the developing organism to produce changes in the subsequent behavior. In designing experiments, it is necessary to be aware of numerous indirect influences the drug might have and to provide proper controls. It is difficult to design studies in which the behavioral response changes as a function of the dose of the drug. This is due in part to the long temporal delay between the time the drug is given and the time the response is observed. With this long time span all of the variables which affect behavior have a high probability of occurring. Fortunately there are systems in which one can use biochemical or morphological markers which are directly related to subsequent behavior. For example, it is well known that drugs such as reserpine alter behavior by an action on catechol- and indoleamine stores in the brain (see Brodie et al., 1957). As discussed by Sparber (this proceedings), one can obtain some indication of the relationship between the drug and the behavioral response by monitoring catecholamine metabolism in the developing animal.

REFERENCES

Beach, F.A., Noble, R.G. and Ordnoff, R.K., 1969, Effects of perinatal androgen treatment on responses of male rats to gonadal hormones in adulthood, J. Comp. Physiol. Psychol. 68: 490.

Brodie, B.B., Olin, J.S., Kuntzman, R.G. and Shore, P.A., 1957, Possible interrelationship between release of brain norepinephrine and serotonin by reserpine, Science 125: 1293.

Cowley, J.J. and Griesel, R.D., 1962, Pre- and post-natal effects of a low protein diet on the behaviour of the white rat, Psychologia Africana 9: 216.

Denenberg, V.H. and Whimbey, A.E., 1963, Behavior of adult rats is modified by the experiences their mothers had as infants, Science (Washington) 142: 1192.

Joffe, J.M., 1969, "Prenatal Determinants of Behaviour", Pergamon
    Press, New York.

Kornetsky, C., 1970, Psychoactive drugs in the immature organism,
    Psychopharmacologia 17: 105.

Ordy, J.M., Samorajski, T., Collins, R.L. and Rolsten, C., 1966,
    Prenatal chlorpromazine effects on liver, survival and be-
    havior of mice offspring, J. Pharmacol. Exp. Ther. 151: 110.

Thompson, W.R. and Goldenberg, L., 1962, Some physiological effects
    of maternal adrenalin injection during pregnancy in rat off-
    spring, Psychol. Rep. 10: 759.

Vierck, C.J., King, F.A., and Ferm, V.H., 1966, Effects of prenatal
    hypoxia upon activity and emotionality of the rat, Psychon.
    Sci. 4: 87.

Werboff, J. and Dembicki, E.L., 1962, Toxic effects of tranquilizers
    administered to gravid rats. J. Neuropsychiat. 4: 87.

Werboff, J., Gottlieb, J.S., Havlena, J. and Word, T.J., 1961,
    Behavioral effects of prenatal drug administration in the white
    rat, Pediatrics 27: 318.

Werboff, J. and Havlena, J., 1962, Postnatal behavioral effects of
    tranquilizers administered to the gravid rat, Exp. Neurol. 6:
    263.

Werboff, J. and Kesner, R., 1963, Learning deficits of offspring after
    administration of tranquilizing drugs to the mothers, Nature 197:
    106.

Whalen, R.E., 1969, Differentiation of the neural mechanisms which con-
    trol gonadotropin secretion and sexual behavior. In: "Perspect-
    ives in Reproduction and Sexual Behavior", (Diamond, ed.),
    Indiana University Press, Bloomington.

GONADAL HORMONES AND THE DEVELOPING BRAIN

Richard E. Whalen

Department of Psychobiology, University of California

Irvine, California

Research during the past 15 years has revealed that the developing brain has a sensitivity and response to gonadal hormones which differs from that of the fully mature brain. This age-dependent sensitivity of brain to hormones has been shown in studies of the ontogeny of gonadal function as well as in studies of the development of behavior. Research in these areas has been extensively reviewed in the past few years (Beach, 1971; Gorski, 1971; Goy, 1968; Whalen, 1968). Thus, no attempt will be made here to review all aspects of the hormonal control of sexual development. Rather, we will focus on one species, the rat, and will attempt to illustrate some principles of hormone action as they relate to the development of sexual behavior.

SEXUAL BEHAVIOR AND ITS HORMONAL CONTROL

The mating responses of male and female rats are quite distinctive and can be reliably scored by a trained observer. The male approaches a female and may engage in investigation of the female's genitalia. The male then mounts the female from the rear and palpates her flanks with his forepaws. The male may dismount at this time, or as is more commonly the case, he may begin a rapid series of thrusting responses, moving his hips and directing his penis toward the vagina. The male may dismount following a few seconds of thrusting or he may achieve insertion of the penis into the vagina of the female. If insertion is achieved it is maintained for approximately 300 msec (Peirce and Nuttall, 1961) after which the male dismounts. Following such an intromission response the male almost invariably licks his penis. Following an interval of approximately

15-60 sec the male will reapproach the female and remount. For the
sexually rested male mounting behavior will continue until the male
has achieved about 11 intromissions at which point ejaculation will
occur. The ejaculatory response is characterized by a deep thrust
with insertion being maintained for 1-4 sec. Following ejaculation
the male withdraws from the female for several minutes during which
he emits an ultrasonic "song" (Barfield and Geyer, 1972). The male
then reapproaches the female and initiates a second series of mounts
and intromissions again culminating in ejaculation. Six or seven
such ejaculatory series may occur before the male ceases copulation
for that day (Beach and Jordan, 1956). The point to be emphasized
here is that the copulatory responses of the male rat are distinctive,
and that they can be reliably measured, thereby providing quantitative data concerning this complex behavior.

The sexual responses of the female rat are also distinctive and
can be reliably measured. The rat is a polyestrous species which
displays either a 4 or 5 day estrous cycle. The female is behaviorally receptive to the male for only a limited part of the cycle. Kuehn
and Beach (1963) and Hardy (1972) report that a female will show a
lordosis response, a concave arching of the back exposing the peri-
neum, for only 15 to 21 hours of a four day cycle. At the initiation
of the receptive period the probability that a mount by a male will
elicit lordosis is low. Approximately 12 hours later nearly every
mount by a male will elicit lordosis. Because the probability of
lordosis varies so systematically over the estrous cycle many investigators have used the ratio of lordosis responses to mounts by a male
as an index of the state of a female's receptivity. Other investigators have added quantitative sophistication by rating the intensity
of each lordosis response in addition to assessing its probability
of occurrence. One such measurement system is illustrated in the
work of Hardy and De Bold (1972).

The sexual responses of male and female rats are under gonadal
control. In the male, removal of the testes is followed by a slow,
but progressive decline in sexual performance. The latency to mount
and to achieve intromission increases as does the interval between the
first intromission and the occurrence of the first ejaculation (Beach
and Holz-Tucker, 1949; Davidson, 1966; Whalen and Luttge, 1971).
Early studies (e.g. Beach and Holz-Tucker, 1949) indicated that mating
responses could be maintained by the administration of testosterone
propionate and that the degree of maintenance is dose dependent. More
recently we (Luttge and Whalen, 1970a) have found that the free al-
cohol form of both testosterone and androstenedione are capable of
restoring mating responses to preoperative levels in castrated male
rats which had ceased to mate. These two steroids showed almost
identical dose-response relationships. Dihydrotestosterone, the
5α-reduced form of testosterone, is incapable of maintaining mating
in the male rat even though this steroid is extremely potent in

maintaining peripheral androgen target tissues such as the prostate (Whalen and Luttge, 1971).

In the female removal of the ovaries results in the disappearance of all sexual responses. If the ovaries are removed during the diestrous phase of the cycle, the female will not come into a state of receptivity one or two days later as expected (Schwartz, 1969). If the ovaries are removed following the period of endogenous estrogen secretion but before progesterone is released, that is, approximately 12 hours before expected mating, the probability of lordosis is reduced but not eliminated. If the ovaries are removed 6 hours after the period of progesterone secretion, intense lordosis behavior is seen at the expected time. Thus, unlike the male, sexual responses in the female disappear rapidly following castration and they seem to be dependent upon the presence of both estrogen and progesterone. This latter conclusion is also supported by studies in which estrogen and progesterone, alone or in combination are administered to ovariectomized females (Beach, 1942; Edwards et al., 1968). The response of female rats to estrogen and progesterone is dose dependent (Powers and Valenstein, 1972; Whalen and Hardy, 1970).

SPECIFICITY OF HORMONAL RESPONSE

The studies outlined above demonstrate that the sexual responses of male and female rats are under gonadal control and that one can maintain mating responses in castrated males by administering testosterone or androstenedione, the natural secretory products of the testis. Similarly, mating responses in the ovariectomized female can be maintained by administering estradiol and progesterone, the natural secretory products of the ovary. These studies do not, however, reveal the potential of the animal to respond to hormonal stimulation. The question remains as to whether the behavior which is displayed, mounting or lordosis, is specific to the sex of the animal or whether the behavior is specific to type of hormonal stimulation provided. Investigators have attempted to answer this question by administering estrogen and progesterone to males and by administering testosterone to females. In early work on this problem Beach (1941, 1942, 1945; Beach and Rasquin, 1942) showed that female rats often exhibit male-like mounting responses, but rarely intromission and ejaculation-type patterns. The administration of testosterone increases the frequency of mounting responses and the probability that a mount will resemble an intromission type response. Beach also reported that males could show lordosis responses, although such behavior was not common.

Contemporary work has clarified the relationships which exist between hormones and the display of sexual responses and has added one truly significant finding about the genesis of the hormonal control of behavior. Following the pioneering work of Phoenix et al., (1959)

on the guinea pig, Harris and Levine (1962, 1965) demonstrated that
the administration of testosterone propionate to newborn female rats
would permanently inhibit their response to estrogen and progesterone
in adulthood. Such females would neither show lordosis spontaneously
nor following hormone treatment. Feder and Whalen (1965) and Grady
et al. (1965) further demonstrated that castration of the newborn
male rat permitted the male to display lordosis in adulthood in response to estrogen and progesterone treatment. These studies suggested that sex differences in adult sexual behavior were influenced
by the presence or absence of hormonal stimulation of the developing
brain.

     To test this hypothesis further we (Whalen and Edwards, 1967)
gonadectomized male and female rats within 12 hours of birth; sham
operated rats were maintained as controls. Some of the gonadectomized animals were administered testosterone propionate at the time
of surgery, and some were oil treated. When these animals were mature they were again administered testosterone propionate and tested
for the display of masculine sexual behavior. Hormonal manipulation
at birth had little effect upon the display of mounting responses.
Both males and females mounted; animals treated with androgen at birth
mounted at the same frequency as untreated animals. This was not
true, however, for the display of intromission-type responses. These
were displayed most frequently by males which were sham operated at
birth and castrated in adulthood. Males which were castrated at birth
showed few intromission responses and these occurred at about the
same frequency as that shown by sham-operated females or females
ovariectomized at birth. Both males and females which were gonadectomized and administered androgen at birth displayed intromission-
type responses more frequently than was shown by animals deprived of
hormonal stimulation at birth. Thus, early hormone stimulation facilitated the display of intromission behavior while having little effect
upon the frequency of mounting.

     Since early postnatal hormonal stimulation facilitated intro-
mission behavior but not mounting behavior we concluded that the hormonal stimulation of the developing brain is not required to prime a
"neural motivational system" for the control of masculine sexual responses. We felt that if early androgen stimulation did activate a
motivational system this should be reflected by increased mounting
behavior. We further felt that the increased intromission behavior
which was observed could be accounted for by the peripheral effects
of the androgen stimulation. Neonatal castration inhibits normal
phallic development while early androgen treatment facilitates phallic
development. Beach et al. (1969) have shown that there is a strong
correlation between phallic size and the probability of intromission
behavior in rats.

Our conclusion that early androgen stimulation does not activate
a motivational system was strengthened when we were unable to demonstrate that any of a variety of pre- and postnatal androgen treatments would facilitate the occurrence of mounting behavior in female
rats (Whalen et al., 1969). Recent evidence, however, forces us to
reevaluate that conclusion. Clemens and Coniglio (1971) have reported
that the probability that a female rat will display mounting behavior
in adulthood is directly related to the number of male sibs in the
litter. This finding suggests that a neural system subserving mounting behavior does exist and is dependent upon hormonal stimulation
prior to birth. These exciting findings deserve extensive replication
because they have important implications for our understanding of the
capacity of the female rat to respond to androgen treatment with the
display of mounting.

The development of the capacity to show lordosis behavior is
strongly determined by the presence or absence of postnatal hormonal
stimulation. Males raised to maturity with their testes in situ
rarely displayed lordosis behavior following estrogen and progesterone
priming. Males castrated at birth, and females castrated at birth
or in adulthood all displayed intense lordosis responses and these
groups did not differ from each other in the probability of lordosis
behavior. Males and females both castrated and hormone treated at
birth failed to show lordosis (Whalen and Edwards, 1967). Thus, the
capacity to display lordosis developed in both males and females if
they grew to maturity without hormonal stimulation. Hormonal stimulation of the developing brain either endogenously by the secretions
of the male testes or exogenously by administered hormones permanently
limits the capacity of the rat to respond to estrogen and progesterone.
These findings are summarized in Table I.

Our conclusion from the above studies was that the major effect
of early postnatal hormonal stimulation in the rat was a "defeminization" of those neural systems which control sexual responses. Thus,
males and androgenized females fail to respond behaviorally to estrogen and progesterone. The question remained as to whether defeminization represented an inhibition of response to estrogen, to progesterone or to both hormones. Clemens et al. (1969) and Davidson
and Levine (1969) presented evidence which suggested that a primary
effect of neonatal androgen stimulation was an inhibition of responsiveness to progesterone. More recently we (Whalen et al., 1971) compared
the response to estrogen alone of male rats which were either castrated at birth or in adulthood and of female rats which were either
androgenized or untreated at birth. Both the untreated females and
the neonatally castrated males responded to estrogen with the display
of lordosis while the androgenized females and the males castrated
in adulthood did not. Thus it would appear that early androgen stimulation desensitizes the neural systems which respond to estrogen
as well as those which respond to progesterone in the control of
behavior.

TABLE I

RELATIONSHIPS BETWEEN HORMONAL CONDITIONS DURING DEVELOPMENT
AND SEXUAL RESPONDING OF THE RAT IN ADULTHOOD

| Hormonal Condition During Critical Period | Hormonal Condition During Adulthood | | | Estrogen and Progesterone |
| | Androgen | | | |
	Mounts	Intromission Responses	Ejaculation Responses	Lordosis Responses
MALE				
Testes Intact	+ + +	+ + +	+ + +	—
Castration at Birth	+ + +	+	—	+ + +
Castration at Birth + TP[1]	+ + +	+ + +	+ +	—
FEMALE				
Ovaries Intact	+ + +	+	—	+ + +
Ovariectomized at Birth	+ + +	+	—	+ + +
TP at Birth	+ + +	+ +	+	—
TP Pre- and Post-natally	+ + +	+ + +	+ + +	—

[1]TP = testosterone propionate

Finally, we have asked which androgens are involved in the defeminization process. In all of the early studies investigators treated newborn animals with the potent long acting synthetic androgen, testosterone propionate. We were concerned that this synthetic agent might not be acting in a physiological manner. We therefore decided to treat animals with the free-alcohol form of the naturally occurring androgens, testosterone and androstenedione, and with the potent androgenic metabolite, dihydrotestosterone (Whalen and Rezek, unpublished). In order to mimic natural conditions of stimulation, these steroids were implanted subcutaneously in silastic capsules which allowed for a slow continuous release of the hormone. Female rats were implanted on the day of birth and the capsules were removed ten days later. Testosterone completely inhibited the display of lordosis in adulthood, androstenedione was partially effective and dihydrotestosterone had no effect upon later behavior. Thus, the defeminization which normally occurs in the male because of the presence of the testes during the first few days after birth is induced by the naturally occurring steroids.

MECHANISM OF ACTION

Since males and neonatally androgenized females fail to respond to estrogen, a number of investigators have hypothesized that the brains of these animals may fail to accumulate and retain estrogen in the manner shown by females. To test this hypothesis on normal males and females as well as neonatally androgenized females, several groups of investigators have administered tritiated estradiol to rats and have determined the retention of hormone in various brain regions. The results have been variable. Some investigators have found that early androgenization inhibits the uptake of estrogen into relevant brain regions, others have not (Eisenfeld and Axelrod, 1966; Flerko et al., 1971; McEwen and Pfaff, 1970; McGuire and Lisk, 1969). In our laboratory we found initially that the brains of female rats accumulated the greatest amount of estrogen and the brains of males the least with neonatally androgenized female falling in between. This relationship, however, did not hold when males and females were equated for body weight (Green et al., 1969). In subsequent work a similar finding was obtained, namely, that male and female rats did not differ in their ability to concentrate estradiol in selected brain regions (Whalen and Luttge, 1970). In still further work on this problem we (Luttge and Whalen, 1970b) found that following the administration of tritiated estradiol both estradiol and estrone could be found in the brain, but that males and females did not differ in this regard. Thus, although males and females differ dramatically in their behavioral response to estrogen the evidence is not strong that they do so by a differential brain accumulation of hormone. Estradiol gets into the brain of the male as it does in the female.

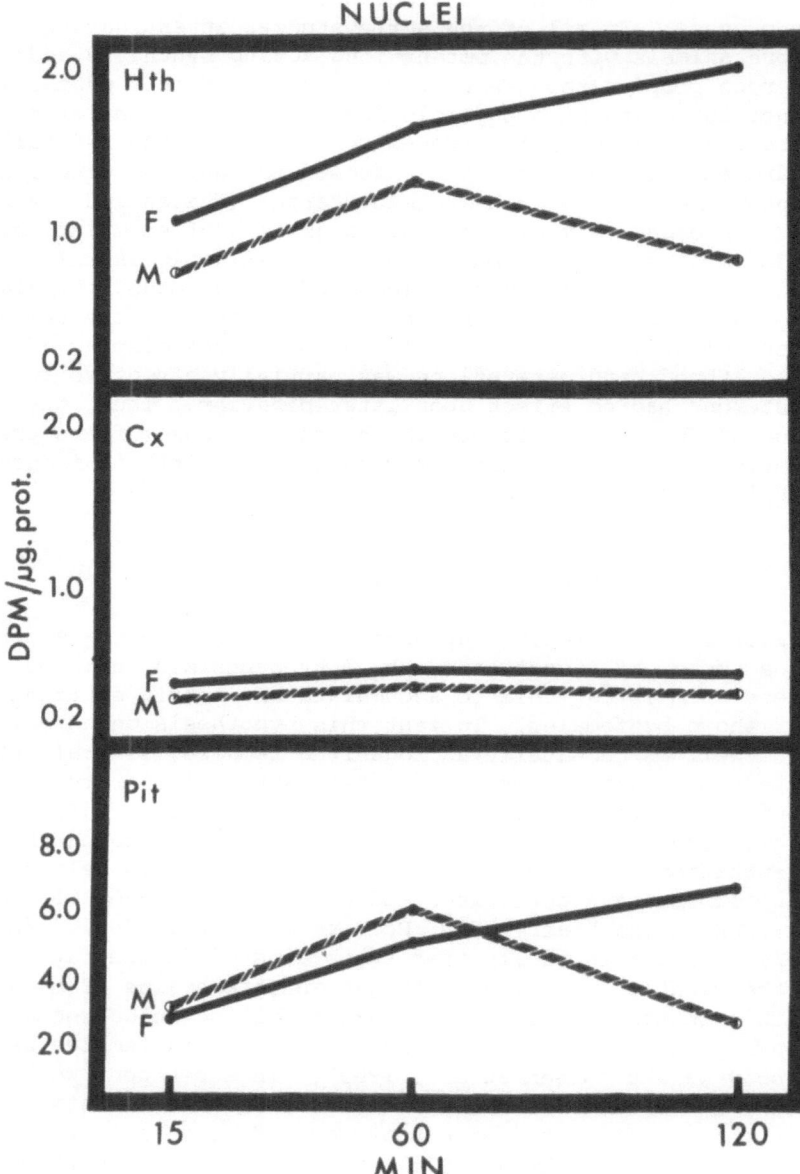

Fig. 1. Uptake and retention of radioactivity in hypothalamic, cortical and pituitary nuclei of male and female rats gonadectomized in
adulthood. The animals were administered 80 μCi tritiated estradiol
intraperitoneally and sacrificed 15, 60 or 120 min later. The nuclei
were isolated using the method of Zigmond and McEwen (1970). N = 5
at each point. Mean body weights: Males - 223.5 gm; Females - 223.2 gm.
Tissue proteins (μg protein/mg tissue): Males - Hth - 2.06; Cx - 2.05;
Pit - 8.96. Females - Hth - 2.06; Cx - 2.06; Pit - 9.23.

The fact that estrogen is accumulated by cells in the brain of males and androgenized females may be insufficient evidence for the hypothesis that early androgenization does not alter cellular response to hormones. Hormones pass through the cell membrane where they are bound by cytoplasmic macromolecules (Eisenfeld, 1970). The hormone is then transferred to the nucleus where it remains in bound form (Zigmond and McEwen, 1970). Studies of whole tissue uptake, as those mentioned above, may fail to reveal critical changes induced by androgenization in cytoplasmic or nuclear binding. To test this hypothesis we recently compared the nuclear binding of estradiol in the hypothalamus of male and female rats (Fig. 1.). Significant sex differences in the nuclear binding kinetics were found. The nuclei from females accumulated more estradiol than did the nuclei from males and retained it for a longer period. If we assume that nuclear binding is critical for the action of estradiol these findings could indicate the source of the functional difference between males and females in their response to estrogen. However, since we know so little about hormone binding and hormone function in the brain this conclusion must be considered tentative at this time.

SUMMARY

Male and female rats differ in their behavioral response to gonadal hormones. The primary difference appears to be an insensitivity of males to estrogen. This differential responsiveness develops because males are stimulated by gonadal secretions, presumably testosterone and androstenedione, during a critical period of development which in the rat occurs perinatally. The biological basis for this sex difference in hormone responsiveness is still unclear, although recent evidence indicates that hypothalamic nuclei from males bind less estradiol than do such nuclei from females, a difference which could underlie the functional difference in hormone response.

REFERENCES

Barfield, R.J. and Geyer, L.A., 1972, Sexual behavior: Ultrasonic postejaculatory song of the male rat, Science 176: 1349.

Beach, F.A., 1942, Importance of progesterone to induction of sexual receptivity in spayed female rats, Proc. Soc. Exp. Biol. Med. 51: 369.

Beach, F.A., 1941, Female mating behavior shown by male rats after administration of testosterone propionate, Endocr. 29: 409.

Beach, F.A., 1942, Execution of the complete masculine copulatory pattern by sexually receptive female rats, J. Genet. Psychol. 60: 137.

Beach, F.A., 1942, Male and female mating behavior in prepuberally castrated female rats treated with androgens, Endocr. 31: 673.

Beach, F.A., 1945, Bisexual mating behavior in the male rat: Effects of castration and hormone administration, Physiol. Zool. 18: 390.

Beach, F.A., 1971, Hormonal factors controlling the differentiation, development and display of copulatory behavior in the ramstergig and related species. In: "The Biopsychology of Development", (Tobach, Aronson and Shaw, eds.), Academic Press, New York.

Beach, F.A. and Holz-Tucker, A.M., 1949, Effects of different concentrations of adrogen upon sexual behavior in castrated male rats, J. Comp. Physiol Psychol. 42: 433.

Beach, F.A. and Jordan, L., 1956, Sexual exhaustion and recovery in the male rat. Quart. J. Exp. Psychol. 8: 121.

Beach, F.A., Noble, R.G. and Orndoff, R.K., 1969, Effects of perinatal androgen treatment on responses of male rats to gonadal hormones in adulthood. J. Comp. Physiol Psychol. 68: 490.

Beach, F.A. and Rasquin, P., 1942, Masculine copulatory behavior in intact and castrated female rats. Endocr. 31: 393.

Clemens, L.G., Hiroi, M., and Gorski, R.A., 1969, Induction and facilitation of female mating behavior in rats treated neonatally with low doses of testosterone propionate, Endocr. 84: 1430.

Clemens, L.G. and Coniglia, L., 1971, Influence of prenatal litter composition on mounting behavior of female rats, Am. Zool. 11: 617.

Davidson, J.M., 1966, Characteristics of sex behaviour in male rats following castration, Anim. Behav. 14: 266.

Davidson, J.M. and Levine, S., 1969, Progesterone and heterotypical sexual behavior in male rats, J. Endocr. 44: 129.

Edwards, D.A., Whalen, R.E. and Nadler, R.D., 1968, Induction of estrus: Estrogen-progesterone interactions, Physiol. Behav. 3: 29.

Eisenfeld, A.J., 1970, ^{3}H-estradiol: In vitro binding to macromolecules from the rat hypothalamus anterior pituitary and uterus,
Endocr. 86: 1313.

Eisenfeld, A.J. and Axelrod, J., 1966, Effect of steroid hormones,
ovariectomy estrogen pretreatment, sex and immaturity on the
distribution of ^{3}H-estradiol, Endocr. 79: 38.

Feder, H.H. and Wahlen, R.E., 1965, Feminine behavior in neonatally
castrated and estrogen-treated male rats, Science 147: 306.

Flerko, B., Illei-Donhoffer, A. and Mess, B., 1971, Oestrodiol-bind-
ing capacity in neural and non-neural target tissues of neonatally adrogenized female rats, Acta Biol. Acad. Sci. Hung.
22: 125.

Gorski, R.A. Gonadal hormones and the perinatal development of endocrine function. In: "Frontiers of Neuroendocrinology",
(Martini and Ganong, eds.), Oxford Univ. Press, New York.

Goy, R.W. Organizing effects of androgen on the behaviour of rhesus
monkeys. In: "Endocrinology and Human Behaviour", (Michael,
ed.), Oxford Univ. Press, London.

Grady, K.L., Phoenix, C.H. and Young, W.C., 1965, Role of the developing rat testis in differentiation of the neural tissues mediating male behavior, J. Comp. Physiol. Psychol. 59: 176.

Green, R., Luttage, W.G. and Whalen, R.E., 1969, Uptake and retention
of tritiated estradiol in the brain and peripheral tissues of
male, female, and neonatally adrogenized female rats, Endocr.
85: 373.

Hardy, D.F., 1972, Sexual behavior in continuously cycling rats.
Behaviour 41: 288.

Hardy, D.F. and De Bold, J.F., 1972, Effects of coital stimulation
upon behavior of the female rat, J. Comp. Physiol. Psychol.
78: 400.

Harris, G.W. and Levine, S., 1962, Sexual differentiation of the brain
and its experimental control, J. Physiol. (Lond) 163: 42P.

Harris, G.W. and Levine, S., 1965, Sexual differentiation of the brain
and its experimental control, J. Physiol. (Lond.) 181: 379.

Kuehn, R.E. and Beach, F.A., 1963, Quantitative measurement of sexual receptivity in female rats, Behaviour 21: 282.

Luttge, W.G. and Whalen, R.E., 1970a, Dihydrotesterone, androstene-
      dione, testosterone: Comparative effectiveness in masculiniz-
      ing and defeminizing reproductive systems in male and female
      rats, Horm. Behav. 1: 265.

Luttge, W.G. and Whalen, R.E., 1970b, Regional localization of estro-
      genic metabolites in the brain of male and female rats, Steroids
      15: 605.

McEwen, B.S. and Pfaff, D.W., 1970, Factors influencing sex hormone
      uptake by rat brain regions. 1. Effects of neonatal treatment,
      hypophysectomy, and competing steroid on estradiol uptake,
      Brain Res. 21: 1.

McGuire, J.L. and Lisk, R.D., 1969, Oestrogen receptors in androgen
      or oestrogen sterilized female rats, Nature 221: 1068.

Peirce, J.T. and Nuttall, R.L., 1961, Duration of sexual contract in
      the rat, J. Comp. Physiol. Psychol. 54: 585.

Phoenix, C.H., Goy, R.W., Gerall, A.A. and Young, W.C., 1959, Organ-
      izing action of prenatally administered testosterone propionate
      on the tissues mediating mating behavior in the female guinea
      pig, Endocr. 65: 369.

Powers, J.B., 1970, Hormonal control of sexual receptivity during the
      estrous cycle of the rat, Physiol. Behav. 5: 831.

Powers, J.B. and Valenstein, E.V., 1972, Individual differences in
      sexual responsiveness to estrogen and progesterone in ovari-
      ectomized rats, Physiol. Behav. 8: 673.

Schwartz, N.B., 1969, A model for the regulation of ovulation in the
      rat, Rec. Prog. Horm. Res. 25: 1.

Whalen, R.E., 1968, Differentiation of the neural mechanisms which
      control gonadotropin secretion and sexual behavior. In:
      "Perspecitves in Reproduction and Sexual Behavior", (Diamond,
      ed.), Indiana Univ. Press, Bloomington.

Whalen, R.E. and Edwards, D.A., 1967, Hormonal determinants of the
      development of masculine and feminine behavior in male and
      female rats, Anat. Rec. 157: 173.

Whalen, R.E., Edwards, D.A., Luttge, W.G. and Robertson, R.T., 1969,
      Early androgen treatment and male sexual behavior in female
      rats, Physiol. Behav. 4: 33.

Whalen, R.E. and Hardy, D.F., 1970, Induction of receptivity in female
      rats and cats with estrogen and testosterone, Physiol. Behav.
      5: 529.

Whalen, R.E. and Luttge, W.G., 1970, Long-term retention of triti-
    ated estradiol in brain and peripheral tissues of male and
    female rats, Neuroendocrinology 6: 225.

Whalen, R.E. and Luttge, W.G., 1971, Testosterone, androstenedione
    and dihydrotestosterone: Effects on mating behavior of male
    rats, Horm. Behav. 2: 117.

Whalen, R.E., Luttge, W.G. and Gorzalka, B.B., 1971, Neonatal andro-
    genization and the development of estrogen responsivity in male
    and female rats, Horm. Behav. 2: 83.

Zigmond, R.E. and McEwen, B.S., 1970, Selective retention of oestra-
    diol by cell nuclei in specific brain regions of the ovari-
    ectomized rat, J. Neurochem. 17: 889.

POSTNATAL BEHAVIORAL EFFECTS OF IN UTERO EXPOSURE TO DRUGS WHICH

MODIFY CATECHOLAMINES AND/OR SEROTONIN

Sheldon B. Sparber

Department of Pharmacology, University of Minnesota

Minneapolis, Minnesota

The past twenty years has witnessed an information explosion in the developmental psychobiology literature, encompassing experiments designed to determine those important variables whose manipulation early in life would result in long-lasting, perhaps permanent effects upon brain function and ultimately behavior. The scope of the interdisciplinary nature of this rediscovered area of endeavor has emerged from an emphasis upon structure and function in various species, including man (Minkowski, 1922; Coghill, 1929; Windle, 1930; Kuo, 1932) through interactions between genetic and environmental factors (Thompson et al., 1962; Joffe, 1965) to an emphasis upon biochemical bases for genetic expression of control mechanisms in intermediary metabolism and transmitter function. (This symposium).

Although the work of Werboff and coworkers (see Werboff and Gottlieb, 1963) on effects of various psychoactive drugs, injected into pregnant rats, upon postnatal behavior of their offspring was intriguing, there were inconsistencies in their data from one experiment to another and it seemed that a number of pre and postnatal maternal variables might have accounted for the behavioral consequences observed (see Joffe, 1969 for a critical review). Some of these variables may reflect whether or not the injected drugs affected biochemistry and/or physiology of the developing organism in a way similar to the pharmacological responses seen in more mature members of the species used or whether they were having their effect upon the mother and thereby indirectly affecting the offspring through altering uterine muscular activity (Koren et al., 1966) altering placental blood flow (Young, 1963; Robson and Sullivan, 1966) or in other ways. Although there are questions regarding the specific effects upon variables used to measure postnatal behavioral consequences in studies that have used reserpine in mammals (Werboff et al., 1961; Werboff

81

and Dembicki, 1962; Jewett and Norton, 1966) there appears to be no doubt that this drug produces at least some behavioral changes in offspring after injection into pregnant rats. In addition, reserpine is capable of depleting biogenic amines in offspring at term under these conditions (injection into the mother) as Kovacic and Robinson (1966) have shown. Our own logitudinal series of experiments with the domestic chicken (Sparber, 1972) showed that a direct effect upon an organism's biochemical and/or behavioral development was a plausible interpretation of effects reported for rats. We are still using the developing chick to get at some fundamental questions regarding drug effects on long-term transmitter control mechanisms during development (Lydiard and Sparber, 1972), an area which will no doubt be reviewed in detail in this symposium (Nair; Waymire).

As a departure from our predilection toward an avian species for studies of drugs and behavioral development, some preliminary data on the effects of three different compounds, administered to rats early in pregnancy, upon several measures of postnatal behavior of their offspring will be presented. One of these compounds (para-chlorophenylalanine, PCPA) has been used in the past few years to study the inborn error of metabolism resulting in phenylketonuria (PKU) because of its ability to inhibit phenylalanine and tryptophan hydroxylases (Koe and Weissman, 1966). Another of the compounds (alpha-methyl-p-tyrosine, α MT) owes its current popularity to its ability to fairly selectively lower catecholamine levels by inhibiting the rate limiting enzyme in their synthetic pathway, tyrosine hydroxylase (Spector et al., 1965). Many studies of this type on postnatal behavior have used the longer-acting depletor of catecholamines and serotonin, reserpine. It was therefore thought desirable to use a shorter acting reserpine-like compound. Tetrabenazine (TBZ) was chosen for this purpose. It produces fewer peripheral autonomic effects and has a much shorter duration of action than reserpine, (Pletscher et al., 1962) ensuring a drug exposure closer to the time of administration, with less likelihood of a protracted action across many more days of the gestational period.

In addition to allowing comparison between data obtained in the past with reserpine with a drug in the same class pharmacologically, the main rationale for the use of TBZ was to partially test the original hypothesis of the experiment under discussion. Based upon regional distribution studies, histofluorescence studies, behavioral and temperature regulation studies, as well as neuroendocrine releasing factor studies, the emerging picture suggests that the catecholamines and serotonin might be functionally antagonistic in the CNS. It was therefore hypothesized that this oversimplified analogy could be tested developmentally, modifying in one way or another (in this case presumably depleting to some extent) either or both the catecholaminergic and serotonergic stores early in development with the idea that examination of function later in life would show divergent effects between PCPA and α MT treatment groups, with a

reversal on mixture of effects when metabolism of both amines is
modified with TBZ.

Since it would be a monumental task to control for the important
time variables (i.e., critical period question) and direct versus
indirect and genetic factors (i.e., fostering and cross-fostering
procedures) and still call this an exploratory study, it was decided
to control for some variables and not others with the idea in mind
that future experiments could be done to tease apart mechanisms.

METHODS

Animals and Treatment

A group of young adult, sexually naive, presumably randomly bred,
female (approximately 275 gm at the time of mating) and male (approximately 350 gm at the time of mating) rats of the Sprague-Dawley variety
(Holtzman Laboratories, Wisconsin) were used. During the month of
acclimation to our laboratory housing quarters and routine, four
females, randomly assigned, lived together in the community cages
where they would subsequently be bred. The males were also housed
in community cages (two per cage) until placed with their randomly
chosen harem for breeding. Identification was maintained with suitable codes utilizing an ear-punch at the time of cage (treatment and
mating) assignments. In order to at least partially control for
genetic factors, it was decided to keep the paternal genetic material
as evenly distributed as possible. As a consequence, no two females
in the same community cage were injected with the same compound.
Daily vaginal smears were examined for the presence of sperm cells
and if even questionably positive (smears were done extremely gently
to avoid pseudopregnancy or mechanically modified estrus cycles) that
day was considered day zero of pregnancy. On days 4,5 and 6 of pregnancy each of the rats, thought to be pregnant, was injected with
either the suspending medium (corn oil, 1 ml/kg) tetrabenazine methane-
sulfonate (TBZ, 2 mg base/kg), d,1-p-chloro-phenylalanine (PCPA,
200 mg/kg) or α-methyl-p-tyrosine (α MT, 100 mg/kg) subcutaneously,
at three different sites near the back of the neck. Of the forty
females (ten community cages), twenty eventually gave birth, after
being placed several days before term (20-21 days) into individual
nesting pans containing pine sawdust. Two to three females per community cage eventually gave birth, resulting in a fairly even distribution of paternal genetic material in those offspring eventually
delivered and subsequently tested for drug effects. No attempt was
made to examine the uteri of females thought to be pregnant via vaginal smears. From the fact that several of the males did not father
any litters, it was decided that the assumption of pregnancy, if
smears were positive, was probably not valid.

Measures of Drug Effects

At the time of birth and within one day after delivery, litters
were examined for size, number of offspring dead and whether or not
pups were killed or devoured by mothers, an observation suggestive
of screening behavior to eliminate abnormal pups.

At 25 days of age the pups were weaned and again litter size and
sex distribution were determined. During the period between birth
and weaning there was little or no handling of litters except for
standard care (food, water and change of bedding or cage washing) and
one transference from the delivery pans to larger cages at two weeks
after birth. Since it has been reported that no observable behavioral
differences could be demonstrated between offspring from litters of
2 or 3 compared to litters of 9, i.e., the extremes of moderate size
litters (Broadhurst and Levine, 1963), all offspring that survived
the initial insults remained with their litter mates prior to weaning
and used in the experiment for measurements of unconditioned locomotor
behavior, regardless of litter size. However, in one case a sole
survivor of a TBZ litter was not considered for operant behavior
measures and therefore the rats chosen for that part of the study
from the TBZ treatment group eventually came from three litters (one
of each sex per litter, the fourth member of each sex randomly chosen
from the remaining rats after the initial randomized-block choice).

Between 48 and 50 days of age all offspring were run in an activity cage (Pickens and Crowder, 1967) for six minutes. The apparatus
used for this measure of unconditioned motor activity was a circular,
enclosed (1/4 inch galvanized hardware cloth) runway with four photo-
electric sensors located at 90° arcs around the periphery of the runway, illuminated by a single bulb located in the center. The cir-
cuitry was such that the subject had to break two contiguous light
beam-sensor combinations to record one unit of activity. This configuration prevented the subjects scoring high on this activity measure as a consequence of simply rocking back and forth or swishing
their tails in front of a single photocell.

After being run in the circular apparatus (within 1-2 days),
four offspring of each sex from each of the treatment groups were
randomly chosen for operant behavior tests to be initiated at approximately 100 days of age. The remaining rats (offspring) were chosen
randomly from the entire remaining pooled population, for studies on
open-field behavior or a sex-linked liver microsomal metabolic study
to determine if peripheral, as well as central factors, could possibly
account for drug related modifications. This last mentioned study
was undertaken after it was discovered that PCPA injection resulted
in what appeared to be an increase in the number of females relative
to males at the time of weaning, with no apparent decrease in litter
size. Examination of external genitalia was the only index used to
determine sex, no attempt was made to examine visceral organs for

possible hermaphroditism.

Open-field behavior, consisting of measures on grooming, lines crossed, rearing on hind quarters and defecation in the novel environment, was determined at 75 days of age. The ability of liver microsomal mixed-function oxidases to N-demethylate ethylmorphine (Anders and Mannering, 1966) was determined in 4 offspring of each sex from PCPA, α MT and control groups at approximately 60 days of age. Since in the rat there are significant differences in the ability to metabolize drugs, males showing greater capacity than females, and these enzymes have been shown to metabolize steroid hormones as well as drugs (Tephly and Mannering, 1968), this assay should be a good index of determining possible changes in sex-linked (genetic) liver function, as well as phenotypic modification of steroid metabolism, if present. This last point is rather pertinent in view of the findings of Ordy et al. (1966), that the livers of offspring, born to pregnant mice injected with chlorpromazine, were modified in enzyme activity (increased leucine aminipeptidase and decreased alkaline phosphatase activity) and glycogen content (decreased).

The open-field apparatus was fashioned so that its 3x3 ft. field was separated into 16 squares of 9x9 in. dimensions. Activity counts during 5 minutes in the arena were determined. One count was defined as a response when all four paws crossed a line.

At 90 days of age the offspring chosen for the operant behavioral study were weighed, placed into separate cages and put on a food deprivation schedule and gradually decreased in body weight to 85% of their initial weight. At the appropriate time, shaping of bar-pressing behavior in a standard two bar operant chamber was initiated, using the method of successive approximation. Within two sessions all subjects were bar-pressing for Noyes (45 mg) pellets on a continuous reinforcement schedule (CRF). Within one or two sessions, when CRF responding appeared stable, they were switched to a schedule of reinforcement which required 3 responses/food pellet (Fixed Ratio-3, FR-3). After 2 FR-3 sessions in which every subject received 50 reinforcers/session they were switched to a discrimination schedule. The discrimination training required that the subject bar-press twice for each pellet (FR-2) during a 3 min. interval signalled by a light over the appropriate bar (the other bar was inoperative) and a clicking tone. The next 6 min. was the time out period, indicated by an absence of the tone and light; a period during which bar-pressing had no consequences (i.e., no food pellets delivered). Each session was 27 min. long so that the subject was exposed to a total of 9 min. during which responding was reinforced and a total of 18 min. during which responding was not reinforced. All subjects were run on this paradigm for 8 sessions and measures of reinforced responding during the discriminative stimuli (S^D) and amount of responding during the time-out period (S^Δ) were made. Programming and recording was accomplished with standard electromechanical logic components located in an adjacent room.

TABLE I

DRUG EFFECTS ON LITTERS AT TERM[a]

Group	N	Litter Size	Dead (Term + 1 Day)	Devoured
Control	6	11.5 ± 0.8[b]	1.0 ± 0.5	0.3 ± 0.2
PCPA	5	10.4 ± 0.4	0.6 ± 0.4	0
α MT	4	10.0 ± 1.6	0.5 ± 0.5	0
TBZ	5	8.2 ± 1.5	1.8 ± 1.3	1.2 ± 0.3

[a]See methods for drug dosages, route of administration, etc.

[b]Mean ± SE

TABLE II

SEX DISTRIBUTION AT WEANING

Group	N	Females	Males
Control	6	5.3 ± 0.6[a]	4.5 ± 0.6
PCPA	5	6.8 ± 0.4	3.0 ± 0.5
α MT	4	4.8 ± 1.1	4.8 ± 0.9
TBZ	4	2.3 ± 1.3	4.3 ± 1.2

[a]Mean ± SE

RESULTS AND DISCUSSION

Viability and Growth

From the results presented in Table I it is apparent that TBZ, at the dose employed, was having at least a partial effect upon the outcome of pregnancy and subsequent behavior of the mothers toward the offspring. At term (approximately 21 days, no measure of delay in the gestational period was made) litter size of the corn oil control, PCPA and α MT groups were averaging 10-11 pups while the 5 litters born to mothers injected with TBZ averaged slightly less (8.2). Within one to two days of the birth of the offspring one of the TBZ mothers died but not before she partially ate at least one pup in her litter. As a consequence, there remained only 4 litters in the TBZ group for the remainder of the study, one of which contained only one pup, since the mother of this litter likewise devoured 2 of her 3 pups. Four of the 5 TBZ mothers partially or completely ate at least one pup from their litters. Only 2 of the six control mothers ate 1 pup while none of the 5 PCPA or 4 α MT mothers ate their pups. It is interesting to note that a salient feature of the study of Werboff and Dembicki (1962) was an increased incidence of devouring of pups by rats injected with either reserpine, chlorpromazine or meprobamate during pregnancy. It cannot be determined from their or the present data whether or not it was due to abnormal behavior of the mother or whether the pups were abnormal and the mothers destroyed them. Since cross-fostering to control mothers of mice born to mothers injected with chlorpromazine did not result in enhanced survival of the drug exposed pups, nor was there decreased survival of control pups fostered to chlorpromazine treated mothers (Ordy et al., 1966), the effect on devouring in rats induced by reserpine, chlorpromazine and meprobamate (and now apparently TBZ) may be due to prenatal drug effects upon the pups. However, a complete factorial experimental design with fostering and cross-fostering manipulations would be required to answer this question more precisely.

At the time of weaning (25 days of age) the average size of the litters decreased from 10.5 for the control, PCPA and α MT groups to about 9.5, while the TBZ litters decreased likewise by about one pup from 8 to 7, indicating no further differences in offspring survival. A rather unexpected distribution of males and females within the PCPA litters was observed (Table II), females outnumbering males by a margin of 2:1, without a difference in litter size when compared to the control and α MT groups. The apparent difference between the distribution of males and females in the TBZ group should not be viewed with equal interest, since the variability between litters and decreased size of the litters could have accounted for that difference. These findings suggest that whatever drug effects emerge on further examination might be sex dependent, a possibility which is supported by previous reports (Ordy et al., 1966).

TABLE III

TWO-WAY ANALYSIS OF VARIANCE OF RUNWAY ACTIVITY, 48-50 DAYS

Source of Variation	SS	df	MS	F	Est. P
Drug	3,315.58	3	1,105.19	4.586	.005
Sex	2,191.25	1	2,191.25	9.093	.003
Interaction	1,832.85	3	610.95	2.535	.058
Error	38,075.53	158	240.98		

TABLE IV

TWO-WAY ANALYSIS OF VARIANCE OF BODY WEIGHT, 48-50 DAYS

Source of Variation	SS	df	MS	F	Est. P
Drug	4,915.09	3	1,638.36	4.340	.007
Sex	174,677.20	1	174,677.20	462.752	<.001
Interaction	2,696.46	3	898.82	2.381	.075
Error	27,555.65	73	377.47		

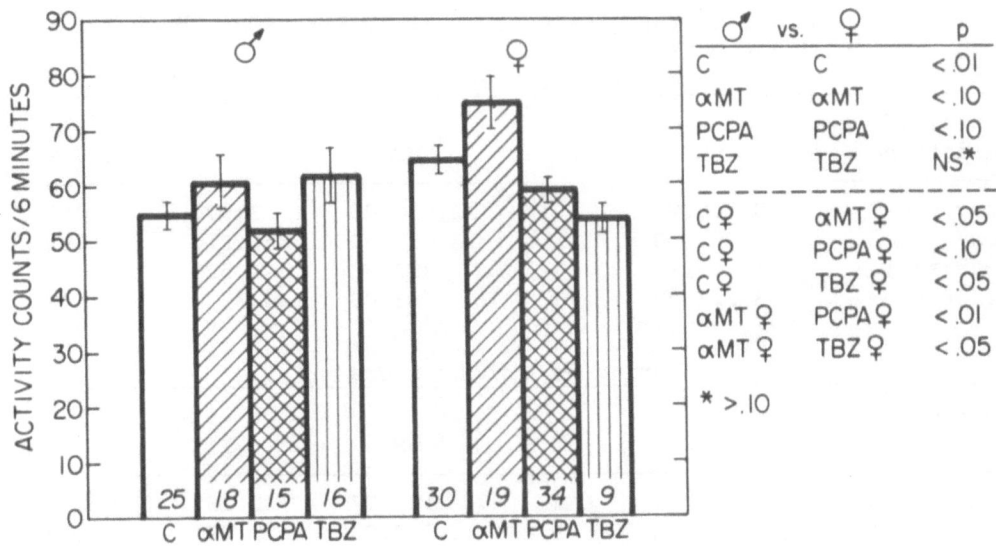

Fig. 1. Effects of prenatal α MT, PCPA or TBZ upon Circular Runway Locomotor activity at 48-50 days of age. Bars represent the group mean for individual sexes and vertical lines the SEM. Values within the bars represent the number of offspring used for each determination.

Unconditioned Behavior

A two-way analysis of variance of the circular runway locomotor activity data revealed an overall significant drug and sex effect with the interaction effect approaching significance (Table III). Figure 1 shows the mean (± SEM) locomotor activity for the males and females of all four groups in histogram form, along with some of the post-analysis of variance Student t-test comparisons. Although the estimated P values include those at the <.10 α level (2-tailed tests in all comparisons), they are included for comparison purposes and should not be construed as suggesting a significant difference between the groups compared. I would tend to choose the more conservative α level of <.01 as definitely showing a significant difference, since there are multiple comparisons made. Using these criteria, the expected activity differences between males and females were observed only for the control groups, all drug treatments obviating that sex difference. It is likewise interesting to note that the only significant difference between female groups was between the α MT and PCPA females, each deviating in opposite directions from the control females, consistent with the original hypothesis under which this experiment was initially undertaken.

TABLE V

TWO-WAY ANALYSIS OF VARIANCE OF OPEN-FIELD BEHAVIOR, 75 DAYS

A-Lines Crossed

Source of Variation	SS	df	MS	F	Est. P
Drug	8,745.87	3	2,915.29	3.977	.011
Sex	14,081.60	1	14,081.60	19.210	<.001
Interaction	1,149.91	3	383.30	.523	.672
Error	53,511.02	73	733.03		

B-Rearing on Hind Quarters

Source of Variation	SS	df	MS	F	Est. P
Drug	545.91	3	181.97	2.252	.088
Sex	1,582.83	1	1,582.83	19.591	<.001
Interaction	138.43	3	46.14	.571	.640
Error	5,897.95	73	80.79		

The analysis of variance of body weights at 48-50 days of age (Table IV) with subsequent t-test comparisons revealed little in terms of unexpected results. Although a highly significant sex difference was shown for all groups, males being much heavier than females at this age, a small but significant difference (P<.01) appeared between the control males and TBZ males, the TBZ males averaging 275 gm compared to the body weight average of 311 gm for controls. This difference, however, was much less than the male-female control differences (a 116 gm difference) or the 80 gm difference between the TBZ males and TBZ females. Since the TBZ females weighed the same as the control females (0.8 gm difference), the (drug) effect upon the body weight is from the TBZ male group (Table IV). (The interaction estimate of F reflects this in the approach to significance value of .075). Of the 4 measures taken in the Open-Field at this age, only Lines Crossed and Rearing on Hind Quarters showed significant drug and/or sex effects, again without interactions. The Defecation and Grooming measures did not show any overall differences and therefore were not analyzed further. The 2-way analysis of variance statistics for Lines Crossed and Rearing is shown in Table V. The group means (± SEM) and P values from subsequent t-test comparisons are presented in Figures 2 and 3. Generally speaking, it appears that locomotor activity in the Runway and activity in the Open-Field (Lines Crossed) may reflect similar sex differences for non-drug treated groups, both measures showing significant differences (P<.01) between control males and females. On the other hand, while no difference between males and females showed

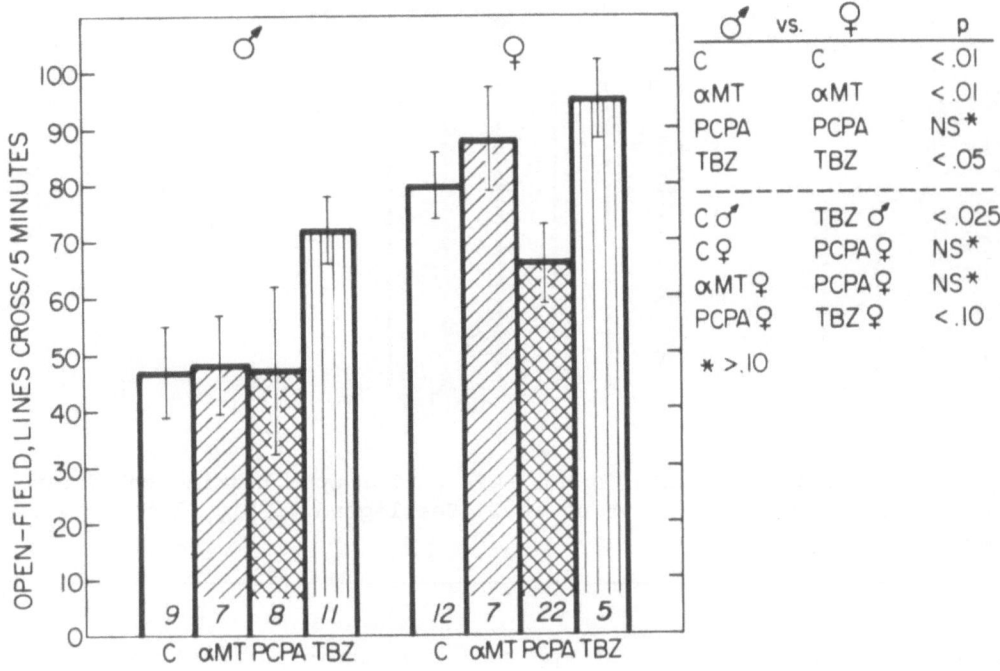

Fig. 2. Effect of prenatal α MT, PCPA and TBZ upon Open-Field locomotor activity at 75 days of age. See legend to Fig. 1 for further
explanations.

in the Circular Runway for the α MT group at 48-50 days of age, a
definite significant sex difference appeared in this group (α MT) at
75 days of age in the Open-Field. PCPA and TBZ groups continued to
show no or marginal sex differences at this age. While α MT males
are definitely significantly lower than α MT females on the Rearing
measure, the differences between control and PCPA males and their
respective females only approach significance. However, the TBZ
males and females show no such difference. In addition, comparison
of TBZ males with the other treatment males likewise shows significant or near significant differences (Fig. 3).

N-demethylation of Ethylmorphine

If treatment of pregnant rats with α MT or PCPA was affecting
the levels of circulating steroids in offspring postnatally or otherwise altering the functional capacity of the liver to metabolize

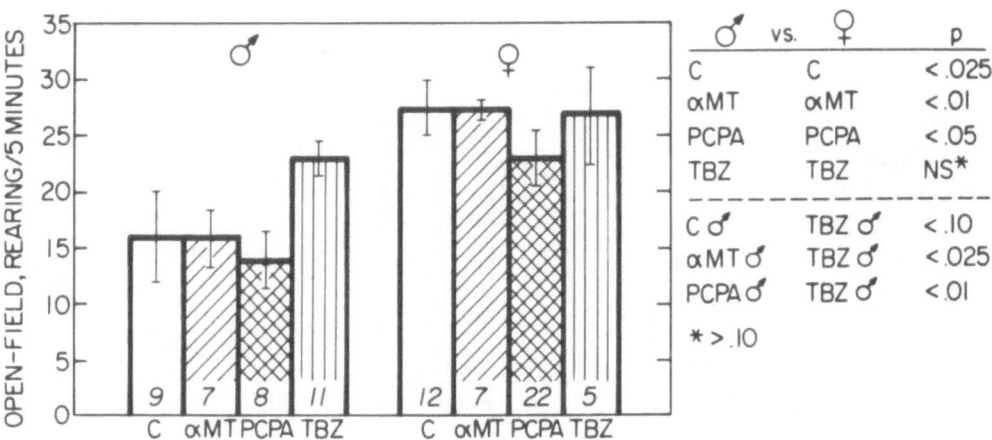

Fig. 3. Effect of prenatal α MT, PCPA or TBZ upon Rearing behavior in the Open-Field at 75 days of age. See legend to Fig. 1 for further explanations.

steroids or drugs, it was not apparent from the experiment on N-demethylation of ethylmorphine. The liver weights and the number of micromoles of formaldehyde formed from the demethylation reaction per gram of liver per hour are shown in Table VI. Although the expected sex differences emerged, there was no hint that either of the two drugs altered either variable.

Operant Behavior

At 90 days of age, the animals chosen for the operant discrimination experiment showed no difference in body weights across treatments. All females were significantly lighter than males within their respective groups as well as across groups. Their rate of acquisition of the operant response during the shaping procedure did not appear grossly different, all rats learning within 1-2 sessions. Since the behavior chosen for study is fairly resistant to external manipulation and quite stable once acquired, it was predicted that subtle changes produced by prenatal drug treatment would probably not show up as a decrement in learning but rather a difference between groups in terms of their overall patterning. Examination of the raw data measure of discrimination ($S^{\Delta}/S^{D} \times 100$) indicated that the rate of learning was a negatively accelerating descending function which could best be described as a first order rate. A natural log transformation of the data followed by a linear regression analysis by the method of least squares produced the family of 8 log-linear curves presented in Fig. 4.

TABLE VI

EFFECTS OF α MT AND PCPA UPON LIVER WEIGHT AND ABILITY OF
LIVERS FROM 60 DAY-OLD OFFSPRING TO N-DEMETHYLATE ETHYLMORPHONE[a]

Group	Sex	Liver Wt. M + SEM	HCHO/gm/hr M + SEM
Control	M	12.7 ± 1.0	11.97 ± 1.09
Control	F	8.0 ± 0.2	2.56 ± 0.32
α MT	M	13.3 ± 0.6	12.71 ± 1.07
α MT	F	8.4 ± 0.4	2.61 ± 0.20
PCPA	M	13.5 ± 0.4	13.45 ± 0.88
PCPA	F	9.0 ± 0.2	2.61 ± 0.25

[a]Formaldehyde was measured by the method of Nash as modified
by Anders and Mannering (1966). Four animals were used for
each sex in each group. Units of measure for liver weights
are grams and for formaldehyde, micromoles.

Although both males and females in all groups showed no overall
significant difference in the apparent rate of learning the discrimination, the data from this experiment shows significant drug effects
upon session to session variability of responding. For example, when
the rats learn the discrimination, as a group, the mean percentage
error (S^Δ/S^D X 100) as well as the variance of the measure should
diminish from session to session; the control males start with large
error scores and large variance but end with small error scores and
small variance (Fig. 5). Cochran's test for homogeniety of variance
across sessions indicates a significant (P<.05) difference in variances, 907.9 at the first session to a low of 2.65 at the last session.
On the other hand, although female controls on the average, likewise
eventually learned the discrimination almost as well as males between sessions 1 and 8, their day to day variability showed no orderly relationship and this was reflected as a fairly homogeneous set
of variances (Fig. 6); initial group variance started at 1232.7,
never getting lower than 302.3 and terminating (session 8) at 1797.6.
Since a natural log transformation resulted in a reversal of the outcome of Cochran's test, it was still not feasible to compare the common variance of the males with the common variance of the females to
test the hypothesis that the females were significantly more variable
than males, as a group. The Mann-Whitney U test allowed this comparison, since the assumption of homogeniety of variance within
groups was not necessary. This test showed the difference to be significant at the P=.028 level (2-tailed). Although the α MT males
likewise showed a significant reduction in the group's variability

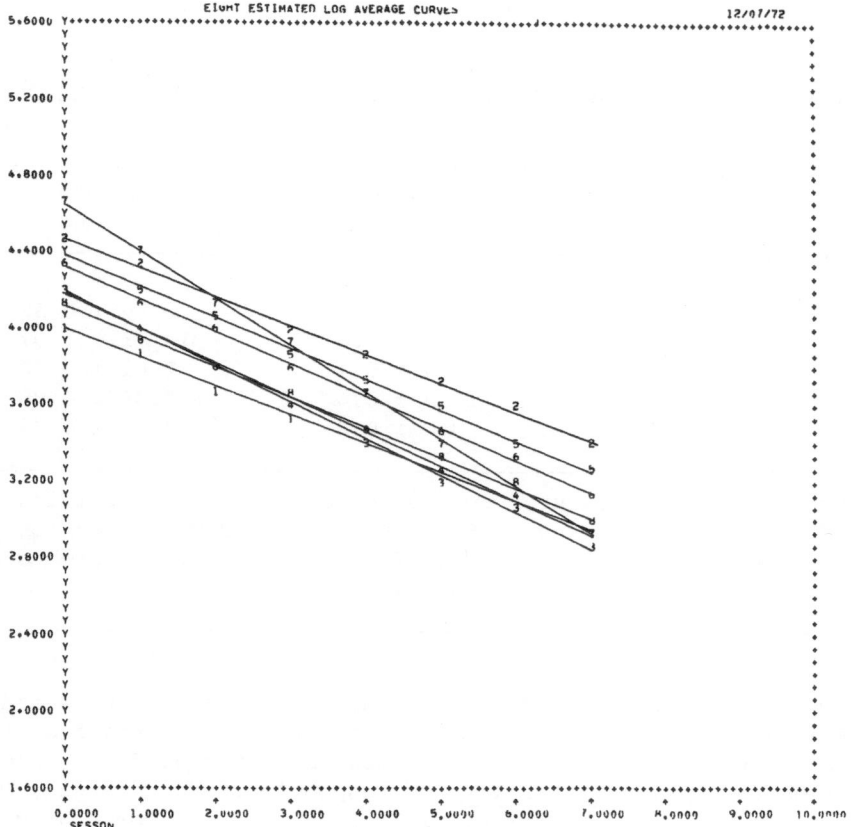

Fig. 4. Learning rates (curves) of the operant discrimination task
plotted as the best fit lines of a linear regression, least squares
method, of natural log transformed error scores (S^{Δ}/S^{D} X 100). Each
line represents one sex for each group. No significant differences
in the rate of acquisition were seen.

---

across sessions, while the α MT females showed no such effect by
Cochran's test, a log transformation was done and this resulted in
a group of data that had homogeniety of variances within both groups
across sessions. This suggested that the α MT females were behaving
somewhat like both the α MT males as well as the control males (borne
out by the raw data distribution in Fig. 6). F tests as well as Mann-
Whitney U tests revealed that all three groups shared a common variance, indicating that α MT females were behaving more like males and
had lost much of their periodicity. When a comparison between α MT
females and control females was done, the resulting F ratio was great
enough to show a significant difference in variability at the P<.01
level, further supporting the above interpretation.

The data from PCPA males and females are likewise shown in
Figures 5 and 6. The females in the PCPA group performed almost
identically to control males. Since log-transformed data of both
groups passed Cochran's test for homogeniety of variance, an F test
was performed and the results indicated what was expected, no difference between control males and PCPA females. On the other hand,
examination of the data in Fig. 6 reveals a totally unexpected effect,
if the unconditioned behavior measures were used as a guide. While
no indication of an effect of PCPA on males was suggested at that
time, the discrimination behavior of the group of PCPA males appears
identical to that of the control females and different from control
males. Appropriate tests reveal such a difference, the variability
(periodicity) of the PCPA males being highly significantly greater
than both PCPA females and control males.

Lastly, whatever TBZ is doing prenatally, it appears to have
produced a group of both males and females that learn as well as the
rest, but in addition show significant changes in variability across
sessions (Cochran's test) for both males (like control males) and
females (unlike control females or any other females). The Mann-
Whitney U test was the only way to compare these two groups with each
other and other groups. Unlike the control males and females, whose
variabilities were statistically different, the males and females of
the TBZ groups showed no such difference. In addition there were no
differences between any allowable contrasts, indicating in a round-
about way, that TBZ "averaged" out normal differences seen in controls,
mostly at the expense of the females, whose great variability was
significantly reduced across sessions.

The experimental data suggest that sex differences seen in control (normal) animals can be significantly modified by prenatal exposure to the drugs used in this study. For example, PCPA caused an
apparent shift in the male to female ratio in litters at weaning,
resulting in many more females per litter than expected. In addition,
none of the measures of unconditioned behavior resulted in significant sex differences in this group. Likewise, the operant measure
of discrimination behavior indicated that PCPA males showed periodicity
or extremely great variability from session to session while the PCPA
females showed little session to session variability. This is completely opposite of the data generated by control males and females.
On the other hand, α MT seemed to produce only marginal effects upon
unconditioned behavior as well as upon the conditioned behavior.

The TBZ group showed the most striking effects on unconditioned
behavior measures; in two cases (both Open-Field measures) the males
behaved more like females while in the Circular Runway the females
behaved more like males. This merging of sex-specific behavior
characteristics was further suggested by their operant discrimination
performance. During the first several sessions both males and females

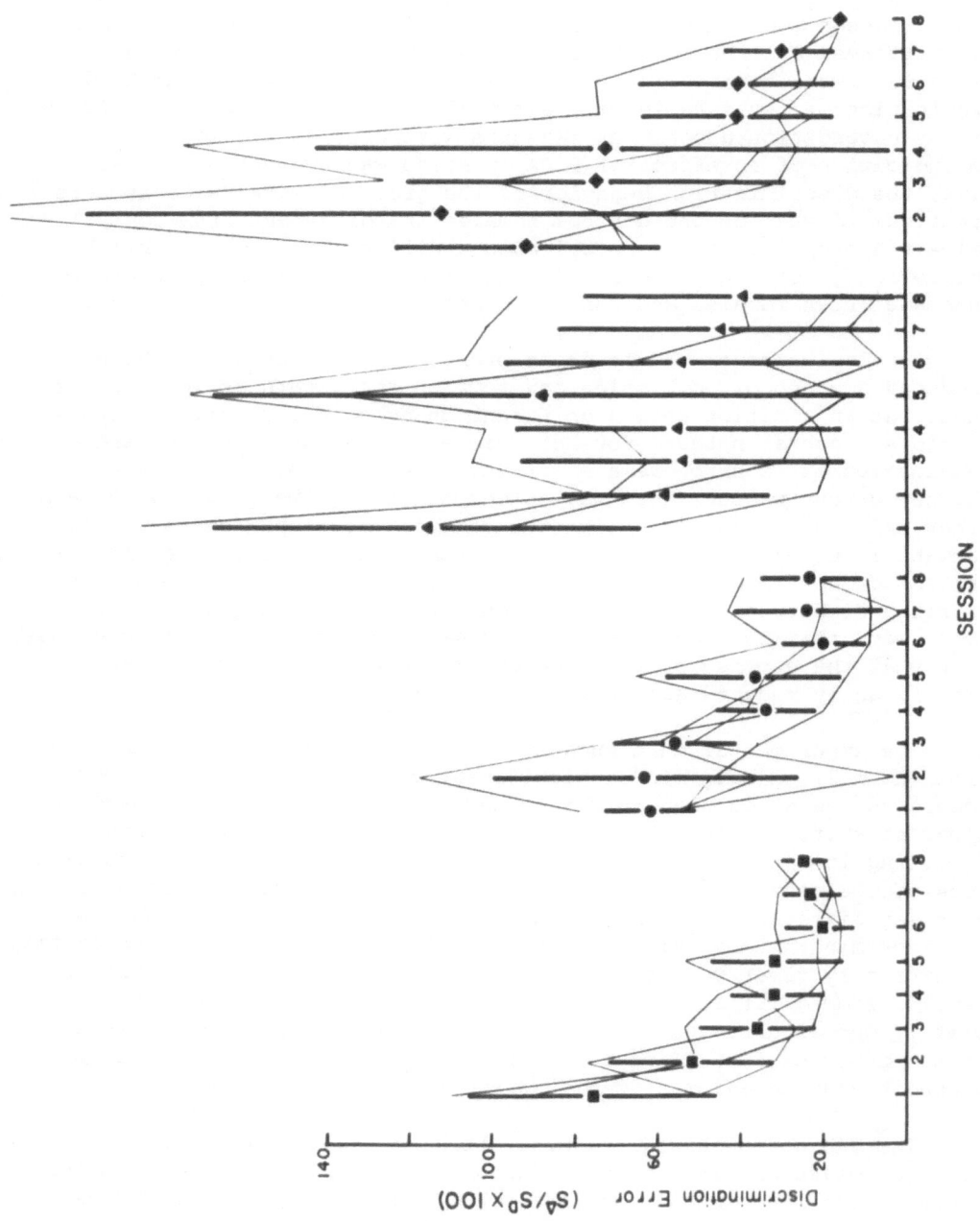

showed fairly large variability within their group (like control females) but their final sessions were more reliable, with little or
no periodicity for either males or females.

Recently Harris and Heistad (1970) found that ovariectomy suppressed the periodic fluctuations in the FR-10 response, while injection of estradiol and progesterone reinstated the significant change
in bar-pressing behavior seen during the different periods of estrus.
While I would question their interpretation regarding a change in
reinforcing properties of food specifically, rather than an overall
effect upon the schedule control of the behavior, our data are very
consistent with theirs in terms of normal (periodic) operant behavior
in control females (Fig. 6) and extends and contrasts it with control
males, whose behavior from session to session did not show these
great fluctuations (Fig. 5).

Although several investigators have used drugs similar or identical to drugs used in this study, they usually administered more drug,
over longer periods of time and/or at a different stage of development of the animal (postnatally). For this reason, it is difficult
to make direct comparisons between the data reported herein and those
presented by others. For example, Hole (1972) injected 200 mg PCPA/kg
(i.p.) every fourth day between days 3 and 14 postnatally and every
other day thereafter until the offspring were 50 days old. His conclusion that treatment of rats during the first weeks of life results
in brain damage, as evidenced by significantly reduced brain weights
in the PCPA treated rats, immediately casts doubt on his behavioral
data showing direct drug treatment related differences described as
reduced arousal. His conclusions that there was no evidence of any
learning defect, in spite of the "damaged" brains, probably due to
undernourishment during the early postnatal period, questions the
use of the standard methods of assessing learning deficits or retardation. It is probable that they are just not sensitive enough to pick
up subtle effects of short-term exposure to drugs, let alone the
greater insult of weeks of high dose drug administration. Further
comparison is even more difficult, since Hole used only males for his
behavior studies and therefore could have missed any sex-specific
effect upon females.

Fig. 5. Mean discrimination error scores for control (■), α MT (●),
PCPA (▲) and TBZ (◆) males for all 8 sessions. Heavy vertical lines
represent ± S.D. while their connecting lines show session to session
variability (performance) for each of the four individual rats/group.
While the figure shows standard deviation estimates, analysis was performed upon the square of these values, which were too great to include in the figure.

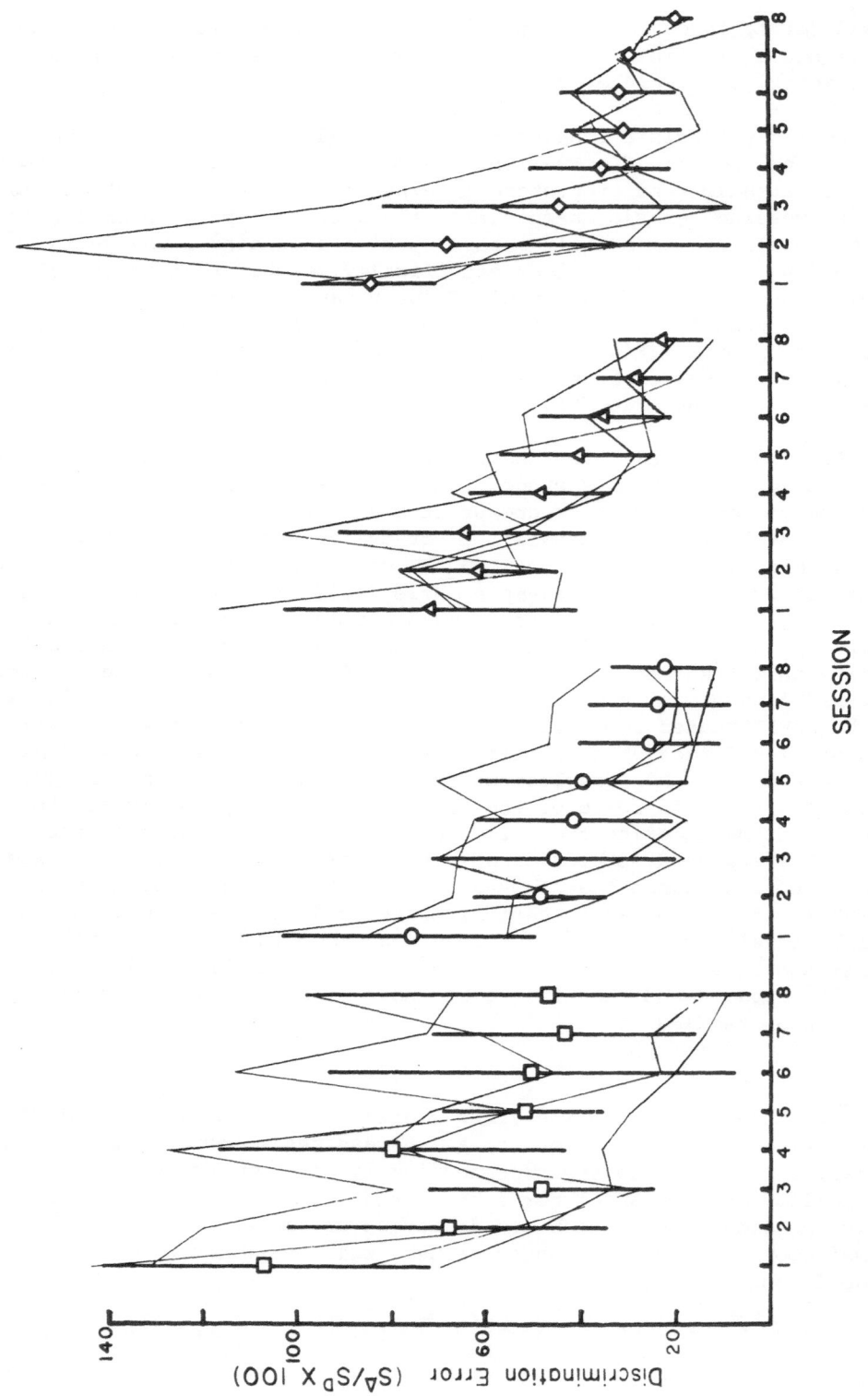

In their study on brain serotonin-behavior interactions, Rosecrans and Schechter (1972) found significant sex differences and
strain differences. Highly active female rats tended to show greater
CNS 5-HT levels than less active female rats but male rats did not
show the high 5HT levels, regardless of activity. They suggest that
"variability between strain or sex could be related to the quantity
of decarboxylase synthesized and/or rate of axonal transport. This
would also suggest that enzyme levels would be under the control of
a genetic code via cell body RNA and DNA." These authors also speculate on individual and intersexual differences to be related to
expression of the genetic code.

It would be extremely tempting to latch onto the above interpretation by Rosecrans and Schechter (1972), since it supports some
of the data presented here for PCPA and elsewhere (Sparber and Luther,
1970) on levels of behavioral activity and monamine function determined genetically and modified during or after development. However,
the recent interest in and information on biogenic amines as con-
trollers or modulators of releasing factors, in the hypothalamus, for
pituitary function (Schneider and McCann, 1970; Wurtman, 1970; Schneider, 1972) suggests that I have unearthed a "bag of worms" and that
the simplistic approach to test the original hypothesis is much more
complex than ever imagined.

In conclusion, although the study reported here was undertaken
to gain information on the normal function of catecholamines and
serotonin in the CNS of the mature organism by manipulating these
systems during development so that consequences could be analysed in
the absence of drugs (no drugs are "pure" or 100% selective), these
data, in conjunction with data by others, indicate that the so-called
critical period for sexually-related behaviors (Levine and Mullins,
1968) may extend further back to an earlier period in development
than heretofore thought.

Furthermore, from a therapeutic standpoint, although society is
finally recognizing that administration of drugs to or exposure to
chemicals of the pregnant woman may lead to unpredictable and bizarre
consequences in offspring, there has recently been reported the
"successful" use of a serotonin blocking agent, cyproheptadine, for
treatment of spontaneous abortion of so-called psychogenic origin
(Sadovsky et al., 1972). No mention was made of any factors which
would indicate that postnatal development has been or will be monitored, I presume other than in the usual manner. If cyproheptadine
does get through the placenta to the embryo or fetus, and there is

Fig. 6. Mean discrimination error scores for control (□), α MT (O),
PCPA (Δ) and TBZ (◇) females for all 8 sessions. See legend to
Figure 5 for further explanations.

no reason to assume it is different from most other drugs, the effects produced by the drug, if any, may be subtle enough to pass gross observation. In addition, it is always possible to assume that these offspring were developing abnormally and therefore the high incidence of wastage in the population prior to drug treatment. This Darwinian philosophy allows me to state my belief that any significnat deviation from normal (control), no matter the direction, should be viewed as deleterious until proven otherwise. This implies that even "enhanced" performance should be viewed in such a manner.

REFERENCES

Anders, M.W. and Mannering, G.J., 1966, Inhibition of drug metabolism. I. Kinetics of the inhibition of the N-demethylation of ethylmorphine by SKF 525-A and related compounds, Molec. Pharmacol. 2: 319.

Broadhurst, P.L. and Levine, S., 1963, Litter size, emotionality, and avoidance learning, Psychol. Rep. 12: 41.

Coghill, G.E., 1929, "Anatomy and the Problems of Behavior", The University Press, Cambridge.

Harris, W.C. and Heistad, G.T., 1970, Food-reinforced responding in rats during estrus, J. Comp. Physiol. Psychol. 70: 206.

Hole, K., 1972, Behavior and brain growth in rats treated with p-chlorophenylalanine in the first weeks of life, Develop. Psychobiol. 5: 157.

Jewett, R.E. and Norton, S., 1966, Effects of tranquilizing drugs on postnatal behavior, Expl. Neurol. 14: 33.

Joffe, J.M., 1965, Genotype and prenatal and premating stress interact to affect adult behavior in rats, Science 150: 1844.

Joffe, J.M., 1969, "Prenatal Determinants of Behavior", Pergamon Press, Oxford, England.

Koe, B.K. and Weissman, A.J., 1966, p-Chlorophenylalanine: a specific depletor of brain serotonin, J. Pharmacol. Exp. Ther. 154: 499.

Koren, Z., Pfeifer, Y. and Sulman, F.G., 1966, Distribution and placental transfer of C-14-serotonin in pregnant rats, Amer. J. Obstet. Gynec. 95: 290.

Kovacic, B. and Robinson, R.L., 1966, The effects of reserpine on catecholamine levels in the gravid rat and its offspring, J. Pharmacol. Exp. Ther. 152: 37.

Kuo, Z.Y., 1932, Ontogeny of embryonic behavior in aves: I. The chronology and general nature of the behavior in the chick embryo, J. Exp. Zool. 61: 395.

Levine, S. and Mullins, R.F. Jr., 1968, Hormones in infancy. In: "Early Experience and Behavior. The Psychobiology of Development", (Newton and Levin, eds.), Charles C. Thomas, Springfield.

Lydiard, R.B. and Sparber, S.G., 1972, Possible induction of tyrosine hydroxylase in chick embryo brain from reserpine administration prior to incubation. Fifth Intl. Congr. Pharmacol. 144.

Minkowski, M., 1922, Uber Fruhezeitige Bewegungen, Reflexe, und muskulare Reactionen bei menschilchen Foetus, and ihre Beziehungen zum foetalen Nerven and Muskelsystem, Schweiz. Med. Woch. 3: 721.

Ordy, J.M., Smorajski, T., Collins, R.L. and Rolsten, Cl., 1966, Prenatal chlorpromazine effects on liver, survival and behavior of mice offspring, J. Pharmacol. Exp. Ther. 151: 110.

Pickens, R.W. and Crowder, W.F., 1967, A photocell-type recorder of locomotor activity, Amer. J. Psychol. 80: 442.

Pletscher, A., Brossi, A. and Gey, K.F., 1962, Benzoquinolizine derivatives: a new class of monoamine decreasing drugs with psychotropic action, Int. Rev. Neurobiol. 4: 275.

Quinn, G.P., Shore, P.A. and Brodie, B.B., 1959, Biochemical and pharmacological studies of RO 1-9569 (tetrabenazine), a nonindole tranquilizing agent with reserpine-like effects, J. Pharmacol. Exp. Ther. 127: 103.

Robson, J.M. and Sullivan, F.M., 1966, Analysis of actions of 5-hydroxytryptamine in pregnancy, J. Physiol. (Lond.) 184: 717.

Rosecrans, J.A. and Schechter, M.D., 1972, Brain 5-hydroxytryptamine correlates of behavior in rats: strain and sex variability, Physiol. and Behav. 8: 503.

Sadovsky, Pfeiffer, Y., Polishuk, W.A. and Sulman, F.G., 1972, The use of anti-serotonin-cyproheptadine HCl in pregnancy: an experimental and clinical study. In: "Drugs and Fetal Development", (Klingeberg, Abramovici and Chemke, eds.), Plenum Press, New York.

Schneider, D., 1972, BIS Conference Report #26, IV International Congress of Endocrinology, HPG Symposia.

Schneider, H.P.G. and McCann, S.M., 1970, Mono- and indoleamines and control of LH secretion, Endocr. 86: 1127.

Sparber, S.B. and Luther, I.G., 1970, Dopamine concentrations in the brainstem-mesencephalon of active rats as compared with passive rats, Neuropharmacol. 9: 243.

Sparber, S.B., 1972, Effects of drugs on the biochemical and behavioral responses of developing organisms, Fed. Proc. 31: 74.

Spector, S., Sjoerdsma, A. and Udenfriend, S., 1965, Blockade of endogenous norepinephrine synthesis by α-methyl-tyrosine, an inhibitor of tyrosine hydroxylase, J. Pharmacol. Exp. Ther. 147:86.

Tephly, T.R. and Mannering, G.J., 1968, Inhibition of drug metabolism. V. Inhibition of drug metabolism by steroids, Molec. Pharmacol. 4: 10.

Thompson, W.R., Watson, J. and Charlesworth, W.R., 1962, The effects of prenatal maternal stress on offspring behavior in rats, Psychol. Monogr. 76 (Whole No. 38).

Werboff, J. and Dembicki, E.L., 1962, Toxic effects of tranquilizers administered to gravid rats, J. Neuropsychiat. 4: 87.

Werboff, J. and Gottlieb, J.S., 1963, Drugs in pregnancy: behavioral teratology, Obstet. Gynec. Survey 18: 420.

Werboff, J., Gottlieb, J.S., Havlena, J. and Word, T.J., 1961, Behavioral effects of prenatal drug administration in the white rat, Pediatrics 27: 318.

Windle, W.F., 1930, The earliest fetal movements in the cat correlated with the neurofibrillar development of the spinal cord, Anat. Rec. 45: 249.

Wurtman, R.J., 1970, The role of brain and pineal indoles in neuroendocrine mechanisms. In: "The Hypothalamus", (Martini, Motta and Fraschini, eds.), Academic Press, New York.

Young, R.D., 1963, Effect of prenatal maternal injection of epinephrine on postnatal offspring behavior, J. Comp. Physiol. Psychol. 56: 929.

DEVELOPMENTAL ASPECTS OF NEUROTRANSMISSION
Norman Weiner, Chairman

NEUROTRANSMITTER SYSTEMS IN THE CENTRAL NERVOUS SYSTEM

Norman Weiner

Department of Pharmacology, University of Colorado

School of Medicine, Denver, Colorado

In a simplistic fashion, one might surmise that the entire
purpose of neuronal development is to construct the mechanisms
for interneuronal communication. Since interneuronal communication
in mammalian systems involves chemical transmission, one might
reason further that the ultimate purpose of central nervous system
development is to develop mechanisms for the synthesis, storage and
release of the substances which effect this interneuronal communication, the transmitters. The dynamics of neurotransmitter
metabolism in the adult peripheral nervous system is quite well
understood. At least in some systems we are beginning to develop
very considerable knowledge of neurotransmitter mechanisms in the
adult central nervous system. In this introduction to our session
on development of neurotransmission, I shall briefly review the
dynamics of neurotransmitter metabolism in, and the neuropharmacology of, a few of these systems. The development of these
systems will be discussed in more detail by the principal speakers
of this session.

General Mechanisms of Drug Actions on the Brain

Before discussing specific neurotransmitters, let us consider, in a general way, how drugs may affect central nervous
system function. In Table 1 are listed five general categories
of how drugs might act on the brain. First of all, drugs may act
to influence the energy metabolism of neurons. If a drug affects
the production of energy in the brain, one might expect that the
agent will have a rather non-specific effect and will produce rather
gross, and frequently irreversible, deleterious effects upon brain
function. Therefore, it is not likely that one will find in this

TABLE 1

POSSIBLE SITES OF DRUG - CNS INTERACTION

1. Energy metabolism of neurons

2. Excitability of neuronal membranes

3. Vascular supply to brain

4. Supporting glial cells

5. Transmitter metabolism or postsynaptic
    receptors

---

group of drugs agents which are selectively useful in modifying
brain function.

A second group of agents affect the excitability of neuronal
membranes. Here again, a fundamental property of all neuronal
membranes is their ability to be depolarized, and to conduct action
potentials. There are a very limited number of drugs which might
in a selective way affect brain function by affecting the excitability of neuronal membranes. Local anesthetics, by inhibiting the enhanced permeability to sodium which occurs in the
initial phase of membrane depolarization, block the propagation of
the action potential down the neuron (Ritchie and Greengard, 1966).
Although these agents exhibit a quantitative selectivity of action,
depending on the diameter of the nerve fiber and the degree of
myelination, in sufficient concentrations they block conduction
down all axons. Their specificity of action chiefly results from
the manner in which they are administered. The drugs are applied
locally to the particular neurons that one desires to anesthetize.

Another group of agents that acts by modifying membrane excitability are some of the antiepileptic drugs, and notably
diphenylhydantoin. Although its precise mechanism of action is not
fully clarified, this agent appears to reduce the spread of
seizure discharge by activating the $Na-K^+$-ATPase pump in membranes,
thus stabilizing membrane potentials in a hyperpolarized state
(Woodbury, 1969).

Affecting the vascular supply to the brain might also be a
means of altering brain function, although this is not likely to
produce specific, selective modifications in behavior. Generally
such drugs are useful only in conditions where cerebral vasospasm
is a major factor in producing disturbances in brain function.

The fourth category, agents which may affect the supporting glial cells, is one about which we know virtually nothing, since we know relatively little about the function of glial cells. It has been estimated that there are probably ten times as many glial cells as there are brain cells and these cells probably play a supportive role, both anatomically and nutritionally, in brain function. No agents are yet available that are known to selectively affect these cells and thus alter brain function.

Lastly, drugs which affect transmitter metabolism, or postsynaptic receptors, are among the agents which possess the greatest potential for selectively affecting brain function. There are many different neurons in the brain which contain specific chemicals which are released on nerve stimulation from nerve endings and which act in some way upon specific postsynaptic receptor sites. If one can modify selectively the metabolism of these transmitter substances, one can then affect one group or class of neurons in the brain and therefore one may be able to modify selectively brain function. Indeed, although definitive evidence is not available as yet that the behavioral effects of most drugs are due to their effects on neurotransmitter metabolism, there is much evidence indicating that most drugs which have profound central nervous system actions also modify the metabolism or the effects of one or more of the neurotransmitter substances in the brain.

Neurotransmitters in the Central Nervous System

One problem which is still being examined for many substances normally present in the brain which modify interneuronal communication concerns whether that substance is a neurotransmitter, or whether it is simply playing some other role in neuronal function. The following is a list of criteria which should be satisfied to provide at least minimal credentials for stating that a particular substance is a respectable candidate as a neurotransmitter: (1) The substance should be synthesized and stored in specific neurons. (2) It should not be uniformly distributed throughout the central nervous system, but should be present in certain specific neuronal pathways. (3) The enzymes involved in the synthesis of the transmitter should be present in the neurons. (4) Neurons operate intermittently and may be required to fire very intensively for a variable duration, or they may remain quiescent for different intervals. Neurons which fire very frequently and intensively must have the potential for restoring the neurotransmitter substance which they release and which, at least to some extent, is metabolized or degraded upon release. Thus, the synthesis of neurotransmitter should be regulated and should be sensitive to neural activity. (5) The substance must be released on nerve stimulation. (6) When the substance is applied to the brain tissue, it must act upon specific postsynaptic

receptor sites to produce the appropriate neurophysiological effect. (7) The action of the applied putative neurotransmitter,
as is true for effects of nerve stimulation, should be rapidly
terminated in some manner.

There are at least a half dozen substances in the brain which
are respectable candidates as neurotransmitters; including
acetylcholine, norepinephrine, dopamine, 5-hydroxytryptamine,
γ-aminobutyric acid and glycine. We certainly have no idea as to
the number of unknown transmitter substances that function in the
brain, but it is fair to estimate that we have only defined the
neurotransmitter substance in a small fraction of the total number
of neurons in the brain. The implication therefore would be that
there are many other unknown neurotransmitter substances waiting
to be discovered.

Acetylcholine

Acetylcholine is a well known neurotransmitter in the peripheral
nervous system. It is present in the somatic nerves which terminate
on skeletal muscle, in the preganglionic and postganglionic neurons
of the parasympathetic nervous system and in the preganglionic
fibers of the sympathetic division of the autonomic nervous system.
Acetylcholine is present in the brain, and the enzyme for its
synthesis, choline acetyltransferase, is also present in brain, as
is the enzyme responsible for its degradation by hydrolysis,
acetylcholinesterase (Quastel, 1962).

In Table 2 is presented the distribution of acetylcholine and
the distribution of the enzymes involved in its synthesis and
degradation in the brain. The distribution of acetylcholine in the
brain is non-uniform, implying that not all neurons contain
acetylcholine. There is a fairly good correlation between the
distribution of acetylcholine and choline acetyltransferase. For
example, there is a fairly high concentration of acetylcholine and
choline acetyltransferase in the motor cortex; there is a very high
concentration of these substances in the anterior roots of the
spinal cord, which contain the axons of the cholinergic motor neurons
originating in the anterior horn of the spinal cord. In addition,
there is a fair amount of acetylcholine and choline acetyltransferase in the thalamus, and a moderate amount of these substances
in the hypothalamus and in the basal ganglion. In contrast, the
dorsal roots of the spinal cord, the cerebellum and the optic
nerve contain very much smaller quantities of both choline acetyltransferase and this putative neurotransmitter substance.

As I shall elaborate upon somewhat later, if acetylcholine
metabolism is modified in the brain, behavior may be profoundly
affected. Thus, alteration in acetylcholine metabolism can

Table 2

DISTRIBUTION OF ACETYLCHOLINE (ACh), CHOLINE
ACETYL TRANSFERASE (ChAc) AND
ACETYLCHOLINESTERASE (AChE) IN BRAIN

Brain Region	ACh nmol/g tissue	ChAc	AChE[a]
		nmoles product per hr per g tissue	
Cerebral Cortex	30.8	5,000	40,000
Caudate nucleus	23.2	20,000	900,000
Thalamus	21.7	21,200	100,000
Hypothalamus	20.5	13,600	9,000
Cerebellum	4.1	600	100,000
Ventral roots	103.0	30,000	30,000
Dorsal roots	0.3	20	8,000
Optic nerve	2.0	20	2,500

Modified from Campbell and Jenden (1970); Hebb and Krnjević (1962); Robson
and Stacey (1962); and Aprison et al (1968). In several cases major discrepancies exist; the most reasonable value was selected for the table.
[a] Acetyl-β-methylcholine was employed as substrate.

markedly affect central nervous system function. Furthermore, it
is well established that if specific regions of the brain are
stimulated, acetylcholine is released. Acetylcholine is very
rapidly hydrolyzed by the enzyme cholinesterase, which is present
in high concentrations in many regions of the brain (Hebb and
Krnjević, 1962).

Norepinephrine, Dopamine and 5-Hydroxytryptamine

Three important putative neurotransmitter substances in the
brain are ethylamine derivatives; two are catechol compounds,
norepinephrine and dopamine, and the third is an indole amine,
5-hydroxytryptamine (serotonin). Dopamine and norepinephrine are
formed from tyrosine, and dopamine itself is a precursor of norepinephrine. The pathway involves conversion of tyrosine to 3,4-di-
hydroxyphenylalanine (dopa) by the enzyme tyrosine hydroxylase,
followed by decarboxylation of dopa to the primary amine, dopamine.
This latter reaction is catalyzed by L-aromatic amino acid decarboxylase, an enzyme with rather broad substrate specificity
that also catalyzes the conversion of 5-hydroxytryptophan to
5-hydroxytryptamine. The enzymes tyrosine hydroxylase and L-aromatic
amino acid decarboxylase (dopa decarboxylase) are presumed to be
present in both dopamine containing and norepinephrine containing
neurons. The enzyme which catalyzes the conversion of dopamine to
norepinephrine, dopamine-β-hydroxylase, is presumably present only
in norepinephrine containing neurons (Weiner, 1970.

Tryptophan hydroxylase catalyzes the aromatic hydroxylation
of tryptophan to 5-hydroxytryptophan (Ichiyama et al, 1970). This
enzyme is presumably exclusively localized in 5-hydroxytryptamine
containing neurons. The decarboxylation of 5-hydroxytryptophan
to 5-hydroxytryptamine is catalyzed by a decarboxylase. There is
some dispute regarding whether this enzyme is identical to the
enzyme which catalyzes the decarboxylation of dopa (Bender and
Coulson, 1972; Christenson et al, 1972; Sims et al, 1973).

The pathways for the biosynthesis of these 3 amines from
aromatic amino acids are thus quite analogous, and, in the case of
dopamine and norepinephrine, the first two steps in the biosynthesis
are identical. Their similarities extend beyond the routes of
synthesis. The pathway for degradation of dopamine, norepinephrine
and 5-hydroxytryptamine is again similar. It involves the enzyme
monoamine oxidase, which carries out oxidative deamination of each
of these substances to an aldehyde metabolite (Weiner, 1960). In
addition, norepinephrine and dopamine may be converted to their
respective 3-O-methylated derivatives by the enzyme catechol-O-
methyl transferase (Axelrod, 1959).

The distribution of norepinephrine in brain is non-uniform.
In Table 3 is shown the distribution of this amine in mammalian
brain, most notably in rat brain. Some values for bovine brain
are also included since one can more precisely separate brain
regions in this organ (Kindwall and Weiner, 1966). A similar
distribution pattern is found in human brain as well as in brains
of other species. The highest concentration of norepinephrine is
found in the hypothalamic region. In this region are located
autonomic centers for both parasympathetic and sympathetic
functions and the central neurons of the sympathetic nervous
system are presumed to be the norepinephrine-containing neurons
which are present in this region. There is also a considerable
amount of norepinephrine present in other regions of the brain
stem, particularly in the reticular formation. Norepinephrine
is also present in the locus coeruleus, the limbic system and the
brain stem. The distribution of dopamine in the brain is
strikingly different from that of norepinephrine (Kindwall and
Weiner, 1966). There is an extremely high concentration of
dopamine in the caudate nucleus and in the putamen, and a small
but significant amount of the material in the substantia nigra.
In addition, dopamine is present in the retina, in the median
eminence and in regions of the limbic system (Table 3) (Holzbauer
and Sharman, 1972). 5-Hydroxytryptamine has a somewhat similar
distribution to that of norepinephrine, although the indole amine
is generally distributed in the brain more medial to norepinephrine (Table 4).

Biochemical analysis of amines in various brain regions only
provides us with a rather gross knowledge of the distribution of
these amines. It does not indicate precisely where these substances are, and it does not even demonstrate that the substances
are in neurons. Conceivably, they could be in glia of different
types in different regions of the brain. A number of years ago,
Falck et al (1962) in Sweden developed an elegant histochemical
fluorescence technique for identifying and localizing the monoamines,
particularly dopamine, norepinephrine and 5-hydroxytryptamine.
This has enabled us to learn in considerable detail the precise distribution of these neurons in the brain (Hillarp et al, 1966).

The method these workers developed is based upon the conversion of these compounds to isoquinoline derivatives, in the
case of catecholamines, or to a carboline derivative, in the case
of 5-hydroxytryptamine. These products are formed at elevated
temperatures in the presence of paraformaldehyde and water vapor.
The formaldehyde condensation products are highly fluorescent and,
since the reaction can be carried out under relatively anhydrous
conditions with fresh frozen tissue, the problems of fixation arti-
facts and diffusion of the amine in the tissue are minimized (Falck
and Owman, 1965). With the catecholamines, a green fluorescence
is observable through the fluorescence microscope. One can
distinguish dopamine from norepinephrine by special reactions; e.g.,
by selective dehydration of dopamine in the presence of anhydrous

Table 3

DISTRIBUTION OF NOREPINEPHRINE (NE), DOPAMINE (DA), TYROSINE (TYR) HYDROXYLASE, DOPAMINE-β-HYDROXYLASE (DBH), AND AROMATIC AMINO ACID DECARBOXYLASE (AADC) IN BRAIN

Brain Region	NE nmoles/g tissue	DA nmoles/g tissue	Tyr Hydroxylase nmoles product per hr per g tissue	AADC[a]	DBH[b]
Cortex	1.1	0.6	8	2500	54
Midbrain	3.3	–	–	–	–
Striatum	2.0	40.0	410	18,700	14
Hippocampus	1.2	0.8[c]	–	2400	–
Hypothalamus	9.0	0.9[c]	61	8600	117
Pons–Medulla	3.6	0.6	16	4500	–
Cerebellum	1.0	<0.6[c]	4	1600	41
Brain Stem	–	<0.6	–	–	149
Mesencephalon	2.4	1.6	85	–	–
Diencephalon	4.5	–	65	–	–
Telencephalon	1.4	1.9	29	–	–
Substantia Nigra	–	2.5[c]	–	–	–

Modified from: Holzbauer and Sharman (1972); Kindwall and Weiner (1966); Porcher and Heller (1972); Coyle and Axelrod (1972 a,b), Sims et al (1973).

[a]Substrate employed was dopa.

[b]Substrate employed was octopamine.

Most values are taken from rat brain studies; some of dopamine and norepinephrine values are taken from bovine brain (c).

Where discrepant values were reported, the most reproducible values reported were selected. In some cases discrepancies are probably due to differences in brain dissection.

Table 4

DISTRIBUTION OF 5-HYDROXYTRYPTAMINE(5-HT), TRYPTOPHAN (TRP)
HYDROXYLASE AND L-AROMATIC AMINO ACID DECARBOXYLASE (AADC)
IN BRAIN

Brain Region	5-HT[a] nmoles/g	TRP Hydroxylase [a] nmoles 5-HTP formed per hr per g tissue	AADC [b] nmoles 5-HT formed per hr per g tissue
Cerebral cortex	1.76	0.89	400
Midbrain	3.46	3.35	-
Striatum	2.22	1.14	200
Hippocampus	1.59	0.58	340
Hypothalamus	4.60	4.81	1,200
Pons-Medulla	2.84	2.83	900
Cerebellum	0.34	0.08	700

Modified from Deguchi and Barchas (1972)[a] and Sims et al (1973)[b].
Values were selected from assays of rat brain.
[b]Substrate employed was 5-hydroxytryptophan (5-HTP)

HCl which results in alterations in the fluorescence spectrum for
the modified dopamine derivative which is distinct from the fluo-
resence of the more stable isoquinoline derivative of norepinephrine (Björklund et al, 1968). 5-Hydroxytryptamine is also
converted to a fluorescent derivative by exposure to formaldehyde
gas, but in this case the color of the derivative is yellow rather
than green. One can thus identify each of these putative neurotransmitters in various brain regions by this technique.

Figure 1 is a histochemical fluorescence picture of the mouse
vas deferens. It shows the diffuse innervation of the smooth
muscle of the vas deferens preparation by norepinephrine-containing
terminals. It is apparent from this section that one has, with
this technique, a very nice means of defining the distribution of
norepinephrine-containing cells or nerve terminals.

In Figure 2 is shown the fluorescence pattern in the rat
mesentery. The (green) norepinephrine-containing fibers may be
seen within the blood vessels of the rat mesentery. The mast cells
in the rat mesentery are intensely fluorescent (yellow) because of
their content of 5-hydroxytryptamine.

Now let us consider the central nervous system. In the
reticular formation or locus coeruleus, for example, there are a
number of cells in whose cytoplasm is concentrated a material which
fluoresces after exposure to formaldehyde. These are norepinephrine-
containing neuronal cells (Hillarp et al, 1966). In the substantia
nigra there is a smaller number of fluorescent cell bodies, which
are confined to the pars compacta. These cells contain dopamine.
These cells are important modulators of the activity of the extrapyramidal motor system. This dopaminergic pathway from the substantia nigra to the neostriatum was elucidated by this histochemical technique and its elucidation was crucial to our full
understanding of the role of dopamine neurons in extrapyramidal
motor function.

In many other regions of the brain, nerve terminals of
catecholamine neurons are found. Fuxe and coworkers and Ungerstedt
have carried out a systematic analysis of the distribution of
monoamine fluorescent fibers in the brain, and have been able to
map many of the neuronal pathways containing these monoamines in
the central nervous system (Hillarp et al, 1966; Ungerstedt, 1971;
Livett, 1973).

Some of the major results of their studies regarding the origin
and distribution of catecholamine and 5-hydroxytryptamine containing
neuronal pathways may be briefly summarized as follows: Many norepinephrine-containing fibers originate in the brain stem area, some
of them proceeding caudally to spinal cord, others projecting through

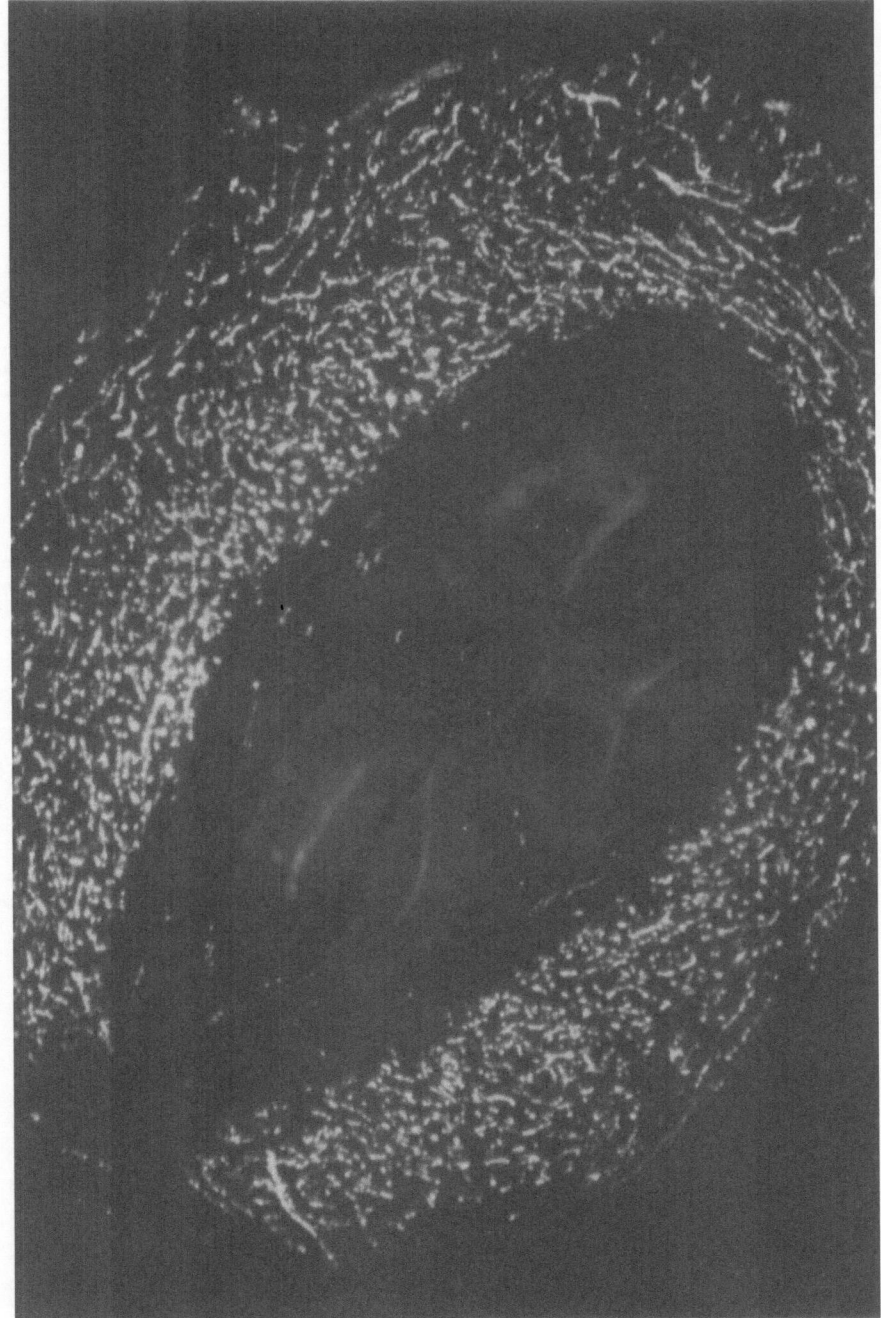

Fig. 1. Histochemical fluorescence pattern of mouse vas deferens.
The fluorescent noradrenergic neurons are distributed throughout
the muscle layer of this organ. (x 40)

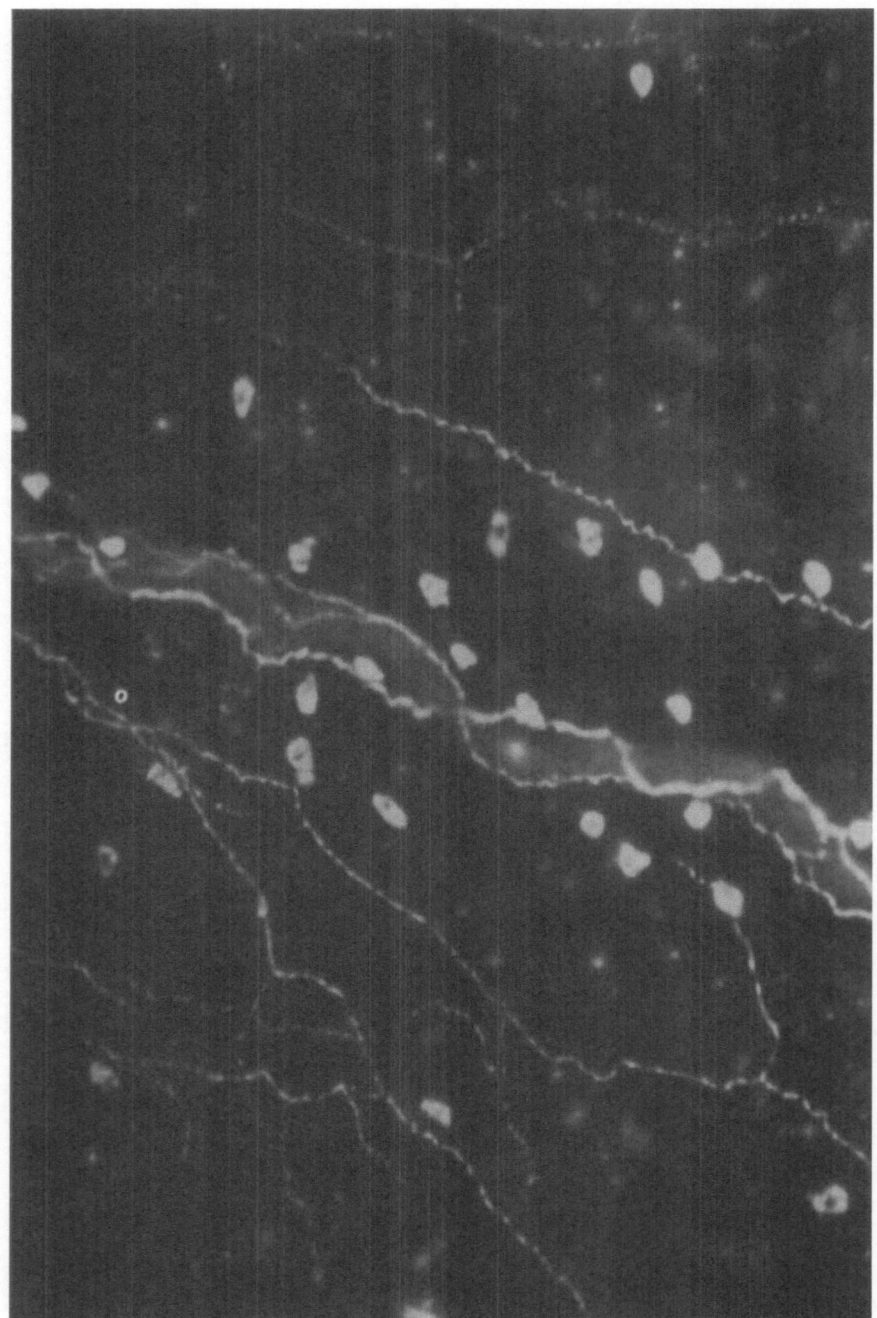

Fig. 2. Histochemical fluorescence pattern of rat mesentery. The
(green) noradrenergic neurons are associated with the blood vessels
of this tissue. Mast cells (yellow) also are highly fluorescent
due to the presence of 5-hydroxytryptamine. The diffuse fluoresent
background (blue) is "autofluorescence" which is visible in the
absence of the paraformaldehyde condensation reaction. (x 10)

the median forebrain bundle to the thalamus, hypothalamus, neocortex, and to the limbic system of the brain. Dopamine neurons
are more sparsely distributed. The most abundant of these neurons
comprise the nigro-striatal pathway, those fibers originating in
the substantia nigra and terminating in the neostriatal region.
Other dopamine neurons originate in the brain stem and project to
the forebrain. There are small groups of dopamine containing
neurons present in the retina and some dopamine neurons which run
from the median eminence to the hypothalamus. The latter group of
neurons appears to regulate the release of hypothalamic releasing
factors: notably LRF and perhaps FRF (Schneider and McKann, 1969;
Kamberi et al, 1971). 5-Hydroxytryptamine neurons, in general,
exhibit a pattern of distribution similar to norepinephrine neurons,
but are located medial to the norepinephrine tracts (Hillarp et al,
1966).

In addition to the distribution of monoamines in different
neurons, we know a considerable amount about the intracellular
localization of these monoamines. By combined centrifugation and
biochemical techniques, vesicles, which have been identified in
nerve terminals by electron microscopy, have been isolated and it
has been demonstrated that these organelles house the neurotransmitter substances. Cholinergic vesicles appear translucent under
the electron microscope, whereas the characteristic feature of
norepinephrine-containing vesicles is their dense or granulated
centers.

All neurons appear to contain the enzymatic machinery for
synthesis of their particular neurotransmitter substance. Both
the biosynthetic enzymes and the storage particles are believed
to be synthesized in the cell body. From this site of macromolecular synthesis and organelle formation, enzymes and vesicles
are transported down the axon to the nerve terminals. The neurotransmitter substances apparently are synthesized largely in the
nerve ending; they are either transferred to the storage particle
after synthesis (as in the case of dopamine, 5-hydroxytryptamine
and acetylcholine) or are synthesized in the storage particles
(norepinephrine) (Weiner, 1970; Dahlström, 1970). On nerve stimulation the neurotransmitter and some of the soluble contents
of the storage particle are released into the synaptic cleft where
the neurotransmitter is able to act upon the postsynaptic receptor.
After stimulating rather briefly the postsynaptic receptor, the
transmitter is removed from the receptor site either by a neuronal
uptake process (norepinephrine) or by degradation (acetylcholine)
and by diffusion from the synaptic region (Weiner, 1970).

This is an extremely brief summary of the complex series of
events which describe neurotransmitter dynamics. It should be apparent that one can in many ways affect the various processes involved in neurotransmission; e.g., with appropriate drugs. As-

suming the availability of such agents, one might be able to modify any one of a number of metabolic processes which relate to the neurotransmitter. Indeed, there are many drugs which are known to affect a variety of these processes; synthesis, storage, uptake, degradation, and release of some of these substances. These drugs may have different effects on the function of the nervous system, depending upon the type of neuron they modify and the manner in which the function of that neuron is altered. We thus have means not only of selectively affecting certain classes of neurons, but we are even able to dissect out and modify specific aspects of neurotransmitter metabolism within each type of neuron.

The Negative Feedback Concept as it Relates to Neurotransmitter Metabolism

Before examining in more detail a few drugs which can affect neurotransmitter metabolism and which do affect behavior, pre-sumably as a consequence of affecting neurotransmitter metabolism, I should like to introduce the concept of negative feedback as it relates to neuronal activity and neurotransmitter metabolism. It is important to realize that the metabolism, or the turnover, of the neurotransmitters of the brain can be markedly affected in an indirect way by a variety of drugs. Unless one appreciates this concept, this may produce much confusion in terms of analyzing the mechanisms of action of drugs. Let us examine a hypothetical neuronal pathway with neurons A and B in series in this pathway. Let us further suppose that neuron A is directly or indirectly excitatory to neuron B. If we affect the more distal neuron B, for example, by directly stimulating that neuron with a drug so that it fires at a considerably greater rate than formerly, feed-back mechanisms or servomechanisms are activated in the brain which in some manner try to restore the homeostasis of the neural process. Neuron A presumably receives messages from a recurrent collateral system which indicates to it that neuron B is firing at an accelerated rate. This message directs neuron A to reduce its spontaneous firing to help curb the activity of overactive neuron B. Thus, a negative feedback system is activated which leads to a marked reduction in the activity of neuron A. As a consequence of that, the neurotransmitter in neuron A is no longer released, and it tends to accumulate in the vesicles of the neuron, resulting in increased levels and reduced turnover of neurotrans-mitter A in the brain.

Now, the converse of this phenomenon is equally applicable. Let us now suppose that, instead of introducing into this nervous system a stimulant of neuron B, we administer a blocker of neuron B. Neuron B will not fire, because it is no longer susceptible to synaptic stimulation. With this situation, the negative feedback mechanism is turned down or off, and neuron A receives a message

from the recurrent collateral system downstream which directs
neuron A to become more active in an effort to increase the firing
of neuron B. Neuron A tries to restore the activity of neuron B to
normal levels by markedly increasing its activity. The neuron A
transmitter is released at a considerably increased rate, and the
turnover of transmitter in neuron A is increased. In turn, the
level of transmitter in neuron A falls because of this accelerated
release and metabolism.

   In both cases one arrives at what might seem superficially to
be a paradox, that is, one achieves a lowered neurotransmitter
level which is associated with increased synthesis and turnover of
the transmitter. The steady state is modified to yield either
higher turnover and lower levels, or, conversely, higher levels associated with reduced turnover of neurotransmitter. Perhaps a
simple analogy would be a consideration of the hydrodynamics of
a bucket with a hole in the bottom into which one pours water in
order to maintain a given level of water in the container. If
the neuron is markedly increased in its activity, this is analogous
to enlarging the hole in the bucket so more water (transmitter)
exits. If the hole is opened up considerably so that there is a
marked increase in the egress of water, the level of water falls
and the input (transmitter synthesis) must increase in order to
try to restore the water level back to the resting height, or
until a balance between input and loss is achieved. The increase
in input would not be completely restorative, so one will achieve
a water level intermediate between that of a bucket with no hole
(resting neuron) and that which one would obtain if the hole were
enlarged but the input remained constant (synthesis is not increased). (Since, for a constant hole diameter, the rate of water
loss is proportional to the logarithm of the height of the water
level in the bucket, the water level will fall until the egress
diminishes to a level which equals the input.) The resultant of
these two effects of increased loss and a partially compensatory
increased input would be increased "water turnover". There would
be enhanced flow of water in and out of the bucket, but a reduced
level in the bucket. This level would be intermediate between the
lowest level possible without increased input and the highest level
possible in the presence of minimal release or loss.

   The concept of negative feedback as it relates to neurotransmitter metabolism may thus be summarized in the following
manner: With stimulation of a postsynaptic receptor, there is
negative feedback to the neuron (or neurons) preceding the affected
receptor, which reduces the activity of the proximal neurons, resulting in increased levels and reduced turnover of the neurotransmitters in the presynaptic neurons. Conversely, there is
reduced negative feedback of the proximal neurons when inhibition
of the postsynaptic receptor occurs, leading to increased activity

of the presynaptic neurons and reduced levels and increased turnover of the transmitters in the presynaptic neurons. One can
therefore have profound effects on the metabolism of one or several
neurotransmitters as a result of administration of a drug which
has no direct effect on the neurons containing those neurotransmitters. The lack of consideration of this fundamental point can
lead to considerable confusion in terms of how drugs act and how
they might affect neurotransmitter metabolism without exhibiting
any direct action on classes of neurons containing the neurotransmitters (Table 5).

TABLE 5

CONCEPT OF NEGATIVE FEEDBACK AND
NEUROTRANSMITTER METABOLISM

STIMULATION OF POSTSYNAPTIC RECEPTOR

Negative feedback of neurons preceding
affected receptor.

Increased levels and reduced turnover of
neurotransmitter in presynaptic neuron.

INHIBITION OF POSTSYNAPTIC RECEPTOR

Reduced negative feedback of neurons
preceding affected receptor.

Reduced levels and increased turnover of
neurotransmitter in presynaptic neuron.

Effects of Psychoactive Drugs on Neurotransmitter Metabolism

Let us briefly examine the actions of a variety of drugs
which influence the neuronal systems containing either acetylcholine or the ethylamines mentioned. Table 6 lists drugs which
affect norepinephrine metabolism. A variety of agents will affect
norepinephrine metabolism, both peripherally and in the central
nervous system. Phenoxybenzamine and phentolamine are agents which
block α-adrenergic postsynaptic receptors. These agents to some
degree produce sedation in man. Blockade of norepinephrine receptors, by reducing negative feedback to the adrenergic neurons
actually leads to an increase in norepinephrine turnover in adrenergic tissue (Dairman et al, 1968). Reserpine, an agent which
was commonly used at one time to treat certain psychiatric
disturbances, produces marked sedation. It produces this effect

TABLE 6

DRUGS AFFECTING NOREPINEPHRINE METABOLISM

Phenoxybenzamine, Phentolamine

    Block norepinephrine α-receptors
    Increase norepinephrine turnover

Reserpine

    Depletes norepinephrine stores by
    block of vesicle amine uptake pump
    Intraneuronal metabolism of amine
    enhanced

Amphetamine, Methamphetamine

    Release norepinephrine from stores
      into extraneuronal space
    Block norepinephrine uptake

Tricyclic Antidepressants, Methylphenidate

    Inhibit norepinephrine uptake into neurons

Monoamine Oxidase Inhibitors

    Inhibit norepinephrine catabolism
    Reduce norepinephrine turnover

Levodopa

    Norepinephrine precursor

α-Methyl-p-tyrosine, α-Methyldopa, Disulfiram

    Inhibit norepinephrine synthesis

---

presumably because of its ability to deplete norepinephrine stores by impairing uptake of the amine into the storage site. The norepinephrine is therefore metabolized within the neuron and is not able to exit from the neuron intact to interact with the receptor site (Rutledge and Weiner, 1967). Amphetamine and methamphetamine release norepinephrine from stores and block norepinephrine uptake into neurons. These actions presumably will produce an effect opposite to that of phenoxybenzamine or reserpine; that is by enhancing the release of norepinephrine from these stores they in-

directly activate the postsynaptic site (Rutledge et al, 1972;
Weiner, 1972). They produce effects opposite to those of reserpine
or phenoxybenzamine in terms of their behavioral actions, and these
drugs are classified as psychomotor stimulants. Agents which block
the amine uptake process, which ordinarily leads to the recapture
of norepinephrine back into the nerve terminal, increase the level
of norepinephrine at the receptor site. These agents would also
be expected to increase the level of central nervous system
activity, and agents in this class include imipramine, protriptyline
and related compounds which are collectively termed tricyclic antidepressants. As this term implies, these blockers of neuronal uptake are useful in the treatment of certain types of depression.
Agents which block the metabolism of norepinephrine also would be
expected to produce stimulation, and among these are the monoamine
oxidase inhibitors, which are classified as antidepressants or
psychomotor stimulants. Blockers of norepinephrine synthesis; e.g.,
α-methyl-p-tyrosine, deplete brain norepinephrine and depress
behavior. Thus, many agents which affect norepinephrine metabolism
have important and, in general, predictable effects on behavior.

Table 7 summarizes the actions of drugs which affect dopamine
metabolism. Apomorphine directly stimulates dopamine receptors.
Phenothiazines and haloperidol, which are important antipsychotic
agents, block dopamine receptors, and increase dopamine turnover
in the brain (O'Keeffe et al, 1970). Again, the increased turnover may be explained by blockade of postsynaptic receptors and
reduction of negative feedback to the dopamine neurons. Therefore
the presynaptic dopamine neuron will increase its activity in an
effort to overcome the blockade. Reserpine depletes dopamine
stores, as it does those of norepinephrine. Amphetamine, similar
to its actions on the norepinephrine neuron, will release dopamine
from stores and will block dopamine uptake, although at somewhat
higher concentrations than are required to produce analogous effects on norepinephrine neurons (Rutledge et al, 1972). Agents
which affect dopamine synthesis and metabolism affect dopamine
neurons in a manner analogous to their effects on norepinephrine
neurons.

Table 8 lists drugs which affect 5-hydroxytryptamine metabolism.
These are perhaps the least understood of the groups of drugs
which affect monoamine metabolism. Lysergic acid diethylamide (LSD)
and other indole ethylamine hallucinogenic agents, have biochemical
effects centrally which suggest that they may stimulate 5-hydroxy-
tryptamine receptors (Aghajanian et al, 1970; Freedman et al,
1970). By stimulating 5-hydroxytryptamine receptors located on
the neuron distal to the 5-hydroxytryptamine neuron, activation of
a negative feedback system might be expected and the electrical
activity of the 5-hydroxytryptamine neurons would therefore be
reduced. Thus, one might anticipate reduced 5-hydroxytryptamine

TABLE 7

DRUGS AFFECTING DOPAMINE METABOLISM

Apomorphine

   Stimulates dopamine receptors

Phenothiazines, Haloperidol

   Block dopamine receptors
   Increase dopamine turnover

Reserpine

   Depletes dopamine stores by block of
      vesicle amine uptake pump
   Intraneuronal metabolism of amine enhanced

Amphetamine

   Releases dopamine from stores into
      extraneuronal space
   Blocks dopamine uptake

Monoamine Oxidase Inhibitors

   Inhibit dopamine catabolism
   Reduce dopamine turnover

Levodopa

   Dopamine precursor

α-Methyl-p-tyrosine, α-Methyldopa

   Inhibit dopamine synthesis

TABLE 8

DRUGS AFFECTING 5-HYDROXYTRYPTAMINE (5-HT) METABOLISM

Lysergic acid diethylamide, psilocybin, Other tryptamines?

    Stimulate 5-HT receptors
    Reduce 5-HT turnover

Reserpine

    Depletes 5-HT stores by blocking vesicle amine uptake
     pump
    Intraneuronal metabolism enhanced

Amphetamine and Analogs

    Release 5-HT from stores into extraneuronal space
    Block 5-HT uptake

Monoamine Oxidase Inhibitors

    Inhibit 5-HT metabolism

5-Hydroxytryptophan

    5-HT precursor

p-Chlorophenylalanine

    Inhibits tryptophan hydroxylase and 5-HT synthesis

---

turnover and increased levels of 5-hydroxytryptamine after administration of LSD. Biochemical studies in animals appear to
support this hypothesis and suggest that LSD and related compounds
exert some of their effects by stimulating 5-hydroxytryptamine
receptor sites (Freedman et al, 1970). Reserpine depletes 5-hy-
droxytryptamine store, as it does the catecholamine stores.
Amphetamine, at higher concentrations than those required to affect catecholamine neurons, will release 5-hydroxytryptamine from
5-hydroxytryptamine neurons and will also block the reuptake of
this amine into the neuron (Rutledge et al, 1972). Both of these
effects would lead to responses which should mimic increased
5-hydroxytryptamine neuron activity. Indeed, high doses of
amphetamine will produce hallucinations and psychotic behavior in
man (Weiner, 1972). p-Chlorophenylalanine, an inhibitor of 5-hy-
droxytryptamine synthesis, also has important, although poorly

understood, effects with regard to the 5-hydroxytryptamine system
and behavior (Koe and Weissman, 1966; Tenen, 1967).

There are many drugs which affect acetylcholine metabolism
(Table 9). Atropine, scopolamine and the piperidyl glycolates
block cholinergic receptors. Again, by blockade of these receptors,
the activity of the negative feedback system is reduced, and the
cholinergic neuron activity is increased markedly in an effort to
overcome the cholinergic blockade. Increased acetylcholine turnover and lowered acetylcholine levels in brain would thus be
expected, observations which have been validated in experimental

---

TABLE 9

DRUGS AFFECTING ACETYLCHOLINE METABOLISM

Atropine, Scopolamine, Piperidyl Glycolates

    Block cholinergic, muscarinic receptors
    Lowered acetylcholine levels
    Increased acetylcholine turnover

Oxytremorine, Tremorine

    Stimulate cholinergic receptors
    Increased acetylcholine levels
    Decreased acetylcholine turnover

Physostigmine, Organophosphorus Cholinesterase
    Inhibitors

    Inhibit acetylcholine hydrolysis
    Increased acetylcholine levels
    Reduced acetylcholine turnover

---

animals given blockers of cholinergic receptors (Holmstedt and
Lundgren, 1966; Campbell and Jenden, 1970). These agents produce
profound effects on behavior, ranging from sedation to convulsions
and coma. Very severe and frightening deliriums and hallucinations
are produced, particularly by the piperidyl glycolates. Oxytremorine and tremorine produce effects opposite to those of the
atropine-like compounds. They stimulate cholinergic receptors, and
this is associated with increased levels of acetylcholine and decreased acetylcholine turnover. The organophosphorus cholinesterase inhibitors and physostigmine, which block the metabolism

of acetylcholine, increase acetylcholine levels and in this way
lead to a marked increase in cholinergic effects. Profound behavioral effects ranging from stimulation to convulsions and
ultimately CNS depression and coma may ensue.

The Effect on the Immature Nervous System
of Drugs which Modify Neurotransmitter Metabolism

The mature central nervous system is both anatomically and
biochemically extremely complex. It would be expected that the
development of this complex organ and the regulation of this development would be extremely delicate and would be highly susceptible to environmental or exogenous perturbations. Many drugs
which influence neurotransmitter metabolism in the mature central
nervous system have been found to affect behavior in later life
when these agents are administered to developing organisms. Increasing attention therefore is being directed toward the development of neurotransmitter systems in the brain and the
modification of this development by drugs and other chemicals,
since modification of neurotransmitter metabolism during maturation
may have important effects on ultimate CNS development and
behavior. Aspects of this challenging problem will be discussed
in detail by the principal speakers of this session.

In addition to the possible significance to development of
the acute effects of drugs on neurotransmitter metabolism and
turnover in the immature brain, there are prolonged effects of
drugs on neurons. Prolonged modification of the electrical
activity of neurons, which may be directly or indirectly a consequence of drug effects or may be related to other environmental
imputs, may markedly affect CNS maturation. In the mature adrenergic system, chronic increase of adrenergic nervous activity
ultimately leads to increased levels of tyrosine hydroxylase and
dopamine-β-hydroxylase in these neurons; i.e., a biochemical
hypertrophy of these neurons occurs. Conversely, chronic de-
centralization of adrenergic neurons leads to a reduction in
levels of tyrosine hydroxylase and dopamine-β-hydroxylase in adrenergic neurons; which might be described as biochemical atrophy.
One could well imagine that chronic alterations in inputs such as
drugs may produce; e.g., by perturbing feedback systems,when
superimposed on the complex and delicate development of immature
central nervous system pathways, might affect the rate or extent
of development of these pathways. Indeed, apparent examples of
this have already been described. Marchisio (1969) demonstrated
that deafferentation of the optic lobes of the chick embryo at
day 3 leads to a marked reduction in the normal developmental
increase in choline acetyltransferase in the contralateral deafferented optic centers by day 17 of incubation. It is of interest
that the difference in choline acetyltransferase levels between

the control side and the deafferented side does not appear until
at least 8 days after the deafferentation.

Finally, I should like to raise a question about the mechanism
by which drugs which influence neurotransmitter metabolism affect the development of the immature nervous system. Can agents
which affect neurotransmitter metabolism affect development of
the immature organism by their known actions if these drugs are
administered prior to the development and the functional maturation of these systems? That is, can such drugs affect these systems before the full expression of their differentiated state
with regard to the process of neurotransmission? Many examples
of the effects of psychoactive drugs on later behavior have been
reported, even when these substances are injected into developing organisms before the development of the neurotransmitter
systems which these drugs affect in the adult organism. However,
there is no definitive demonstration that this effect on later
behavior is causally related to an effect on the neurotransmitter
systems that are known to be perturbed in the mature organism.
In this regard, I would like to mention a study reported by
Brimijoin and Molinoff (1971). Mueller et al (1969) had shown
that reserpine administration leads, after a few days, to an increase in tyrosine hydroxylase and dopamine-β-hydroxylase in
adrenal gland and in the superior cervical ganglia of mature rats.
Brimijoin and Molinoff showed that, if instead of simply giving
reserpine, either the axon is sectioned or 6-hydroxydopamine is
administered at the time reserpine is given, no enzyme induction
results. It is possible that the reparative processes which are
triggered by section of the neuron or by administration of 6-hy-
droxydopamine take precedence over the synthesis of neurotransmitter
enzymes and neurotransmitter substances. Speculating still further,
this may imply that normal structural growth may precede, and take
precedence over, the expression of the differentiated state, as
manifested by the development of enzymes involved in neurotransmitter metabolism and the process of neurosecretion. If so, it may
be difficult to modify the development of these neuronal systems
by attempting to affect the metabolism of the neurotransmitter
prior to the full development of these systems, and any predictable
effect of these agents may occur only subsequent to the maturation
of the neurons and the initiation of neurosecretion and synaptic
transmission. Perhaps our speakers during this session may provide some insight into this question as the session progresses.

REFERENCES

Aghajanian, G.K., Foote, W.E. and Sheard, M.H., 1970, Action of psychotogenic drugs on single midbrain raphe neurons. J. Pharmacol. Exp. Ther. 171: 178-187.

Aprison, M.H., Hariya, T., Hingtgen, J.N. and Toru, M., 1968, Neuro-chemical correlates of behavior. Changes in acetylcholine, norepinephrine and 5-hydroxytryptamine concentrations in several discrete brain areas of the rat during behavioral ex-citation. J. Neurochem. 15: 1131-1139.

Axelrod, J., 1959, Metabolism of epinephrine and other sympatho-mimetic amines. Physiol. Rev. 39: 751-776.

Bender, D.A. and Coulson, W.F., 1972, Variations in aromatic amino acid decarboxylase activity towards dopa and 5-hydroxytryptophan caused by pH changes and denaturation. J. Neurochem. 19: 2801-2810.

Björklund, A., Ehinger, B. and Falck, B., 1968, A method for dif-ferentiating dopamine from noradrenaline in tissue sections by microspectrofluorometry. J. Histochem. Cytochem. 16: 263-270.

Brimijoin, S. and Molinoff, P.B., 1971, Effects of 6-hydroxydopamine on the activity of tyrosine hydroxylase and dopamine-β-hy-droxylase in sympathetic ganglia of the rat. J. Pharmacol. Exp. Ther. 178: 417-424.

Campbell, L.B. and Jenden, D.J., 1970, Gas chromatographic eval-ulation of the influence of oxotremorine upon the regional distribution of acetylcholine in rat brain. J. Neurochem. 17: 1697-1699.

Christenson, J.C., Dairman, W. and Udenfriend, S., 1972, On the identity of DOPA decarboxylase and 5-hydroxytryptophan de-carboxylase. Proc. Natn. Acad. Sci., U.S.A. 69: 343-347.

Coyle, J.T. and Axelrod, J., 1972a, Dopamine-β-hydroxylase in rat brain: Developmental characteristics. J. Neurochem. 19: 449-459.

Coyle, J.T. and Axelrod, J., 1972b, Tyrosine hydroxylase in rat brain: Developmental characteristics. J. Neurochem. 19: 1117-1123.

Dahlström, A., 1970, The effects of drugs on axonal transport of amine storage granules. In: New Aspects of Storage and Release Mechanisms of Catecholamines. Bayer Symposium II (H.J. Schümann and G. Kroneberg, Eds.) Springer-Verlag, Berlin, pp. 20-36.

Dairman, W., Gordon, R., Spector, S., Sjoerdsma, A. and Udenfriend, S., 1968, Increased synthesis of catecholamines in the intact rat following administration of α-adrenergic blocking agents. Molec. Pharmacol. 457-464.

Deguchi, T. and Barchas, J., 1972, Regional distribution and developmental change of tryptophan hydroxylase in rat brain. J. Neurochem. 19: 927-929.

Falck, B., Hillarp, N.-Å., Thieme, G. and Torp, A., 1962, Fluorescence of catecholamines and related compounds condensed with formaldehyde. J. Histochem. Cytochem. 10: 348-354.

Falck, B. and Owman, Ch., 1965, A detailed methodological desscription of biogenic monoamines. Acta Univ. Lund II 7: 1-23.

Freedman, D.X., Gottlieb, R. and Lovell, R.A., 1970, Psychotomimetic drugs and brain 5-hydroxytryptamine metabolism. Biochem. Pharmacol. 19: 1181-1188.

Hebb, C.O. and Krnjević, K., 1962, The physiological significance of acetylcholine. In: Neurochemistry (K.A.C. Elliott, I.H. Page and J.H. Quastel, Eds.) Charles C Thomas, Springfield pp. 452-521.

Hillarp, N.-Å., Fuxe, K. and Dahlström, A., 1966, Demonstration and mapping of central neurons containing dopamine, noradrenaline and 5-hydroxytryptamine and their reactions to psychopharmaca. Pharmacol. Rev. 18: 727-741.

Holmstedt, B. and Lundgren, G., 1966, Tremorigenic agents and brain acetylcholine. In: Mechanisms of Release of Biogenic Amines. (Euler, U.S. v., Rosell, S. and Uvnas, B., Eds.) Pergamon Press, Oxford, pp. 439-468.

Holzbauer, M. and Sharman, D.F., 1972, The distribution of catecholamines in vertebrates. In: Catecholamines (H. Blaschko and E. Muscholl, Eds.) Springer-Verlag, Berlin, pp. 110-185.

Ichiyama, A., Nakamura, S., Nishizuka, Y. and Hayaishi, O., 1970, Enzymic studies on the biosynthesis of serotonin in mammalian brain. J. Biol. Chem. 245: 1699-1709.

Kamberi, I.A., Mical, R.S. and Porter, J.C., 1971, Hypophyseal portal vessel infusion: In vivo demonstration of LRF, FRF and PIF in pituitary stalk plasma. Endocrinology 89: 1042-1046.

Kindwall, E.P. and Weiner, N., 1966, The distribution and rates of formation of catecholamines in several regions of bovine brain. J. Neurochem. 13: 1523-1531.

Koe, B.K. and Weissman, A., 1966, p-Chlorophenylalanine. A specific depletor of brain serotonin. J. Pharmacol. Exp. Ther. 154: 499-516.

Livett, B.G., 1973, Histochemical visualization of adrenergic neurones. Brit. Med. Bull. 29: 93-99.

Marchisio, P.C., 1969, Choline acetyltransferase (ChAc) activity in developing chick optic centres and the effects of monolateral removal of retina at an early embryonic state and at hatching. J. Neurochem. 16: 665-671.

Mueller, R.A., Thoenen, H. and Axelrod, J., 1969, Increase in tyrosine hydroxylase activity after reserpine administration. J. Pharmacol. Exp. Ther. 169: 74-79.

O'Keeffe, R., Sharman, D.F. and Vogt, M., 1970, Effect of drugs used in psychoses on cerebral dopamine metabolism. Brit. J. Pharmacol. 38: 287-304.

Porcher, W. and Heller, A., 1972, Regional development of catecholamine biosynthesis in rat brain. J. Neurochem. 19: 1917-1930.

Quastel, J.H., 1962, Acetylcholine distribution and synthesis in the central nervous system. In: Neurochemistry (K.A.C. Elliott, I.H. Page and J.H. Quastel, Eds.) Charles C Thomas, Springfield, pp. 431-451.

Ritchie, J.M. and Greengard, P., 1966, On the mode of action of local anesthetics. Annu. Rev. Pharmacol. 6: 405-430.

Robson, J.M. and Stacey, R.S., 1962, Recent Advances in Pharmacology, Third Ed., Little Brown & Co., Boston, pp. 1-41.

Rutledge, C.O., Azzaro, A.J. and Ziance, R.J., 1972, The role of monoamine oxidase in determining the amount of monoamines released by drugs in the central nervous system. In: Monoamine Oxidases - New Vistas. (E. Costa and M. Sandler, Eds.) Raven Press, New York, pp. 379-392.

Rutledge, C.O. and Weiner, N., 1967, The effect of reserpine upon
    the synthesis of norepinephrine in the isolated rabbit heart.
    J. Pharmacol. Exp. Ther. 157: 290-302.

Schneider, H.P.G. and McKann, S.M., 1969, Possible role of dopamine
    as transmitter to promote discharge of LH-releasing factor.
    Endocrinology, 85: 121-132.

Sims, K.L., Davis, G.A. and Bloom, F.E., 1973, Activities of
    3,4-dihydroxy-L-phenylalanine and 5-hydroxy-L-tryptophan
    decarboxylases in rat brain: Assay characteristics and
    distribution. J. Neurochem. 20: 449-464.

Tenen, S.S., 1967, The effects of p-chlorophenylalanine, a
    serotonin depletor, on avoidance acquisition, pain sensitivity
    and related behavior in the rat. Psychopharmacologia
    10: 204-219.

Ungerstedt, U., 1971, Stereotaxic mapping of the monoamine path-
    ways in the rat brain. Acta Physiol. Scand. Suppl. #367,
    1-48.

Weiner, N., 1960, Substrate specificity of brain amine oxidase of
    several mammals. Arch. Biochem. 91: 182-188.

Weiner, N., 1970, Regulation of norepinephrine biosynthesis. Annu.
    Rev. Pharmacol. 10: 273-290.

Weiner, N., 1972, Pharmacology of central nervous system stimulants,
    In: International Symposium on Drug Abuse, ed. by C.J.D.
    Zarafonetis, Lea and Febiger, Phila. pp. 243-251.

Woodbury, D.M., 1969, Mechanisms of action of anticonvulsants.
    In: Basic Mechanisms of the Epilepsies. (Jasper, H.H.,
    Ward, A.A., Jr. and Pope, A., Eds.) Little, Brown and Company,
    Boston, pp. 647-681.

UPTAKE AND STORAGE OF ^{3}H-NOREPINEPHRINE IN THE CEREBRAL HEMISPHERES

AND CEREBELLUM OF CHICKS DURING EMBRYONIC DEVELOPMENT AND EARLY

POSTHATCHING

Antonia Vernadakis

Departments of Psychiatry and Pharmacology, University of

Colorado School of Medicine, Denver, Colorado

INTRODUCTION

Intercommunication between neurons involves neurotransmitter substances which: (a) are synthesized and stored in the presynaptic neuron, (b) are released by the arrival of the impulse; and (c) act on the postsynaptic neurons. The molecular events occurring pre- synaptically, at the synaptic cleft, or on the postsynaptic membrane are among the most intensively studied subjects in neurobiology. Whereas considerable knowledge exists about the adult CNS, informa- tion concerning the differentiation of neurotransmisstion mechanisms during development has only recently begun to accumulate.

The studies reported here are concerned with the maturation of noradrenergic neurotransmission in the cerebellum and cerebral hemi- spheres of chicks from embryonic age up to 3 months after hatching. The chick embryo has been one of the most extensively used prepara- tions in the study of morphological, biochemical and functional neural maturation (Corner et al., 1967; Vos et al., 1967; Corner and Bot, 1967; Vernadakis and Burkhalter, 1965; Vernadakis and Burkhalter, 1967).

The maturational profile of endogenous norepinephrine (NE) levels was studied. Noradrenergic development was studied further by in- vestigating two processes which are involved in the storage of nore- pinephrine. Prior to storage within noradrenergic nerves, exogenous NE is taken up across the neuronal membrane and subsequently taken up across the membrane of the storage granule in which it is ulti- mately stored. In the brain of the adult rat it is possible to

133

demonstrate the neuronal uptake of NE in vitro in slices (Dengler
et al., 1962; Rutledge and Jonason, 1967; Rutledge, 1970), in isolated synaptosomes (Davis et al., 1967) and in homogenates (Snyder
and Coyle, 1969).

MATERIALS AND METHODS

Animals

All experiments were performed on chick embryos or chicks after
hatching. Fertile eggs from White Leghorn hens were incubated at
37°-38^oC. At 10, 14, 16, 18 and 20 days of embryonic age, chicks
were removed from their shell, rapidly decapitated and the cerebral
hemispheres and cerebellum quickly removed. In experiments using
chicks after hatching, the chicks were decapitated and cerebral
hemispheres and cerebellum were quickly removed. For the determination of NE levels the tissues were frozen immediately over dry ice
and stored at -20^oC until analysed; for the uptake and storage of
NE, tissue slices were prepared (approx. 0.3 mm thick) from these
brain areas by slicing free-hand, and the slices immersed in Krebs-
Henseleit solution at 4^oC.

Uptake of ^{3}H-Norepinephrine

A modification of the procedure of Snyder et al. (1968) was
followed and is described in detail elsewhere (Kellogg et al., 1971).
Tissue slices of the cerebral hemispheres or cerebellum were incubated
in a Dubnoff metabolic shaker for 10 min in 2 ml of Krebs-Henseleit
solution at 37^oC in an atmosphere of 95% O_2-5% CO_2. In some samples
cocaine (3 x $10^{-5}M$) or reserpine ($10^{-6}M$) were added to the incubation
medium prior to the 10 min incubation. Then DL-(^{3}H)NE (0.78 Ci;
specific radioactivity, 3.8 Ci/mmol) was added to a final concentration of $10^{-7}M$, and the incubation was continued for 5-20 min. A control sample in which the tissues were incubated at 0° under 95% O_2-
5% CO_2, was included with each experiment. NE was extracted by ethanol and aliquots of the medium and the extract were counted as described in detail elsewhere (Kellogg et al., 1971). Tissue to medium
ratios of tritium were calculated as the ratio of dpm/g wet tissue
to dpm/ml of medium.

Extraction of Biogenic Amines

Endogenous norepinephrine (NE) was extracted by the method of
Maickel et al. (1968) as modified in our laboratory (Vernadakis, 1973a).
Brain samples were homogenized in 10 volumes of acidified n-butanol
(to a total volume of 2.8 ml). Duplicate standards of 1 µg NE in

100 λ of 0.1 N HCl were similarly prepared. An aliquot (2.5 ml) of
the butanol was then transferred to a 13 ml glass-stoppered centri-
fuge tube containing 5 ml of n-heptane and 0.2 ml of 0.1 N HCl. After
being shaken for 5 min on a mechanical shaker, the tubes were centrifuged for 5 min at 2,000 RPM. The organic phase was removed by as-
piration and discarded. Aliquots of 0.1 ml of the acid phase were
then transferred to 12x75 mm test tubes for the determination of NE.

Norepinephrine Analysis

Norepinephrine was determined according to the method of Maickel
et al. (1968). To: a) 0.1 ml aliquot of the acid phase of both samples and standards and; b) 0.1 ml of unextracted standard (1 μg) and
to 0.1 ml of 0.1 N HCl for unextracted blanks was added 0.2 ml of
1 M sodium acetate (pH 7) containing 0.1 M disodium ethyldiamine
tetraacetate (EDTA). Then 0.1 ml of 0.1 N iodine prepared in absolute
ethanol was added. After mixing and allowing to stand for 10 min at
room temperature, 0.2 ml of a freshly prepared alkaline sulfite solution was added. One-and-one-half min later 0.2 ml of 5 N acetic acid
was added and samples and standards were boiled for 2 min in a boiling
water bath. After cooling in tap water, the fluorescence was measured
at activation and emission wavelengths of 385 nm and 485 nm respectively. Using the values for the extracted tissue standards and blanks
and unextracted standards and blanks, the percent recovery was calculated and each sample was corrected accordingly.

Butyrylcholinesterase Analysis

The activity of butyrylcholinesterase (BuChE) was determined
colorimetrically by means of a Beckman DU spectrophotometer, using
the rate of hydrolysis of butyrylthiocholine according to the method
of Ellman et al. (1961). The selective acetylcholinesterase (AChE)
inhibitor, 1,5-bis-(4-tri-methylammonium-phenyl) pentan-3-one di-
iodide (62c47) was used. At a final concentration of $2x10^{-5}M$, the
AChE inhibitor has been shown to inhibit AChE activity 100% but BuChE
activity very slightly (Bayliss and Todrick, 1956). The determination
of enzyme activity was carried out at 37°C. The final reaction mixture for determining BuChE activity consisted of 1.2 ml of pH 8.0
buffer, (0.07 M Na_2HPO_4 and 0.07 M KH_2PO_4), 0.8 homogenate (1 mg/ml),
100 μl (0.01M) dithiobisnitrobenzoid acid, 0.5 ml BuTCh iodine (0.033M)
and 0.5 ml 62c47 $(6x10^{-5}M)$.

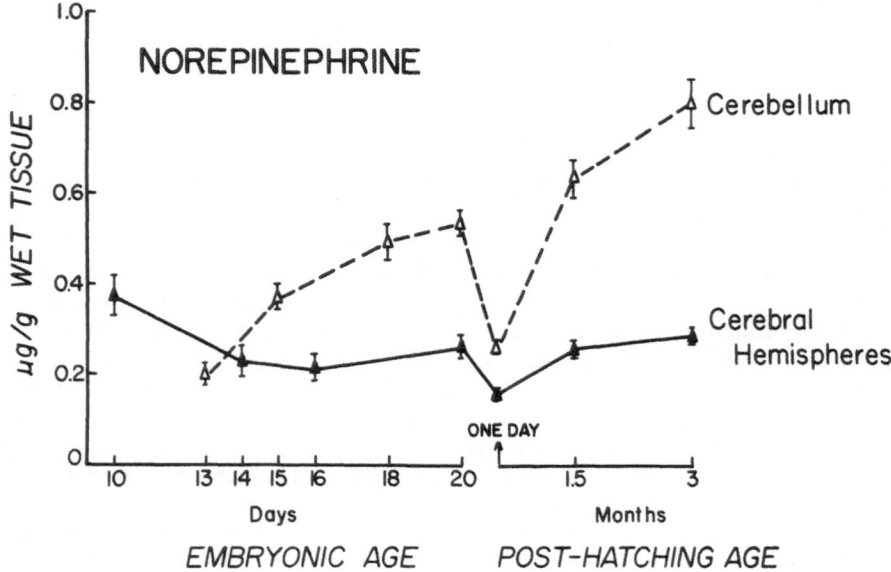

Fig. 1. Changes in endogenous norepinephrine expressed as μg per g
wet tissue in the cerebral hemispheres and cerebellum of chicks
during embryonic age and post-hatching up to 3 months. Points with
vertical lines represent mean ± S.E. for 4-8 samples.

RESULTS AND DISCUSSION

Endogenous Levels of Norepinephrine

        In the cerebral hemispheres NE content was at a high level at
10 days of embryonic age, dropped at 14 days, leveled off up to 20
days of embryonic age, dropped again at one day after hatching and
gradually increased up to 3 months (Fig. 1). In contrast to the
cerebral hemispheres, in the cerebellum NE content increased from 13
days up to 20 days of embryonic age, again NE declined at one day
after hatching and then markedly and progressively increased up to
3 months (Fig. 1).

The high levels of NE in the cerebral hemispheres and cerebellum during early embryonic development (between 10 and 14 days of embryonic age) when functional activity has not yet matured (Corner et al., 1967) is interpreted to indicate a functional role of NE other than the classical proposed neurotransmission role. Monoamines have been proposed to be involved in biochemical cellular differentiation (Renson, 1971) and the presence of high levels of NE in the cerebral hemispheres prior to electrical activity is supporting evidence for this role. Preliminary findings from this laboratory (Vernadakis and Gibson, 1973a) have shown that in neural embryonic explants cultured in the presence of either L-dopa, dopamine or NE, the activities of acetylcholinesterase, an enzyme associated with neural growth (Filogamo and Marchisio, 1971) and butyrylcholinesterase, an enzyme associated with glial cells (Giacobini, 1964), were higher than controls. Moreover, we found that ^{3}H-uridine incorporation into RNA is increased in neural embryonic explants cultured in the presence of these substances (Vernadakis and Gibson, 1973a).

The drop in NE at 1 day after hatching in both the cerebral hemispheres and cerebellum is interpreted to reflect an adaptation phenomenon occuring in several systems. For example, Dr. Waymire (this proceedings) has found the same drop in the activity of enzymes involved in catecholamine metabolism.

The increase in endogenous norepinephrine from 1 day after hatching up to 3 months (especially prominent in the cerebellum) may reflect both a continuous maturation of adrenergic neurons and the accumulation of these substances in other cells which are becoming functionally mature during this age period. It is possible, for example, that glial cells also accumulate NE. Recent studies by Fritz and Hamberger (1971) show that glial cell-enriched fractions of brain tissue accumulate NE. Glial cells markedly proliferate after 16 days of embryonic age in chicks (Hanaway, 1967). If the glial cells, for example, accumulate norepinephrine but do not metabolize it as rapidly as neurons, then an increase in levels of NE can involve extraneuronal (glial) uptake as well as increase storage capacity of neurons during maturation.

Uptake of ^{3}H-norepinephrine in Cerebral Hemispheres and Cerebellum

There was a marked increase in the rate of accumulation of ^{3}H-NE in the cerebral hemispheres from chicks 1-day after hatching in comparison to the cerebral hemispheres from 10-day-old chick embryos; also, there was a marked increase between 1 day after hatching and 3 months after hatching (Fig. 2). Incubation of the tissue slices in the presence of cocaine (3×10^{-5}M) resulted in a marked inhibition of the accumulation of ^{3}H-NE at both embryonic and post-hatching ages. When 10^{-6}M reserpine was added to the incubation media there was

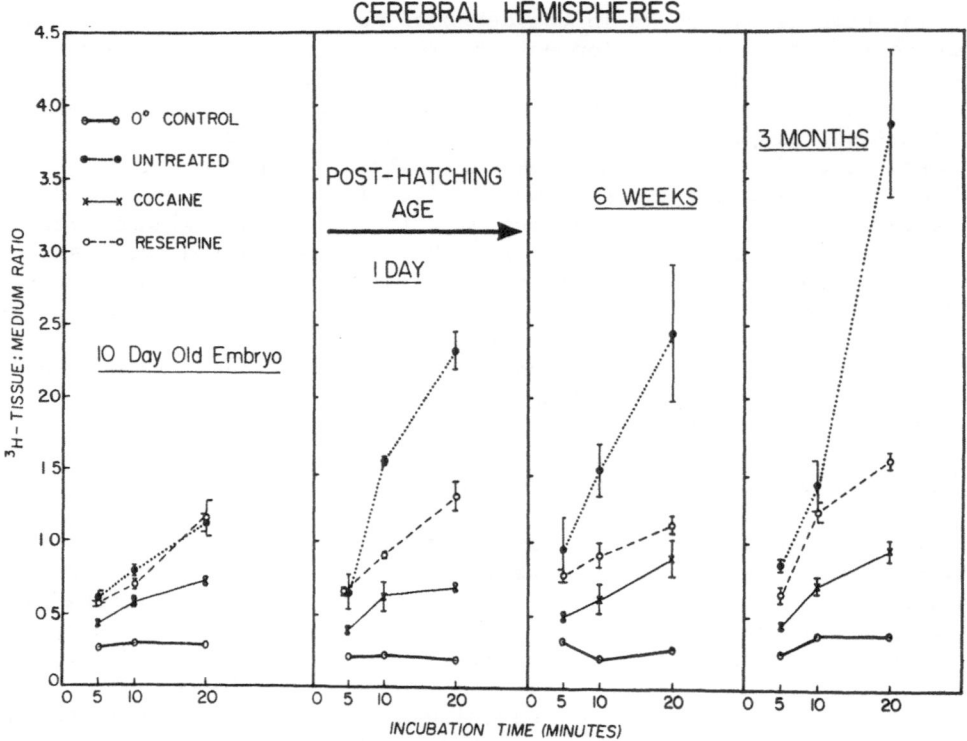

Fig. 2. Uptake of ^{3}H-NE into slices of cerebral hemispheres taken from chick embryos at 10 days of age and from chicks at 1 day, 6 weeks and 3 months after hatching. The effects of cocaine (3×10^{-5}M) and reserpine (10^{-6}M) are illustrated. Points with vertical lines represent mean ± S.E. for 5-6 determinations.

---

marked inhibition of ^{3}H-NE in the 20-day embryo, not shown in Fig. 2, (Kellogg et al., 1971) and in the chicks after hatching. In another study we (Kellogg et al., 1971) found that the inhibition by reserpine of the accumulation of ^{3}H-NE was much less prominent in tissues from 10-day-old embryos (Fig. 2). It is concluded from these data that uptake processes in the cerebral hemispheres develop earlier than the mechanisms for storage of NE.

Uptake of ^{3}H-NE by cerebellar slices occurred in chicks at 15 days of embryonic age (the earliest age tested) and reached mature levels by 20 days of embryonic age (Fig. 3). Moreover, the storage of ^{3}H-NE, as indicated by reserpine inhibition, was present in the cerebellum of chick embryos as early as 15 days of age. Thus, it appears from these data that adrenergic mechanisms reach maturation earlier in the cerebellum than in the cerebral hemispheres in chicks.

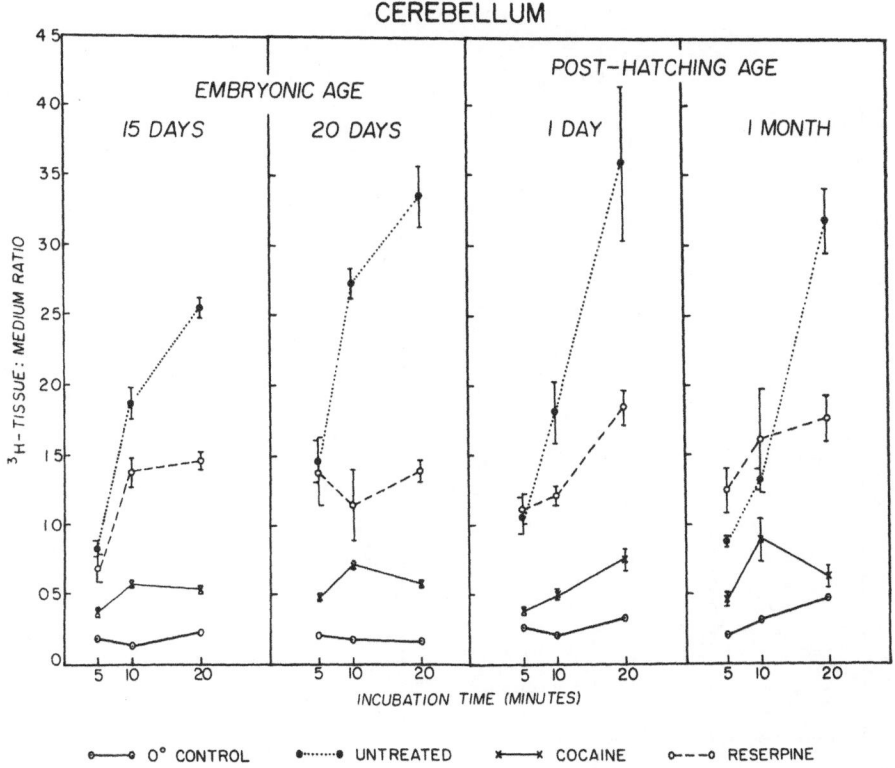

Fig. 3. Uptake of ^{3}H-NE into slices of cerebellum from chick embryos at 15 and 20 days of age and from chicks at 1 day, and 1 month after hatching. The cocaine and reserpine effects are illustrated as in Fig. 2.

To test further the development of the ability to accumulate NE in the cerebral hemispheres, two drugs, amphetamine and chlorpromazine, were used. Amphetamine has been shown to inhibit neuronal uptake of NE and also to enhance its release (Rutledge, 1970; Ziance and Rutledge, 1972); chlorpromazine has been shown to inhibit neuronal uptake of NE and also block the postsynaptic adrenergic receptor (Hornykiewicz, 1966).

Accumulation of ^{3}H-NE was inhibited by amphetamine in tissue slices from cerebral hemispheres of all chick embryos (Fig. 4). However, in the 15- and 20-day-old embryos the percent of inhibition increased as the dose of amphetamine increased, whereas in the 10-day-old, the percent of inhibition was the same with 10^{-4}M, 10^{-5}M, or 10^{-6}M amphetamine. In view of the fact that amphetamine also enhances the release of NE (Rutledge, 1970; Ziance and Rutledge, 1972)

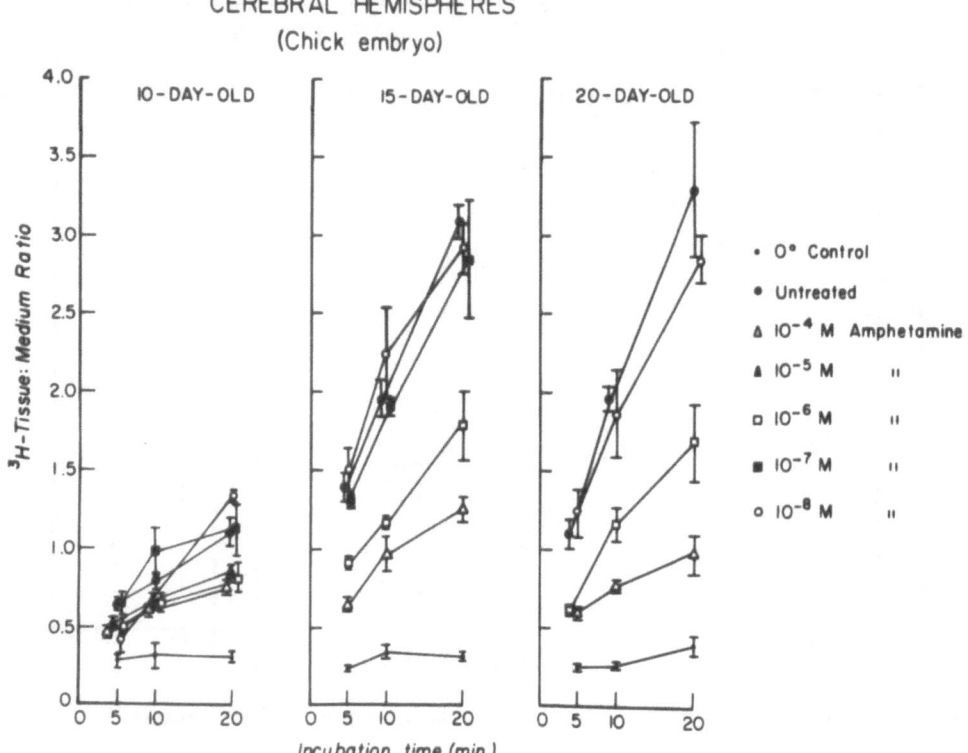

Fig. 4. Effects of amphetamine on the uptake of ^{3}H-NE into slices of cerebral hemispheres taken from chick embryos at 10, 15 and 20 days of age. Points as in Fig. 2.

---

the present findings may also reflect amphetamine release of NE. The ontogenesis of the release process of NE as yet has not been investigated.

Chlorpromazine at 10^{-3}M markedly inhibited the accumulation of ^{3}H-NE in the cerebral hemispheres of 15-day-old chick embryos, but 10^{-7}M did not. In the 20-day-old chlorpromazine at 10^{-3}M and 10^{-5}M inhibited accumulation of ^{3}H-NE, but 10^{-7}M did not (Fig. 5). These data indicate that the uptake processes, although present in the cerebral hemispheres of 10-day-old chick embryos, are at a very early stage of maturation.

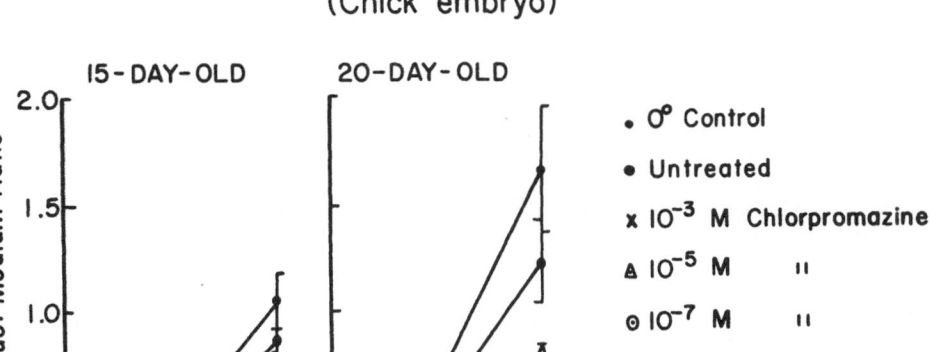

Fig. 5. Effects of chlorpromazine on the uptake of ^{3}H-NE into slices
of cerebral hemispheres taken from chick embryos at 10 and 15 days
of age. Points as in Fig. 2.

Role of Glial Cells in Neurotransmission

The continuous increase in the accumulation of ^{3}H-NE in the
cerebral hemispheres in chicks up to 3 months after hatching (Fig. 2)
together with the increase in endogenous NE (Fig. 1) are consistent
with the speculation that NE may be present in glial cells known to
proliferate during brain maturation (Vernadakis, 1973b), as well as
neurons.

In an attempt to correlate changes in the uptake of NE in brain
tissue with glial proliferation during maturation, changes in butyrylcholinesterase (BuChE) activity was studied in the cerebral hemispheres and cerebellum of chick embryos and chicks up to 3 months
after hatching. Butyrylcholinesterase is predominantly localized in
glial cells, as shown by early studies of Giacobini (1964). We
(Vernadakis and Gibson, 1973b) also have found that the activity of
BuChE in glial fractions obtained from cerebral hemispheres of chicks

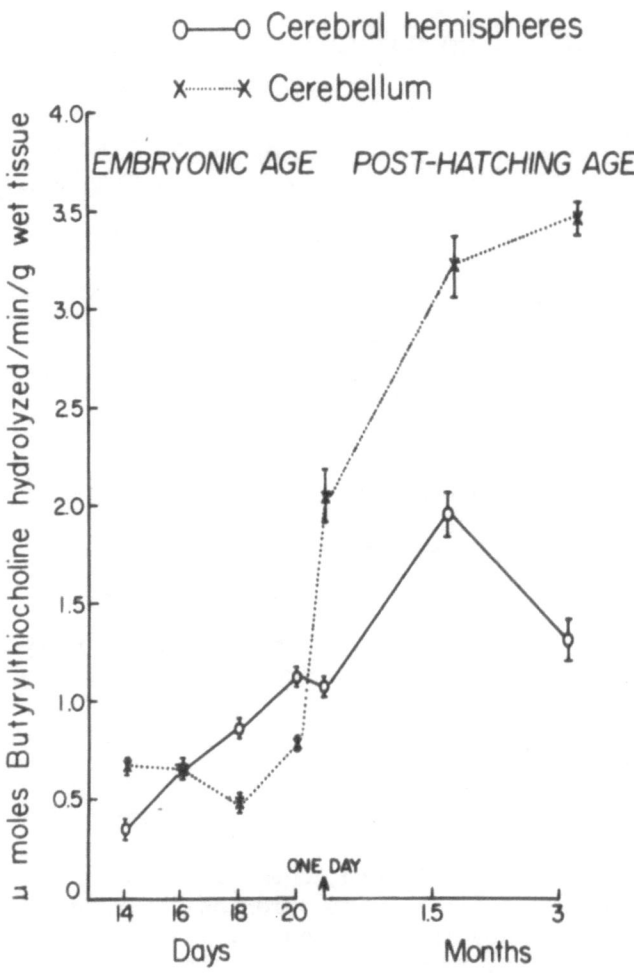

Fig. 6.   Changes in the activity of butyrylcholinesterase expressed
as μmoles of butyrylthiocholine hydrolysed per min per g wet tissue
in the cerebral hemispheres and cerebellum of chicks during embryonic
age and posthatching up to 3 months.   Points as in Fig. 1.

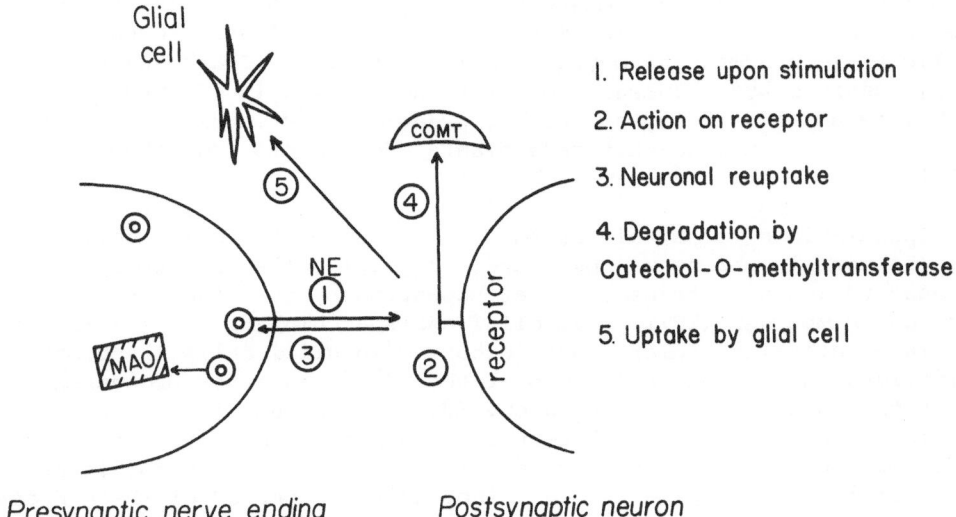

Fig. 7. A diagramatic representation of the fate of norepinephrine
in the central nervous system (see text for details).

at early posthatching is double that found in the neuronal fractions.

There is a marked increase in the activity of BuChE in both the
cerebral hemispheres and cerebellum between 20 days of embryonic age
and 1 day to 6 weeks after hatching (Fig. 6). This increase in BuChE
activity correlates with the marked proliferation of glial cells
during this age period (Hanaway, 1967). That this increase could
also represent an increase in the specific activity of the enzyme in
the glial cells cannot be excluded.

The role of glial cells in neurotransmission mechanisms is specu-
lative at present. The fate of NE in the CNS and the proposed role
of glial cells in NE metabolism is illustrated in Fig. 7. When NE
is released upon stimulation (Step 1 in Fig. 7), NE acts on the postsynaptic receptor (Step 2); NE may be inactivated by the reuptake
process (Step 3); NE may be degraded by catechol-O-methyltransferase
(Step 4); the proposal is put forward here that NE also may be taken
up by the glial cells (Step 5). Evidence supporting Step 5 may be

summarized as follows: extraneuronal uptake (Uptake$_2$) occurs in peripheral tissues (Iversen, 1971); glial cell-enriched brain fractions accumulate NE (Fritz and Hamberger, 1971); and NE stimulates a number of substances in glial cells, i.e., adenosine 3',5'-monophosphate (cyclic AMP) in human astrocytoma cells in culture (Clark and Perkins, 1971), lactic dehydrogenase in C-6 rat tumor cells in culture (De Vellis et al., 1971), and BuChE, predominantly localized in glial cells, in neural tissue culture explants (Vernadakis and Gibson, 1973a).

Speculations for a role of norepinephrine in the glial cells are: (1) norepinephrine may be stored in glial cells and subsequently released to act as a transmitter as supported by the findings of Fritz and Hamberger (1971) that glial cells accumulate NE; (2) NE may stimulate several cellular events occuring in glial cells which may be involved in the general growth of the CNS or in other processes. Recent findings from this laboratory (Vernadakis and Gibson, 1973a) have shown that NE increases ^{3}H-uridine incorporation into RNA in neural explants removed from 20-day-old chick embryos but not in explants from earlier age embryos. Since this age period of chick brain development is characterized by active proliferation of glial cells, we suggest that the increased ^{3}H-uridine incorporation by NE represents primarily glial cell RNA; (3) finally, glial cells may act as a safety valve to limit high extracellular concentrations of NE that may occur under stressful conditions.

Glial cells may act to modulate the level of brain excitability. For example, it is known that cortisol increases brain excitability (Vernadakis and Woodbury, 1971a, 1971b). The effect may be mediated via the action of cortisol on accumulation of NE in glial cells. Preliminary studies from this laboratory (unpublished) have shown that cortisol inhibits the uptake of norepinephrine in neural explants removed from 16-day-old chick embryos and maintained in culture. We speculate that cortisol may affect extraneuronal uptake (glial cells) of NE since it occurs only with high concentration of NE in the incubation medium. As shown by Iversen (1971), extraneuronal uptake in the peripheral nervous system occurs with high concentrations of NE, and Iversen and Salt (1970) have reported that cortisol inhibits extraneuronal uptake in the rat heart. Inhibition of NE uptake by cortisol in glial cells would result in high concentration of NE in the synaptic cleft available to act on the postsynaptic receptor with subsequent enhanced effect. Although these findings are preliminary, they support the view that glial cells play an important role in the regulation of CNS activity.

CONCLUSIONS

Endogenous levels of NE are very high in both the cerebral hemispheres and cerebellum of chicks at early embryonic age. This high level of brain NE, when functional (electrical) activity has not yet developed, suggests that this neuro humor substance has other cellular functions than neurotransmission during early brain maturation.

In the cerebral hemispheres, mechanisms for the cellular uptake of NE develop before mechanisms for intraneuronal storage of NE. This can be discerned from the fact that cocaine inhibits accumulation of ^{3}H-NE as early as 10 days, whereas reserpine inhibits storage primarily after 20 days of embryonic age. In contrast to the cerebral hemispheres, in the cerebellum the mechanisms of both uptake and storage of NE appear to reach maturation by 20 days of embryonic age.

The continued increase in accumulation of NE in the cerebral hemispheres of chicks up to 3 months after hatching may be a consequence of the continued growth and maturation of noradrenergic neurons and/or the enhanced uptake activity of glial cells known to actively proliferate during this age period. Evidence suggests that glial cells accumulate NE and it is speculated that glial cells act as regulators of the concentration of NE at the synapse and thus ultimately play an active role in neurotransmission.

ACKNOWLEDGMENTS

This work was supported by U.S. Public Health Service research grant NS-09199, University of Colorado General Research Support GRS 388, 421, 11 and a Research Scientist Development Award KO2 MH-49479 from the National Institute of Mental Health.

REFERENCES

Bayliss, B.J., and Todrick, A., 1956, The use of a selective acetylcholinesterase inhibitor in the estimation of pseudocholinesterase activity in rat brain, Biochem. J. 62: 62.

Clark, R.B. and Perkins, J.P., 1971, Regulation of adenosine 3':5'-cyclic monophosphate concentration in cultured human astrocytoma cells by catecholamines and histamine, Proc. Nat. Acad. Sci. 68: 2757.

Corner, M.A. and Bot, A.P.C., 1967, Developmental patterns in the central nervous system of birds. II. Somatic motility during the embryonic period and its relation to behavior after hatching, Progr. Brain Res. 26: 214.

Corner, M.A., Schadé, J.P., Sedláček, J., Stoeckart, R., and Bot,
    A.P.C., 1967, Developmental patterns in the central nervous
    system of birds. I. Electrical activity in the cerebral
    hemisphere, optic lobe and cerebellum, Progr. Brain Res. 26:
    145.

Davis, J.M., Goodwin, F.K., Bunney, W.E., Murphy, D.L., and Colburn,
    R.W., 1967, Effects of ions in uptake of norepinephrine by
    synaptosomes, Pharmacologist 9: 184.

Dengler, J.J., Michaelson, I.A., Spiegal, H.E. and Titus, E., 1962,
    The uptake of labelled norepinephrine by isolated brain and
    other tissues of the cat, Int. J. Neuropharmacol. 1: 23.

De Vellis, J., Inglish, D., and Galey, F., 1971, Effects of cortisol
    and epinephrine on glial cells in culture, in: "Cellular
    Aspects of Neural Growth and Differentiation", (D. Pease, ed.)
    UCLA Forum in Medical Sciences, University of California Press.

Ellman, G.L., Courtney, K.D., Andres, V., and Featherstone, R.M., 1961,
    A new and rapid colorimetric determination of acetylcholinester-
    ase activity, Biochem. Pharmacology 7: 88.

Filogamo, G. and Marchisio, P.C., 1971, Acetylcholine system and
    neural development, Neurosciences 4: 29.

Fritz, A.H. and Hamburger, A., 1971, Glial cell function: Uptake of
    transmitter substances, Proc. Nat. Acad. Sci. 68: 2686.

Giacobini, E., 1964, Metabolic relations between glia and neurons
    studied in single cells, in: "Morphological and Biochemical
    Correlates of Neural Activity," (Cohen and Snider, eds.),
    Hoeber, New York.

Hanaway, J., 1967, Formation and differentiation of the external
    granular layer of the thick cerebellum, J. Comp. Neurol. 131:1.

Hornykiewicz, O., 1966, Dopamine (3-hydroxytryptamine) and brain
    function, Pharmacol. Rev. 18: 925.

Iversen, L.L., 1971, Role of transmitter uptake mechanisms in synap-
    tic neurotransmission, Br. J. Pharmacol. 41: 571.

Iversen, L.L. and Salt, P.J., 1970, Inhibition of catecholamine
    Uptake$_2$ by steroids in the isolated rat heart, Br. J. Pharma-
    col. 40: 528.

Kellogg, C., Vernadakis, A. and Rutledge, C.O., 1971, Uptake and
    metabolism of ^{3}H-norepinephrine in the cerebral hemispheres
    of chick embryos, J. Neurochem. 18: 1931.

Maickel, R.P., Cox, R.H., Jr., Sailant, J. and Miller, F.P., 1968,
    A method for the determination of serotonin and norepinephrine
    in discrete areas of rat brain, Int. J. Neuropharmacol. 7: 275.

Renson, J., 1971, Development of monaminergic transmission in the
    rat brain in "Chemistry and Brain Development", (Paoletti
    and Davison, eds.), Plenum Press, New York.

Rutledge, C.O., 1970, The mechanisms by which amphetamine inhibits
    oxidative deamination of norepinephrine in brain, J. Pharmacol.
    Exp. Ther. 171: 188.

Rutledge, C.O. and Jonason, J., 1967, Metabolic pathways of dopa-
    mine and norepinephrine in rabbit brain in vitro, J. Pharmacol.
    Exp. Ther. 157: 493.

Snyder, S.H. and Coyle, J.T., 1969, Regional differences in ^{3}H-
    norepinephrine and ^{3}H-dopamine uptake into rat brain homogen-
    ates, J. Pharmacol. Exp. Ther. 165: 78.

Snyder, S.H., Green, A.I. and Hendley, E.D., 1968, Kinetics of ^{3}H-
    norepinephrine accumulation into slices from different regions
    of rat brain, J. Pharmacol. Exp. Ther. 164: 90.

Vernadakis, A., 1973a, Comparative studies of neurotransmitter sub-
    stances in the maturing and aging central nervous system of
    the chicken, in "Neurobiological Aspects of Maturation and
    Aging," (Ford, ed.), Elsevier, Amsterdam, in press.

Vernadakis, A., 1973b, Changes in nucleic acid content and butyryl-
    cholinesterase activity in CNS structures during the life-span
    of the chicken, J. Gerontology: 28: 281.

Vernadakis, A. and Burkhalter, A., 1965, Convulsive responses in
    developing chickens, Proc. Soc. Exper. Biol. & Med. 119: 512.

Vernadakis, A. and Burkhalter, B., 1967, Acetylcholinesterase
    activity in optic lobes of chicks at hatching, Nature 214: 594.

Vernadakis, A. and Gibson, D.A., 1973a, Role of neurotransmitter sub-
    stances in neural growth, in "Conference on The Problems and
    Priorities in Perinatal Pharmacology" sponsored by National
    Institute of Child Health, April 12-14, 1973, Raven Press, in
    press.

Vernadakis, A. and Gibson, D.A., 1973b, Chemical properties of
    neuronal and glial fractions isolated from chicks early post-
    hatching. Abstract of paper presented at the 4th Inter.
    Meeting of the Inter. Soc. for Neurochemistry, Aug. 26-31,
    1973, Tokyo, Japan.

Vernadakis, A. and Woodbury, D.M., 1971a, Influence of cortisol on
    brain and spinal cord excitability in developing rats, in
    "Steroid Hormones and Brain Function", (Sawyer and Gorski, eds.)
    UCLA Forum in Medical Sciences, University of California Press.

Vernadakis, A. and Woodbury, D.M., 1971b, Effects of cortisol on
    maturation of the central nervous system, in "Influence of
    Hormones on the Nervous System", (Ford, ed.), Proc. Intern.
    Soc. of Psychoneuroendocrinology, S. Karger, Basel, New York.

Vos, J., Schadé, J.P., and Van Der Helm, 1967, Developmental patterns
    in the central nervous system of birds. II. Some biochemical
    parameters of embryonic and post-embryonic maturation, Progr.
    Brain Res. 26: 193.

Ziance, R.H. and Rutledge, C.O., 1972, A comparison of the effects
    of fenfluramine and amphetamine on uptake, release and cata-
    bolism of norepinephrine in brain, J. Pharmacol. Exp. Ther.
    180: 118.

STUDIES ON THE DEVELOPMENT OF TYROSINE HYDROXYLASE, MONOAMINE

OXIDASE AND AROMATIC-L-AMINO ACID DECARBOXYLASE IN SEVERAL REGIONS

OF THE CHICK BRAIN

J. C. Waymire*, A. Vernadakis and N. Weiner

Departments of Pharmacology and Psychiatry, University

of Colorado School of Medicine, Denver, Colorado

INTRODUCTION

Noradrenergic and dopaminergic neurons are present in the central nervous system and their distribution has been mapped out in considerable detail in rat brain by histochemical fluorescence procedures (Hillarp et al, 1966; Ungerstedt, 1971). Norepinephrine neurons arise in the medulla oblongata and pons and either descend into the spinal cord to terminate in the ventral horn or ascend in the median forebrain bundle to terminate in the lower brain stem, mesencephalon and diencephalon. A second major norepinephrine pathway arises in the locus coeruleus. Some of the axons from this nucleus descend to innervate lower brain stem nuclei. Others either proceed laterally to terminate on the purkinje cells of the cerebellum, or ascend via the median forebrain bundle to terminate in such diverse regions as the hypothalamus, hippocampus, thalamus and cerebral cortex (Ungerstedt, 1971).

The major dopaminergic pathway in the central nervous system arises in the pars compacta of the substantia nigra and terminates in the neostriatum. This nigrostriatal pathway is involved in extrapyramidal motor function. Destruction of this system is as-sociated with the development of the parkinsonian syndrome. Other dopamine neurons arise in the interpeduncular nucleus and terminate in the accumbens nucleus, the olfactory tubercle and the amygdalus. Dopamine neurons which are involved in the release of hypothalamic releasing factors arise in the median eminence and terminate in the hypothalamus. A small group of dopamine containing neurons also is present in the retina (Ungerstedt, 1971).

---

* Present address: Department of Psychobiology, University of California, Irvine, California.

In recent years, considerable effort has been directed toward understanding the mechanisms for the regulation of the level and activity of the enzymes involved in catecholamine synthesis, most notably tyrosine hydroxylase (Weiner, 1970; Molinoff and Axelrod, 1971). Because of the difficulty of analyzing phenomena which occur in a tissue as heterogeneous and complex as the brain, most investigations of regulation of biosynthesis, metabolism and maintenance of tissue levels of catecholamines have been conducted either with preparations containing peripheral adrenergic neurons or with the adrenal medulla. Unfortunately, although many of the studies in these peripheral systems have led to results that suggest mechanisms of regulation of catecholamine synthesis, several of these results are not quantitatively reproducible in catecholamine systems of the central nervous system. Treatments such as parenteral L-dopa administration (Dairman and Udenfriend, 1972), and reserpine depletion of catecholamine stores, (Mueller et al, 1969), are associated with dramatic changes in levels of tyrosine hydroxylase in peripheral adrenergic neurons. However, prolonged depletion of catecholamines with reserpine is associated with only a modest increase in the level of this enzyme in the central nervous system (Segal et al, 1971). It may be that the regulatory mechanisms for controlling the level of tyrosine hydroxylase in the central nervous system are not identical to those in the periphery. Problems such as the complexity of the CNS, the determination of the electrical activity of the neurons under study, and the existence of the blood-brain barrier make interpretation of experiments on the brain difficult.

An approach we have taken to study the regulatory neurochemistry of tyrosine hydroxylase and other adrenergic enzymes in the central nervous system is to examine these processes in the developing organism (Waymire et al, 1972a). This approach has the possible advantage that these enzymes are undergoing change during this period and this may provide a more sensitive model for determining whether any predictable process, such as substrate induction or end-product feedback inhibition of enzyme synthesis, is operating.

The chick embryo brain appears to be an excellent preparation for such developmental studies. A considerable amount of information is available concerning many aspects of development in this organism. The preparation is especially suitable for examining the effects of chemicals in the environment of the organism, since, in the embryonic stages, the chick embryo is enclosed in its shell and the egg represents virtually a closed system which is easily entered without destroying the organism. Since the blood-brain barrier does not develop until several weeks after hatch, drug studies can be carried out in the developing chick more easily than in other organisms (Lajtha, 1957).

In employing the developing organism as an experimental model for the study of tyrosine hydroxylase regulation, we have attempted first to examine the course of development of the biochemical machinery (enzymes) necessary for the disposition of catecholamines. By coupling these studies with the determination of the changes in the level of the various substrates and end products of catecholamine biosynthesis in several brain regions, we are attempting to determine the factors which may trigger the development of these enzymes. Ignarro and Shideman (1968) have shown, for example, that the appearance of each enzyme necessary for catecholamine synthesis in the embryonic chick heart is directly preceded by the appearance of its respective substrate. In studies of the serotonin synthesizing pathway in chick brain, Eiduson has found evidence that the activity of the rate limiting enzyme in this pathway, tryptophan hydroxylase, may be depressed by experimentally increasing serotonin levels (Eiduson, 1966). Since the regulatory studies must be preceded by a thorough analysis of the normal developmental pattern for the catecholaminergic enzymes under investigation, much of our efforts thus far have been directed to defining these developmental changes.

The maturation of catecholamine neurons in rat brain has been examined in detail by Coyle and Axelrod who measured the development of neuronal uptake of norepinephrine (1971) and the development of the enzymes tyrosine hydroxylase (1972b) and dopamine-β-hydroxylase (1972a). They observed that these three indices of noradrenergic neuron development increased in a coordinated fashion from the fifteenth day of gestation to adult life. Regions which contained noradrenergic and dopaminergic cell bodies (pons-medulla and midbrain-hypothalamus) acquired tyrosine hydroxylase levels at earlier stages of development than did regions in which nerve terminals of these systems predominate (striatum, cortex and cerebellum)(Coyle and Axelrod, 1972b). Over 90% of the total dopamine-β-hydroxylase and tyrosine hydroxylase activities and of the uptake and storage capability of the rat brain developed after birth (Coyle and Axelrod, 1972b).

Kellogg et al (1971) examined the uptake of ^{3}H-norepinephrine into chick brain slices at different stages of development and observed that, whereas the uptake capability of the 20-day old chick brain approximated that of the brain from the adult hen, the storage capability of the brain continues to develop after birth. Although the methods employed by Kellogg et al (1971) and Coyle and Axelrod (1971) differed somewhat, and therefore make comparisons difficult, it would appear that the norepinephrine uptake mechanisms develop more slowly in rat brain than in the chick brain.

We have initiated a study of the development of several enzymes related to catecholamine metabolism in the developing

chick brain in order to determine the mechanisms which trigger
and determine the rate and sequence of maturation of the
catecholamine biosynthetic and degradative enzymes. In these
studies, the development of tyrosine hydroxylase, aromatic-L-amino
acid decarboxylase and monoamine oxidase have been examined in
several regions of the chick brain at different stages of
maturation.

METHODS

General Procedure

Eggs from white leghorn chickens were incubated at 37-38° C.
After 10, 14, 16, 17, 18, 20, and 21 days of incubation, chick
embryos were separated from the egg and decapitated. One- and
three-day old chicks (post-hatch) were also studied. The brains
were quickly removed, divided into optic lobes, cerebral hemispheres, cerebellum and diencephalon-midbrain, and homogenized
in four volumes of 100 mM imidazole HCl buffer at pH 7.0.

Assay of Tyrosine Hydroxylase

The recently developed procedure of Waymire et al (1971) was
used for the assay of tyrosine hydroxylase. This procedure
involves the recovery and assay of $^{14}CO_2$ after quantitative
decarboxylation with hog kidney aromatic-L-amino acid decarboxylase of carboxyl labeled dopa formed from carboxyl labeled
tyrosine. A 200 µl incubation included 40 µmole sodium acetate
pH 6.1, 0.2 µmole ferrous sulfate, 0.4 µmole 2-amino-4-hydroxy-6,
7-dimethyl-5,6,7,8-tetrahydropteridine hydrochloride (DMPH$_4$),
10 µmole mercaptoethanol, 20 nmole 1-^{14}C-L-tyrosine (10 mCi/mmol)
and 10 units hog kidney aromatic-L-amino acid decarboxylase
containing 5 nmole pyridoxal phosphate. After 20 min incubation
at 37° C the reactions are stopped by the injection of 200 µl
10% trichloroacetic acid (TCA). A plastic well (Kontes Glass
Company) containing 200 µl NCS solubilizer is used to trap $^{14}CO_2$.
The radioactivity is counted in toluene scintillation fluid
containing 0.5 gm 1,4-bis [2(4-methyl-5-phenyloxazolyl)] benzene
(dimethyl POPOP) and 4.0 g 2,5-diphenyloxazole (PPO) per liter.

Assay of Aromatic-L-Amino Acid Decarboxylase

Enzyme activity was determined by measurement of the rate of
$^{14}CO_2$ evolution from carboxyl labeled L-dihydroxyphenylalanine
(L-dopa). The assay contained in 200 µl: 20 nmole imidazole-HCl
buffer, pH 7.0, 2 nmole pyridoxal phosphate and 50 µl enzyme preparation. The contents were incubated 5 min at 37° C, after which
400 nmole 1-^{14}C-L-dopa (0.25 µCi/mmole) was added to begin the re-

action. Tubes are capped and 200 µl NCS solubilizer contained in
a Kontes plastic well is used to trap $^{14}CO_2$. Reactions are stopped
with 200 µl 10% TCA after a 10 min incubation. Radioactivity was
counted as described above.

Assay of Monoamine Oxidase

Monoamine oxidase activity was measured by toluene extraction
of ^{14}C-indole acetic acid formed from ^{14}C-tryptamine. Purified
aldehyde dehydrogenase was included in the incubation to convert
all the indole aldehyde to acid since the aldehydes are known to
extract poorly into toluene and often adhere to protein, resulting
in variable extraction. The assay contained in 200 µl: 20 mmole
phosphate buffer, pH 7.4, 200 nmole nicotinamide adenine dinucleo-
tide, purified beef liver aldehyde dehydrogenase, 100 nmole
^{14}C-tryptamine (0.4 µCi/mmole) and 100 µl enzyme preparation. Contents are incubated 10 min at 37° C, the reaction is stopped with
the addition of 100 µl 16% perchloric acid, and ^{3}H-indole acetic acid
(8.8×10^5 DPM) is added to determine recovery. Protein is removed by centrifugation and the labeled indole acetic acid is extracted with 3 ml toluene. Tubes are immersed in dry ice-acetone
to freeze out dissolved water and the toluene is decanted into a
scintillation vial containing 7 ml of a concentrated toluene
scintillation fluid (4.0 g PPO and 0.5 g dimethyl POPOP dissolved
in 700 ml toluene. ^{3}H- and ^{14}C-5-hydroxyindole acetic acid radioactivity is counted and the results are corrected for incomplete
recovery of the ^{3}H-indole acetic acid.

Norepinephrine was extracted and determined by the method of
Maickel et al (1968);(Vernadakis, this Symposium). DNA was extracted and analyzed according to Geel and Timiras (1967).

RESULTS

Tyrosine Hydroxylase

Tyrosine hydroxylase activity could not be demonstrated in
the optic lobes, cerebral hemispheres, cerebellum and diencephalon-
midbrain at 10 days of embryonic age (Figures 1-4). The enzyme
was detectable in all areas studied by day 14. A large increase
in activity takes place in all areas between days 16 and 18. The
rise in enzyme level is greatest in the cerebellum, optic lobes
and cerebral hemispheres (over 3-fold). The diencephalon-midbrain
region, which exhibits the highest enzyme level, increases more
slowly during this early period, but continues to rise until the
day of hatching (day 21). The activity in the optic lobes and
cerebellum does not increase further between day 18 and hatching.
In contrast, tyrosine hydroxylase activity in the cerebral
hemispheres rises continuously from the 16th to the 20th day of

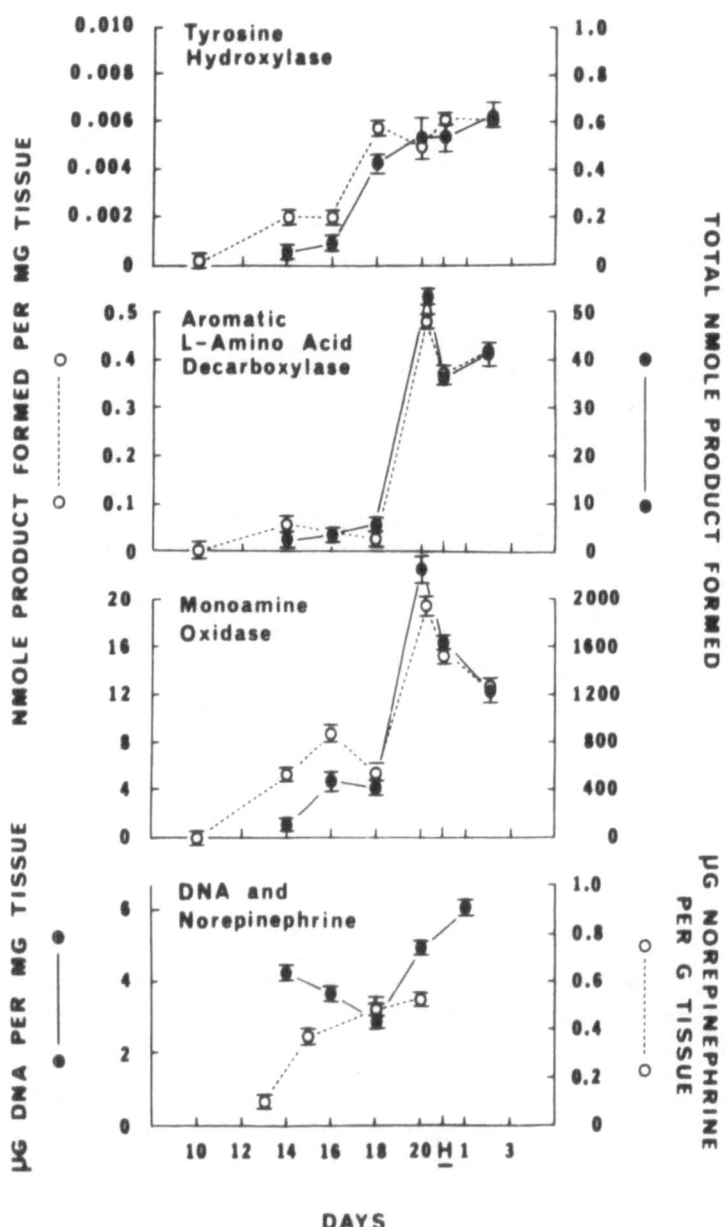

Fig. 1.   Development of tyrosine hydroxylase, aromatic-L-amino acid decarboxylase, monoamine oxidase, norepinephrine and DNA in the cerebellum.

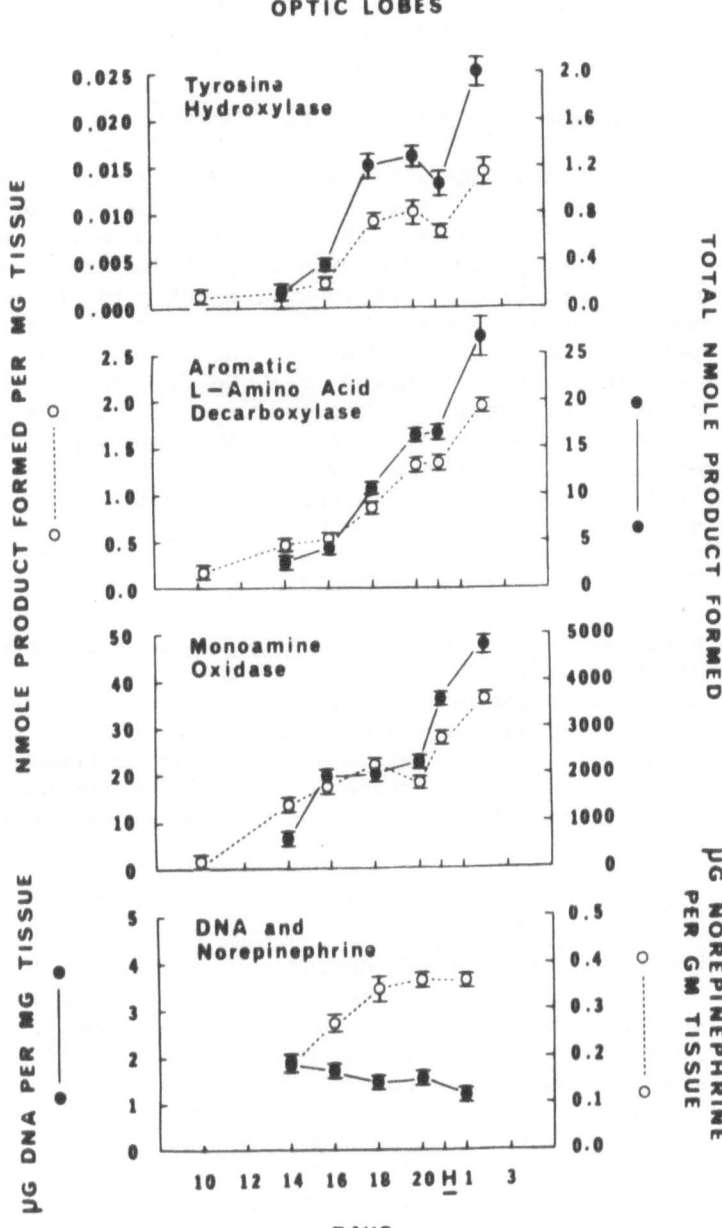

Fig. 2. Development of tyrosine hydroxylase, aromatic-L-amino acid decarboxylase, monoamine oxidase, norepinephrine, and DNA in the optic lobes.

incubation. The rate of increase in the cerebral hemispheres is
greatest between days 16 to 18 and immediately prior to hatch. In
the diencephalon-midbrain and in the optic lobes, tyrosine hydroxylase levels continue to increase during the three days post-
hatch.

Aromatic-L-Amino Acid Decarboxylase

Aromatic amino acid decarboxylase activity was detectable in
all areas studied at day 14 (Figures 1-4). The cerebellum exhibited
little enzyme activity until day 20, just prior to hatch, when the
level rose approximately 10-fold. The activity in the cerebellum
decreased slightly at birth. Decarboxylase activity in the
cerebral hemispheres and optic lobes increased steadily throughout
the development of the embryo and during the early post-hatch
period. A 4-fold increase occurred over the five day period prior
to hatch in both brain regions. The increase in decarboxylase
activity was more gradual in the diencephalon-midbrain with the most
rapid increase occurring between days 18 to 21. The level of the
enzyme did not increase further in this region during the immediate post-hatch period.

Monoamine Oxidase

Monoamine oxidase activity was measurable in all brain regions
at day 14 (Figures 1-4). The activity of the enzyme in the cerebral
hemispheres and diencephalon-midbrain rose steadily between day 14
of incubation and 2 days post-hatch. The increase in activity of
monoamine oxidase in the cerebellum and optic lobes appeared to be
biphasic with the greatest increases occurring between days 14 and
16 and in the period just prior to (cerebellum) or at (optic lobes)
hatching.

DNA Changes

The changes in level of DNA during day 16 through 20 were
similar in the cerebral hemispheres and cerebellum. In these
regions a decrease in the level of DNA per gram tissue was observed
at day 18, which is probably due to increases in cell size and
proliferation of neuronal processes. The levels rise above that
seen prior to day 18 in both tissues on day 20, apparently re-
flecting a spurt of glial cell proliferation.

DNA levels in the optic lobe do not change or decrease slightly
during the period measured. This may reflect a balance between cell
division and cell growth. In the diencephalon-midbrain region, DNA
content per gram tissue rises slightly between days 16 and 20.

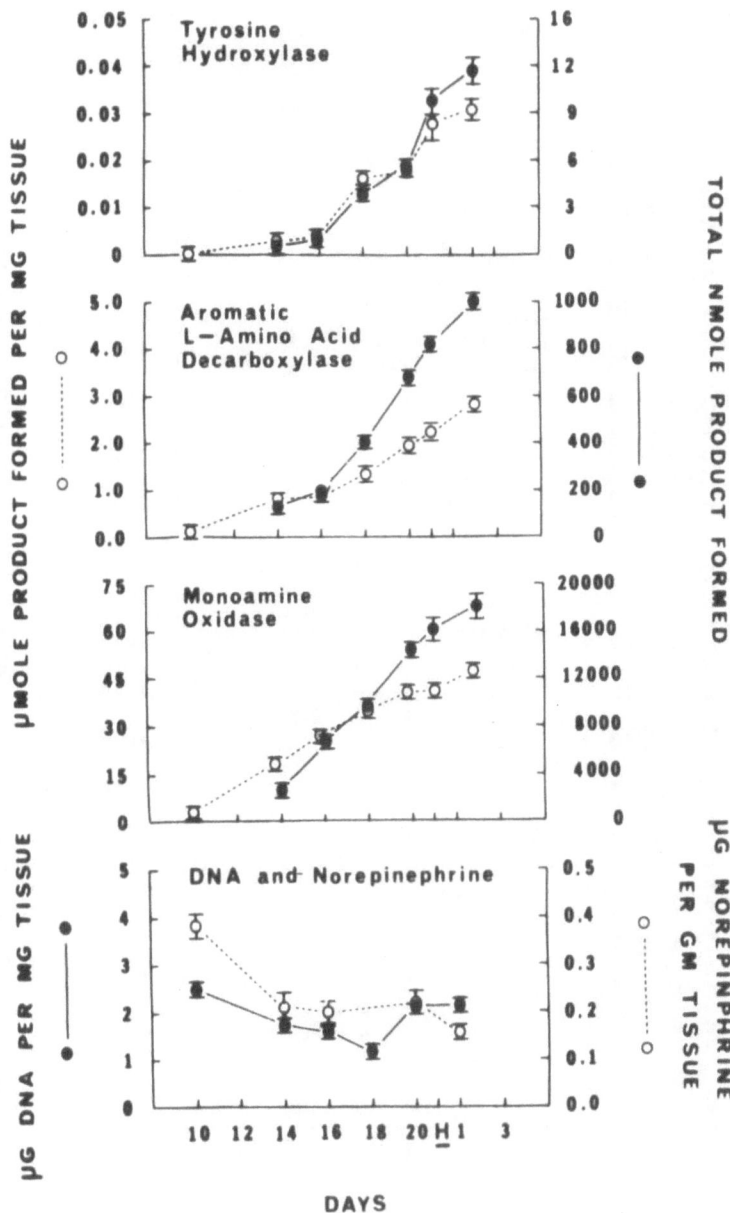

Fig. 3. Development of tyrosine hydroxylase, aromatic-L-amino acid decarboxylase, monoamine oxidase, norepinephrine, and DNA in the cerebral hemispheres.

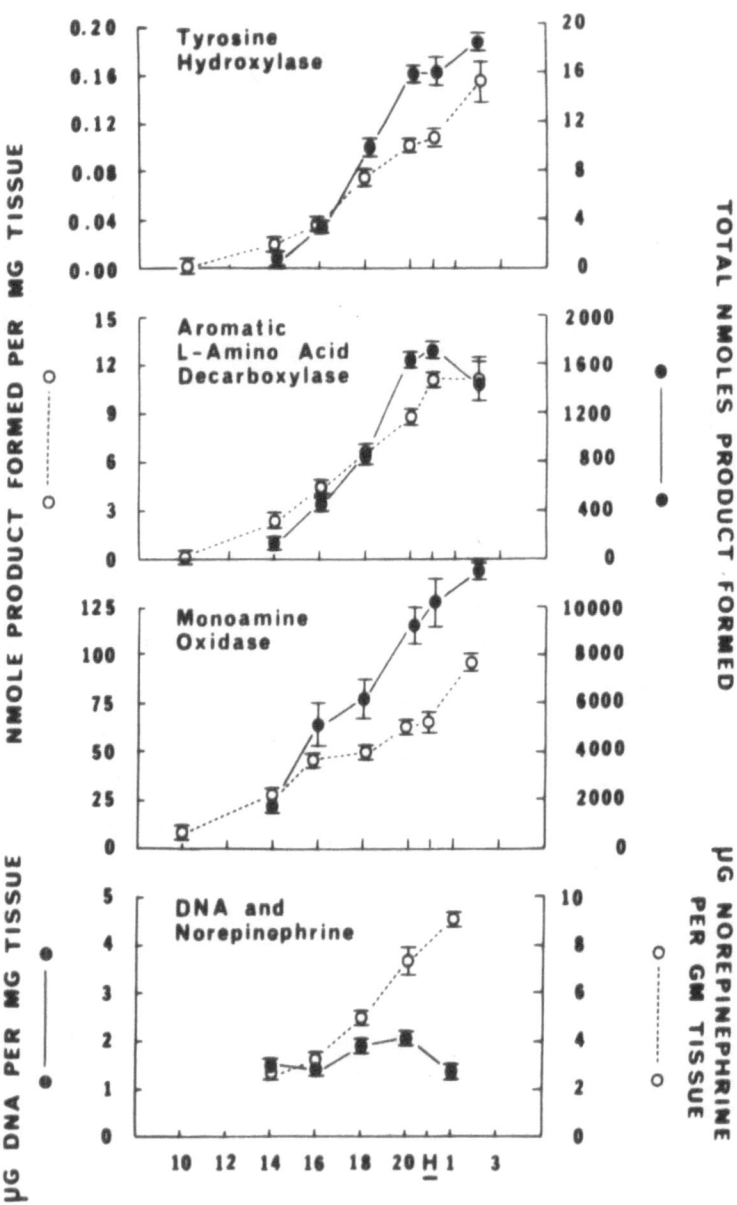

Fig. 4. Development of tyrosine hydroxylase, aromatic-L-amino acid
decarboxylase, monoamine oxidase, norepinephrine, and DNA in the
diencephalon-midbrain.

Norepinephrine Levels

Norepinephrine levels in the diencephalon-midbrain increase steadily from day 14 to one day post-hatch. An increase in levels of catecholamine is also observed between days 14 and 18 in the cerebellum and optic lobes. In contrast norepinephrine levels are highest in the cerebral hemisphere at day 10 and decline about 40% by day 14. Thereafter, the level of norepinephrine in the cerebral hemispheres of the embryo remains fairly steady. A slight further decline is apparent one day post-hatch.

Effect of Dibutyryl Cyclic AMP and Phosphodiesterase Inhibitors on Tyrosine Hydroxylase Levels in Chick Brain

Dibutyryl cyclic AMP, 0.05 and 0.1 mmoles per kg egg, was injected into the air sac of the eggs on days 10, 12 and 14 of incubation. The chick embryo brains were analyzed for tyrosine hydroxylase activity on day 16. No change in tyrosine hydroxylase levels in any region of the chick brain was demonstrable (Table 1). These experiments were repeated by injecting the cyclic AMP on day 8 and analyzing the enzyme in 10- and 12-day old chick brains. Similar negative results were obtained.

In an analogous series of experiments, papaverine or theophylline, 0.1 and 0.5 mmoles per kg egg, were injected into eggs on days 10 and 12 and the chick brains were removed for tyrosine hydroxylase assay on day 16. Again, no effect of these treatments on tyrosine hydroxylase levels in any region of the chick brain was observed (Table 2). Higher doses of these substances were lethal to the eggs and could not be employed.

Effect of Dopa, Catecholamines and Pargyline on Chick Brain Tyrosine Hydroxylase, Aromatic-L-Amino Acid Decarboxylase and Norepinephrine

Pargyline, 0.5 mg; L-dopa, 1.2 mg; dopamine, 1.2 mg; or L-norepinephrine, 1.7 mg; was injected into eggs at days 12, 14 and 16 of incubation, and the chick brains were assayed at 18 days of incubation for norepinephrine, tyrosine hydroxylase and aromatic-L-amino acid decarboxylase. None of these treatments had any effect on the development of the two enzymes involved in catecholamine biosynthesis. However, since none of these treatment affected the brain norepinephrine content, no firm conclusions regarding end-product regulation of the development of these enzymes can be drawn (Table 3).

TABLE 1

TYROSINE HYDROXYLASE ACTIVITY
IN FOUR AREAS OF CHICK BRAIN ON
DAY 16 AFTER TREATMENT WITH
DIBUTYRYL cAMP ON DAY 10, 12 AND 14

Brain Areas

Treatment	Cerebellum	Optic Lobes	Cerebral Hemispheres	Diencephalon- Midbrain
Control (vehicle)	1.48 ± .16[a]	2.80 ± .40	4.46 ± .65	29.79 ± 6.0
DBcAMP (0.1 mM)	1.45 ± .17	2.79 ± .39	4.45 ± .14	32.12 ± 5.9
DBcAMP (0.05 mM)	1.50 ± .18	2.81 ± .41	4.47 ± .59	34.00 ± 5.8

[a] nmole $^{14}CO_2$ formed per gram per hour ± S.E.

n = 5

TABLE 2

TYROSINE HYDROXYLASE ACTIVITY IN
FOUR AREAS OF CHICK BRAIN ON DAY
16 AFTER TREATMENT WITH PHOSPHODIESTERASE INHIBITORS
ON DAY 10 AND 12

Treatment	Brain Areas			
	Cerebellum	Optic Lobes	Cerebral Hemispheres	Diencephalon-Midbrain
Control (vehicle)	$1.44 \pm .20^a$	$2.78 \pm .40$	$4.45 \pm .88$	32.0 ± 7.9
Papaverine (0.1 mM)	$1.38 \pm .28$	$2.69 \pm .36$	$4.32 \pm .72$	29.8 ± 5.4
Papaverine (0.5 mM)	$1.52 \pm .25$	$2.53 \pm .51$	$4.81 \pm .58$	32.2 ± 3.8
Theophylline (0.1 mM)	$1.32 \pm .17$	$2.81 \pm .42$	$4.29 \pm .69$	31.8 ± 5.4
Theophylline (0.5 mM)	$1.41 \pm .19$	$2.62 \pm .48$	$4.29 \pm .59$	28.8 ± 8.1

[a] nmole $^{14}CO_2$ formed per gram per hour ± S.E.

n = 5

TABLE 3

TYROSINE HYDROXYLASE (TH) ACTIVITY, AROMATIC-L-AMINO ACID
DECARBOXYLASE (AADC) ACTIVITY AND NOREPINEPHRINE LEVEL IN
18 DAY EMBRYONIC CHICK BRAIN AFTER DRUG TREATMENTS
ON DAY 12, 14, AND 16

Treatments	TH[a] Activity	AADC[a] Activity	Norepinephrine[b]
Control (vehicle)	74.4 ± 5.1	6914. ± 281.	.28 ± .04
L-DOPA (1.2 mg)	76.3 ± 3.7	6713. ± 274.	.27 ± .02
Dopamine (1.2 mg)	79.4 ± 2.1	6873. ± 314.	.25 ± .03
Norepinephrine (1.7 mg)	78.9 ± 4.0	5819. ± 292.	.26 ± .03
Pargyline (0.5 mg)	79.4 ± 4.8	6433. ± 314.	.27 ± .03

[a] nmole $^{14}CO_2$ formed per gram per hour ± S.E.

[b] µg/gram ± S.E.

Effect of 3-Hydroxy-4-bromobenzyloxyamine Phosphate (NSD-1055)
and Reserpine on Chick Brain Tyrosine Hydroxylase,
Aromatic-L-Amino Acid Decarboxylase and Norepinephrine

Reserpine, 10 µg, or NSD-1055, 1.5 mg, was injected into one-
day old chick eggs and the brains were removed at day 18 of incubation and assayed for tyrosine hydroxylase, aromatic-L-amino acid
decarboxylase and norepinephrine. Reserpine did not affect the
development of the catecholamine biosynthetic enzymes, and NSD-1055
did not influence the level of tyrosine hydroxylase at day 18.
Aromatic amino acid decarboxylase was lower after NSD-1055, but this
may be due to persistence of the inhibitor in the egg. Only the
administration of reserpine was associated with a significant
reduction in brain norepinephrine at day 18 of incubation (Table 4).

DISCUSSION

Development of Tyrosine Hydroxylase, Aromatic Amino Acid
Decarboxylase and Monoamine Oxidase in Chick Brain

The levels of tyrosine hydroxylase, aromatic amino acid decarboxylase and monoamine oxidase all increase during the development of the chick brain although the pattern of development of each
of these enzymes appears to be distinct in the several brain regions
examined. With the exception of the cerebral hemispheres, there is
a rough correlation in each brain region between the development
of the biosynthetic enzymes and the levels of norepinephrine.
Highest levels of both norepinephrine and tyrosine hydroxylase are
found in the diencephalon-midbrain just prior to hatch. However,
cerebral hemispheres, which exhibit considerable tyrosine hydroxylase activity, contain the lowest concentration of norepinephrine
during the later stages of embryonic development. It is possible
that the turnover of norepinephrine in this region, which contains
predominantly nerve terminals, is higher than in the other regions
examined, and that the steady-state level of the amine is therefore
low.

For all areas of the brain examined, the most rapid rate of
tyrosine hydroxylase increase occurs between the 16th and 18th day
of embryonic age. The only region of the chick brain in which
tyrosine hydroxylase does not exhibit a sustained increase in
activity after this time is in the optic lobes. Here the rate of
increase in enzyme activity decreases shortly prior to hatch and
there is an absolute decline in activity at hatch. Between hatch
and three days post-hatch, the activity in the optic lobes almost
doubles. The rise in tyrosine hydroxylase post-hatch suggests
that the adrenergic neurons in the optic lobes might be influenced
by the changes in the environment consequent to hatch. The afferent visual stimulation associated with hatching may result in
increased input into the optic lobes which may be responsible for
the abrupt rise in tyrosine hydroxylase levels in this region of

TABLE 4

TYROSINE HYDROXYLASE ACTIVITY, AROMATIC-L-AMINO ACID
DECARBOXYLASE ACTIVITY AND NOREPINEPHRINE LEVEL IN 18 DAY
WHOLE CHICK BRAIN TREATED ON DAY ONE WITH RESERPINE OR NSD-1055

Treatment	Tyrosine[a] Hydroxylase	Aromatic Amino Acid[a] Decarboxylase	Norepinephrine[b]
Control	75.4 ± 3.8	6124. ± 274.	.22 ± .04
Reserpine (10 µg)	76.4 ± 3.9	6437. ± 248.	.01 ± .005
NSD-1055 (1.5 mg)	74.4 ± 4.0	1042. ± 100.	.23 ± .05

a nmole $^{14}CO_2$ formed per gram per hour ± S.E.

b µg/gram ± S.E.

the brain after hatch. To evaluate this, we initiated experiments where we attempted to hatch the chickens in the dark to determine whether exposure to light at hatch time had any influence on the post-hatch tyrosine hydroxylase levels. Hatching in the dark did not depress the increases in tyrosine hydroxylase at this period. We plan to evaluate this possibility further by deafferentation of the optic lobes to see if this has any effect on enzyme development, since the spontaneous firing in the dark of the receptors in the eye may be sufficient to produce the effect observed. Norepinephrine levels in this region do not reflect the changes in enzymes up to hatch date.

With the exception of the cerebellum, the development of aromatic-L-amino acid decarboxylase occurs at approximately the same time as does that of tyrosine hydroxylase. In cerebellum, decarboxylase activity increases most rapidly at the period of time directly before hatch. In both the cerebellum and the diencephalon-midbrain, the activity abruptly levels off after hatch. Since the measured level of this enzyme probably reflects enzyme from serotoninergic as well as adrenergic cells, the significance of these findings is difficult to interpret. Measurement of the levels of the adrenergic intermediates should help in the analysis of these changes.

Interpretation of changes in DNA levels in various areas of the brain gives some means of evaluating whether the changes in enzyme and amine levels are due to the maturation of cells, in which case DNA concentration should decline or remain unchanged. Conversely, if the changes in levels are due to an increase in cell number, the DNA level would be expected to increase. The difficulty in interpreting such results lies in the fact that the regions being studied are heterogeneous and the changes in DNA levels may not reflect accurately changes in the number of catecholamine containing neurons. With this reservation in mind, the following generalizations in the four brain areas studied may be made. Tyrosine hydroxylase undergoes the greatest rate of increase in all areas studied, except the diencephalon, during a period when DNA levels are falling. This may represent the invasion and development of nerve endings in these areas. This inverse relationship is not so apparent with aromatic-L-amino acid decarboxylase, perhaps because this enzyme is more ubiquitous than is tyrosine hydroxylase, being present in both adrenergic and serotoninergic cells and perhaps in other cells as well. Similarly, changes in monoamine oxidase levels cannot be correlated with changes in DNA levels, since this enzyme undergoes a steady increase throughout the maturation period studied. As noted above, because a number of other types of neurons are developing during the maturation period, it is difficult to evaluate definitively these correlations.

The level of the three enzymes at the time of hatching is
very nearly that which is found in the mature chicken. This is in
sharp contrast to the development of these enzymes in the rat brain
reported by Coyle and Axelrod (1972a,b) who observed that tyrosine
hydroxylase levels increased about 3-fold between birth and the
adult stage. These differences in development might be expected
in view of the fact that chicks are much more mature at time of
hatch than are rats at birth.

Analysis of the time course of the appearance and levels of
each of the enzymes studied reveals that the phenomenon that
Ignarro and Shideman observed in the developing chick heart; that
is, the sequential appearance of each of the catecholamine precursors or intermediates and their respective enzymes, may be
occurring only in the case of the cerebellum. In this region,
tyrosine hydroxylase appears first, slightly before the development of aromatic-L-amino acid decarboxylase. A complication to an
analysis of this kind of study in the brain is that serotoninergic
neurons also contain both aromatic-L-amino acid decarboxylase and
monoamine oxidase. Perhaps the decarboxylase and monoamine
oxidase associated with these neurons develop at a time which differs from the development of catecholamine neurons. For this
reason the levels of the catecholamine intermediates must be
determined before one can critically evaluate the theory of sequential substrate induction of enzymes. These studies have not
yet been completed. Conclusions about the existence of substrate
induction of the enzymes in the biosynthetic pathway for catecholamines awaits this further information. Our studies in which
norepinephrine or its precursors, or pargyline, a monoamine
oxidase inhibitor, were injected into eggs in order to determine
their effect on the development of the catecholamine biosynthetic
enzymes were inconclusive, since no changes in the levels of brain
catecholamines were produced (Table 3).

Influence of Drugs on the Development of Adrenergic Enzymes

A second approach to the study of the regulation of enzymes
concerned in the synthesis and degradation of catecholamines is to
study the level of these enzymes in developing chicks after alterations have been made in either substrates or products of the
biosynthetic sequence. These alterations can be produced by the
administration of these substances (vide supra) or by the use of
drugs known to alter the levels of these substances in the chick
brain.

Reserpine, a drug known to deplete granular catecholamine
stores in both peripheral and central adrenergic neurons in adult
animals is effective as a depletor of norepinephrine levels in the
developing chick embryo (Table 4). In spite of the alteration in

norepinephrine content, there is no change in tyrosine hydroxylase
levels. This is in contrast to the reported increase in tyrosine
hydroxylase levels after reserpine treatment in peripheral neurons
(Mueller et al, 1969). In the study summarized in Table 3, 10 μg
of reserpine was injected into the yolk sac at day one of incubation.
Norepinephrine levels were still totally depleted by 18 days of
embryonic age, but no change in tyrosine hydroxylase was apparent.
These results are in contrast to those of Lydiard and Sparber
(1972) who have found that a similar treatment prior to incubation is associated with a significant increase in tyrosine
hydroxylase levels in the brains of 15 and 20 day old chick
embryos.

Another means by which norepinephrine levels may be lowered is
to block its synthesis at one of the biosynthetic steps. We
selected for this study the decarboxylase inhibitor, 3-hydroxy-4-
bromobenzyloxyamine phosphate (NSD-1055). However, this drug apparently was not effective in blocking totally the decarboxylase,
since norepinephrine levels were unaffected by the drug. Higher,
or more frequent doses of NSD-1055 were also not effective in
lowering norepinephrine levels so that no conclusion could be
drawn from this study.

Cyclic AMP and Tyrosine Hydroxylase

Evidence is accumulating in support of the concept that
cyclic 3',5'-adenosine monophosphate (cAMP) may be involved in
some way in the regulation of tyrosine hydroxylase levels. The
dibutyryl derivative of cAMP has been found to restore tyrosine
hydroxylase levels in the adrenal medullae of animals in which a
decrease has been produced by hypophysectomy (Kvetnansky et al,
1971). Studies with neuroblastoma cells grown in culture have
demonstrated that cAMP analogs such as dibutyryl- or 8-methylthio-
cAMP or phosphodiesterase inhibitors will markedly increase
tyrosine hydroxylase activity in three days in cells that have
progressively lost the enzyme over a course of previous cultur-
ing (Waymire et al, 1972b).

Attempts to elevate tyrosine hydroxylase in the brains of
adult rats with treatment of cAMP analogs or phosphodiesterase inhibitors have been unsuccessful. The treatments have therefore
been applied to the study of tyrosine hydroxylase in developing
chick embryonic brains. There appears to be no effect of either
dibutyryl cyclic AMP or the phosphodiesterase inhibitors on the
level of tyrosine hydroxylase. Treatment of embryos on days 10,
12, and 14, times immediately prior to the anticipated natural increases in tyrosine hydroxylase in chick brain, did not reveal any
alteration in the rate of increase of tyrosine hydroxylase levels
(Tables 1 and 2). Doses of these drugs higher than those reported

could not be used since they were lethal to the embryos. In other experiments the drugs were given either earlier (day 8) or for longer periods of time (until day 16) with no detectable change in tyrosine hydroxylase levels. These results suggest that tyrosine hydroxylase levels in the developing CNS may not be regulated by a mechanism related to cAMP. The possibility that the levels of tyrosine hydroxylase in the adult chick may not be influenced by cAMP must also be considered.

In conclusion, we have presented a description of the development of three of the enzymes participating in catecholamine metabolism but have not as yet been able to elucidate any controlling mechanism acting during this developmental period. It is possible that hormones such as glucocorticoids or growth hormone or other neurotransmitters, such as acetylcholine, may act in some way to modulate increases in these catecholamine synthesizing and catabolizing enzymes; or that perhaps nerve growth factor or other peptides may influence this development. Alternatively, it may well be that the information necessary for development of biosynthetic systems is preprogrammed into the cell and that it is difficult to change this developmental pattern.

ACKNOWLEDGMENTS

This work was supported by the U.S. Public Health Service research grants NS-07642, NS-09199, NS-07927 and a Research Scientist Development Award K02 MH-49479 from the National Institute of Mental Health to Dr. A. Vernadakis.

REFERENCES

Coyle, J.T. and Axelrod, J., 1971, Development of the uptake and storage of L-[^{3}H]norepinephrine in the rat brain. J. Neurochem. 18: 2061-2075.

Coyle, J.T. and Axelrod, J., 1972a, Dopamine-β-hydroxylase in rat brain: Developmental characteristics. J. Neurochem. 19: 449-459.

Coyle, J.T. and Axelrod, J., 1972b, Tyrosine hydroxylase in rat brain: Developmental characteristics. J. Neurochem. 19: 1117-1123.

Dairman, W. and Udenfriend, S., 1972, Studies on the mechanism of the L-3,4-dihydroxyphenylalanine-induced decrease in tyrosine hydroxylase activity. Molec. Pharmacol. 8: 293-299.

Eiduson, S., 1966, 5-Hydroxytryptamine in the developing rat brain: its normal and altered development and possible control by end-product repression. J. Neurochem. 13: 923-932.

Geel, S. and Timiras, P.S., 1967, The influence of neonatal hypothyroidism and of thyroxine on the ribonucleic acid and deoxyribonucleic acid concentrations of rat cerebral cortex. Brain Res. 4: 135-142.

Kvetnansky, R., Gewirtz, G.P., Weise, V.K. and Kopin, I.J., 1971, Effect of dibutyryl cyclic-AMP on adrenal catecholamine synthesizing enzymes in repeatedly immobilized hypophysectomized rats. Endocrinology 89: 50-55.

Hillarp, N.-Å., Fuxe, K. and Dahlström, A., 1966, Demonstration and mapping of central neurons containing dopamine, noradrenaline and 5-hydroxytryptamine and their reactions to psychopharmaca. Pharmacol. Rev. 18: 727-741.

Ignarro, L.J. and Shideman, F.E., 1968, Appearance and concentrations of catecholamines and their biosynthesis in the embryonic and developing chick. J. Pharmacol. Exp. Ther. 159: 38-48.

Kellogg, C., Vernadakis, A., and Rutledge, C.O., 1971, Uptake and metabolism of [^{3}H]norepinephrine in the cerebral hemispheres of chick embryo. J. Neurochem. 18: 1931-1938.

Lajtha, A., 1957, Development of the blood-brain barrier. J. Neurochem. 1: 216-227.

Lydiard, R.B. and Sparber, S.B., 1972, Possible induction of tyrosine hydroxylase in chick embryo brain from reserpine administration prior to incubation. Fifth International Congress on Pharmacology, p. 144 (Abstract 861).

Maickel,R.P., Cox, R.H., Jr., Saillant, J. and Miller, F.P., 1968, A method for the determination of serotonin and norepinephrine in discrete areas of rat brain. Int. J. Neuropharm. 7: 275-281.

Molinoff, P.B. and Axelrod, J., 1971, Biochemistry of catecholamines. Annu. Rev. Biochem. 40: 465-500.

Mueller, R.A., Thoenen, H. and Axelrod, J., 1969, Increase in tyrosine hydroxylase activity after reserpine administration. J. Pharmacol. Exp. Ther. 169: 74-79.

Segal, D.S., Sullivan, J.L. III, Kuczenski, R.T. and Mandell, A.J., 1971, Effect of long-term reserpine treatment on brain tyrosine hydroxylase and behavioral activity. Science 173: 847-849.

Ungerstedt, U., 1971, Stereotaxic mapping of the monoamine pathways in the rat brain. Acta Physiol. Scand. Suppl. #367, 1-48.

Vernadakis, A., Uptake and storage of ^{3}H-norepineprine in the cerebral hemispheres and cerebellum of chicks during embryonic development and early posthatching. (This Symposium).

Waymire, J.C., Bjur, R. and Weiner, N., 1971, Assay of tyrosine hydroxylase by coupled decarboxylation of dopa formed from 1-^{14}C-L-tyrosine. Anal. Biochem. 43: 588-600.

Waymire, J.C., Vernadakis, A. and Weiner, N., 1972a, Maturation of monoamine oxidase, aromatic-L-amino acid decarboxylase, and tyrosine hydroxylase in four CNS areas in chick embryos. Fed. Proc. 31: 920 Abs.

Waymire, J.C., Weiner, N. and Prasad, K., 1972b, Regulation of tyrosine hydroxylase activity in cultured mouse neuroblastoma cells: Elevation induced by analogs of adenosine 3',5'-cyclic monophosphate. Proc. Natn. Acad. Sci., U.S.A., 69: 2241-2245.

Weiner, N., 1970. Regulation of norepinephrine biosynthesis. Annu. Rev. Pharmacol. 10: 273-290.

PRENATAL EXPOSURE TO DRUGS: EFFECT ON THE DEVELOPMENT OF BRAIN MONOAMINE SYSTEMS

Velayudhan Nair

Department of Pharmacology, The Chicago Medical School

University of Health Sciences, Chicago, Illinois

Numerous clinical and experimental studies of recent years (Millen and Woollam, 1963; Brill and Forgotson, 1964; Medearis, 1964; Peckham and King, 1963; Nora et al., 1967; Bleyer et al., 1970) have indicated that exposure to a wide variety of agents (radiation, drugs, viruses, etc.) during specific stages of pregnancy can result in various morphologic and behavioral anomalies in the offspring. Much of the previous work in this area has been concerned with teratologic effects. Equally important and yet, relatively less understood are the subtler molecular effects. Unlike the gross abnormalities and malformations, these are not readily evident and may be revealed only by specific tests or when challenged by environmental stresses. The molecular or biochemical lesion may remain dormant and manifest it-self later in life as a functional impairment, behavioral disorder or abnormal reaction to drugs. Presently, we have little information about these events and there are few systematic studies directed towards the sequelae. In a sense, these are more insidious than the teratologic effects because the latter are evident early enough for appropriate corrective measures to be taken.

With these considerations in mind, we have initiated a systematic multispecies investigation on the effects of maternal exposure to drugs in pregnancy on the biochemical and functional development of the offspring. We began these studies in rats and are extending them now in rabbits.

There are two major facets to our study. One is that which per-tains to the practical aspects, i.e., the identification of the varied effects of prenatal drug exposure. Second, and perhaps more important in our view, is that dealing with the basic and fundamental aspects of biochemical differentiation. By this we mean the process by which the various organs acquire their characteristic - qualitative and quantitative - pattern of enzyme systems in the course of prenatal and early postnatal development. During this period, the various biochemical systems appear in a definite and orderly sequence. The fundamental process underlying this phenomenon is that of gene expression.

Can we induce or evoke the premature formation of an enzyme? What are the factors, physiologic or other, which regulate their orderly appearance? Are there critical periods when these systems are extremely vulnerable, i.e., when exposure to drugs or chemicals, etc. could permanently influence their development? Some partial answers to these questions have become available with respect to liver, in the recent studies of Greengard and others (1969). But we know very little with respect to brain.

In the present investigation, we have studied both brain and liver, but this report describes our findings in brain. Specifically, our objective was: 1) to elucidate the normal developmental pattern of the brain monoamine systems 5-hydroxytryptamine (5HT) and norepinephrine (NE) in control rats; 2) to study the influence of prenatal exposure to drugs on the development of these amine systems; 3) to identify the critical periods, if any, in development when the amine systems are vulnerable to environmental influences; and 4) to study the relationship between the brain amine changes and functional and behavioral alteration.

The drugs studied include: chlorpromazine (CPZ), lysergic acid diethylamide (LSD), dextroamphetamine (DA), imipramine (IMP), Δ^9-tetrahydrocannabinol (THC).

The above mentioned amine systems were selected because there is evidence from other studies, totally unrelated to the present topic, implicating 5HT and NE in behavioral and mental disorders (Sjoerdsma et al., 1970; Schildkraut and Kety, 1967). Page (1968) has listed 18 conditions in which serotonin may be involved. It was felt that if a positive effect on any of the amine systems was identified, then this would provide another experimental model to study the correlation between brain biochemistry and function.

In this report is described: 1) the normal development pattern of brain 5HT and NE systems in rats and rabbits; 2) the effect of prenatal chlorpromazine, LSD, dextroamphetamine, imipramine, and THC on the development of the brain amine systems in rats; 3) response of the drug exposed offspring to certain behavioral and functional tests; and 4) the factors underlying the suppression of brain 5HT.

RAT STUDIES

Materials and Methods

The subjects for this study were Sprague-Dawley rats. They were housed under controlled environmental conditions (temperature, 70°F, light 5AM to 7PM, relative humidity 50%). Food and water were given ad libitum. Female rats in estrus were housed overnight with males (2:1) and the following morning, vaginal smears were taken and examined. If the smears were positive for sperm, that day was taken as day 1 of pregnancy. The animals were divided into different groups and each group received the drug (CPZ or LSD)* daily for the selected period of gestation as follows: 1) days 1-4; 2) days 5-8; 3) days 9-12; 4) days 13-15; 5) days 16-17; 6) days 18-21; and 7) days 1-21. Controls received the vehicle. After drug treatment, the animals were allowed to deliver and raise their offspring. The offspring were examined daily from day of birth until weaning for gross malformations and they were also weighed periodically during this time. They were weaned at 21 days of age and separated according to sex. At 1, 20, 40 and 80 days of age, 6-8 animals from each group were sacrificed by decapitation, brain and liver were removed rapidly, blotted free of blood and tissue fluids and weighed. They were then frozen on a bed of dry ice and stored frozen at -20°C until ready for the assay.

Drugs

All drugs were administered subcutaneously. Chlorpromazine (Thorazine, 25 mg/cc) was given at two dose levels (10 and 30 mg/kg); LSD (Delysid, supplied by the National Institute of Mental Health, Batch No. 88601) at dosages of 1, 10, 100 and 1000 µg/kg; and dextroamphetamine at 1 mg/kg; Imipramine at 10 mg/kg and Δ^9-THC (in tween 80) at 10 mg/kg dosages. Control animals received the respective vehicles.

---

*For DA, IMP, and THC, this report describes only the results of drug exposure during gestation days 18-21.

Brain 5HT and NE

      Brain was homogenized in 4 volumes of 0.01N HCl using a teflon-
glass homogenizer. 5HT and NE were determined in the same sample
according to the method of Mead and Finger (1961). From the sodium
chloride saturated homogenate, 5HT was extracted into n-butanol and
then heptane and finally into 0.01N HCl. Concentrated HCl was added
to the acid extract and the fluorescence measured in an Aminco-Bowman
spectrophotofluorometer; activation at 295 nm and fluorescence read
at 545 nm. The spectrophotofluorometer was fitted with a Kodak pola-
screen polarizing filter in number 4 slit position. Norepinephrine
was determined in an aliquot of the acid (0.01N) extract after oxidation with potassium ferricyanide in phosphate buffer (pH 6.3).
Freshly prepared alkaline ascorbate solution was then added and the
fluorescence of the solution measured; activation at 408 nm and fluorescence read at 508 nm.

5-Hydroxyindoleacetic Acid (5HIAA)

      5HIAA, the oxidative metabolite of 5HT was determined in the
same sample of brain tissue as used for 5HT and NE, according to a
modification of the method of Miller et al., (1970).

Statistical Analysis

      Analysis of variance procedures were used to evaluate the sig-
nificance of differences.

                         Results and Discussion

                      Gross and Biochemical Effects

Chlorpromazine

      Gross Effects. There were no significant differences between
the control and the drug (10 mg/kg body weight) treated groups with
respect to the duration of pregnancy and litter size (Table I). There
was an increased incidence of infant deaths (within the first three
weeks of life) in the offspring of groups receiveing drug on gestation days 1-4, 9-12, or 18-21 (P<0.01).

      Body Weight. A significant supression of the normal development-
al increase in body weight was noted in all the drug exposed groups,
this effect being maximal in those receiving drug during the last
few days of gestation (18-21) or throughout pregnancy (Fig. 1).

TABLE I

GROSS EFFECTS OF PRENATAL CHLORPROMAZINE IN RATS

	Control	Days of Drug Treatment[a]								All Time Periods
		1-4	5-8	9-12	13-15	15	16-17	18-21	1-21	
Number of Animals	30	9	9	13	9	2	3	16	6	67
Number Not Pregnant or Not Delivered	2	0	2	1	1	0	1	3	1	9
Duration of Pregnancy (days)	21.9	22.0	21.8	21.9	21.8	22.0	21.5	21.8	22.2	21.9
Number of Offspring	270	76	79	116	74	24	19	137	41	566
Average Litter Size	9.6	8.4	11.3	9.7	9.3	12.0	9.5	10.5	8.2	9.8
% Deaths	7.0	18.4	0	13.8	5.8	0	0	15.5	0	9.8

[a]Chlorpromazine (10 mg/kg body weight) was administered to pregnant rats during various days of pregnancy.

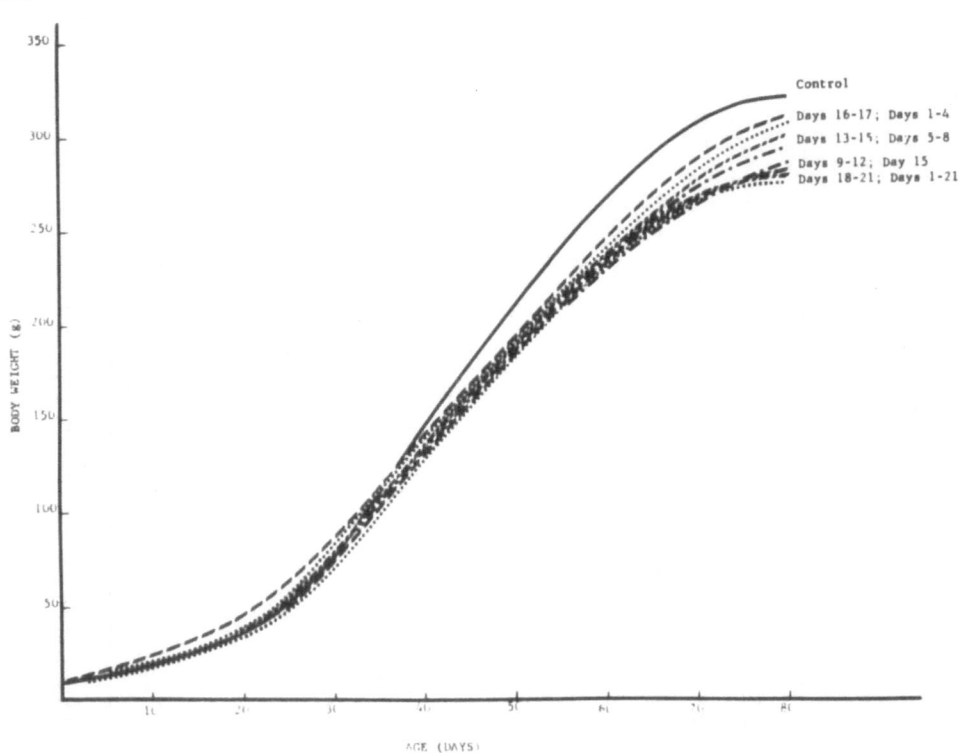

Fig. 1. Effect of prenatal CPZ (10 mg/kg) on body weight of rats.
The days refer to the gestation time.

Brain Weight. In general (with the exception of two groups),
there were no significant changes in brain weight of the drug exposed groups. Female rats from the groups receiving CPZ on gestation
days 13-15 or 18-21 showed an increase in brain weight when examined
at 80 days of age (P<0.02).

Brain 5HT. In control rats (data derived from over 200 rats)
there were no significant differences between brain 5HT levels in
the two sexes at all ages tested. This was true for NE also. Therefore, we had pooled the data from the two sexes (except in cases
where there were significant differences) in comparing the drug
treated rats with the controls. The development of brain 5HT was
suppressed in all the groups receiving CPZ prenatally and this effect
was maximal in the animals exposed to CPZ on gestation days 18-21
and 1-21 (Fig. 2).

Brain NE. In contrast to the effects on 5HT, brain NE development was not significantly altered except in the group receiving drug
on days 18-21. In these animals, there was an elevation in brain NE

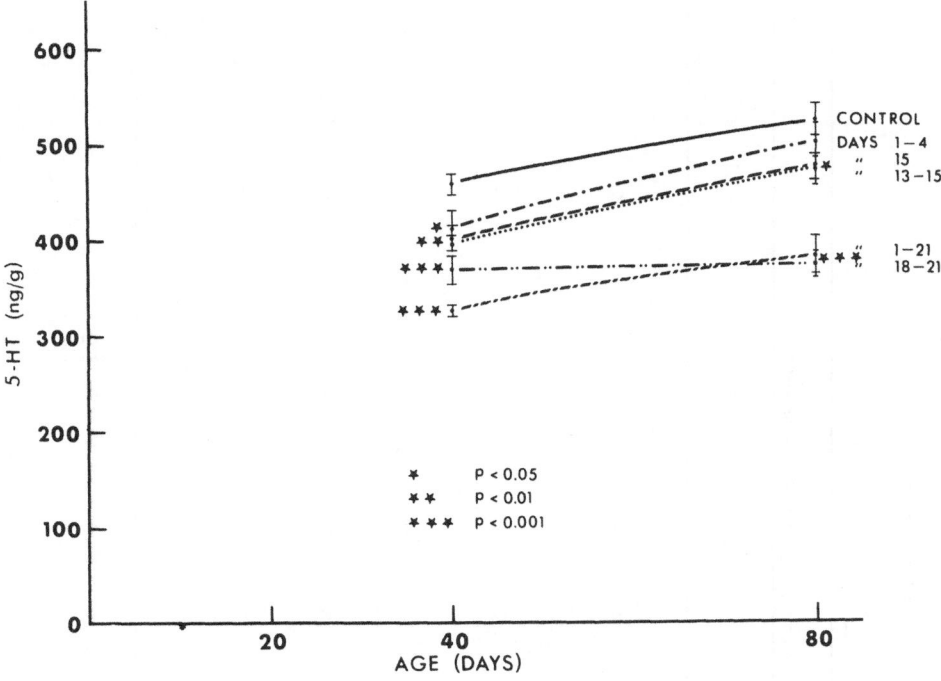

Fig. 2. Effect of prenatal CPZ (10 mg/kg) in rats on development of
brain 5HT. The days refer to the gestation time. Each point represents the mean of 8-10 animals; vertical bars denote standard
errors.

---

at both 40 and 80 days of age (Fig. 3).

Lysergic Acid Diethylamide

Gross Effects. To date, we have not observed any gross organ
malformations or anomalies in the offspring of LSD treated rats.
Drug was given at a relatively high dose level (100 μg/kg) in comparison
to the human psychoactive dosage. Furthermore, we have covered the
whole duration of pregnancy by administering the drug at selected
intervals from day 1 through day 21 of gestation. An increased incidence of early death was noted in all the drug exposed groups (Table II).
This effect was more pronounced in the groups receiving drug on gestation days 1-3, 9-12 and 13-15.

Body Weight. A significant suppression of the normal developmental increase in body weight was noted in all the drug exposed
groups, except the day 8 group, this effect being maximal in those

TABLE II

GROSS EFFECTS OF PRENATAL LSD IN RATS

	Control	Days of Drug Treatment[a]							All Time Periods
		1-3	4	8	9-12	13-15	18-21	1-21	
Number of Animals	34	6	3	4	6	6	6	2	33
Number Not Pregnant or Not Delivered	3	1	0	1	1	1	0	0	4
Duration of Pregnancy (days)	21.9	22	22	21.7	22	21.6	22.3	22	21.9
Number of Offspring	289	59	22	23	47	49	65	18	283
Average Litter Size	9.3	11.8	7.3	7.6	9.4	9.8	10.8	9	9.8
% Deaths	5.9	27.1	9.1	8.7	44.7	32.3	13.8	16.7	24.4

[a] LSD (100 µg/kg body weight) was administered to pregnant rats during various days of pregnancy.

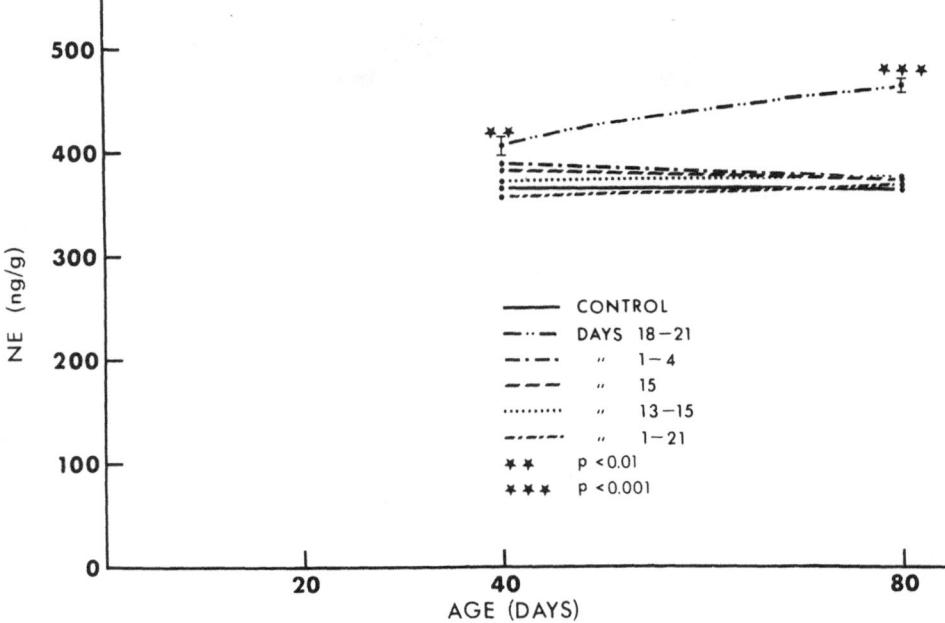

Fig. 3. Effect of prenatal CPZ (10 mg/kg) in rats on development of brain NE. The days refer to the gestation time. Each point refers to the mean of 8-10 animals; other symbols as in Fig. 2.

receiving drug during the last few days of gestation (18-21) or throughout pregnancy (Fig. 4).

Brain Weight. There were no significant changes in brain weight in comparison to the controls.

Chromosomal Effects. The chromosomal effects of LSD were studied in pregnant rats and their offspring. Drug (100 µg/kg) was given during implantation and during the period of differentiation and chromosome analysis were performed in the embryo and bone marrow cells from the mother and the adult offspring. Our results showed that exposure to pure LSD in pregnancy, at the dosages used, did not damage the chromosomes of the mother, embryos or adult offspring.

Brain 5HT. Significant decreases in brain 5HT were noted in the groups exposed to the drug on gestation days 1-3, 9-12, 13-15, and 18-21 (Fig. 5). In the last group, suppression of brain 5HT development was evident both at 40 and 80 days of age in the males, while

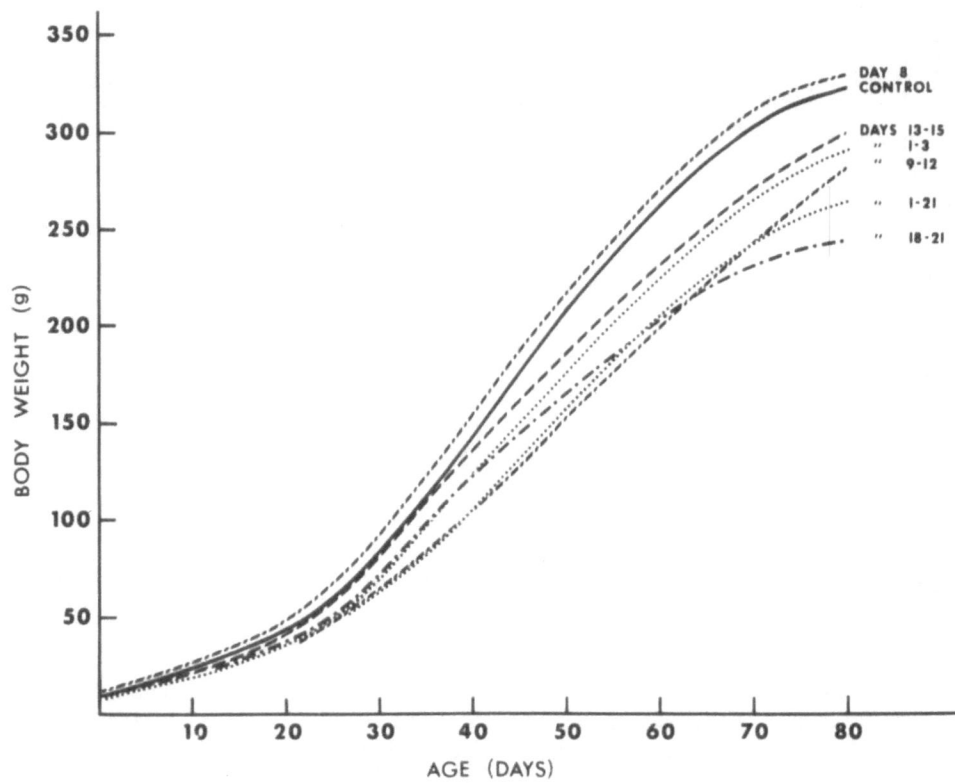

Fig. 4. Effect of prenatal LSD (100 µg/kg) on body weight of rats. The days refer to the gestation time.

in the females, the amine level has returned to control levels by 80 days of age.

Brain NE. In the group exposed to drug on gestation days 18-21, brain NE levels were lower than that in the controls (Fig. 6). In the other groups, even though the level was frequently lower at 40 days of age, it was the same as in controls by 80 days, except in the males from 9-12 days group, which showed increased brain levels of NE.

The most significant finding of the studies with CPZ and LSD is the suppression of brain 5HT development in the offspring of rats exposed to either of these drugs in pregnancy. Since the same response is produced by two drugs, which are pharmacologically dissimilar, the question arises whether this is a specific effect or just a nonspecific effect which may be produced by any chemical given during the corresponding gestation periods. In order to answer this question, we studied the effects of three other drugs under similar conditions: 1) dextroamphetamine, a central nervous system stimulant;

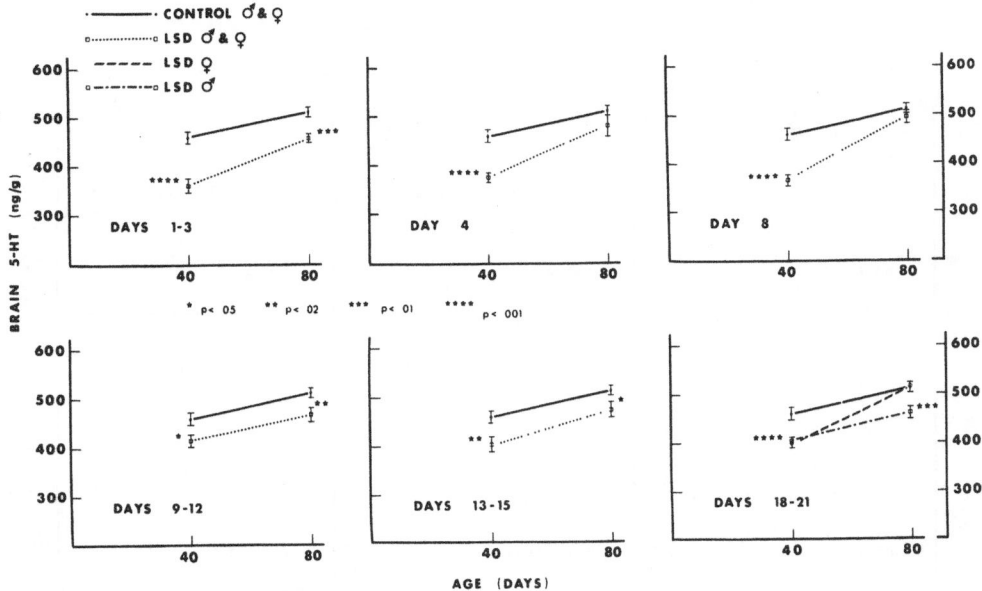

Fig. 5. Effect of prenatal LSD (100 µg/kg) in rats on the development of brain 5HT. Each point represents the mean of 8-10 animals;
vertical bars denote standard errors. Days refer to the gestation
time.

2) imipramine, an antidepressant; and 3) Δ^9-THC, a psychotropic agent.
They were administered (see methods) daily for 4 days during the
gestation period 18-21, the time when maximal suppression of brain
5HT was noted with CPZ.

Dextroamphetamine produced no significant alterations in brain
5HT development (Fig. 7). No changes were noted in either NE or
5HIAA levels also. On the other hand, administration of Δ^9-THC resulted in a suppression of brain 5HT development which was evident
at birth and also at 40 days of age (Fig. 8). It is noteworthy that
all three drugs, CPZ, DA, and THC produced weight loss in the pregnant rat presumably due to decreased food consumption. However, the
effects on 5HT systems were dissimilar. In contrast, there was an
increase in brain 5HT, at birth, in the offspring of rats exposed to
imipramine (Fig. 8). The 5HT levels appeared to return to that of
controls by 20 days of age. These results indicate that the effects
of CPZ and other drugs on brain 5HT development are specific effects.

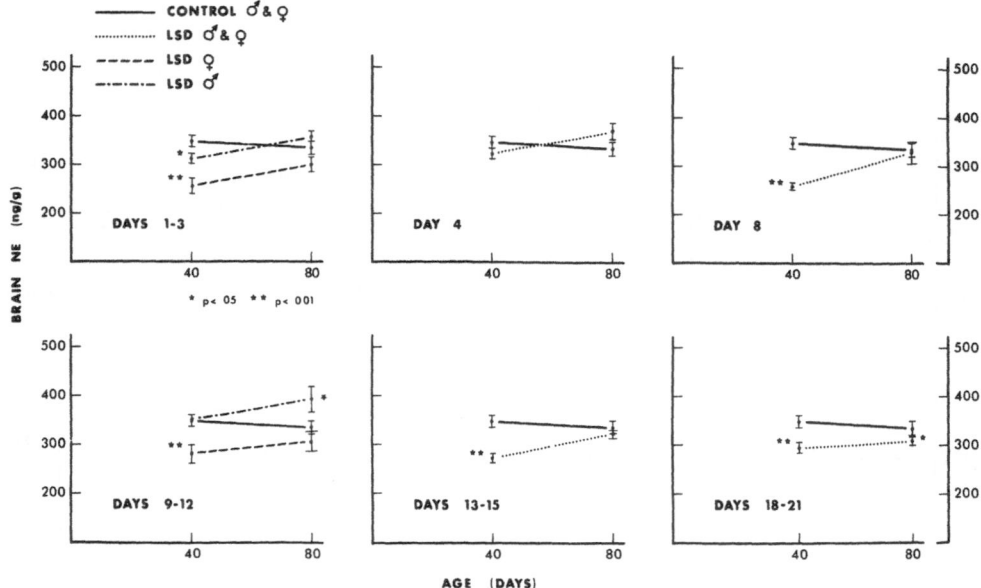

Fig. 6. Effect of prenatal LSD (100 µg/kg) in rats on the development of brain NE. Symbol as in Fig. 5.

Factors Underlying the Suppression of Brain 5HT Development in Rat Offspring Exposed to Chlorpromazine in Pregnancy

Our attention was next turned to the elucidation of the mechanisms underlying the suppressive effect on 5HT system.

In theory, this could result from an effect of CPZ on any one of the following steps in the metabolism of 5HT. 1) On the synthesis of 5HT, possibly through inhibiting the enzyme tryptophan hydroxylase (which is generally believed to be the rate limiting step in the overall reaction); 2) On the breakdown of 5HT, accelerating the degradation by the enzyme monoamine oxidase; and/or 3) On the transport and storage mechanisms.

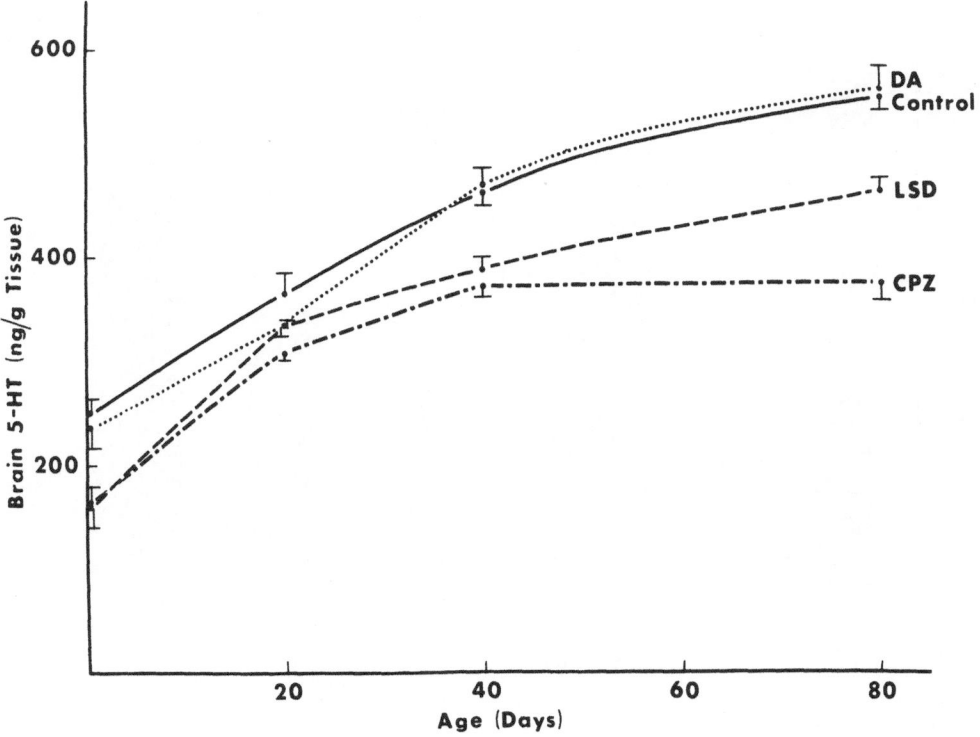

Fig. 7. Comparison of the effects of prenatal exposure to DA (dex-troamphetamine, 1 mg/kg), LSD (100 µg/kg) and CPZ (10 mg/kg) in rats, on brain 5HT development. Each point represents the mean of 8-10 animals; vertical bars denote standard errors. The drugs were ad-ministered daily for 4 days during gestation days 18-21.

Determination of Brain Tryptophan Hydroxylase Activity

We employed the method of Lovenberg et al. (1967), a radioassay which consisted basically of the following steps: L-tryptophan-2-C^{14} is incubated with brain tissue containing the enzyme, cofactors, and a monoamine oxidase inhibitor. After the reaction has proceeded, a portion of 5-hydroxytryptophan (5HTP) is enzymatically decarboxy-lated with partially purified aromatic-L-amino acid decarboxylase. The 5HT formed is isolated by column chromatography and its specific radioactivity determined. The preparation and purification of the aromatic-L-amino acid decarbozylase proved to be a lengthy and la-borious procedure. Moreover, this enzyme could not be stored for any length of time because it lost 40% of its activity in 10 days. These difficulties led us to introduce a modification.

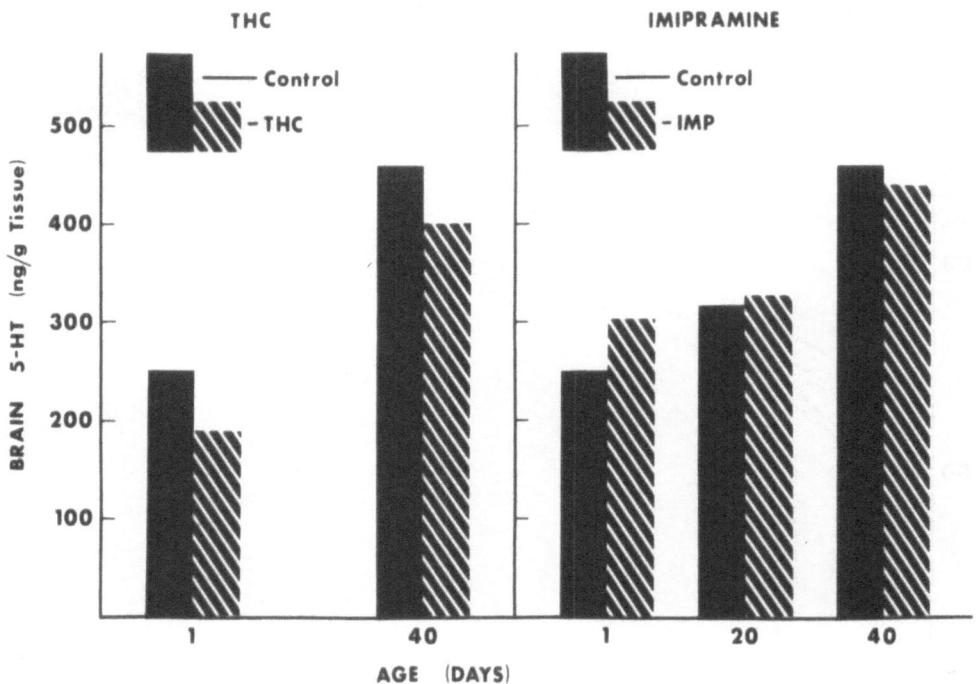

Fig. 8. Effect of Δ^9-THC (10 mg/kg) and imipramine (10 mg/kg) in rats on brain 5HT development. Drugs were administered daily for 4 days on gestation days 18-21. Each value is the mean of 8-10 animals. The values at 1 and 40 days for THC and 1 day for IMP treated animals were significantly different from the corresponding controls ($P<0.05$).

_____

The method of Peters <u>et al.</u> (1968), which utilizes the decarboxylase from cat brain was tried, substituting rat brain for cat tissue. Our results indicated that rat brain tissue preparation did not contain high enough enzyme activity for utilization in the assay. In fact, a commercially prepared bacterial decarboxylase was slightly more active than our rat brain decarboxylase preparation.

As we were mainly interested in the hydroxylating step from tryptophan to 5HTP, we then attempted to determine the enzyme activity by isolating 5HTP. In a series of experiments, we added different combinations of cofactors based on the studies of Ichiyama <u>et al.</u> (1968), and Robinson <u>et al.</u> (1968), and isolated the formed 5HTP by paper chromatography and radioassay. The enzyme activity as measured by isolating 5HTP was very low and could not be used with confidence, for a quantitative assay.

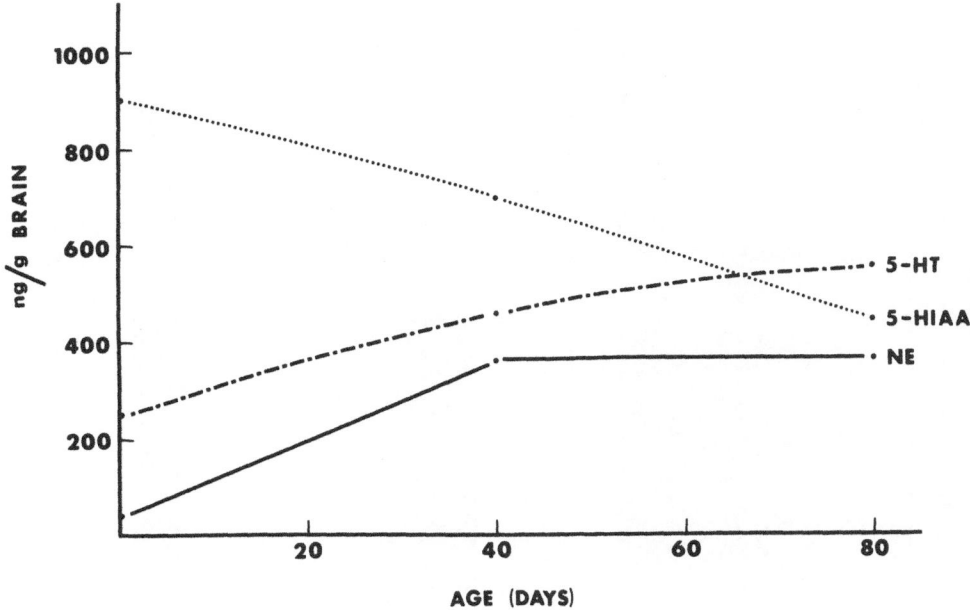

Fig. 9. Ontogenetic changes in control rats of brain 5HT, 5HIAA,
and NE. Each point represents the mean of 8-10 animals.

Metabolism of Brain 5HT

We then proceeded to study the metabolism of brain 5HT in the
control and CPZ aminals. First, we determined the 5HT and 5HIAA
levels in the whole brain of both groups of animals at various ages.
In normal controls, brain 5HIAA levels are highest at birth and progressively decline with age, while 5HT levels continue to rise after
birth until they reach a plateau about 80 days of age or after
(Fig. 9). In the offspring of CPZ exposed animals (drug was given
during gestation days 18-21), brain 5HIAA levels were significantly
higher than in the corresponding controls. Similar results were
noted in the LSD offspring (drug was given during gestation days
18-21). As mentioned earlier in the text, these animals had low
brain 5HT. A comparison of the pattern of changes in brain 5HIAA
and 5HT in control, CPZ and LSD rats is shown in Fig. 10. It can be
seen that when the data are expressed as a ratio, the values are less
than 1 in adult control rats while in both the drug groups, the ratios
are significantly greater than 1. In other words, there is a greater
amount of 5HIAA in the brain of CPZ and LSD animals both in absolute

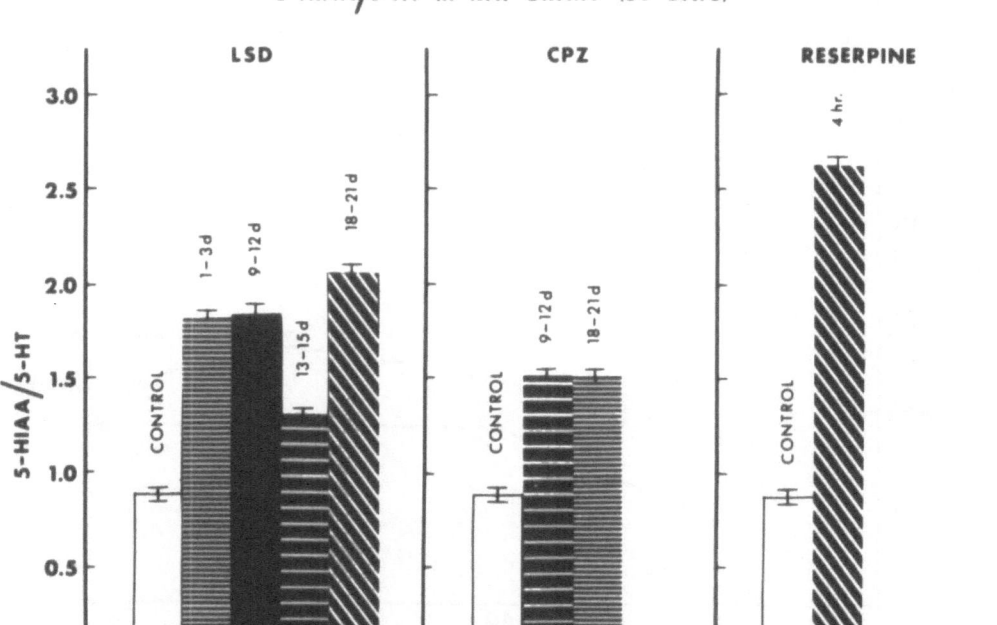

Fig. 10.   Comparison of the effects of prenatal LSD (100 µg/kg) and
CPZ (10 mg/kg) and reserpine (2.5 mg/kg in adult rats) on the ratio
5HIAA/5HT in rat brain.   The time of drug exposure is indicated
above each bar; vertical bars represent standard errors.   Each value
is derived from 8-10 experiments.

amounts and also with respect to the amount of 5HT present.

        Being aware of the limitations of whole brain analysis (Nair
and Roth, 1960, 1965) we also determined the distribution in hypothalamus (Table III).   Again, in CPZ animals, 5HT levels were lower
and 5HIAA levels higher than in the corresponding controls.

        Animals treated with CPZ on gestation days 1-4 are not signifi-
cantly different from the controls with respect to whole brain 5HT
(Fig. 2).   The situation remains the same with respect to hypothalamic 5HT also.   The lack of changes in the 1-4 d group, not only
strengthens the validity of the positive changes noted in 18-21 d
group but also supports the concept of critical periods in development when vulnerability to environmental toxicity is maximal.

TABLE III

LEVELS OF 5HT AND 5HIAA IN HYPOTHALAMUS OF 80 DAYS OLD MALE RATS,
EXPOSED TO CPZ DURING GESTATION

Exposure Time (Days of Gestation)	Hypothalamus[a] 5HT (ng/g)	Hypothalamus 5HIAA (ng/g)	5HIAA/5HT	Number of Experiments
CPZ 18-21	872.1 ± 37[bc]	1259.7 ± 43	1.44	4
CPZ 1-4	1013.4 ± 48	1182.3 ± 49	1.17	4
CONTROLS	1025.5 ± 36[c]	1190.4 ± 33	1.16	6

[a]For the dissection of hypothalamus, the frozen state dissection method, reported earlier was employed (Nair and Bau, 1969). Briefly, this procedure consisted of transferring the decapitated head to a cold room (-10°C), rapid removal of the brain and freezing on a bed of dry ice to the appropriate consistency for sectioning. Serial coronal sections, 2-3 mm in thickness, were then obtained by means of free hand sectioning with a razor blade. The sections containing hypothalamus were then selected and hypothalamus dissected out with the aid of a dissecting lens and scalpel blades. The whole operation including weighing, was performed in the cold room, thereby minimizing the various errors which may result from leaching of the blood, condensation of moisture (when dissection is performed at room temperature on dry ice), water shift, etc. Pooled specimens from 4 brains were used for each experiment.

[b]The values indicated are mean ± S.E.

[c]Significantly different from control ($P < 0.05$).

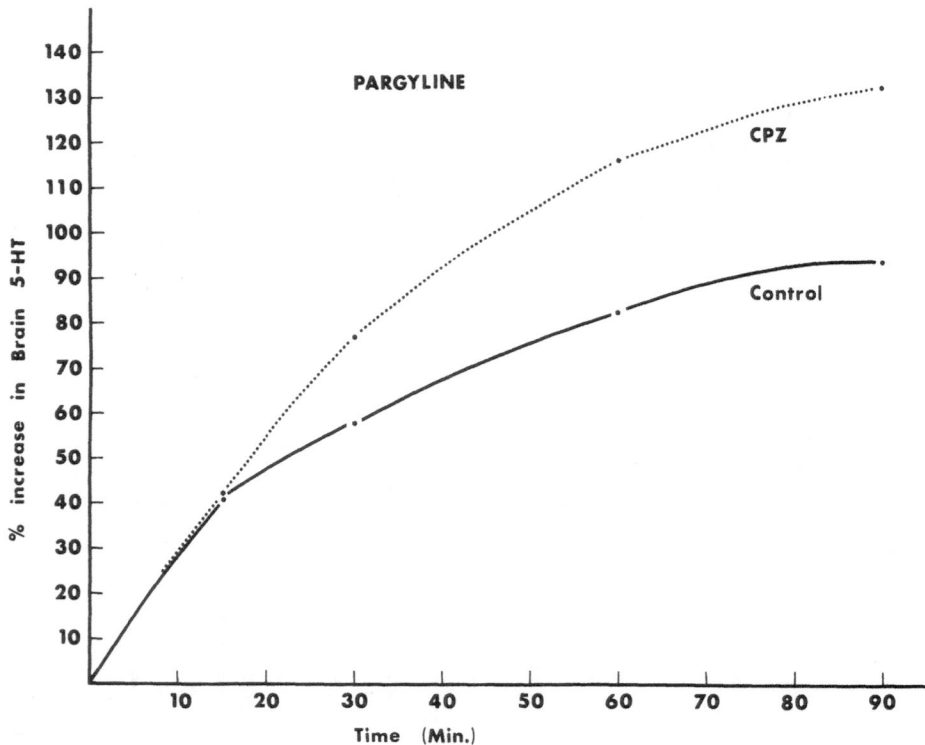

Fig. 11. Brain 5HT levels in 15 day old rats following pargyline
treatment (75 mg/kg). Each point represents the mean of 4-6 experiments. CPZ refers to animals, who have been exposed prenatally to
CPZ (10 mg/kg) during gestation days 18-21. The brain 5HT values,
(mean ± S.E.) at zero time were: control, 300.5 ± 12.3 ng/g brain;
CPZ, 250.0 ± 16.2 ng/g brain.

These findings suggest that increased metabolism of 5HT in the
CPZ animals may be responsible for the lowered brain 5HT values.
However, preliminary studies on brain monoamine oxidase activity
(MAO)* revealed no significant changes from the controls. This means
that CPZ given prenatally, at critical times, might affect such factors as transport and binding associated with the storage of 5HT,
thus making it more vulnerable to the action of MAO. Such a hypothesis would gain credence if it could be shown that a similar metabolic profile is seen in other experimental conditions where binding
or storage of 5HT is impaired.

*Work done in association with Dr. Boris Tabakoff, Department
of Biochemistry. Enzyme activity determined according to the method
of Tabakoff and Alivisatos (1972).

There is considerable evidence to suggest that reserpine inter-
feres with the intracellular storage mechanisms of 5HT. Therefore
we determined the ratio of brain 5HIAA/5HT in rats treated with reserpine (Fig. 10). Indeed in the reserpinised animals, the ratio of
brain 5HIAA/5HT was markedly higher than in controls.

In another experiment, we examined the fate of brain 5HT after
inhibition of MAO by pargyline (75 mg/kg). A similar approach has
been employed by Neff and Tozer (1968) for the in vivo measurement
of brain 5HT turnover. At selected intervals after pargyline administration, animals were sacrificed and brain 5HT determined. The CPZ
animals were found to accumulate more 5HT than the controls (Fig. 11).

Thus in comparing the offspring of rats exposed prenatally to
CPZ with the corresponding controls, 1) brain 5HT levels are considerably decreased; 2) brain 5HIAA levels are markedly elevated; 3) brain
5HT production is significantly greater; 4) brain MAO activity is not
altered, and 5) the ratio of brain 5HIAA/5HT is considerably greater
and is qualitatively similar in pattern to that noted in reserpinised
animals. The apparent paradox of an increased 5HT production but
decreased absolute levels may be explained by an increased turnover
of 5HT in brain. However, since MAO activity is not increased while
5HIAA levels are, it is postulated that prenatal administration of
CPZ has resulted in an impairment of the binding or storage mechanisms
of 5HT, which normally protects the endogenously formed amine from
oxidation by MAO. The impairment in storage mechanisms permits more
5HT to be oxidized thus resulting in higher levels of the acid metabolite and lower levels of the amine.

Our findings also focus attention on the importance of binding
and storage mechanisms in determining the steady state levels of 5HT.
At least in certain situations, binding and storage mechanisms could
be the rate limiting step in the overall production of 5HT.

Acid metabolites are eliminated from the brain by an active
transport mechanism. An impairment of this transport mechanism could
also contribute to the high brain levels of 5HIAA in the CPZ offspring.
The transport kinetics have not been studied in the present investigation and therefore this mechanism cannot be excluded.

It is pertinent to point out here that the above described biochemical effects were not seen in all the offspring. From our results
to date, it is estimated that 70-80% of the progeny showed the biochemical lesion pertaining to 5HT development. Such variations are
not unusual in developmental pharmacology experiments. For example,
normal offspring have been reported along with the malformed after
exposure to potent teratogens such as thalidomide (Somers, 1963) and
cyclopamine (Keeler, 1970). This variability could be found within
the same litter or in different litters. In a study conducted on the

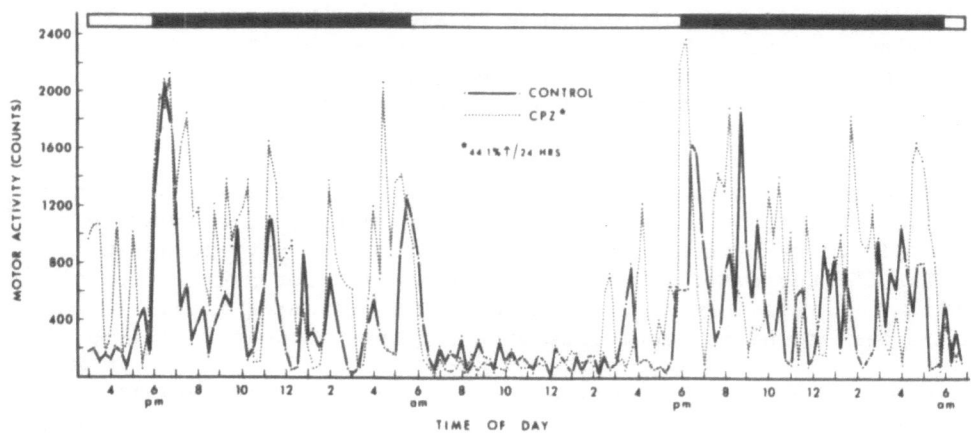

Fig. 12. Effect of prenatal CPZ (10 mg/kg) on the locomotor activity
of rats. The dark bars indicate the periods without light. The data
were obtained using an Animex activity meter (Farad Electronics,
Stockholm). The animals were 80 days of age. There was a 44.1%
increase in activity per 24 hours in the CPZ group.

---

effect of prenatal LSD, Alexander et al. (1967) found that of five
litters exposed to the drug one was completely normal, 7/8 normal in
another litter, and all stillborn in one litter. One can assume that
drug effects on the biochemical level may vary to a similar degree.
Furthermore some of the discrepancies might be a reflection of differing levels of drug and/or its metabolite in the fetus during the
critical gestation period. Even though it is known that CPZ crosses
the placental barrier (Ordy et al., 1966), it would be worthwhile to
measure the actual plasma drug levels in the mother and in the fetus.
Recent studies in psychiatric patients with tricyclic antidepressant
drugs have revealed considerable individual differences in plasma
drug levels (Hammer et al., 1969) and the therapeutic response has
been related to the plasma drug levels. Among the many factors which
may contribute to the variability are the genetic makeup, metabolic
profile, drug absorption and disposition.

Functional and Behavioral Tests in the Offspring
of Rats Exposed to Chlorpromazine or LSD

Locomotor Activity

The locomotor activity of the animals was measured at two ages,
30 and 80 days, both in groups of 3-6 animals as well as individually.
The group activity was recorded by means of a sensitive microphone

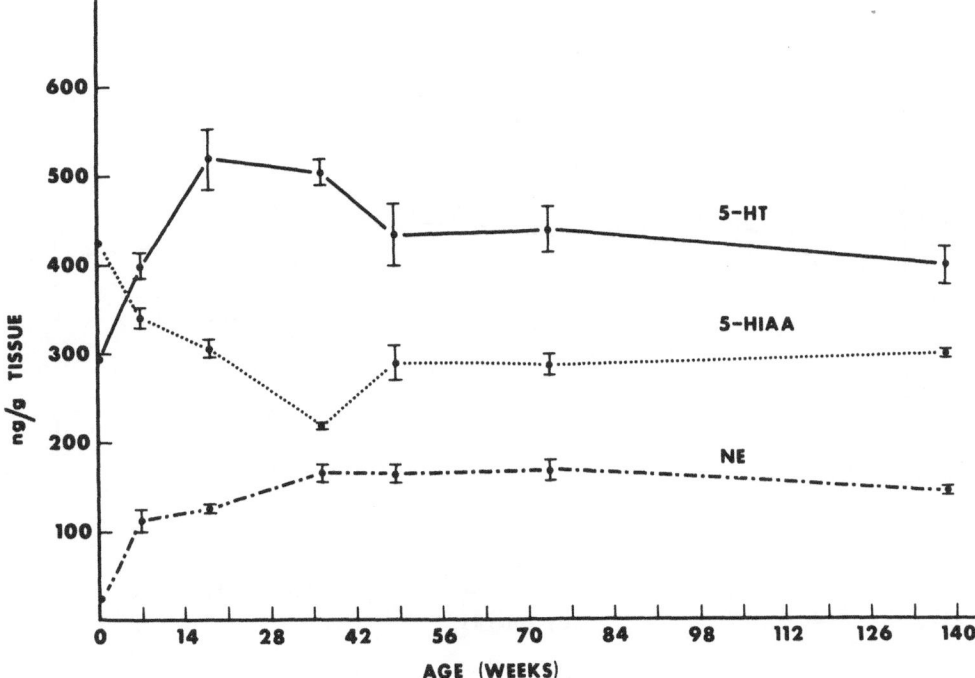

Fig. 13. Ontogenetic changes in brain 5HT, 5HIAA, and NE in control rabbits. Each point represents the mean of 6-8 animals; vertical bars denote standard errors.

mounted in close proximity to the cages. All the noise emanating from the room (the room was provided with a double door to minimize outside interferences) was picked up by the microphone and was amplified and fed into a recorder which operated continuously. The recordings were made for 3 days. Individual activity was measured by the use of Animex activity meter (Farad Electronics, Stockholm). Our results indicate that the locomotor activity was increased in the CPZ offspring both at the group and individual levels (Fig. 12). A similar although smaller increase was seen in the LSD offspring.

Openfield Behavior

There was considerable overlap in the data and the results, to date, do not point to any significant difference between the control and experimental animals.

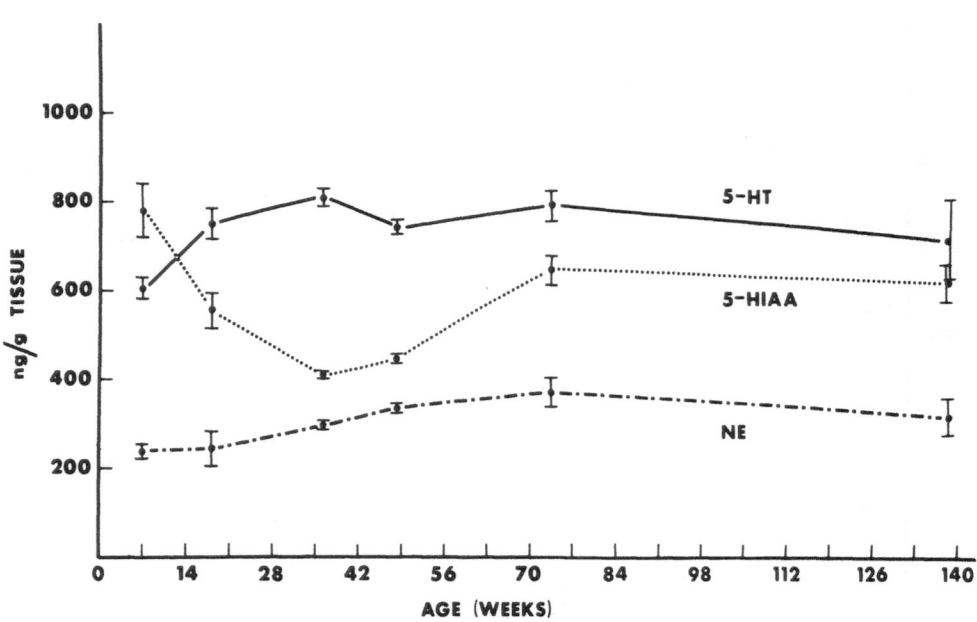

Fig. 14. Ontogenetic changes in brain stem 5HT, 5HIAA, and NE in control rabbits. Symbols as in Fig. 13.

Aggressive Behavior and Sexual Behavior

Only preliminary studies have been done so far. In one batch of LSD offspring, we noted a hypersexual behavior in the males. There was increased frequency of mounting, intromission and ejaculation. However, another batch of LSD offspring did not show any significant differences in sexual behavior with respect to the controls.

To date, no agressive behavior was noted in either the CPZ or LSD offspring. The test was conducted according to the procedure of Sheard (1969).

RABBIT STUDIES

New Zealand white rabbits were used in these studies. The normal developmental patterns of the biochemical systems under study here have been examined from day of birth to over 2½ years of age in both male and female rabbits. The results are summarized in Figures 13 and 14 for brain 5HT,5HIAA and NE.

TABLE IV

GROSS EFFECTS OF PRENATAL CHLORPROMAZINE IN RABBITS

	Control	Chlorpromazine[a]
Number of Animals	23	7
Duration of Pregnancy (days)	33.1	33.3
Number of Offspring	178	58
Average Litter Size	7.7	8.3
% Deaths	23.6	65.5

[a]Chlorpromazine (10 mg/kg body weight) was administered daily for 4 days on gestation days 27-30.

Chlorpromazine (10 mg/kg, subcutaneously) was administered daily for 4 days to pregnant rabbits on gestation days 27-30.* The animals were allowed to complete their pregnancy, deliver and raise their offspring. The gross effects observed in a typical series are summarized in Table IV. What is striking here is the significantly greater incidence of infant deaths in comparison to the observations in rats. Exposure to higher doses of CPZ resulted in an even greater incidence of infant deaths. The body weight of the surviving offspring was slightly lower than their controls up to about 10 weeks of age after which, there was no significant difference.

Brain/body weight ratios were also determined and there were no significant differences between the controls and CPZ offspring.

No sifnigicant differences were observed in the development of 5HT or NE in the CPZ offspring. The amines were determined in the whole brain as well as in the brain stem. With respect to 5HIAA, the whole brain values did not show any changes from the control. However, when the brain stem was assayed, a significant increase in 5HIAA levels was noted in the older CPZ offspring. A similar increase in brain 5HIAA was seen in the offspring of rats exposed to CPZ.

---

*The average gestation period in rabbits was 33.1 days. The gestation days 27-30 were selected for drug treatment because in rats, maximal effect on brain 5HT was noted when CPZ was given during the last few days of pregnancy.

The findings, to date, in rabbits exposed to CPZ prenatally, are in contrast to that of rats. 1) The most conspicuous effect in rabbits was the significantly greater incidence of infant deaths in the CPZ offspring. 2) In rats, we noted a suppression of the increase in brain 5HT in the CPZ exposed group, which was not detected in the rabbit. This may be a reflection of the species difference in sensitivity of response. It may also be that the biochemically malformed ones were eliminated in the early deaths in rabbits and those surviving were the normal ones. This would explain the absence of any significant effect on the biochemical systems examined.

SUMMARY

The effects of prenatal exposure to certain psychotropic drugs (chlorpromazine, lysergic acid diethylamide, dextroamphetamine, imipramine and Δ^9-tetrahydrocannabinol) on the development of brain 5HT and NE systems were studied in rats and rabbits. The most conspicuous finding was the lowered brain 5HT levels in the offspring of rats exposed to chlorpromazine or LSD. This appeared to be a permanent effect since, in general, the amine levels remained low at all ages examined from birth until adulthood. Even though our results to date do not indicate well defined critical periods in prenatal development for the vulnerability of the amine systems, relatively speaking, maximal effects on growth and brain 5HT were observed when drug exposure took place during the last few days of gestation (18-21 d).

In behavioral tests, these animals with low brain 5HT were found to be markedly hyperactive. No clear cut results were obtained with respect to their sexual behavior or aggression.

Regarding the mechanisms underlying the suppression of brain 5HT development using CPZ offspring as models, it is speculated that prenatal exposure to chlorpromazine may have resulted in an impairment of the 5HT binding and storage mechanisms within the neuron thereby making it more vulnerable to the oxidative action of MAO. Our findings also focus attention on the importance of binding and storage mechanisms in determining the steady state levels of brain 5HT.

The ontogenetic changes in brain 5HT, 5HIAA and NE in rabbits from day of birth to $2\frac{1}{2}$ years of age show that in contrast to the response in rats, prenatal chlorpromazine administration did not produce any significant changes in brain amines in rabbits. Some of the factors underlying the species differences in sensitivity are discussed.

ACKNOWLEDGMENTS

This investigation was supported by grants from the State of Illinois Department of Mental Health (233-12-RD-105), the Easter Seal Research Foundation (N-7040), and General Research Support Grant (FR-05366-11) from NIH. I wish to acknowledge the excellent technical assistance of Mr. David Bau and Miss Francine Sanes. My thanks are due to Dr. Sebastian P. Grossman for discussions on the behavioral test.

REFERENCES

Alexander, G.J., Miles, B.E., Gold, G.M., and Alexander, R.B., 1967, LSD: Injection early in pregnancy produces abnormalities in offspring of rats, Science 157: 459.

Bleyer, W.A., Au, W.Y.W., Lange, W.A., and Raisz, L.G., 1970, Studies on the detection of adverse drug reactions in the newborn, J. Am. Med. Ass. 213: 2046.

Brill, A.B., and Forgotson, E.H., 1964, Radiation and congenital malformations, Am. J. Obstet. Gynec. 90: 1149.

Greengard, O., 1969, Enzymic differentiation in mammalian liver, Science 163: 891.

Hammer, W., Martens, S., and Sjoquist, I., 1969, A comparative study of the metabolism of desmethylimipramine, nortriptyline, and oxyphenylbutazone in man, Clin. Pharmacol. and Therap. 10: 44.

Ichiyama, A., Nakamura, S., Nishizuka, Y., and Hayaishi, O., 1968, Tryptophan-5-hydroxylase in mammalian brain, in "Advances in Pharmacology", (S. Garattini and P.A. Shore, eds.), Vol. 6A, pp. 5-17, Academic Press, New York.

Keeler, R.F., 1970, Teratogenic compounds of veratrum californicum (durand). X. Cyclopia in rabbits produced by cyclopamine, Teratology 3: 175.

Lovenberg, W., Jequier, E., and Sjoerdsma, A., 1967, Tryptophan hydroxylation: Measurement in pineal gland, brain-stem, and carcinoid tumor, Science 155: 217.

Mead, J.A.R., and Finger, K.F., 1961, A single extraction mentod for the determination of both norepinephrine and serotonin in brain, Biochem. Pharmac. 6: 52.

Medearis, D.N., 1964, Viral infections during pregnancy and abnormal
    human development, Am. J. Obstet, Gynec., 87: 609.

Millen, J.W., and Woollam, D.H.M., 1963, Congenital malformations of
    the skeletal system, in "Effects of Drugs on the Fetus". Pro-
    ceedings of the European Society for the study of Drug Toxicity,
    Vol. 1, pp. 9-24, Excerpta Med. Found., Amsterdam.

Miller, F.P., Cox, R.H. Jr., Snodgrass, W.R., and Maickel, R.P.,
    1970, Comparative effects of p-chlorophenylalanine, p-chloro-
    amohetamine and p-chloro-N-methylamphetamine on rat brain nore-
    pinephrine, serotonin and 5-hydroxyindole-3-acetic acid, Biochem.
    Pharmac., 19: 435.

Nair, V., and Bau, D., 1969, Effects of prenatal x-irradiation on the
    ontogenesis of acetylcholinesterase and carbonic anhydrase in
    rat central nervous system, Brain Research 16: 383.

Nair, V., Palm, D., and Roth, L.J., 1960, Relative vascularity of
    certain anatomical areas of the brain and other organs of the
    rat, Nature 188: 497.

Nair, V., and Roth, L.J., 1965, Penetration of substances into the
    brain, in "Isotopes in Experimental Pharmacology", (L.J. Roth,
    ed.), pp. 219-228, Univ. Chicago Press, Chicago.

Neff, N.H., and Tozer, T.N., 1968, In Vivo measurement of brain sero-
    tonin turnover, in "Advances in Pharmacology", (S. Garattini and
    P.A. Shore, Eds.), Vol. 6A, pp. 97-109, Academic Press, New York.

Nora, J.J., Nora, A.H., Sommerville, R.J., Hill, R.M., and McNamara,
    D.G., 1967, Maternal exposure to potential teratogens, J. Am.
    Med. Ass. 202: 1065.

Ordy, J.M., Samoragiski, T., Collins, R.L., and Rolsten, C., 1966,
    Prenatal chlorpromazine effects on liver survival and behavior
    of mice offspring, J. Pharmac. Exp. Therap. 151: 110.

Page, I.H., 1968, "Serotonin", Year Book Medical Publishers, Inc.,
    Chicago.

Peckham, C.H., and King, R.W., 1963, Study of intercurrent conditions
    observed during pregnancy, Am. J. Obstet. Gynec. 87: 609.

Peters, D.A.V., McGeer, P.L., and McGeer, E.G., 1968, The distribution
    of tryptophan hydroxylase in cat brain, J. Neurochem. 15: 1431.

Robinson, D., Lovenberg, W., and Sjoerdsma, A., 1968, Subcellular
    distribution and properties of rat brain stem tryptophan hydroxy-
    lase, Arch. Biochem. Biophys. 123: 419.

Schildkraut, J.J., and Kety, S.S., 1967, Biogenic amines and emotion, Science, 156: 21.

Sheard, M.H., 1969, The effect of p-chlorophenylamine on behavior in rats: relation to brain serotonin and 5-hydroxyindoleacetic acid, Brain Res., 15: 524.

Sjoerdsma, A., Lovenberg, W., Engelman, K., Carpenter, W.T., Wyatt, R.J., and gessa, G.L., 1970, Serotonin now: Clinical implications of inhibiting its synthesis with para-chlorophenylalamine, Am. Intern. Med. 73: 607.

Somers, G.F., 1963, The foetal toxicity of thalidomide, in "Effects of Drugs on the Foetus", Proceedings of the European Society for the Study of Drug Toxicity, pp. 49-58, Excerpta Medica Found., Amsterdam.

Tabakoff, B., and Alivisatos, S.G.A., 1972, Modified method for spectrophotometric determination of monoamine oxidase activity, Analyt. Chem., 44: 427.

CHROMOGRANINS AND NEUROTRANSMITTER RETENTION DURING DEVELOPMENT OF

THE ADRENERGIC NEURON

Bernard L. Mirkin

Division of Clinical Pharmacology, Departments of

Pharmacology and Pediatrics, University of Minnesota,

Minneapolis, Minnesota

INTRODUCTION

Functional maturation within the sympathetic nervous system is reflected by the ability of the neuron to synthesize, retain, release and metabolize adrenergic neurotransmitter. The ontogenetic patterns of catecholamine biosynthesis (Friedman et al., 1968; Friedman, 1969; Ignarro and Shideman, 1968a, 1968b), uptake (Iversen et al., 1967; Mirkin, 1972), release (Iversen et al., 1967) and metabolism (Brunjes et al., 1964; Glowinski et al., 1964; Ignarro and Shideman, 1968b) have been reasonably well, if not completely, defined. A major un-resolved question is how adrenergic neurotransmitter is bound and re-tained within the neuron ready to be released in an active form upon neuronal activation. The relationship between neuronal binding of catecholamines and the presence of specific soluble proteins in the adrenergic vesicle has been studied in the developing adrenergic neuron. Data derived from these investigations will be presented in this report.

INTRACELLULAR LOCALIZATION OF ADRENERGIC MEDIATOR

The initial subcellular fractionations of neural crest deriva-tives such as the adrenal medulla (Blaschko and Welch, 1953; Hillarp and Nilson, 1954) and the post-ganglionic adrenergic neuron (von Euler and Hillarp, 1956) suggested that a large proportion of the catechol-amine present in these tissues was localized in discrete organelles which were readily isolated by differential ultracentrifugation pro-cedures (Potter and Axelrod, 1963). Precise quantitative estimation of the percentage of tissue catecholamine residing in these vesicles

199

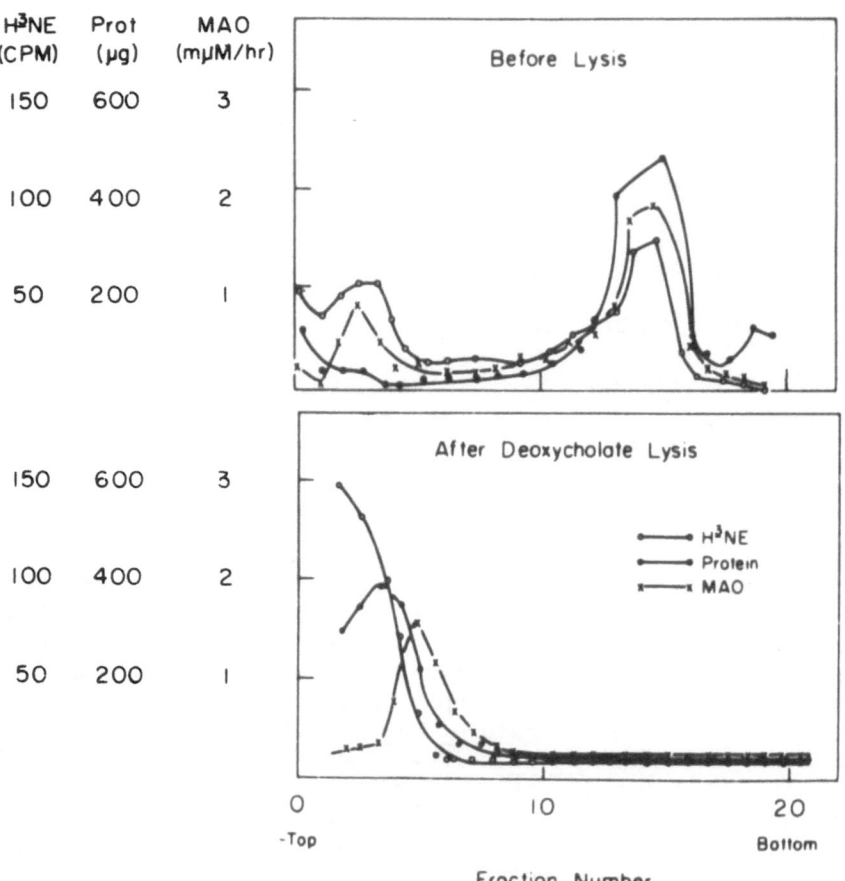

Fig. 1. Sucrose density gradient distribution of ^{3}H-norepinephrine, monoamine-oxidase activity and protein in microsomal fractions of rat heart prepared two hours after administering ^{3}H-norepinephrine (100 μC i.v.) to the whole animal. Density gradient: 0.25M to 1.7M. (A) Washed heart microsomes prior to lysis; (B) Washed heart microsomes after lysis in 0.5% desoxycholate. Note shift in ^{3}H-norepinephrine peak from more dense to less dense portions of gradient associated with loss of function of vesicle as storage organelle.

under physiological conditions remains a vexing problem since arti-
facts caused by homogenization and other analytical procedures probably modify the distribution pattern (Lundborg, 1967). Nonetheless,
most reports suggest that about 60% of rat heart norepinephrine
(Potter and Axelrod, 1963), 35% of the norepinephrine in splenic
nerve press juice (von Euler and Lishjako, 1961), 59% of the rat vas
deferens content of norepinephrine and 57% of cat spleen norepinephrine are vesicle bound (Bisby and Fillenz, 1971). Disruption of
the vesicles by osmotic shock, freeze-thawing or desoxycholate is
associated with an egress of catecholamine into the extravesicular
milieu and subsequent loss of function as a storage organelle (Mirkin
and Mueller, 1968; Fig. 1). Electron micrographic studies of these
subcellular organelles have shown them to be non-homogeneous in nature
consisting of small as well as large dense-cored vesicles (with
differing sedimentation characteristics) both of which are able to
take up and store norepinephrine (Roth et al., 1968; Bisby and
Fillenz, 1971).

ADRENERGIC VESICLES: COMPOSITION AND AMINE BINDING CHARACTERISTICS

     The chemical make-up of the mature adrenergic vesicle has been
intensively studied and a rather complex array of substances have
been isolated from these structures. The major non-catecholamine
materials include the following: adenine nucleotides (ATP), nucleic
acids, divalent cations (calcium, magnesium), soluble proteins (chromogranins), enzymatically active proteins (dopamine-beta-hydroxylase,
ATPase) and lipids (cholesterol, phospholipid, lysolecithin, phos-
phatidylethanolamine, lecithin). The role any of these constituents
may have in the vesicular retention or binding of adrenergic neurotransmitter is not clear, despite evidence that the molar ratio of
catecholamines to ATP in the vesicular sap ranges consistently between three and four in many, but not all species (Hillarp, 1960;
De Potter, 1970). Other qualitative similarities between the nerve
trunk amine-containing particles and the adrenomedullary catecholamine
storage granules have been collated by Lagercrantz (1971).

     Additional support for the significance of this relationship
has been provided by the demonstration that a stable catecholamine-
ATP complex is formed when these compounds are allowed to interact
under in vitro conditions (Berneis et al., 1972). Further studies
suggest that the storage of catecholamines in the adrenal chromaffin
granule is dependent upon the formation of high molecular weight
aggregates not only between ATP and norepinephrine but the intra-
granular proteins as well (Berneis et al., 1971, 1972, personal
communications). Complexes between catecholamines, ATP and chromogranins with a catecholamine to ATP ratio of three have also been
described by Banks and Helle (1971). Some in vivo experiments have
demonstrated the maintenance of stoichiometric relationships between
catecholamine, ATP and soluble proteins both prior to and following

discharge of the amine from its vesicular locus in the adrenal medulla (Banks and Helle, 1965; Sage et al., 1967). The release of
chromogranins (Geffen et al., 1969) and dopamine-beta-hydroxylase
(Gewirtz and Kopin, 1970) into splenic venous effluents following
sympathetic nerve stimulation has been clearly demonstrated. These
data not only support the view that an exocytotic process is involved
in neurotransmitter release but also suggest a very close functional
relationship between intravesicular soluble proteins and catecholamines.

While several investigators have shown that catecholamines are
bound to chromogranins under in vitro and in vivo conditions the
physiologic significance of these observations is not at all clear.
Smith and Kirschner (1967), utilizing equilibrium dialysis (at pH 6.4)
concluded that the amount of isotopic catecholamine bound to adrenal
chromogranins under in vitro conditions was so low that it could not
explain the high intravesicular concentrations of catecholamines
observed in vivo. In contrast, Mirkin and Mueller (1968) employing
gel-filtration on sephadex G-25 as their basic technique, clearly
demonstrated the binding of ^{3}H-norepinephrine (^{3}H-NE) to soluble
proteins (chromogranins) present in the intravesicular sap of mature
adrenergic vesicles isolated from the heart. These studies indicated
that one hour after administering ^{3}H-NE (intraveneously) between 15
and 30% of the isotope isolated from the myocardial adrenergic vesicle fraction was bound to soluble proteins. Comparable experiments
performed with adrenal medullary vesicles revealed only about 3% of
the total vesicular isotope (the isotope was rigorously characterized
and found to consist of 65 to 70% ^{3}H-NE) to be protein bound (Mirkin
and Mueller, unpublished data; Mirkin, 1972).

ONTOGENESIS OF THE ADRENERGIC NEURON

The adrenergic neuron undergoes dramatic biochemical and functional changes during maturation making it a useful model with which
to study the potential relationship between chromogranins and neurotransmitter retention. Several aspects of this problem have been
investigated and will be considered in the ensuing discussion.

Catecholamine Uptake and Binding

The concentrations of endogenous norepinephrine in adrenergically
innervated tissues of the fetal and neonatal mammal are much lower
than those present in the adult (Iversen et al., 1967; Mirkin, 1972).
The uptake of exogenously administered ^{3}H-NE by neonatal rats is also
significantly reduced in the heart and spleen (relative to the adult)
but not in the salivary glands and intestinal tract which resemble
the adult in this respect (Iversen et al., 1967). The uptake and
subcellular distribution patterns of ^{3}H-NE in fetal rat heart also

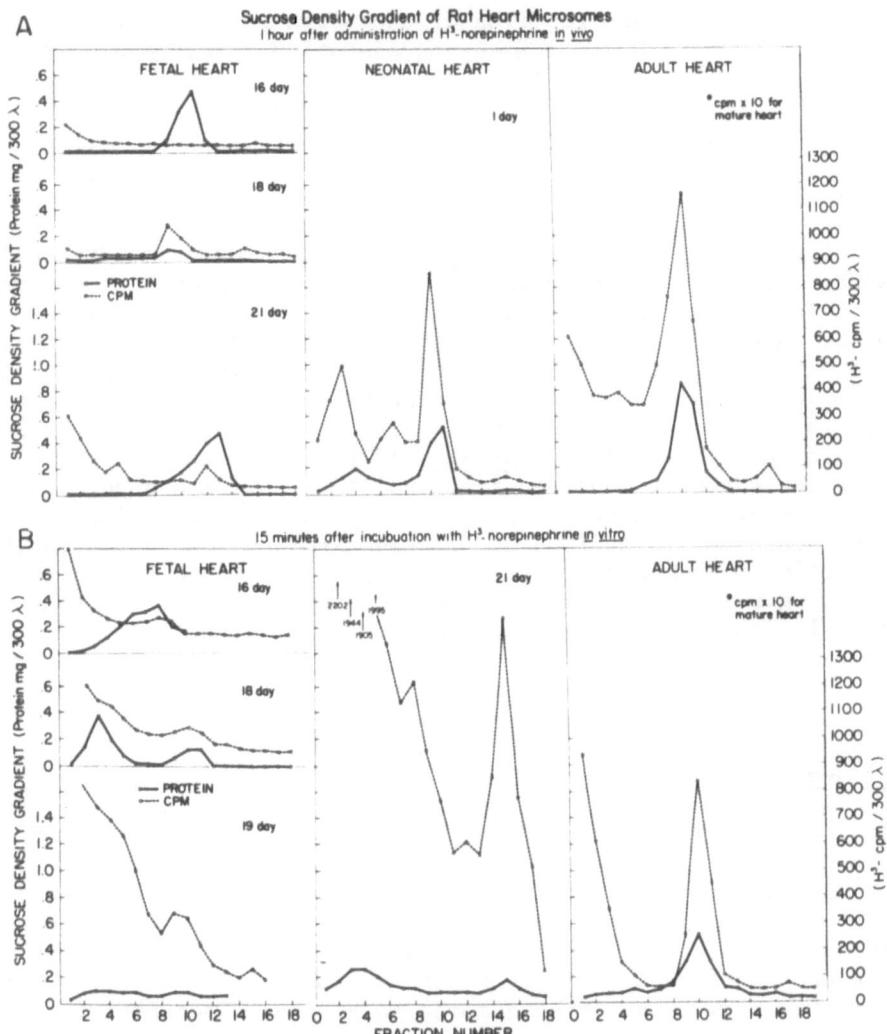

Fig. 2. A - In vivo uptake of ^{3}H-norepinephrine by fetal, neonatal and adult rat hearts. ^{3}H-norepinephrine was administered to pregnant rats (100 μC i.v.) and neonatal rats (0.1 μC/g i.p.). Animals were sacrificed one hour after injection. Sucrose density gradients (0.27M to 1.7M) used for subcellular fractionation. Ordinate, left: protein mg/300 μl (0——0); right: counts per minute ^{3}H/300 μl (0---0); Abscissa: density gradient fraction number.

B - In vitro uptake of ^{3}H-norepinephrine by fetal, neonatal and adult rat hearts. Tissues were incubated in oxygenated Nasmyth solution containing 1 μC/ml of ^{3}H-norepinephrine at 37°C. Assays were carried out after a 15 min. incubation. Sucrose density gradient, ordinate and abscissa as above. (From Mirkin, 1972).

suggests that the storage function of the adrenergic vesicle is not
manifest until the 19th or 21st day of gestation (Fig. 2A,B; Mirkin,
1972).

Ultrastructural Morphology

Fluorescence microscopy techniques have demonstrated the presence of catecholamine containing neurons in the rat heart (Schiebler
and Heene, 1968) and in the myenteric plexus of the rat gastrointesti-
nal tract (Reed and Burnstock, 1969) on the 12th and 15th days of
gestation, respectively. The histochemical fluorescence pattern of
the developing adrenergic neuron undergoes marked changes between the
15th and 21st days of gestation which probably indirectly reflects
alterations in its functional capacity for neurotransmitter synthesis, uptake and binding (Sachs et al., 1970). Electronmicrophoto-
graphs of the adrenergic neuron indicate that there are generally
more small, dense-cored vesicles in the terminal arborizations of
the neuron than in its cell body. It has also been demonstrated that
the proportion of osmiophilic to empty appearing organelles in the
adrenergic neuron is low during prenatal development and increases
substantially throughout postnatal existence (Elfvin, 1967).

Intravesicular Constituents

Nucleotides

The 18 day-old fetal rat adrenal gland has a low catecholamine
and ATP content. The levels of catecholamine in the adrenal gland
increase by a factor of 10 from day 18 to day 21 (parturition)
of gestation and about 150 times from birth to the 80th post-gesta-
tional day (O'Brien et al., 1972). In sharp contrast, the ATP concentration is constant from the 18th day of gestation until birth
and increases by only 19 fold from that period until adulthood. As
a consequence, the molar catecholamine to ATP ratio detected in the
adrenal glands are less than one prior to birth, achieves equivalency
at birth and increases to greater than one in the adult.

Intravesicular Soluble Proteins (Chromogranins)

While the life cycle of adrenergic vesicles has not been completely defined it appears as if they probably originate in the cell
body of the axon and move down the neuron via axoplasmic transport,
undergoing maturation enroute. The presence of enzymatically active
and inactive soluble proteins in the cytosol of mature adrenergic
vesicles has been clearly established by lysis of the vesicle and
analysis of its released contents. The antigenic potency of these
proteins differs. Some of them are extremely effective antigens
capable of developing antibodies with relatively high degrees of
specificity and of providing thereby a sensitive and selective method
for detecting small quantities of these proteins in tissue extracts
(Helle, 1966; Schneider et al., 1967).

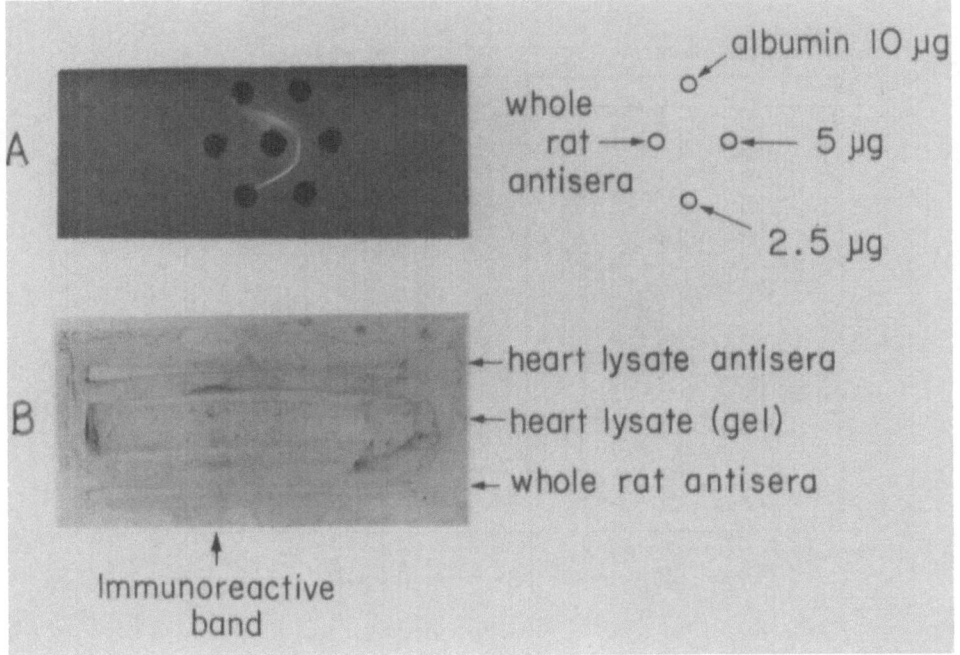

Fig. 3. Immunodiffusion patterns of serum albumin and heart lysate antigen reacted against whole rat antisera and heart lysate antisera. A: whole rat antisera versus serum albunim. B: unstained acrylamide electrophoretic gel of heart lysate antigen versus heart lysate antisera (upper trough) and whole rat antisera (lower trough). Note difference in intensity of immunoprecipitin line formed to each antisera.

The dominant protein in lysate preparations obtained from rat heart migrates anodally during immunoelectrophoresis in a manner similar to the albumins (Mirkin, 1972) but differs distinctly from serum albumin in its immunologic characteristics. The soluble protein in these lysates reacts strongly with its specific antibody in heart lysate antisera but extremely weakly or not at all to the antibodies in whole rat antisera (Fig. 3B). It should be noted that rat albumin forms a sharp precipitin line with whole rat antisera (Fig. 3A) demonstrating thereby the distinction between serum albumin and the immunoreactive protein in the rat heart lysates.

The temporal relationship between catecholamine uptake by the adrenergic neuron and the presence of immunoreactive intravesicular

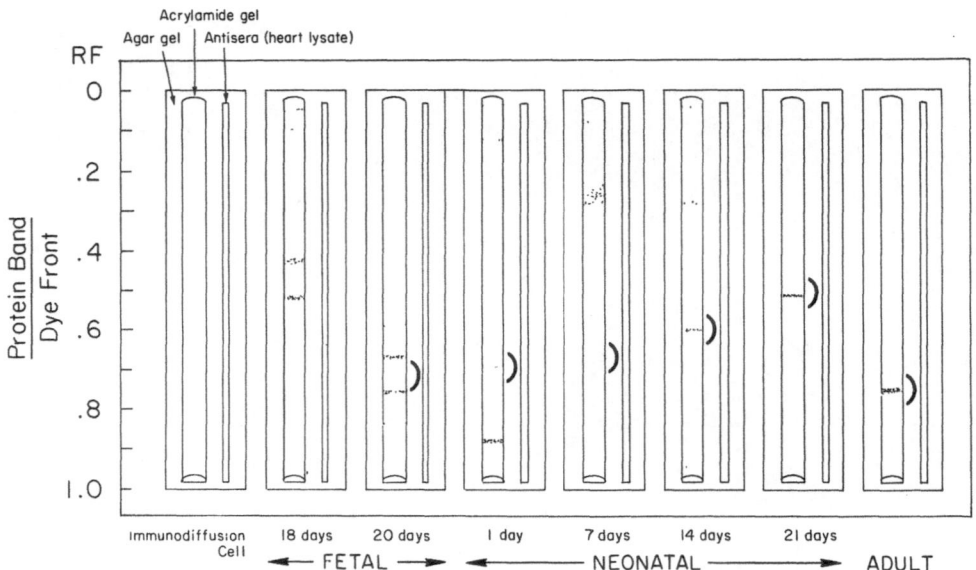

Fig. 4. Ontogenetic development of immunoreactive proteins in heart
lysates. Immunodiffusion pattern of acrylamide electrophoretic gels
of heart lysates from fetal, neonatal and adult rats reacted against
adult heart lysate antisera. Schematic diagram derived from experiments in which one-half of gel was stained and remainder utilized for
immuno-diffusion reaction. Only one immunoprecipitin band was detected at a point corresponding to an Rf of 0.65-0.70 (exception
21 day neonate). Heart lysate protein applied to each gel ranged
from 50 to 100 µg/gel.

soluble proteins has been studied during pre- and postnatal development. Adrenergic vesicles isolated from the rat heart were lysed and
the soluble proteins in the supernatant fluid (intravesicular sap)
initially electrophoresed on acrylamide gel. The gels were then reacted, by standard immunodiffusion techniques, against antisera prepared to chromogranins isolated from mature adrenergic vesicles. This
type of analysis permitted the detection of specific immunoreactive
bands in the lysates of subcellular fractions (adrenergic vesicles)
isolated from different tissues at various times in development.

These data indicate that the total number of soluble proteins
in vesicle lysates increases with advancing gestational and neonatal
age. However, only a single major immunoprecipitin band could be

identified under the experimental conditions of this study. Lysates prepared from 18 day-old fetal hearts did not form any detectable precipitin line whereas the 20 day-old fetal heart did react (Fig. 4). This corresponds to the stage in ontogenesis when uptake of ^{3}H-NE was initially demonstrable in the isolated fetal heart (Fig. 2B). The Rf of this immunoreactive band ranged between 0.65 and 0.70 with some variations noted in the 21 day-old neonate (Fig. 4). The striking temporal correlation between the presence of a specific immunoreactive protein in the lysates of adrenergic vesicles and the onset of catecholamine retaining capacity suggests that amine binding to intraneuronal organelles may require not only an intact, membrane-bound vesicle, but specific intravesicular constituents, amongst which are the chromogranins and probably ATP.

Reserpine administration markedly reduces the content of vitamin B_{12}-binding protein in gastric enterochromaffin-like cells (Hakanson et al., 1971), suggesting that an analogous situation might exist with respect to the adrenergic vesicle. Following treatment with reserpine, the uptake and binding of exogenous ^{3}H-NE by rat heart was virtually abolished; however, chromogranin could still be detected in adrenergic vesicle lysates prepared from these tissues. Since the immunologic assay employed was qualitative in nature, the actual amount of chromogranin present after the administration of reserpine could not be determined at this time (Mirkin, unpublished data). The continued presence of chromogranin in the reserpinized animal and its apparent immunologic similarity to chromogranin isolated from untreated controls (based upon their joint recognition by the same antibody) suggests that the attenuation of catecholamine binding produced by this drug may occur independently of an effect upon chromogranin.

Alternatively, it is possible that reserpine does alter the chromogranins in a manner not detectable by the methodology used in this study. Reserpine may incompletely deplete the adrenergic vesicle of its chromogranin content so that immunoprecipitin reactions are still present. If reserpine acts at an intravesicular site the alteration in molecular configuration or characteristics of the protein may be insufficient to prevent interaction with antibodies prepared to the original chromogranin.

The primary reason for proposing a long term influence by reserpine upon intravesicular components of the adrenergic vesicle stems from the report of Norn and Shore (1971), demonstrating that the binding of reserpine to rat heart consists of two distinct phases; an early reversibly bound phase temporally related to inhibition of the active intraneuronal amine-transport system; and a longer-lasting phase designated as irreversible, which appears to be associated with the sustained modification of storage mechanisms within the adrenergic vesicle. It is tempting to consider the latter interaction as

one occurring between reserpine and the intravesicular soluble proteins (chromogranins). Clarification of this issue must await the
development of immunologic or pharmacologic techniques which will
allow modification of adrenergic vesicular chromogranins during ontogenesis so that alterations in catecholamine binding can be correlated with qualitative and quantitative changes in the chromogranins.

ACKNOWLEDGEMENT

The investigations of the author were supported by USPHS
Grants NS-07255 and GM 01988.

REFERENCES

Banks, P. and Helle, K., 1971, Chromogranins in sympathetic nerves,
    Philos. Trans. R. Soc. Lond. B. Biol. 261: 305.

Banks, P. and Helle, K., 1965, The release of protein from the
    stimulated adrenal medulla, Biochem. J. 97: 40c.

Berneis, K.H., Goetz, U., Da Prada, M. and Pletscher, A., 1972,
    The binding of aggregated catecholamines and nucleotides to
    intragranular proteins, in press.

Berneis, K.H., Pletscher, A. and Da Prada, M., 1971, Interaction of
    proteins with aggregates of catecholamines and nucleotides:
    Possible biological implications, Agents and Actions 2: 65.

Berneis, K.H., Pletscher, A., Da Prada, M., 1969, Mental-dependent
    aggregation of biogenic amines: A hypothesis for their storage
    and release, Nature 224: 281.

Bisby, M.A. and Fillenz, M., 1971, The storage of endogenous nor-
    adrenaline in sympathetic nerve terminals, J. Physiol. 215:
    163.

Blaschko, H. and Welch, A.D., 1953, Localization of adrenaline in
    cytoplasmic particles of the bovine adrenal medulla, Arch.
    Exp. Path. Pharmacol. 219: 17.

Brunjes, S., Castner, E. and Hodgman, J., 1964, Catecholamine
    metabolism in newborn infants, Clin. Research 12: 88.

De Potter, W.P., Smith, A.D., De Schaepdryver, A.F., 1970, Subcell-
    ular fractionation of splenic nerve: ATP, chromogranin A and
    dopamine β-hyrdoxylase in noradrenergic vesicles, Tissue and
    Cell 2: 547.

Elfvin, L.G., 1967, The development of the secretory granules in the rat adrenal medulla, J. Ultrastruc. Res. 17: 45.

Euler, U.S.V., and Hillarp, N.A., 1956, Evidence for the presence of noradrenaline in submicroscopic structures of adrenergic axons, Nature, Lond. 177: 44.

Euler, U.S.V. and Lishajko, F., 1961, Noradrenaline release from isolated nerve granules, Acta. Physiol. Scand. 51: 193.

Friedman, W.F., 1969, Influence of the autonomic nervous system on the developing myocardium, adress presented to The Society for Pediatric Research, Proc. Ped. Research Soc.

Friedman, W.F., Pool, P.E., Jacobowitz, D., Seagren, S.C., and Braunwald, E., 1968, Sympathetic innervation of the developing rabbit heart, Circulation Res. 23: 25.

Geffen, L.B., Livett, B.G. and Rush, A.A., 1969, Immunological localization of chromogranins in sheep sympathetic neurones and their release by nerve impulses, J. Physiol. (Lond) 204: 58.

Gewirtz, G.P. and Kopin, I.J., 1970, Release of dopamine-beta-hydroxylase with norepinephrine during cat splenic nerve stimulation, Nature 227: 406.

Glowinski, J., Axelrod, J., Kopin, I.J., and Wurtman, R., 1964, Physiological disposition of ^{3}H-norepinephrine in the developing rat, J. Pharmacol. Exp. Ther. 146: 48.

Hakanson, R., Londstrand, K., Nordgren, L. and Owman, C., 1971, Reserpine-induced mobilization of histamine and vitamin B_{12}-binding proteins from a special type of endocrine cell in rat stomach, Biochem. Pharm. 20: 1259.

Helle, K.B., 1966, Some chemical and physical properties of the soluble protein fraction of bovine adrenal chromaffin granules, Mol. Pharmacol. 2: 298.

Hillarp, N.A., 1960, Different pools of catecholamine stored in the adrenal medulla, Acta. Physiol. Scand. 50: 8.

Hillarp, N.A. and Nilson, B., 1954, The structure of the adrenaline and noradrenaline containing granules in the adrenal medullary cells with reference to the storage and release of the sympathomimetic amines, Acta. Physiol. Scand. 31: supp. 113, 79.

Ignarro, L.J. and Shideman, F.E., 1968a, Appearance and concentra-
    tions of catecholamines and their biosynthesis in the embryo-
    nic and developing chick, J. Pharmacol. Exp. Ther. 159: 38.

Ignarro, L.J. and Shideman, F.E., 1968b, The requirement of sym-
    pathetic innervation for the active transport of norepineph-
    rine by the heart, J. Pharmacol. Exp. Ther. 159: 59.

Iversen, I., De Champlain, J., Glowinski, J. and Axelrod, J., 1967,
    Uptake, storage and metabolism of norepinephrine in tissues of
    the developing rat brain, J. Pharmacol. Exp. Ther. 157: 509.

Lagercrantz, H., 1971, Isolation and characterization of sympath-
    etic nerve trunk vesicles, Acta. Physiol. Scand. supp. 366: 1.

Lundborg, P., 1967, Studies on the uptake and subcellular distribu-
    tion of catecholamines and their α-methylated analogues,
    Acta. Physiol. Scand. suppl. 302.

Mirkin, B.L., 1972, Ontogenesis of the adrenergic nervous system:
    Functional and pharmacologic implications, Fed. Proc. 31: 65.

Mirkin, B.L. and Mueller, R., 1968, Binding of ^{3}H-norepinephrine
    to soluble proteins in adrenergic storage vesicles, Fed. Proc.
    27: 467.

Norn, S. and Shore, P., 1971, Further studies on the nature of per-
    sistent reserpine binding: Evidence for reversible and ir-
    reversible binding, Biochem. Pharm. 20: 1291.

O'Brien, R.A., Da Prada, M. and Pletscher, A., 1972, The onto-
    genesis of catecholamines and adenosine-5'-triphosphate in
    the adrenal medulla, Life. Sci. 11: 749.

Potter, L. and Axelrod, J., 1963, Properties of norepinephrine
    storage particles of the rat heart, J. Pharm. Exp. Ther.
    142: 299.

Reed, J.B. and Burnstock, G., 1969, A method for the localization
    of adrenergic nerves during early development, Histochemie
    20: 197.

Roth, R.H., Stjarne, L., Bloom, F.E. and Giarman, N.J., 1968, Light
    and heavy norepinephrine storage particles in the rat heart
    and in bovine splenic nerve, J. Pharmacol. Exp. Ther. 162: 203.

Sachs, C., De Champlain, J., Malmfors, T., and Olson, L., 1970,
    The postnatal development of noradrenaline uptake in the
    adrenergic nerves of different tissues from the rat, Eur. J.
    Pharmacol. 9: 67.

Sage, H., Smith, W. and Kirschner, N., 1967, A microquantitative
    immunologic assay for bovine adrenal catecholamine storage
    vesicle protein and its application to studies of the secre-
    tory provess, Mol. Pharmacol. 3: 81.

Schiebler, T.M. and Heene, R., 1968, Nachweis von katecholaminen in
    rattenherzen wahrend der entwicklung, Histochemie 14: 328.

Schneider, F.H., Smith, A.D. and Winkler, H., 1967, Secretion from
    the adrenal medulla: Biochemical evidence for exocytosis, Brit.
    J. Pharmacol. Chemother. 31: 94.

Smith, A.D., De Potter, W.P., Moerman, E.J. and De Schaepdryver, A.F.,
    1970, Release of dopamine-β-hyrdoxylase and chromagranin upon
    stimulation of the splenic nerve, Tissue Cell 2: 2547.

Smith, W.J. and Kirschner, N., 1967, A specific soluble protein
    from the catecholamine storage vesicles of bovine adrenal
    medulla, Mol. Pharmacol. 3: 52.

DRUG ACTIONS: BIOCHEMICAL DEVELOPMENT:
(Enzymes, Amino Acids, Proteins and Nucleic Acids)
Abel Lajtha, Chairman

ALTERATIONS OF PROTEIN METABOLISM DURING DEVELOPMENT OF THE BRAIN

Abel Lajtha and David Dunlop

New York State Research Institute for Neurochemistry

and Drug Addiction, Ward's Island, New York, N.Y.

Clearly development and the metabolism of macromolecules are closely linked phenomena, since growth is necessarily the result of altered protein and nucleic acid synthesis; similarly, mechanisms that control growth and those that control macromolecular metabolism must be closely linked, if not identical. Not surprisingly, this problem has attracted the interest of a number of laboratories during recent years, and many important findings are now available on the nervous system. Nevertheless, details of any mechanisms controlling sequence, regional variations, or functional organization of the development process still escape us. It is timely therefore to briefly discuss our present knowledge on changes in protein turnover during development.

CHANGES IN THE FREE AMINO ACID POOL

In measurements of protein turnover, the free amino acid pool has to be taken into account in estimating the specific activity of the precursor. Also it has been suggested that protein metabolism in the brain can be influenced by changes in amino acid levels (Roberts and Morelos, 1965; Roberts, 1968); thus it is important to keep in mind that great and complex changes occur in the level and possibly the distribution of cerebral amino acids during development. Changes in amino acid concentrations in brain during growth have been studied in some detail (Davis and Himwich, 1973; Agrawal et al., 1968), and it was shown that the concentrations go through maximal or minimal values nonlinearly during development (Vernadakis and Woodbury, 1962; Piccoli et al., 1971).

215

TABLE I

PERINATAL CHANGES IN THE FREE AMINO ACID POOL IN BRAIN*

	Foetus		Newborn		Adult
	15 d	19 d	0 h	24 h	
Taurine	14.1	12.2	14.1	15.6	6.64
Glutamic acid	7.54	5.71	4.81	5.02	10.1
Threonine	4.28	0.90	0.93	0.90	0.70
Alanine	5.08	3.01	4.29	0.80	0.51
Lysine	0.86	0.88	0.91	0.41	0.22
Proline	0.89	0.52	0.66	0.57	0.08

*From Lajtha and Toth (1973).

Freshly excised mouse brain was homogenized in one per cent perchloric acid and an aliquot of the extract was measured in an amino acid analyzer.

Values are expressed as μmoles amino acid per g brain tissue.

The types of changes that occur in the major constituents are illustrated in Table I. Some changes are gradual, as the increase in taurine and the decreases in lysine and proline from newborn to adult. Other changes are more dramatic, as the large decrease in threonine just before birth and in alanine just after birth. Complex patterns are also seen. Glutamic acid decreases in foetal life and then increases postnatally. Although blood amino acid levels also change from intrauterine to extrauterine life, they do not seem to be responsible for most of the changes in brain. The rapid changes in metabolically highly active amino acids such as threonine and alanine indicate changes in the metabolic utilization of these compounds at specific developmental periods, which deserve further detailed study. The general pattern, that glutamic acid and related compounds increase during development along with increasing complexity of metabolism while the concentration of many essential amino acids decreases with decreasing protein metabolism of the brain, shows that changes in metabolic utilization parallel metabolite levels during development; though the complex concentration changes shown in Table I would indicate that this may be an oversimplification.

TABLE II

AMINO ACID UPTAKE IN MICE AT DIFFERENT AGES*

Amino Acid	Age	μmoles amino acid per g tissue			
		Blood		Brain	
		Control	30 min	Control	30 min
Glycine	Newborn	0.61	8.66	3.61	4.86
	Adult	0.69	7.25	2.06	2.88
Aspartic	Newborn	0.08	6.68	1.85	2.22
Acid	Adult	0.14	12.80	3.55	3.93

*From Seta et al. (1972). Adult mice (30-35 g) were injected intraperitoneally with 200 μmoles of neutralized aspartate or glycine at 0 min and with 100 μmoles at 10 min and at 20 min. Newborn mice (2-3 g) received either 10 μmoles of aspartate at 0 min followed by an additional 5 μmoles at 10 min and at 20 min or a single injection of 20 μmoles of glycine at 0 min. At 30 min the animals were sacrificed. Free amino acids were extracted from samples of blood and homogenates of brain with perchloric acid and determined microbiologically.

CHANGES IN THE BRAIN BARRIER SYSTEM

Changes in brain permeability to amino acids, by altering the specific activity of the precursor free amino acid pool, not only influence measurements of protein metabolism, but by influencing the various compartments may affect protein metabolism itself. It has been shown with glutamic acid (Himwich et al., 1957), lysine (Lajtha, 1958), leucine (Lajtha and Toth, 1961), and tyrosine and tryptophan (Guroff and Udenfriend, 1964), that under similar conditions of administration of amino acids there is a larger increase in young than in adult brain. Such findings were interpreted in general to show the absence of any barriers in newborn. We recently reinvestigated differences in uptake between newborn and adults with ten additional amino acids, and in each case uptake by newborn brain was greater (Seta et al., 1972). This, however, does not prove the complete absence of barriers in young. Table II demonstrates the situation with amino acids which penetrate brain with difficulty. Although the increase in glycine is greater in young brain than adult and although higher levels of blood aspartate are required in adult to get a similar increase in brain concentrations, these amino acids do not reach equilibrium between blood and brain in the young. Slices from newborn brain are also capable of active amino acid transport, uptake against a concentration gradient (Levi et al., 1967). We interpreted the findings in vivo and in slices to mean that carriers and transport of metabolites are not absent in newborn brain but that a number of aspects of homeostatic control are not full developed in young animals (Seta et al., 1972).

Barriers exist not only between the brain and the circulation
but also within the brain itself. Many aspects of the distribution
of amino acids are determined not at capillary endothelial membranes
but at cell membranes and at the membranes of particulates within
the cells. A number of studies showed developmental changes in the
compartmentation of glutamic acid in the brain (Berl and Purpura,
1966; Patel and Balazs, 1970). The apparent absence of compartmentation at early stages indicates a weaker functional activity of
the intracellular membranes but does not prove their complete permeability to metabolites. In vitro, nuclear and mitochondrial fractions from newborn brain were capable of amino acid uptake against
a concentration gradient (Navon and Lajtha, 1969), showing the
presence of transport mechanisms at particulate membranes in brain
already at birth. All aspects of cerebral barriers, therefore -
restrictions to uptake, exit by active transport, exchange, regional
and particulate heterogeneity - can be expected to be less manifest
in young but not completely absent.

It has to be emphasized that in addition to quantitative changes
in membrane permeability, transport activity, etc., other developmental alterations may occur in the barrier system. An example of this
is the finding of two transport systems for GABA in young brain, one
of which becomes undetectable in the adult (Levi, 1970). Clearly
many similar complex changes may occur in affinities, specificity,
and metabolism, all of which may affect amino acid distribution.

PROTEIN TURNOVER IN ADULT BRAIN

General problems of protein metabolism of the nervous system
are beyond the scope of the present report, but a brief discussion
of the rate and the extent of protein turnover in adult brain is
necessary in any treatment of developmental changes. The dynamic
state of brain proteins has been well established (Lajtha and Marks,
1971), and several studies have attempted to measure turnover rates.
A major obstacle for precise rate estimates is the uncertainty in
measuring the true specific activity of the precursor. It seems
that, because of the heterogeneity of the intracellular free amino
acid pool, average acid soluble radioactivity in the tissue taken as
precursor is misleading. Recently Adamson et al. (1972) indicated
that the precursor amino acid for protein synthesis in embryonic
chick cartilage may be from the extracellular rather than the intracellular amino acid pool.

Recently we reexamined turnover rates in rats using continuous
intravenous infusion of labeled amino acids for up to nine hours
(Seta et al., 1973). Since slow infusion results in constant
specific activity of the amino acid in the plasma within 15 minutes,

TABLE III

INCORPORATION OF AMINO ACIDS INTO RAT BRAIN PROTEINS DURING INFUSION*

Amino Acid	Infusion (hours)	Incorpora- tion Rate	Amino Acid	Infusion (hours)	Incorpora- tion Rate
Valine	3	0.30	Arginine	2	0.37
	6	0.29		3	0.26
	9	0.30		6	0.25
Lysine	3	0.52	Leucine	3	0.82
	6	0.69		6	0.58
Tyrosine	3	0.67	Glycine	3	0.79
	6	0.70		6	0.80
Glutamic Acid	6	0.68			

*From Seta et al. (1973). A cannula was implanted in the femoral artery and amino acid infused intravenously into the rats at a rate which resulted in an essentially constant plasma specific radioactivity. The plasma specific radioactivity was determined by withdrawing samples of blood at several times during the infusion. At the times indicated the rats were sacrificed and the specific radioactivity of the free and protein bound amino acid determined. Incorporation rates are expressed as percent replacement of the protein bound amino acid per hour and are calculated over each interval of the infusion, i.e., 0-3 h, 3-6 h, and 6-9 h.

the equilibration of the various cerebral pools is more likely with this method than it is with methods involving changing specific activities. In addition we tested the infusion of several different amino acids, since it is not likely that each would have the same compartmentation. We also compared incorporation in the 0-3h period with that of the 3-6h period; since a greater degree of equilibration (lesser manifestation of compartmentation) can be expected in the longer time period. A summary of these infusion experiments (Table III) shows metabolic rates for two amino acids (valine, arginine) to be 0.3% per hour, for the other five tested (lysine, tyrosine, glutamate, leucine and glycine), 0.7% per hour. There was little difference in turnover rates between the 0-3h and 3-6h periods. During the infusion, metabolic conversion of the labeled amino acid is so rapid, that, although it was measured after chromatographic separation, and specific activities were corrected for metabolism, it introduces a 10-15 per cent error in the measurements. The average half-life of brain proteins in adults calculated from the values of Table III would be between 4 and 9 days, with an average of about 5 days. This half-life of 5 days indicates a considerably higher rate of turnover than the 14 days average half-life previously estimated with a single pulse dose (Lajtha, 1959, 1964), showing that in a single pulse experiment incorporation occurs from a pool with lower than average specific activity. A half-life of brain proteins of 4 days was estimated recently with infusion of tyrosine (Garlick and Marshall, 1972), and 3.5 days with several injections of ^{14}C glucose giving a steady specific activity of several cerebral amino acids up to 8h (Austin et al., 1972). It has to be realised that even with a half-life of 4 days, experiments of 6-9 hours measure incorporation into only a small percentage of the total brain proteins. These experiments indicate that metabolically very active fractions with a half-life of less than 3 hours could be only a very low percentage of the total.

We tested in a separate set of experiments the metabolic stability of brain proteins. Mice were fed with a diet that contained ^{14}C lysine of constant specific activity. After about 2 weeks, when plasma lysine reached the specific activity of the diet, the animals were mated. They were fed the same labeled diet throughout pregnancy, and to the offspring, throughout growth, causing all protein-bound lysine to be labeled with the specific activity present in the diet. Then the labeled diet was exchanged for a non-labeled one, and the rate of decay of label was measured (Lajtha and Toth, 1966). Table IV illustrates the results of these experiments, which led to two main conclusions: a) Since all cerebral proteins were labeled at the beginning (0 day) of these experiments and after 150 days very little radioactivity remained, at least 98% of brain proteins are in a dynamic state (are actively turning over); b) The average half-life from decay is 16 days. Decay type experiments measure the lower limit of turnover rate values since they do not measure the part of turnover involving reincorporation of the labeled amino acid released by breakdown. The 16 days half-life calculated from Table IV means therefore that the greater part of brain proteins have a half-life of 16 days or less.

Putting together the results of Tables III and IV demonstrates that the half-life of 90% or more of brain proteins is between 1 and 16 days.

The high rate of protein metabolism in itself may cause an apparent compartmentation of the free amino acid pool. A half-life of 4 days would mean a rate of metabolism that incorporates the total content of the free pool of a number of amino acids in an hour or less. If the rate of exchange between free pools of brain and plasma is lower than this rate (half-life of free pool lower than 30 min), then protein turnover would keep the cerebral pool specific activities below that of plasma for a considerable time. We did observe that even after 6h infusion many amino acids in the brain were not in equilibrium with plasma (Seta et al., 1973).

TABLE IV

DECREASE IN PROTEIN-BOUND RADIOACTIVITY IN MOUSE BRAIN WITH TIME*

Experimental time, days	Counts/min/ μmoles lysine	% of original activity left
0	30	100
30	8.8	29
60	2.1	7.0
150	0.7	2.4

*From Lajtha and Toth (1966).

Mice were fed throughout their development (prenatal and postnatal) with a diet containing ^{14}C lysine of constant specific activity (30 counts/μmole lysine). At the beginning of the experiment (0 day) the diet was replaced by one containing unlabeled lysine and the animals were sacrificed 30, 60 and 150 days later. a 75% drop of label in 28 days corresponds to a decay half-life of 14 days.

DEVELOPMENTAL CHANGES IN PROTEIN METABOLISM

Although changes of incorporation during growth have been investigated in some detail in vivo as well as in vitro (for recent reviews see Roberts et al., 1971; Lajtha and Marks, 1971), we reinvestigated incorporation in vivo in young under such conditions that turnover can be compared to adult infusion experiments. Because it was not possible to use constant infusion in young, an alternative technique was adopted - the intraperitoneal injection of a very large dose of labeled amino acid, well in excess of the total body free amino acid content (Dunlop et al., in preparation). This technique results in a large increase in tissue free amino acids, and the flooding dose keeps specific activities in the tissue free pool fairly constant, since the contribution to dilution from the endogenous pool is small. This method has the disadvantage that increased tissue amino acid could affect the rate of protein metabolism, but its advantage is that the specific activity of the free amino acid pool of the whole body is kept fairly constant with a single intraperitoneal injection. The rate of incorporation of valine measured by this method decreased to about one third from the 8th to the 37th day of age in rats (Table V); in this period, the net deposition of protein in the brain also decreased to very low levels by 37 days of age. By subtracting the net deposition of

TABLE V

CHANGES IN PROTEIN METABOLISM IN RAT BRAIN WITH AGE

(mg protein metabolized per 100 mg tissue protein per hour)

Age (days)	Cerebral Hemisphere			Cerebellum		
	Incorporation	Deposition	Breakdown	Incorporation	Deposition	Breakdown
8	1.71	0.46	1.25	2.06	1.26	0.80
18	0.88	0.18	0.70	1.06	0.28	0.78
37	0.58	0.01	0.57	0.60	0.01	0.59

Incorporation rates were determined following intraperitoneal injection of 15 μmoles valine per g body weight to rats. Deposition rates were determined by measuring the protein content of brain at different ages; the growth curves of protein are relatively straight lines around the ages shown, so that deposition rates can be fairly accurately calculated. Breakdown represents the difference between incorporation and deposition. Values are expressed as per cent change per hour; incorporation was measured in a 60 min period.

TABLE VI

INCORPORATION OF VALINE IN VARIOUS RAT BRAIN AREAS
(n moles valine incorporated per mg protein per hour)

Age (days)	Cortex	Midbrain	Pons-medulla	Cerebellum	Cord
2	8.2	7.6	7.5	9.3	7.8
18	4.4	4.2	4.7	5.2	4.6
37	2.8	2.8	2.8	3.0	2.8

Rats were injected intraperitoneally with 12 μmoles ^{14}C-L-valine per g body weight, sacrificed and the radioactivity incorporated per mg brain protein determined. Hydrolysis and amino acid analysis show that most of the radioactivity in the protein is in valine at incorporation times of 30 to 90 min. Under these conditions the specific activity of the free valine in the brain approaches that of the valine injected. Rates of incorporation are then calculated on the basis of the specific activity of the injected valine. Rates given are averages of determinations at 30, 60 and 90 min.

protein from incorporation, turnover could be calculated. Protein turnover - the amount of synthesis equal to that of breakdown - also decreased with development, which indicates that not only synthesis but also the catabolic portion (breakdown) of turnover is more active in young than in adult brain. The more rapid net deposition of protein in cerebellum than in cerebrum at 8 days seems to be due more to the lower rate of breakdown than to greatly increased synthesis in the cerebellum (Table V). It should be noted that this method measures the disappearance of protein, and if significant amounts of protein are moved out of the cells and leave the organ without being broken down, then the rates measured are not equivalent to degradation.

When the decrease in incorporation with this method was tested in several brain areas, the developmental decrease in protein turnover seemed to be fairly similar in the areas tested, and adult values were reached in all areas by 37 days in rats (Table VI).

Developmental changes in brain protein metabolism can be studied in greater detail in isolated systems. Although the rates of synthesis are greatly diminished in such systems, and control mechanisms are probably altered, in vitro experiments open the possibility of studying each element of protein metabolism separately (Cain et al., 1972; Gilbert et al., 1972). Changes in ribosomal structure and stability were among those found during development (Roberts, 1971); changes in the living brain are now sought, to connect the findings of in vitro systems with in vivo occurrences.

TABLE VII

THE DEPENDENCE OF INCORPORATION OF VALINE IN BRAIN
ON AMBIENT TEMPERATURE

Age, days	n moles valine incorporated/mg protein/h	
	37°	25°
2	7.5	3.7
7	7.2	3.8
14	5.9	5.5
21		4.2

Following the intraperitoneal injection of 15 μmoles ^{14}C
valine per g body weight rats were put in a container that was
placed in a water bath at 25 or $37^{\circ}C$. After 1h the brain was homogenized in 5% trichloroacetic acid, lipids and nucleic acids were
removed from the protein precipitate. The specific activity of
valine was determined with an amino acid analyzer and liquid scintillation counter.

Changes in protein metabolism are probably connected with
changes in composition. Obviously there may be more rapid turnover
in young brain, either because there is a higher proportion of the
metabolically more active proteins in the young brain or because the
same proteins are metabolized faster in young; or these possibilities
may occur simultaneously. Evidence of changes in composition is
accumulating (Cicero et al., 1972) as methods identifying and analyzing specific brain proteins improve. An important finding not pur-
sued in further detail showed that some of the changes in protein
metabolism depend on the date of birth rather than on the stage of
development (Shain et al., 1967), the change from intrauterine to
extrauterine environment having an important influence on protein
turnover rates.

SOME ALTERATIONS OF PROTEIN METABOLISM IN YOUNG BRAIN

Of particular importance to the subject of the present book
is whether protein metabolism in young brain shows a different sensitivity to environmental alterations and drugs than adult. Such
differences can be expected especially in brain, where in the young
there is active cell division and in the adult it is practically
absent. This explains special sensitivity to nutritional deficiencies

TABLE VIII

INCORPORATION OF AMINO ACIDS IN VIVO AND IN BRAIN SLICES

Age (days)	n moles incorporated/mg protein/h in vivo	in slices	Slice % in vivo
3	7.5	6.8	91
7	7.4	5.6	76
9	7.6	5.3	70
14	5.8	3.4	59
Adult	2.5	0.5	20

Incorporation rates in vivo were determined as in Table V. For incorporation in vitro 0.5 mm thick brain slices were incubated in a Krebs Ringer-Hepes buffer medium in 8 mM valine at 37° for 1 h. The specific activity of free and protein bound valine was determined in vivo and in vitro as described in the legends to Table VI.

such as restricted protein diet (Zamenhof et al., 1968), which re- sults in permanent effects if it occurs during the period of active cell division. It seems to be well established that early nutritional deficiency can result in a permanent deficit in brain proteins and in brain cell numbers. In a preliminary study we found a strong temperature dependence of amino acid incorporation into brain pro- teins that disappears with development (Table VII); when 2-day-old rats were kept at 25°, incorporation was only half of that at 37°. Several factors, for example, energy supply, compartmentation, trans- port, or the rate of protein metabolism may be altered directly; but temperature effect has to be kept in mind in any experimentation measuring incorporation in young. The decrease of sensitivity to environmental temperature changes in turn may be the result of better body temperature control in older animals.

Detailed discussion of effects in isolated systems are beyond the scope of this article; however, one observation can be briefly discussed, in view of the usually greatly diminished rates of protein synthesis in isolated systems. If incorporation of amino acids is compared between slices of brain and brain in vivo, differences are much smaller in young than in adult (Table VIII). Incorporation in slices from 3-day-old rats proceeds almost at the rate in the living brain, while in adult incorporation in vitro is only 1/5th of that in vivo. Such differences in development may be very useful for

studying the controls of protein turnover and the development of
these controls; it seems that processes that are damaged upon preparation of slices are not present in young brain.

CONCLUSIONS

In spite of the great interest in cerebral protein metabolism,
and of the several studies measuring rates of synthesis, the accuracy
of our methods of measurement is still open to some question. The
complexity of the various pools of free amino acid in the brain is
yet to be completely unravelled. In a sense, we are still not certain of the precursor specific activity. When one considers development, it is clear that many of the factors that complicate measurements of rates at any given age are undergoing change. It is therefore necessary to exercise caution in the interpretation of experimental data on rates of synthesis, changes in such rates associated
with development, and effects of drugs on the rates measured.

Though the results are not equivocable, different types of
experiments appear to be converging on a rate of incorporation in
the adult of approximately 0.5 to 0.7 per cent per hour, that is
fairly linear up to 9 hours. Although this value represents incorporation into a small fraction (5 to 6 per cent) of brain proteins,
and is an average of many divergent turnover values, it indicates a
dynamic state of brain proteins. In combination with studies that
measured 16 days as an upper limit of turnover for the major portion
of brain proteins, the turnover rate of most proteins appears to be
between one and sixteen days in the adult brain.

Many results converge also on the fact that protein turnover is
more active in the young than in the adult brain. A number of factors
can be analyzed that may be causative, expecially in _in vitro_ systems.
We hope that some of the conclusions we made will also be valid for
the living brain. Because active cell division occurs only in early
stages of development, the brain is more sensitive in these stages,
and some effects on the brain are known to permanently alter cell
numbers and protein content. Since homeostatic controls are not as
well developed in the young, incorporation into brain proteins seems
to be easier to alter. It is not clearly established, however,
whether this indicates a greater sensitivity of the synthetic mechanism.

The data presently available on _in vitro_ rates of protein breakdown depend more on the methods of measuring synthesis than on direct
measurement of degradation, but the indications are that protein
breakdown also shown changes with development.

ACKNOWLEDGMENTS

This work was supported in part by U.S. Public Health Service Research Grant NS-03226 from the National Institute of Neurological Diseases and Stroke.

REFERENCES

Adamson, L.F., Herington, A.L., and Bornstein, J., 1972, Evidence for the selection by the membrane transport system of intra- cellular or extracellular amino acids for protein synthesis, Biochim. Biophys. Acta 282: 352-365.

Agrawal, H.C., Davis, J.M., and Himwich, W.A., 1968, Developmental changes in mouse brain: weight, water content and free amino acids, J. Neurochem. 15: 917-923.

Austin, L., Lowry, O.H., Brown, J.G., and Carter, J.G., 1972, The turnover of protein in discrete areas of rat brain, Biochem. J. 126: 351-359.

Berl, S., and Purpura, D.P., 1966, Regional development of glutamic acid compartmentation in immature brain, J. Neurochem. 13: 293-304.

Cain, D.F., Ball, E.D., and Dekaban, A.S., 1972, Brain proteins: qualitative and quantitative changes, synthesis and degradation during fetal development of the rabbit, J. Neurochem. 19: 2031-2042.

Cicero, T.J., Ferendelli, J.A., Suntreff, V., and Moore, B.W., 1972, Regional changes in CNS levels of the S-100 and 14-3-2 proteins during development and aging of the mouse, J. Neurochem. 19: 2119-2125.

Davis, J.M., and Himwich, W.A., 1973, Amino acids and proteins in the developing brain, in "Biochemistry of the Developing Brain" (W.A. Himwich, ed.) Marcel Dekker, New York.

Garlick, P.J., and Marshall, I., 1972, A technique to measure brain protein synthesis, J. Neurochem. 19: 577-583.

Gilbert, B.E., Grove, B.K., and Johnson, T.C., 1972, Characteristics and products of a cell free polypeptide synthesizing system from neonatal and adult mouse brain, J. Neurochem. 19: 2835-2842.

Guroff, G., and Udenfriend, S., 1964, The uptake of aromatic amino acids by the brain of mature and newborn rats, in "Progress in Brain Research", vol. 9, The Developing Brain, (W.A. Himwich and H.A. Himwich, eds.), pp. 187-197, Elsevier, Amsterdam.

Himwich, W.A., Petersen, J.C., and Allen, M.L., 1957, Hematoencepha-
    litic exchange as a function of age, Neurology (Minneapolis)
    7: 705-710.

Lajtha, A., 1958, Amino acid and protein metabolism of the brain.
    II. The uptake of L-lysine by brain and other organs of the
    mouse at different ages, J. Neurochem. 2: 209-215.

Lajtha, A., 1959, Amino acid and protein metabolism of the brain.
    V. Turnover of leucine in mouse tissues, J. Neurochem. 3:
    358-365.

Lajtha, A., 1964, Protein metabolism of the nervous system, in
    "International Review Neurobiology", vol. 6, (C.C. Pfeiffer
    and J.R. Smythies, eds.), pp. 1-98, Academic Press, New York.

Lajtha, A., and Marks, N., 1971, Protein turnover, in "Handbook of
    neurochemistry", vol. 5, (A. Lajtha, ed.), pp. 551-629, Plenum
    Press, New York.

Lajtha, A., and Piccoli, F., 1971, Alterations related to the cere-
    bral free amino acid pool during development, in "Cellular
    Aspects of Neural Growth and Differentiation", (D.C. Pease,
    ed.), pp. 419-432, University of California Press, Los Angeles.

Lajtha, A., and Toth, J., 1961, The brain barrier system. II. Uptake
    and transport of amino acids by the brain, J. Neurochem. 8:
    216-225.

Lajtha, A., and Toth, J., 1966, Instability of cerebral proteins,
    Biochem. Biophys. Res. Comm. 23: 294-298.

Lajtha, A., and Toth, J., 1973, Perinatal changes in the free amino
    acid pool of the brain in mice, Brain Research, in press.

Levi, G., 1970, Cerebral amino acid transport in vitro during develop-
    ment: a kinetic analysis, Arch. Biochem. Biophys. 138: 347-349.

Levi, G., Kandera, J., and Lajtha, A., 1967, Control of cerebral
    metabolic levels. I. Amino acid uptake and levels in various
    species, Arch. Biochem. Biophys. 119: 303-311.

Navon, S., and Lajtha, A., 1969, The uptake of amino acids by par-
    ticulate fractions from brain, Biochim. Biophys. Acta 173:
    518-531.

Patel, R.J., and Balazs, R., 1970, Manifestation of metabolic com-
    partmentation during the maturation of the rat brain,
    J. Neurochem. 17: 955-971.

Piccoli, F., Grynbaum, A., and Lajtha, A., 1971, Developmental
    changes in Na^+, K^+, and ATP and in the levels and transport
    of amino acids in incubated slices of rat brain, J. Neurochem.
    18: 1135-1148.

Roberts, S., 1968, Influence of elevated circulating levels of amino
    acids on cerebral concentrations and utilization of amino acids,
    in "Brain Barrier Systems", Progress in Brain Research, vol. 29,
    (A. Lajtha and D.H. Ford, eds.), pp. 235-243, Elsevier,
    Amsterdam.

Roberts, S., 1971, Protein synthesis, in "Handbook of Neurochemistry,"
    Vol. 5, (A. Lajtha, ed.) pp 1-48, Plenum Press, New York.

Roberts, S., and Morelos, B.S., 1965, Regulation of cerebral meta-
    bolism of amino acids. IV. Influence of amino acid levels on
    leucine uptake, utilization and incorporation into protein
    in vivo, J.Neurochem. 12: 373-387.

Roberts, S., Zomzely, C.E., and Bondy, S.C., 1971, Developmental
    alterations in cerebral ribonucleic acid and protein synthesis,
    in "Cellular aspects of neural growth and differentiation,
    (D.C. Pease, ed.), pp. 447-471, University of California Press,
    Los Angeles.

Schain, R.J., Carver, M.J., Copenhaver, J.H., and Underdahl, N.R.,
    1967, Protein metabolism in the developing brain: Influence of
    birth and gestational age, Science 156: 984-986.

Seta, K., Sershen, H., and Lajtha, A., 1972, Cerebral amino acid
    uptake in vivo in newborn mice, Brain Research 47: 415-425.

Seta, K., Sansur, M., and Lajtha, A., 1973, The rate of incorporation
    of amino acids into brain proteins during infusion in the rat,
    Biochim. Biophys. Acta 294: 472-480.

Vernadakis, A., and Woodbury, D.M., 1962, Electrolyte and amino acid
    changes in rat brain during maturation, Am. J. Physiol. 203:
    748-752.

Zamenhof, S., van Marthens, E., and Margolis, F.L., 1968, DNA (cell
    number) and protein in neonatal brain: Alteration by maternal
    dietary protein restrictions, Science 160: 322-323.

FREE AMINO ACIDS IN THE DEVELOPING BRAIN AS AFFECTED BY DRUGS

Williamina A. Himwich[1] and Jimmie M. Davis

Thudichum Psychiatric Research Laboratory, Galesburg

State Research Hospital, Galesburg, Illinois

INTRODUCTION

As Nyhan (1961) pointed out, the effects of most drugs in children are sufficiently different from those seen at older ages and in the adult to warrant considerable systematic investigation. Not only are the differences between the young and the adult of importance, but the timing and patterns of changes which occur as the animal matures are also of importance. During the period of rapid brain development the free amino acid pool in the brain serves as a source of building material for the brain proteins, and in addition some members such as glutamate are used for energy, while others such as GABA serve as neurotransmitters. Any disturbance of the delicate balance among the free amino acids can be expected to affect many reactions necessary to the unimpeded development of the brain. How serious these may be, we have as yet no means of determining. The data presented below are the result of some of our efforts to study these factors.

INSULIN

Although many studies have demonstrated that a depletion of glutamic acid occurs in insulin hypoglycemia and is concomitant with an increase in aspartic acid and a decrease in GABA (Cravioto et al., 1951; Dawson, 1950; Massieu et al., 1962), no systematic longitudinal investigations of insulin hypoglycemia had been made up to the time Davis et al. (1970) undertook the following study.

---

[1]Present address: University of Nebraska, College of Medicine,
Omaha, Nebraska 68105

TABLE I

EFFECT OF INSULIN HYPOGLYCEMIA ON SOME RAT BRAIN AMINO ACIDS DURING DEVELOPMENT

Amino Acid	Age (days after birth)							
	6 Day Old		12 Day Old		25 Day Old		Adult	
	Control (6)	Exptl (6)	Control (6)	Exptl (6)	Control (6)	Exptl (6)	Control (6)	Exptl (6)
Glutamic Acid	5.10 ± 0.91[a]	2.98 ± 0.88[b]	11.18 ± 0.76[b]	4.69 ± 0.18[b]	11.19 ± 1.87	10.69 ± 1.17	11.06 ± 0.43	8.28 ± 0.97[b]
Aspartic Acid	1.44 ± 0.15	4.53 ± 0.61[b]	3.30 ± 0.20	3.84 ± 0.64	3.66 ± 0.81	4.43 ± 0.62	2.79 ± 0.20	4.62 ± 0.57[b]
GABA	1.36 ± 0.13	1.05 ± 0.36	1.44 ± 0.14	1.15 ± 0.29	3.36 ± 0.20	3.52 ± 0.16	3.77 ± 0.32	2.89 ± 0.16[b]

[a]values are means ± SEM, expressed as μmoles/g of wet weight tissue; number of rats are given in parentheses.

[b]values significantly different from controls. (Adapted from Davis et al., 1970.)

Wistar strain albino rats maintained under a regimen described elsewhere (Davis et al., 1970) were given 100 U/kg of insulin. Control animals received an equivalent injection(s) of physiological saline. In the experimental animal the end point was considered to be the onset of convulsions 3 to 4 hr postinjection, and if necessary, enough additional insulin was given to produce convulsions. The results therefore embody both the effects of insulin per se and of the resultant convuslions. In all experimental groups the terminal blood sugar levels were between 20 and 15 mg%. Only slight changes were seen in the water and protein contents of the brain, and in body and brain weights. The changes in brain amino acid levels were directly related to age. Glutamic acid was markedly reduced at all ages except 25 days. The reduction was approximately 40% at 6 days, 60% at 12 days, but only 25% in the adult (Table I). Aspartic acid increased to approximately 300, 116, and 160% of the control values in the same age groups respectively. The increases for 6 days and for the adult are both significant (Table I). GABA remained essentially unchanged except in the adult animals, in which it fell to 79% of the control value. These data suggest that in the 6-day-old animal the pathway from glutamic to aspartic acid is well developed, while that to GABA is either not developed or the concentration of GABA is of such importance that it is maintained at a fairly constant level. The nearly threefold increase in GABA in the control animals between 6 days and adult life is especially interesting. Although little effect on the level of aspartic acid was seen at 12 days of age, GABA was also relatively unchanged. In the adult, glutamate was only slightly reduced, aspartic was moderately increased, but GABA was decreased significantly (Table I) - almost a reversal of the picture in the 6-day-old animal. At 25 days of age the effect of insulin hypoglycemia on the concentrations of any of these related metabolites was minimal. On the other hand Dravid and Jílek (1965) found that stagnant hypoxia produced the greatest effect on these metabolites in the 25-day-old animal. These data, taken with those of Davis et al., (1970), suggest that preferred metabolic pathways in the 25-day-old animal may differ significantly both from those in the adult and in the young. Both our data and those of Dravid and Jílek (1965) indicate that this difference probably begins as early as the 12th day of life.

Massieu et al. (1962) suggested on the basis of experiments with animals simultaneously receiving desoxypyridine and a pyrodoxine deficient diet that an important pathway for glutamic acid during insulin hypoglycemia is not via decarboxylation and that the passage of glutamic acid to the TCA cycle during insulin hypoglycemia is mainly via α-ketoglutarate. Although glutamic acid is reduced significantly at all ages except 12 days during insulin hypoglycemia, GABA was reduced significantly only in the adult. Therefore, GABA pathway apparently was unimportant in the infant but of relatively greater importance in the adult. The concomitant increase in aspartate

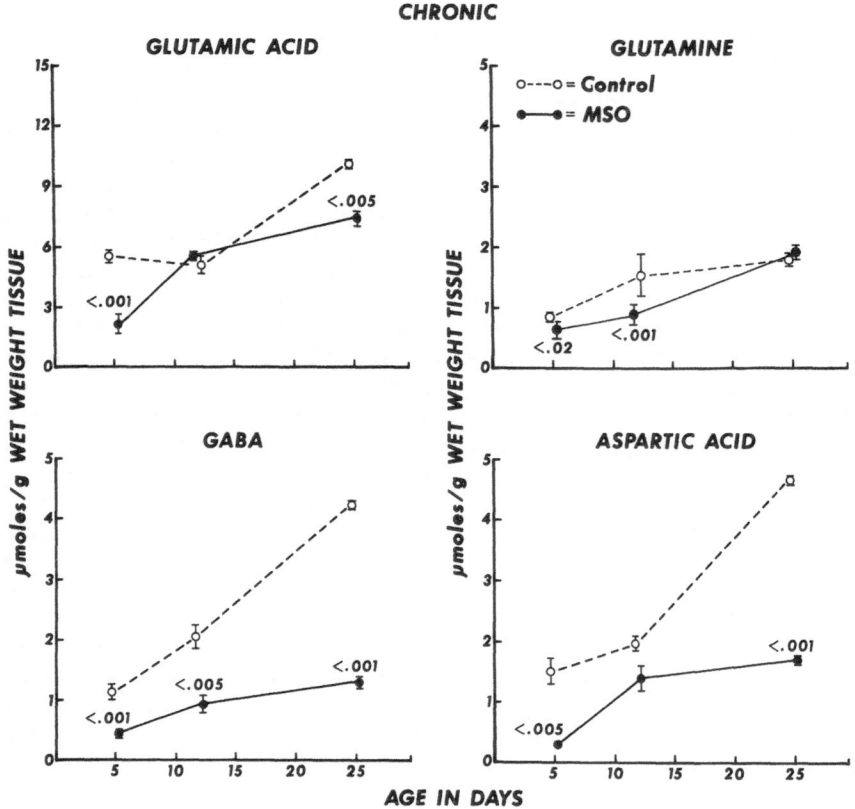

Fig. 1. The effects of the chronic administration of MSO on amino
acid levels in the brain of the young rat. From 1 day of age 40 mg/kg
of MSO wa injected intraperitoneally every other day. Each point
is the mean (± SEM) of 6 determinations. All animals were killed 24
hours after last injection.

is more difficult to explain since the newly formed α-ketoglutarate
would be assumed to be funneled directly into the TCA cycle under
conditions of insulin hypoglycemia. Aspartate arises from the trans-
amination of glutamic acid with pyruvic and oxaloacetic acids and
could presumably enter the cycle through oxaloacetic acid. Even if
this pathway is available, it is not clear why aspartic acid accumulates to a marked degree in the young brain but to a lesser extent in
the adult. Roberts (1960) suggested that the combination of oxaloacetic acid with acetyl CoA leading to citrate is depressed so more
oxaloacetic acid is available for combination with glutamate thus
leading to increased aspartic and α-ketoglutaric acid. Under this
condition aspartic acid is a dead end as the equilibrium appears to
favor its formation but not its metabolism. This situation appears
to be more acute in the young (6-day-old), to be somewhat alleviated

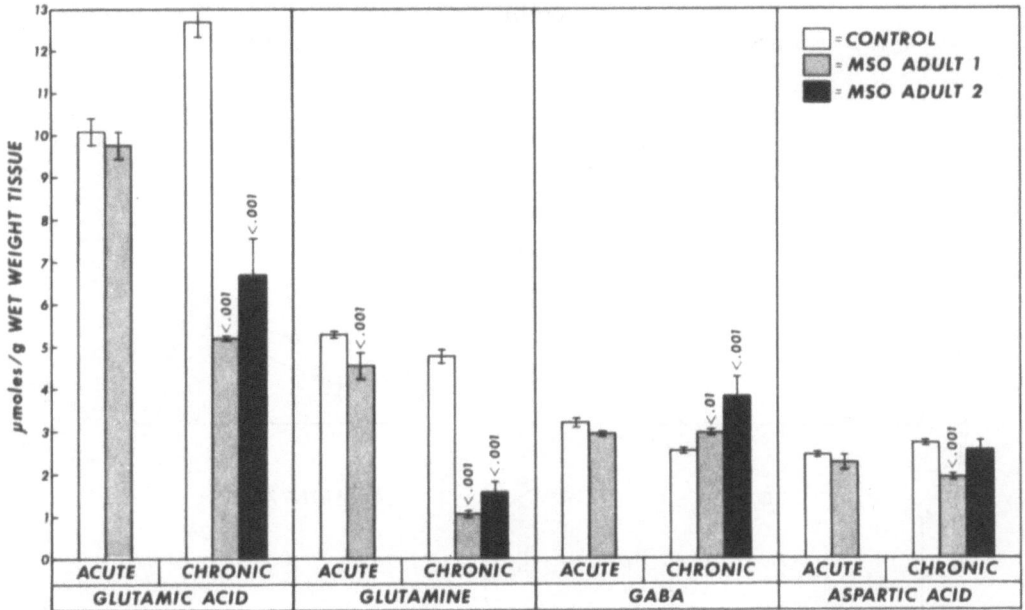

Fig. 2.   The effects of the acute and chronic administration of MSO
on amino acid levels in the brain of the adult rat.   Groups 1 and 2
received three intraperitoneal injections of 40 mg/kg of MSO every
24 and 48 hours respectively; the "acute" group received a single
injection.   The bars represent the means ± SEM of 6 determinations.
All animals were killed 24 hours after last injection.

---

at 12 days of age, and to reoccur to a lesser degree in the adult.
Systematic studies of the enzymes involved would be necessary to
elucidate the reasons for these differences.

METHIONINE SULFOXAMINE

Methionine sulfoxamine (MSO), a known inhibitor of glutamine
synthetase, was studied chronically in young rats of the same strain
and maintained under the same conditions as those given insulin.   From
day one until the day they were killed, a dose of 40 mg/kg was given
intraperitoneally every other day.   Adult animals received 3 injections; in group 1 the drug was administered every 24 hrs, and in
group 2 every 48 hrs.   Control animals received equivalent injections
of physiological saline.

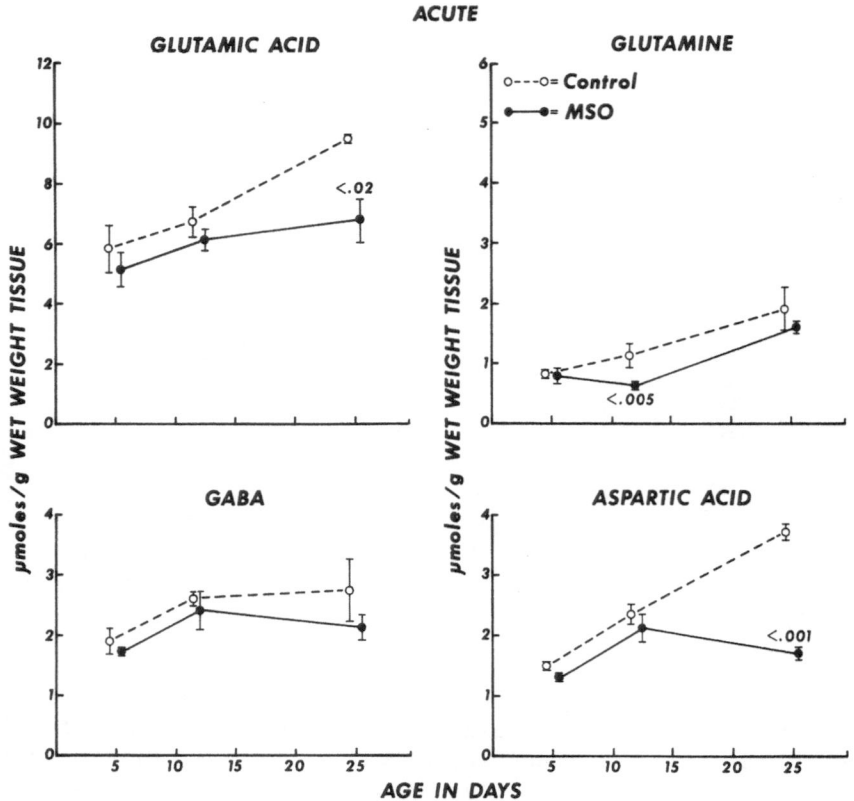

Fig. 3. The effects of a single intraperitoneal injection of MSO on
amino acid levels in the brain of rats 5, 11 and 25 days of age. Each
point (± SEM) is the mean of 6 determinations. All animals were
killed 24 hours after last injection.

The chronic administration of MSO produced depressions in the
levels of GABA and aspartic acid up to 11 days of age. However, less
than the expected effect was seen on glutamine. In the case of this
compound the chronic administration after 12 days apparently had no
effect (Fig. 1). In attempting to interpret these data it is important to remember that the older animals received a greater total
amount of MSO than the younger; for example, animals killed at 26
days received an injection every other day from day one, i.e., 14
injections, while those killed at day 12 received 6 injections.

The effects of MSO on chronically treated adults were very different from those in the young animal (Fig. 2). The drug depressed
both glutamic and glutamine levels, slightly elevated GABA and had
little effect on aspartic acid.

In contrast to the chronically treated young animals, in those
receiving a single injection of MSO on days 5 and 25 the expected
depressant effect on the glutamine level was observed, but differences
from the control values were not significant at day 25 (Fig. 3). At
12 days, however, the values for control and experimental animals
were 1.17 ± 0.02 and 0.67 ± 0.07 with $P < .005$. The glutamic acid level
also fell, but only at 25 days did the difference approach statistical
significance. The decrease in GABA was negligible, but that in aspartic was significant at 25 days. Although the levels of these four
compounds were depressed in general, most of the differences from the
control levels were not significant.

These data suggest that at these low doses, the effects of the
drug in the young and in the adult animal were different. If the
effects of chronic and acute administration in the adult were not
so similar, i.e., depression of glutamine (Fig. 2, all groups)
and of glutamic acid, the explanation could be sought in some physiologic accomodation to the chronic administration. In the case of
aspartic acid the adults receiving 3 injections of MSO 24 hours apart;
i.e., Group I, resembled the animals receiving one injection, i.e.,
acute. However, Group II adults (injections 48 hours apart) did not
show a depression of aspartic acid. The group II animals also showed
a changed pattern in respect to GABA. The relatively small changes
in GABA and the difference for this amino acid between the control
animals for the two groups, however, make it difficult to assign significance to the changes. When the effects in the acute and chronic
animals during development are compared there appears to be, in the
chronically treated animals, some adaptation of glutamine synthetase;
for example, recovery or escape of the enzyme from the drug (compare
Fig. 1, 26-day-old animals and 12-day-old animals - glutamine).

From these data on MSO and those presented on insulin it seems
possible that the preferred pathways for glutamic acid metabolism
may differ at various ages. The changes are most marked from 9 to
21 days of age, the time when compartmentation is rapidly developing
(Patel et al., 1970). An investigation of whether or not changes in
the development of compartmentation occur in young animals treated
with these drugs might yield pertinent data as to the mode of action
of the drug. Another possibility is that MSO may interfere with the
formation of glutamic acid as well as of GABA and aspartic acid.
However, it seems that in the 11-day-old animals at least the depression of GABA cannot be the result of changes of glutamate.

HALOPERIDOL

Our earlier data had shown that in the adult dog the administration of haloperidol at levels of 7.5 mg/kg reduced dopamine significantly in the caudate nucleus associated with characteristic behavioral

TABLE II

EFFECTS OF HALOPERIDOL ON DOPAMINE LEVELS IN CAUDATE
NUCLEUS OF PUPPIES (DOGS)

Group	Dopamine Levels[b] μg/g
Nonhandled (6)	3.55 ± 0.69[c]
Saline Injections (4)	4.02 ± 1.41
Haloperidol, 1 mg/kg[a] (4)	4.84 ± 1.71
Haloperidol, 3 mg/kg[a] (4)	5.19 ± 1.16

[a]Drug injected subcutaneously daily for 27 to 31 days.

[b]Corrected for recovery. Recovery = 80%

[c]Values expressed as μg/g caudate nucleus (wet weight) ± SEM;
number of dogs are given in parentheses.

and EEG responses (Himwich and Glisson, 1967), but had no detectable
effects on serotonin (Himwich et al., 1970). For these reasons we
investigated the effects of this drug when administered subcutaneously
to puppies (dog) daily from the age of 5 to 7 days until they were
33 to 37 or 60 to 70 days of age. Much to our surprise no changes
occurred in the level of dopamine (Table II). Moreover no behavioral
changes were observed. Some statistically significant variations
were observed in the free amino acid pool of the Brain (Table III).
These shifts, however, defy any functional interpretation at the
moment. In contrast to adult dogs haloperidol had no effects on
either dopamine levels of behavior of adult rabbits (Table IV). Recently, however, Lundborg (1972) has published a report on the effects
of haloperidol in rabbits 1 to 8 days of age when the drug was given
to the mother in the drinking water. These animals showed an inability to stand but recovered spontaneously at about 4 weeks of age.
These data suggest that species as well as age differences in the
enzymes responsible for the synthesis and degradation of dopamine
would be worth investigating.

The data presented here have led us to a philosophy of design
for drug experiments in young animals which includes more than one
age level, more than one dosage level and more than one species. Ad-
mittedly such experiments multiply the cost and yield data much more
difficult to interpret. Nonetheless, they forestall broad interpre-
tations of data which are limited to the single experimental situation
being investigated.

TABLE III

EFFECT OF HALOPERIDOL ON DEVELOPING DOG BRAIN AMINO ACIDS AND PHOSPHOETHANOLAMINE

Amino Acid	33 – 37 Day Pups			60 – 70 Day Pups	
	Control (8)	1 mg/kg (9)	3 mg/kg (5)	Control (4)	1 mg/kg (3)
Glutamic Acid	6.17 ± 1.14[a]	7.02 ± 1.20	7.25 ± 0.94	10.55 ± 1.86	6.57 ± 0.67 $p < .05$
Aspartic Acid	1.91 ± 0.21	2.70 ± 0.07 $p < .001$	2.48 ± 0.46	2.80 ± 0.21	2.64 ± 0.38
Valine	0.11 ± 0.02	0.26 ± 0.02 $p < .001$	0.19 ± 0.03	0.16 ± 0.01	0.22 ± 0.03
Leucine	0.26 ± 0.02	0.34 ± 0.04	0.36 ± 0.03	0.14 ± 0.01	0.27 ± 0.01 $p < .001$
Lysine	0.04 ± 0.00	0.14 ± 0.00 $p < .005$	---	0.13 ± 0.10	---
Arginine	0.09 ± 0.01	0.13 ± 0.01 $p < .01$	0.09 ± 0.01	0.16 ± 0.01	0.17 ± 0.02
Phosphoethanolamine	2.24 ± 0.01	3.41 ± 0.25 $p < .005$	3.15 ± 0.27 $p < .02$	2.73 ± 0.37	1.44 ± 0.08 $p < .02$

[a] values expressed as μmoles/g wet weight tissue ± SEM; number of dogs are given in parentheses.

TABLE IV

EFFECTS OF HALOPERIDOL ON DOPAMINE LEVELS IN CAUDATE
NUCLEUS OF ADULT RABBIT

Group	Dopamine Content (μg/g)
Control (4)	4.74 ± 1.37[b]
Haloperidol[a] (6)	4.26 ± 2.38

[a]Drug administered subcutaneously for 5 days daily.

[b]Values are expressed as μg/g caudate nucleus (wet weight) ± SEM; number of rabbits given in parentheses. Samples taken 2 hrs after last injection. (Taken from Himwich et al., 1970

REFERENCES

Cravioto, R.O., Massieu, G., and Izquierdo, J.J., 1951, Free amino-acids in rat brain during insulin shock, Proc. Soc. Exp. Biol. Med. 78: 856.

Davis, J.M., Himwich, W.A. and Pederson, V.C., 1970, Hypoglycemia and developmental changes in free amino acids of rat brain, J. Appl. Physiol. 29: 219.

Dawson, R.M.C., 1950, Studies on the glutamine and glutamic acid content of the rat brain during insulin hypoglycemia, Biochem. 47: 386.

Dravid, A.R. and Jílek, L., 1965, Influence of stagnant hypoxia (oligemia) on some free amino acids in rat brain during ontogeny. J. Neurochem. 12: 837.

Himwich, W.A., and Glisson, S.N., 1967, Effect of haloperidol on caudate nucleus, Int. J. Pharmacol. 6: 329.

Himwich, W.A., Davis, J.M., Leiner, K.Y. and Stout, M., 1970, Biochemical effects of haloperidol in different species, Biol. Psychiat. 2: 315.

Lundborg, P., 1972, Abnormal ontogeny on young rabbits after chronic
     administration of haloperidol to the nursing mothers, Brain Res.
     44: 684.

Massieu, G.H., Ortega, B.G., Syrquin, A. and Tunea, M., 1962, Free
     amino acids in brain and liver of deoxypyridoxine-treated mice
     subjected to insulin shock, J. Neurochem. 9: 143.

Nyhan, W.L., 1961, Toxicity of drugs in the neonatal period, J.
     Pediat. 59: 1.

Patel, A.J., Balázs, R. and Richter, D., 1970, Contribution of the
     GABA bypath to glucose oxidation, and the development of
     compartmentation in the brain, Nature 226: 1160.

Roberts, E., 1960, Free amino acids of nervous tissue: Some aspects
     of metabolism of gamma-aminobutyric acid. In: "Inhibition in
     the Nervous System and Gamma-Aminobutyric Acid", Pergamon Press,
     New York.

EFFECTS OF PRENATAL AND POSTNATAL NICOTINE ADMINISTRATION ON BIO-CHEMICAL ASPECTS OF BRAIN DEVELOPMENT

Doherty B. Hudson, Beverly J. Merrill and Laurie A. Sands

Department of Physiology-Anatomy, University of California

Berkeley, California

It has now been established from a number of studies concerned with the effects of nicotine on the adult brain that, depending on the dose administered, nicotine is capable of facilitating elementary forms of learning (Bovet et al., 1969), stimulating or depressing spontaneous motor activity (Bovet et al., 1967; Larson and Silvetti, 1965), inducing EEG and behavioral arousal (Knapp and Domino, 1962; Yamamoto and Domino, 1965), and inducing seizure discharges (Stümpf, 1965; Stümpf and Gogolák, 1967). Although less work has been conducted on the effects of this noxious agent on the developing brain, work from this laboratory using electroconvulsive tests as a measure of whole brain activity has shown that maturation is delayed in the offspring of nicotine-treated animals and that susceptibility to convulsions is temporarily increased once maturity has been attained (Hudson et al., 1973).

The rat is a useful experimental animal for studies of CNS development because its brain undergoes significant maturational events during the first postnatal month, when it is amenable to systematic functional and chemical investigation. Our long-term studies in this species on the effects of various internal and external environmental conditions on brain development have established that even subtle alterations occurring at critical growth periods can lead to significant immediate and long-term functional deficits (Timiras et al., 1968; Vernadakis and Timiras, 1972).

Our primary concern in the present research is to determine the biochemical alterations which nicotine induces in the developing brain in an effort to elucidate some of the functional changes observed in later postnatal periods. Certain other indices, both with regard to the course of gestation itself and the somatic development

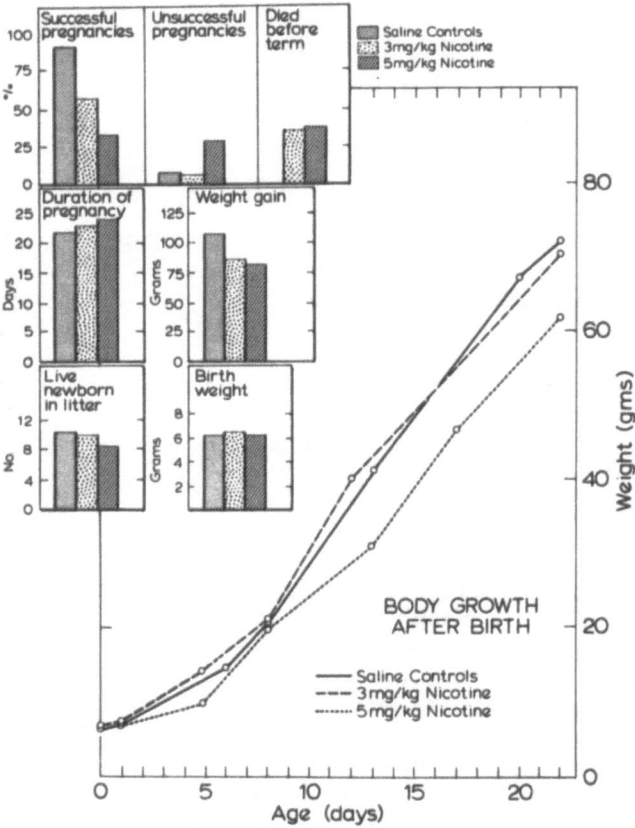

Fig. 1. Effects of nicotine on pregnancy and on growth of offspring.
Nicotine in the doses indicated was administered subcutaneously twice
daily throughout pregnancy. Controls received subcutaneous saline
on the same schedule. Body weight of offspring was measured from
birth to weaning (22 days), each point represents the mean weight
of 9-16 animals.

of the offspring, bear significant correlations to brain development,
and will be briefly summarized. In general, our procedure was to
establish three groups of pregnant rats in which doses of nicotine
(1 mg, 3 mg, 5 mg/kg, respectively) were injected twice daily throughout gestation, and a control group injected with saline on the same
schedule, in order to observe the direct effects upon pregnancy as
well as indirect effects upon development in the offspring (Hudson
and Timiras, 1972).

The average period of gestation in the Long-Evans rat is 22 days.
As shown in Fig. 1, the mean duration of the gestational period was

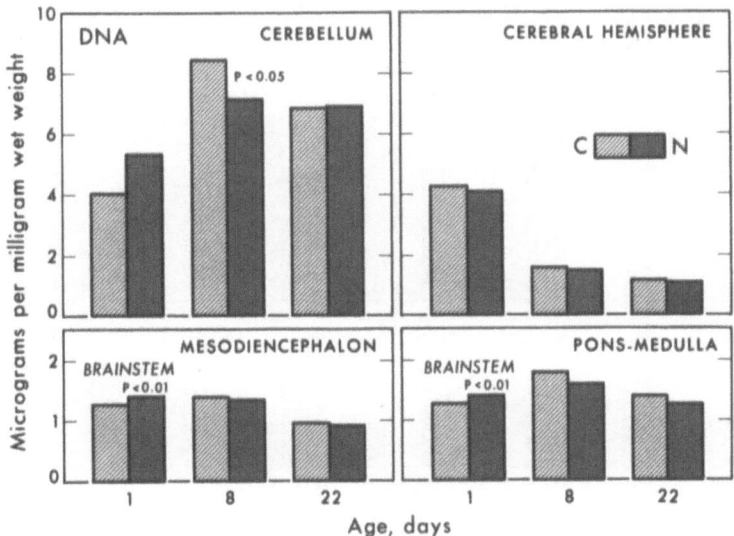

Fig. 2. Regional levels of DNA in the brains of preweanling off-spring of control and nicotine-treated rats. Offspring were sacri-ficed at 1, 8 and 22 days of age. Responses to the three nicotine dose levels used (1, 3 and 5 mg/kg) were pooled for presentation of data. Each group ranged in number from 9-24 animals.

increased to 23 days in animals treated with 3 mg/kg nicotine, and to 24 days in animals treated with 5 mg/kg nicotine, differences which are statistically significant. The 5 mg dose of nicotine also resulted in a reduction of maternal weight gain and in fewer viable litters. To validate that this effect was nicotine-induced and not related to the amount of food intake, weight gain and length of preg-nancy were measured in pair-fed controls and found to be comparable to ad libitum fed controls. Despite the longer period of gestation in nicotine-treated animals, birth weights of all offspring were com-parable; however, when the length of gestation was artificially stan-dardized by delivering all fetuses by caesarean section on day 21 of gestation, the offspring of nicotine-treated animals weighed signi-ficantly less than controls. Normally delivered offspring of 5 mg nicotine-treated mothers compared to controls showed a significant weight reduction by the time of weaning - the 22nd postnatal day. Although body weight of offspring of nicotine-treated mothers was comparable or less than that of controls, wet brain weight of these animals was generally heavier, especially in the offspring of mothers receiving 3 mg/kg nicotine; in these animals, higher brain weights persisted until 22 days, whether delivery was spontaneous or by caesarean section, but the ratio of wet weight to dry weight was higher in the brains of offspring from nicotine-treated mothers.

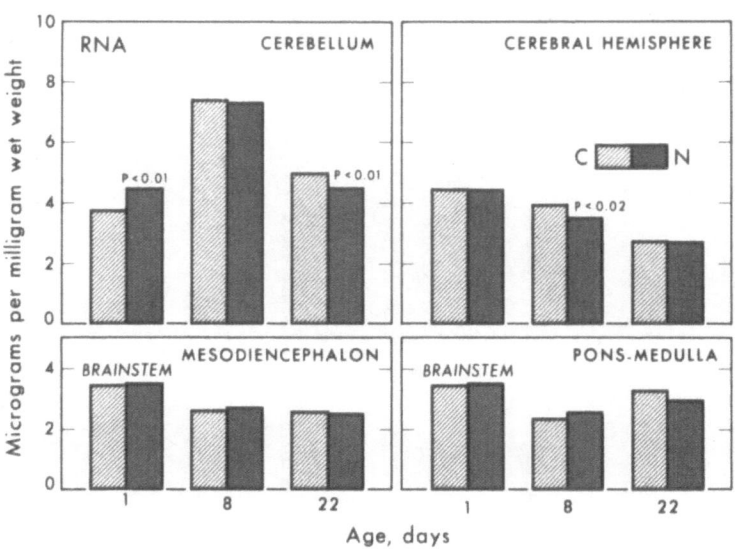

Fig. 3. Regional levels of RNA in the brains of preweanling offspring of control and nicotine-treated rats. Offspring were sacrificed at 1, 8 and 22 days of age. Responses to the three nicotine
dose levels used (1, 3 and 5 mg/kg) were pooled for presentation of
data. Each group ranged in number from 9-24 animals.

To study the effects of nicotine on the biochemical development
of the brain, DNA, RNA and protein levels in four brain areas were
selected as useful indices of cell number, regional growth and cellular activity, respectively. The dose levels utilized in this portion
of the study apparently exerted no quantitative or qualitative effects
on these parameters. The levels of DNA, expressed in µg/mg wet brain
tissue, were measured on the 1st, 8th and 22nd postnatal days in the
cerebral hemispheres, cerebellum, mesodiencephalon and pons-medulla,
each region having its own timetable of maturation (Fig. 2). At one
day of age, the mesodiencephalon and pons-medulla were studied together and designated the brainstem. DNA concentration normally decreases with age in all brain structures except the cerebellum, where
DNA levels increase from birth to 8 days of age, a period when neuro-
blastic proliferation is known to occur in the rat cerebellum and to
continue through the second postnatal week (Altman and Das, 1966).
In the offspring of nicotine-treated rats, DNA levels in the brain-
stem were higher than in controls at one day of age and in the cerebellum were 25-35% higher at this time. At 8 days, however, DNA
concentration in the cerebellum of these animals was 17% lower than
in controls, but by 22 days no apparent differences could be detected.

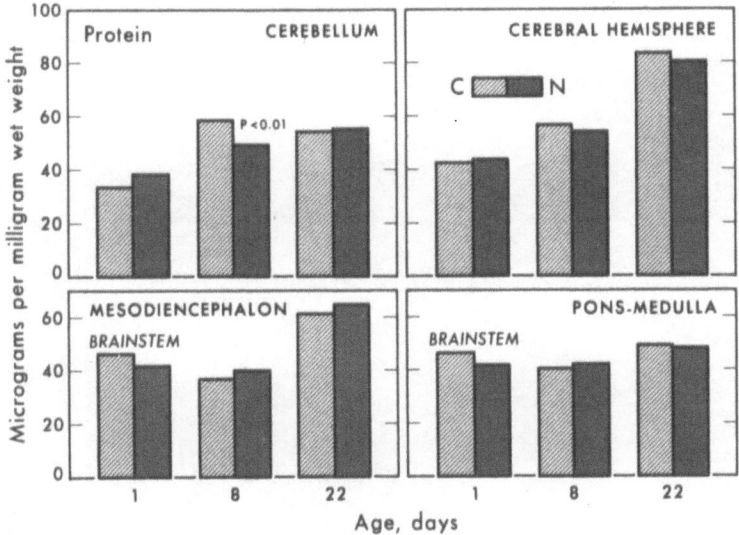

Fig. 4. Regional levels of protein in the brains of preweanling offspring of control and nicotine-treated rats. Offspring were sacrificed at 1, 8 and 22 days of age. Responses to the three nicotine dose levels used (1, 3 and 5 mg/kg) were pooled for presentation of data. Each group ranged in number from 9-24 animals.

We observed tha the RNA concentration in the cerebral hemispheres decreased with maturation in both groups, but that the decrease is more pronounced in 8 day old offspring of nicotine-treated animals (Fig. 3). In the cerebellum of control animals, a peak in RNA levels was observed at 8 days after birth, paralleling the DNA peak and indicating the later maturation of this structure. In the offspring of nicotine-treated rats, however, RNA was higher on day 1 and lower on day 22 than in the cerebellum of controls. These deviations from the normal developmental pattern are far more pronounced in the cerebellum than in other brain areas, and suggest that this structure is more susceptible to the effects of nicotine, perhaps because of its relative immaturity during early postnatal life. Protein levels increased with age in both control and nicotine-treated groups (Fig. 4), however the protein level was significantly lower in the cerebellum of the nicotine-treated group than in controls at 8 days, paralleling the lowered concentration of DNA at that time. In evaluating the DNA, RNA and protein findings presented here, it can be argued that experimental and control animals were uniformly sacrificed at 1, 8 and 22 days after birth, despite their differing time periods <u>in</u> <u>utero</u> and thus, the differences between physiological age and chronological age may explain the disparity in the biochemical findings. However, a similar biochemical pattern was observed in animals uniformly

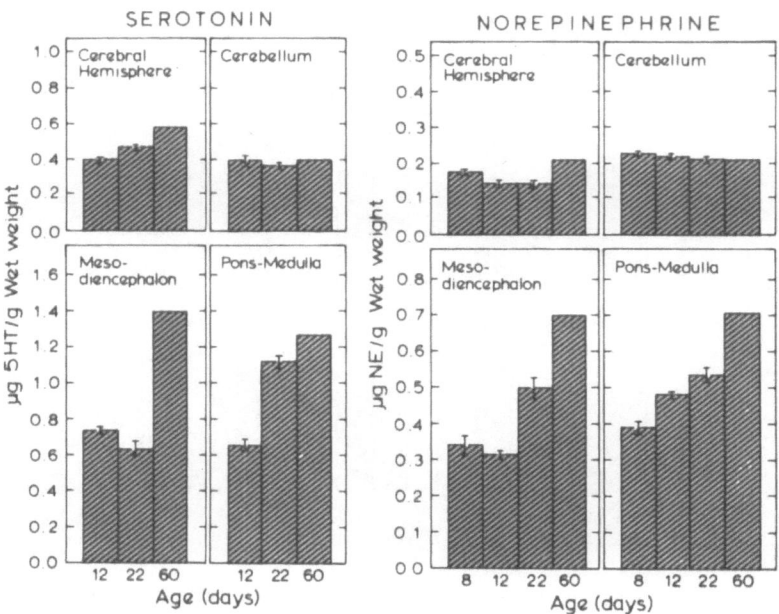

Fig. 5. Regional levels of 5-HT and NE in the brains of control (saline-treated) rats at selected developmental ages. 12 and 22 day-old groups comprised at least 11 animals: 60-day-old group consisted of two animals. Bracketed vertical lines indicate standard error.

delivered by caesarean section at 21 days, indicating that the neuro-chemical differences in offspring of nicotine-treated animals were not merely the consequence of their extended period in utero but rather the direct effect of nicotine on brain growth and metabolism.

These biochemical studies were extended to investigate the effects of nicotine on CNS monoamine levels, specifically on serotonin (5-HT) and norepinephrine (NE), on the basis that these substances, as neurotransmitters, may show closer correlations to the behavioral and functional changes noted in nicotine-treated animals. As shown in Fig. 5, 5-HT reaches adult levels most rapidly in the pons-medulla, followed by the mesodiencephalon - brain regions which contain the cell bodies of most 5-HT and NE-containing neurons. The rate of increase of this system in the cerebral hemispheres (which, together with the cerebellum, contain the axon terminals of 5-HT and NE-containing neurons) is consistent with data from histochemical studies of others (Loizou, 1969; Loizou and Salt, 1970) demonstrating that in the rat, serotonergic neurons begin to project rostrally into the cerebral hemispheres at a constant rate between the first and second postnatal week and that the adult pattern appears to be established by the third week of postnatal life. With respect to NE levels,

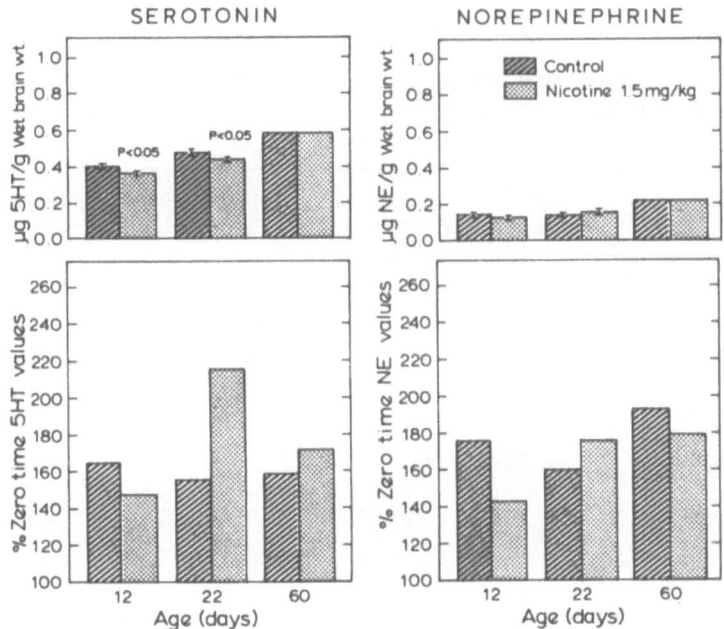

Fig. 6. Developmental changes in levels and turnover of monoamines in cerebral hemispheres of control and nicotine-treated rats. Rats were treated with 1.5 mg/kg nicotine from birth to day 9; control rats treated with vehicle (saline) on same schedule (N = 11-13). Bracketed vertical lines indicate standard error. The percentage of change in 5-HT and NE levels was obtained one hour after injection of pargyline (75 mg/kg). (N = 3-5 at days 12 and 22; 2 at day 60.)

maturation is attained most rapidly in the mesodiencephalon and then in the pons-medulla. NE levels in the cerebral hemispheres show no observable developmental changes during the period studied and this finding is consistent with the fact that the noradrenergic neurons do not undergo the same rostral projection found in serotonergic neurons. NE containing cell bodies and terminals develop slowly over the first two postnatal weeks, after which NE content increases, rapidly attaining its adult pattern by the fourth to fifth week of life. Neither 5-HT nor NE levels show any significant changes with development in the cerebellum.

    The relationship between monoamines and the functional capacity of a region is perhaps more closely related to the turnover of these substances at different ages, rather than to the levels of the monoamines. Synthesizing enzymes of the monoamines are present at birth and start to increase at about 7-10 days of age in the rat (Smith et al., 1962; Robinson, 1968; Schmidt and Sanders-Busch, 1971;

DOHERTY B. HUDSON, BEVERLY J. MERRILL, AND LAURIE A. SANDS

TABLE I

EFFECTS OF STRESS ON MONOAMINE LEVELS IN THE 8-DAY OLD RAT BRAIN BEFORE AND AFTER ADMINISTRATION OF MONOAMINE SYNTHESIS INHIBITORS[a]

Treatment	Pons-Medulla		Meso-Diencephalon		Cerebral Hemispheres		Cerebellum	
	Percent Change from Pre-Stress Levels							
	%	N	%	N	%	N	%	N
SEROTONIN								
Control[b]								
Stressed, saline-injected	+40	(12)	+14	(18)	-3	(16)	+11	(8)
Stressed, PCPA-injected	-2	(8)	+3	(15)	-4	(14)	-9	(8)
Nicotine[b]								
Stressed, saline-injected	+43	(13)	+9	(20)	+1	(21)	-2	(12)
Stressed, PCPA-injected	-18	(10)	-2	(15)	-11	(16)	+6	(6)
NOREPINEPHRINE								
Control[b]								
Stressed, saline-injected	+28	(7)	+19	(9)	+18	(7)	+8	(7)
Stressed, PCPA-injected	-18	(8)	-24	(11)	-7	(10)	-21	(8)
Stressed, αMT-injected	-21	(6)	-19	(9)	0	(11)	+44	(6)
Nicotine[b]								
Stressed, saline-injected	+15	(7)	+21	(10)	+25	(11)	-4	(7)
Stressed, PCPA-injected	-33	(8)	-36	(15)	-19	(13)	-23	(6)
Stressed, αMT-injected	-39	(7)	0	(10)	-6	(10)	+38	(8)

[a]Pre-stress monoamine levels (zero time) used as base for calculating percent change following stress (4 hours separation from mother). Saline, PCPA (400 mg/kg) and αMT (100 mg/kg) injected immediately prior to separation.

[b]Control = offspring of mothers injected with saline twice daily throughout pregnancy. Nicotine = offspring of mothers injected with 3 mg/kg nicotine twice daily throughout pregnancy.

Coyle and Axlerod, 1971, 1972a, 1972b; Deguchi and Barchas, 1972).
To test the responsiveness of the monoamine systems at early ages,
8-day old rats were mildly stressed by removing them from their
mothers for four hours and observing consequent changes in 5-HT and
NE levels. As shown in Table I, with the exception of 5-HT in the
cerebral hemispheres, both monoamines increased in all brain structures studied. Having established the competence of the monoaminer-
gic systems to respond to stress at this age, we elected to use two
experimental approaches to the investigation of monoamine turnover
in the brain: (1) blocking synthesis through the use of selected inhibitors, and (2) blocking catabolic activity. To block the formation of 5-HT, para-chlorophenylalanine (PCPA) was injected intraperitoneally into 8-day old control animals which were killed after 4
hours (corresponding to the stress conditions previously described).
As with mild stress, 5-HT in the cerebral hemispheres did not change
although both 5-HT and NE levels were reduced by PCPA in all other
regions. PCPA, although described as a tryptophan-hydroxylase inhibitor, has been stated by Peters (1972) to inhibit also catecholamine synthesis, and Gal et al. (1970) showed that PCPA induced a
decrease in the transport of aromatic amino acids into neural cells.
Inasmuch as tryptophan-hydroxylase and phenylalanine-hydroxylase are
considered to be identical, the systemic administration of PCPA would
block the formation of tyrosine from phenylalanine in the liver and
reduce the circulating tyrosine, thus limiting the tyrosine available
to the brain for NE synthesis. It is also possible that the brain
is capable of taking up phenylalanine for the synthesis of tyrosine,
but PCPA blocks the synthesis thereby reducing the level of substrate
for NE formation. To block the formation of NE, alpha-methyltyrosine
(αMT) was used (200 mg/kg IP at time zero and again at 2 hours).
After four hours, NE was reduced in all regions except the cerebellum,
where paradoxically, a significant increase occurred.

Having obtained these data on the metabolism of monoamines in
the CNS of normal animals subjected to mild stress, offspring of
nicotine-treated animals (3 mg/kg body weight) were exposed to the
same experimental procedures. Four hours following separation from
mothers, as in control animals subjected to this stress, nicotine-
treated rats showed an increase of 5-HT in the pons-medulla and mesodiencephalon, but not in the cerebral hemispheres (Table I). NE
levels increased in all areas except the cerebellum. In contrast to
controls in which 5-HT and NE increased slightly in the cerebellum,
nicotine offspring showed no change in monoamine levels in this brain
area, suggesting that development of the synthesizing enzyme systems
had perhaps been retarded by nicotine. Continuing with the same experimental procedures, as in controls PCPA had no effect on 5-HT
levels in the cerebral hemispheres of the nicotine group. In the
pons-medulla, however, 5-HT inhibition was 20 per cent higher in
nicotine-treated animals than in controls, whereas in the cerebellum,
treated animals showed an 8 per cent increase in 5-HT in contrast to
the 20 per cent decrease observed in controls. The inhibitory effect

of αMT on NE formation was essentially similar to that in controls, including the same paradoxical increase in NE levels in the cerebellum.

For the investigation of monoamine systems by the alternate approach of inhibiting the catabolism of 5-HT and NE, rats were injected intraperitoneally with nicotine (1.5 mg/kg) twice daily between birth and 9 days of age; a control group was injected with saline on the same schedule. All animals were sacrificed at 12, 22 and 60 days of age, and the absolute levels as well as the rates of synthesis of 5-HT and NE were determined. The 12 and 22 days old rats were kept with their mothers until sacrificed to avoid the stressful effects of maternal separation. Pargyline (75 mg/kg), which inhibits the activity of monoamine oxidase (MAO), was administered to both nicotine-treated and control animals, which were sacrificed at 15 minute intervals up to one hour after administration. As shown in Fig. 6, 5-HT levels were significantly lower than control in the cerebral hemispheres of 12 and 22 day old nicotine-treated animals, and, as revealed by data from corollary studies, the rate of accumulation of 5-HT in this region was also lower at 12 days, but at 22 days, when the level of 5-HT is still significantly lower than in controls, the rate of accumulation is double that of controls. Thus, whereas the lower level of 5-HT may at 12 days reflect an alteration in either its rate of synthesis or of destruction, by 22 days the pronounced increase in the rate of 5-HT accumulation clearly suggests increased 5-HT metabolism. NE turnover after pargyline treatment follows essentially the same pattern as 5-HT turnover - in controls the turnover is similar from 12 to 60 days of age, whereas the nicotine-treated animals have an age-related increase in NE accumulation, although the increase at day 22 is not as striking as with 5-HT.

Comparison of monoamine turnover in the cerebellum of treated and control animal (Fig. 7) shows that at 12 days of age, when this brain structure is in its rapid growth phase, 5-HT levels are comparable but the rate of 5-HT formation is one-sixth that of controls. At 22 days of age, the level of 5-HT is statistically lower ($P<0.05$) in treated animals whereas the rates of formation are almost equal. By 60 days, serotonergic activity is low in both controls and nicotine-treated animals. In both groups, NE levels in the cerebellum are low and do not appear to change with age, although in controls the activity of NE formation does show an age-related increase between 12 and 22 days, whereas there is a slower increase in NE synthesis in the nicotine-treated group. Based on consistent findings that NE levels are low in the rat cerebellum, it had been concluded that NE plays little or no functional role in this brain structure, but Hoffer et al. (1971) were able to show that the input to certain cerebellar neurons was mediated by NE. The present findings in the 3 week-old rat indicating rapid turnover of NE despite low levels, together with similar reports by Iversen and Glowinski (1966) in adult rats, support the hypothesis that this monoamine has a functional

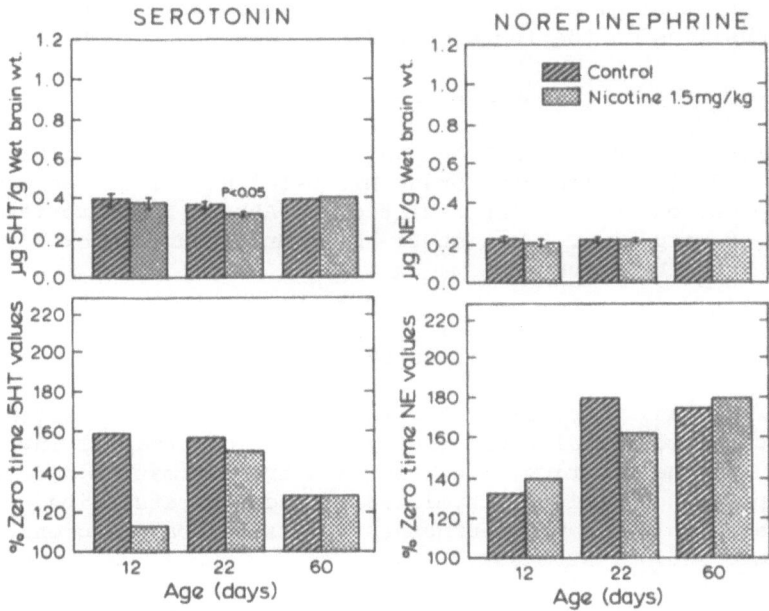

Fig. 7. Developmental changes in levels and turnover of monoamines
in cerebellum of control and nicotine-treated rats. Rats were treated
with 1.5 mg/kg nicotine from birth to day 9; control rats treated
with vehicle (saline) on same schedule. (N = 11-13). Bracketed vertical lines indicate standard error. The percentage of change in
5-HT and NE levels was obtained one hour after IP injection of pargyline (75 mg/kg). (N = 3-5 at days 12 and 22; 2 at day 60.)

role in the cerebellum.

     Among the findings presented here some emerge as more significant
and perhaps functionally important. It appears that those areas onto-
genetically older are less affected by nicotine, regardless of whether
the agent is received indirectly through the mother or directly in
early postnatal life. Specifically, the later developing regions
show lower DNA and lower protein levels in nicotine-treated animals
than in controls, suggesting delayed maturation of these structures.
Furthermore, the lower levels and low turnover of monoamines which
persisted until 12 days of age, as well as the increased turnover of
5-HT at 3 weeks of age in treated rats parallel electrophysiological
alterations previously reported in nicotine-treated rats: low turnover rates corresponding to delayed neuronal maturation and high
turnover rates corresponding to enhanced excitability. Although a
direct causal relationship is not being proposed, it does appear that
nicotine administered during development alters the maturation of

selected neurochemical parameters that may reasonably be expected to
have repercussions on the functional competence of the CNS.

ACKNOWLEDGMENTS

This work was supported by A.M.A. Education and Research Foundation Grant and N.I.H. Training Grant No. 5-T01-HD-00101. We would
like to express our sincere appreciation to Abbott Laboratories for
the supply of pargyline. We wish to thank Mrs. Laurel Cook for her
assistance with the manuscript.

REFERENCES

Altman, J. and Das, G.D., 1966, Autoradiographic and histological
    studies of postnatal neurogenesis. I. A longitudinal investi-
    gation of the kinetics, migration and transformation of cells
    incorporating tritiated thymidine in neonate rats, with special
    reference to postnatal neurogenesis in some brain regions,
    J. Comp. Neurol. 126: 337.

Bovet, D., Bovet-Nitti, F. and Oliverio, A., 1967, Action of nicotine
    on spontaneous and acquired behavior in rats and mice, Ann. N.Y.
    Acad. Sci. 142: 261.

Bovet, D., Bovet-Nitti, F. and Oliverio, A., 1969, Genetic aspects
    of learning and memory in mice, Science 163: 139.

Coyle, J.T. and Axelrod, J., 1971, Development of the uptake and
    storage of L-(^{3}H)norepinephrine in the rat brain, J. Neurochem.
    18: 2061.

Coyle, J.T. and Axelrod, J., 1972a, Dopamine-β-hydroxylase in the
    rat brain: developmental characteristics, J. Neurochem. 19: 449.

Coyle, J.T. and Axelrod, J., 1972b, Tyrosine hydroxylase in rat brain:
    developmental characteristics, J. Neurochem. 19: 1117.

Deguchi, T. and Barchas, J., 1972, Regional distribution and develop-
    mental change of tryptophan hydroxylase activity in rat brain,
    J. Neurochem. 19: 927.

Gal, E.M., Roggeveen, A.E. and Millard, S.A., 1970, DL-(2-^{14}C)p-
    chlorophenylalanine as an inhibitor of tryptophan-5-hydroxylase,
    J. Neurochem. 17: 1221.

Hoffer, B.J., Siggins, G.R. and Bloom, F.E., 1971, Studies on nore-
    pinephrine-containing afferents to Purkinje cells of rat cere-
    bellum. II. Sensitivity of Purkinje cells to norepinephrine and
    related substances administered by microiontophoresis, Brain
    Res. 25: 523.

Hudson, D.B. and Timiras, P.S., 1972, Nicotine injection during gestation: impairment of reproduction, fetal viability, and development, Biol. Reproduc. 7: 247.

Hudson, D.B., Meisami, E. and Timiras, P.S., 1973, Brain development in offspring of rats treated with nicotine during pregnancy, Experientia 29: 286.

Iversen, L.L. and Glowinski, J., 1966, Regional studies of catecholamines in the rat brain -- II. Rate of turnover of catecholamines in various brain regions, J. Neurochem. 13: 671.

Knapp, D.E. and Domino, E.F., 1962, Action of nicotine on the ascending reticular activating system, Int. J. Neurochem. 1: 333.

Larson, P.S. and Silvetti, H., 1965, Tobacco alkaloids and central nervous system functions. In: "Symposium of Tobacco Alkaloids and Related Compounds", (U.S. von Euler, ed.), Macmillan, New York.

Loizou, L.A., 1969, The development of monoamine-containing neurons in the brain of the albino rat, J. Anat. 104: 588.

Loizou, L.A. and Salt, P., 1970, Regional changes in monoamines of the rat brain during postnatal development, Brain Res. 20: 467.

Peters, D.A.V., 1972, Inhibition of brain tryptophan-5-hydroxylase by amino acids - The role of L-tryptophan uptake inhibition, Biochem. Pharmacol. 21: 1051.

Robinson, N., 1968, Histochemistry of rat brain stem monoamine oxidase during maturation, J. Neurochem. 15: 1151.

Schmidt, M.J. and Sanders-Busch, E., 1971, Tryptophan hydroxylase activity in developing rat brain, J. Neurochem. 18: 2549.

Smith, S.E., Stacey, R.S. and Young, I.M., 1962, 5-hydroxytryptamine and 5-hydroxytryptophan decarboxylase activity in the developing nervous system of rats and guinea-pigs. In: "Proceedings of the First International Pharmacology Meeting", (W.D.M. Paton, ed.), Vol. 8, The Macmillan Co., New York, pp. 101-105.

Stümpf, C., 1965, Drug action on the electrical activity of the hippocampus, Intern. Rev. Neurobiol. 8: 77.

Stümpf, C. and Gogólak, G., 1967, Actions of nicotine upon the limbic system, Ann. N.Y. Acad. Sci. 141: 143.

Timiras, P.S., Vernadakis, A. and Sherwood, N.M., 1968, Development and plasticity of the nervous system. In: "Biology of Gestation", (N.S. Assali, ed.), Vol. II, Academic Press, New York, pp. 261-319.

Vernadakis, A. and Timiras, P.S., 1972, Disorders of the nervous system. In: "Pathophysiology of Gestation", (N.S. Assali, ed.), Vol. III, Academic Press, New York, pp. 233-304.

Yamamoto, K. and Domino, E.F., 1965, Nicotine-induced EEG and behavioral arousal, Int. J. Neuropharmacol. 4: 359.

DRUG ACTIONS: BIOCHEMICAL DEVELOPMENT:
(Electrolytes, Acid-Base)
Dixon M. Woodbury, Chairman

MATURATION OF THE BLOOD-BRAIN AND BLOOD-CSF BARRIERS

Dixon M. Woodbury

Department of Pharmacology, University of Utah

College of Medicine, Salt Lake City, Utah

It is important to elucidate in a Symposium on the Effects of
Drugs on the Developing Brain the routes and mechanisms by which
drugs that act on the brain enter and leave this organ. Many
factors determine the concentration of drugs in the brain and it is
the purpose of this paper to describe what these factors are and
what changes occur during maturation. Thus, the volume of distribution of a drug, its pKa, the properties of the cerebral capillary
endothelial cells that constitute the "blood-brain barrier", the
rate of cerebrospinal fluid flow, and the properties of the systems
that transport drugs across the choroid plexus are all important
factors to be discussed. The developing animal is ideal for studying the "blood-brain barrier" because large changes take place in
a short period of time. Thus, the brain of rats is mature by 21
days of age, although certain events (for example, myelination and
glial growth) take place over a longer period of time. (For discussions of the ontogeny of the blood-brain barrier, see Davson,
1973 and Saunders and Bradbury, 1973).

A diagrammatic representation of the anatomical basis for the
"blood-brain" and"blood-CSF" barrier system in adult animals is
shown in Figure 1. In order to enter the brain and CSF a drug must
cross several epithelial cell barriers. These will be discussed in
the order that they are traversed when a substance enters the
central nervous system from the cerebral capillaries.

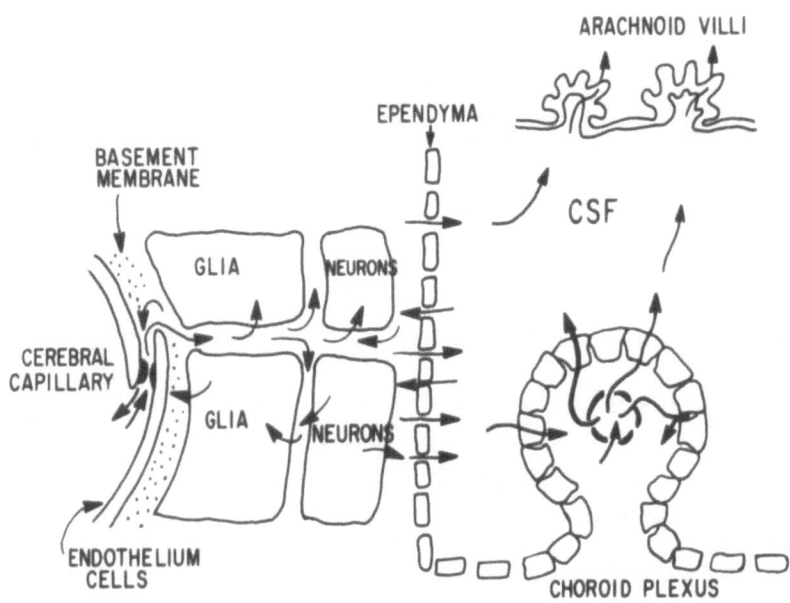

CHANGES WITH MATURATION

1 ↓ PERMEABILITY OF CEREBRAL CAPILLARIES
2 ↓ EXTRACELLULAR SPACE
3 ↑ NUMBER AND VOLUME OF GLIAL CELLS
4 ↑ GROWTH OF NEURONAL PROCESSES
5 ↓ PERMEABILITY OF EPENDYMAL LINING
6 ↑ CSF PRODUCTION AND FLOW
7 ↑ TRANSPORT ACROSS CHOROID PLEXUS

Fig. 1. Schematic representation of the anatomical basis for the
"blood-brain" and "blood-CSF" barrier systems in adult animals.
The pathways by which various substances can enter and leave the
various compartments in the system are also shown. Presented
below the diagram is a list of the changes that take place during
development of the system. The diameter of the pathway for substances moving between the endothelial cells of the cerebral capillaries is thought to be about 15Å. Note also that the capillaries
of the choroid plexus are fenestrated. See text for further discussion.

BLOOD-BRAIN AND BLOOD-CSF BARRIER SYSTEMS IN ADULTS

Cerebral Capallaries

The endothelial cells of the cerebral capillaries constitute
the site of the so-called "blood-brain barrier". The characteristics of these cells have been discussed by Brightman and Reese
(1969), Pappenheimer (1970) and Chrone (1971). Large molecules
such as albumin, trypan blue (largely bound to plasma protein),
horseradish peroxidase and ferritin do not cross the cerebral capillaries, except possibly very slowly and in small amounts by the
process of pinocytosis. This is true even for the capillaries of
fetal animals (Grazer and Clemente, 1957; Olsson, 1968). However, molecules as large as inulin (molecular weight, 5000), ouabain
and sucrose do cross these capillaries, albeit at a slower rate
than these agents traverse capillaries elsewhere in the body.
These data have been interpreted to show that,since molecules like
inulin (which measures extracellular space) presumably cannot enter
cerebral capillary cells, their entrance into the interstitial space
of the brain must be by way of channels between the endothelial
cells. The diameter of the channels is thought to average about
15Å, which is sufficiently large to allow a molecule the size of
inulin to pass through slowly, but is not large enough for the passage of albumin or other large molecules. The basement membrane
that separates the endothelial cells of the capillaries from the
glial endfeet and the interstitial channels of the brain does not
appear to be a barrier to movement of large molecules. For example, Brightman and Reese (1969) have shown that both horseradish
peroxidase and ferritin injected into the cerebrospinal fluid
readily pass through the interstitial space of the brain to the
endothelial cell border without being impeded by the basement
membrane. However, these substances do not cross the endothelial
cells. Therefore, the endothelial cells are impermeable to large
molecules in both directions. Inulin and smaller molecules can
leave the brain by this route through the 15Å pores between the
endothelial cells. The permeability of the cerebral capillaries to
inulin is much greater in fetal and neonatal rats than in adults and
the rate of entrance decreases with increasing age (Ferguson and
Woodbury, 1969). Electron microscopic studies suggest that changes
in capillary structure occur with increasing age and that these
changes may account for the decrease in the permeability of the
capillaries to various molecules (Donahue and Pappas, 1961).

Most drugs are weak electrolytes and as such exist in both
the nonionized and ionized form. The extent of ionization depends
on the pKa of the molecule and the pH of the solution. The nonionized form of drugs readily crosses the cell membrane whereas
the ionized form is impermeable or only slowly permeable. The
rate of penetration of the nonionized form depends on the lipid:

water partition coefficient of the molecule. The greater the lipid
solubility the faster the movement of the nonionized form across
the cell membrane. The rate of movement also depends on the extent
of plasma and tissue binding of the drug.

Ependymal Lining

After crossing the endothelial cells and the basal membrane
(which offers no resistance), a drug enters the narrow interstitial
channels of the brain that constitute the extracellular space.
These are about 150-200 Å in diameter and allow free diffusion of
all size molecules through them, as clearly demonstrated by
Brightman and Reese (1969) by electron miscroscopic determination
of the distribution of horseradish peroxidase of ferritin in brain.
From the interstitial channels the drugs have access to neurons or
their surrounding glial cells or can move into the cerebrospinal
fluid by crossing the ependymal cells lining the ventricular
cavaties. The cells are joined together by gap junctions in many
places and this allows ready movement of all molecules, except for
large protein molecules, between the cells and around the junctions.
Movement across the ependymal cells is mainly dependent on molecular
size. For example in the study of Reed and Woodbury (1963) the
rate of movement of various substances across this border was as
follows: albumin < inulin < sucrose < iodide.

Glial Endfeet and Glial Cells

Few data are available on the movement of drugs into glial
cells or into the glial endfeet bordering on the basal membrane
and the capillary endothelial cells (see Figure 1). Weak electrolytes undoubtedly enter by nonionic diffusion as is the case with
all other cells and their rate, therefore, is dependent on the pH,
pKa and the partition coefficient of the nonionized drug. There is
evidence that Na and K are actively transported across glial cells
and that these cells contain a high K concentration and a relatively
high Na concentration (Kuffler and Nicholls, 1966, for review).
Active uptake of amino acids and some neurotransmitters also appear to occur in glial cells and they are postulated to be sinks
for neurotransmitters to remove them from the synaptic areas after
their release following a nerve impulse. There is also evidence
that the glial cells are a sink for K and thereby maintain a constant extracellular potassium concentration under conditions of
excessive neuronal activity. The latter would tend to increase
extracellular K concentration as a result of leakage of the cation
from the nerve during nervous activity (Orkand, 1969; Pollen
and Trachtenberg, 1970; Trachtenberg and Pollen, 1970; Henn et al.,
1972).

The role of the glial endfeet lining the capillaries (see
Figure 1) is not known but it has been speculated that they function

to exchange various metabolic waste products (collected by the glial
cells from the neurons they surround and then transported down the
glial cell processes to the endfeet) for nutrients and electrolytes
such as K and PO_4. Further work in this area is obviously needed.

Neurons

From the interstitial channels drugs also enter neuronal cells
as depicted in Figure 1. Movement of drugs across neuronal cell
membranes appears to be by the same mechanisms as for other cells,
i.e., by pH-dependent nonionic diffusion and by active transport of
ionized molecules.

Epithelial Cells of the Choroid Plexus

These cells are the site of formation of CSF. This is a
process that involves the active transport of Na across the
choroidal epithelial cells similar to the process that occurs
across the eipthelial cells of frog skin and toad bladder. The
capillaries supplying the choroid plexus differ from the cerebral
capillaries in that there are fenestrations between the endothelial cells and these allow the permeation of large molecules
such as peroxidase and ferritin. However, the choroid plexus cells
are held together by tight junctions and molecules such as peroxidase, ferritin, inulin, and sucrose cannot pass through them into the CSF. Thus the choroid plexus cells are the site of the
"blood-CSF" barrier. Entrance of substances into the CSF via the
choroid plexus cells takes place only by passage through the cells.
Small molecules such as urea, antipyrine, formamide can enter the
CSF by this route by diffusion across both cell membranes. However, their rate of passage is slower than that of water and this
sieving effect can account for the CSF/plasma ratios of these substances of < 1.0. Weak electrolytes enter the CSF across the
choroid epithelial cells, as is the case for other cells, by pH-
dependent nonionic diffusion. Electrolytes such as Na^+ and Mg^{++}
enter the CSF by active transport processes and Cl^- probably also
enters by an active process that involves carbonic anhydrase.
Potassium is maintained constant in the CSF at a value about 0.6
that of plasma by active transport of this ion out of the CSF
across the choroidal epithelial cells into plasma. CSF secretion
is inhibited by ouabain, which blocks active Na transport across
the choroid plexus cells, and by acetazolamide, which probably
blocks Cl and HCO_3^- transport across these cells by inhibiting the
activity of carbonic anhydrase. The potential difference across
choroid plexus cells is sensitive to acid-base changes in the
plasma which, therefore, can alter the distribution of ions between
CSF and plasma and possibly affect CSF secretion. This is discussed in the paper by Dr. Withrow elsewhere in this volume. After
the CSF is formed at the choroid plexus the fluid flows through the

ventricles, enters the subarachnoid space and exits into the
cerebral venous system via the arachnoid villi as shown in Figure 1.
The exit of CSF via the arachnoid villi is a pressure-dependent
filtration process.

Substances that enter the CSF, either by way of the cerebral
capillary--brain interstitial space--ependymal cell pathway or by
crossing the choroid plexus, can exit from the CSF by two routes.
One is by bulk flow of the substance in the CSF and exit via the
arachnoid villi; nonelectrolyte molecules such as inulin and
sucrose, albumin and even red blood cells exit by this pathway.
Small nonelectrolytes, weak electrolytes, and strong electrolytes
can also leave by this mechanism, but they can also leave by the
second mechanism which involves active transport of the substance
across the choroid plexus from CSF to blood. This is the pre-
dominant system for exit of the anionic and cationic forms of
organic electrolytes, the inorganic halide ions, and probably
potassium ion.

The anion system transports inorganic anions such as I^-,
ClO_4^-, SCN^-, Br^- and Tc^- out of the CSF into blood. The system
is similar to the anion transport system in the thyroid. The
choroid plexus cells concentrate these anions as does the thyroid.
This system also transports organic anions and the anionic species
of weak acids out of the CSF. Thus, drugs such as penicillin,
probenecid and PAH and endogenous metabolites, e.g., 5HIAA, homovanillic acid and possibly lactate, leave the CSF by this route.
This is a carrier mediated, energy-dependent system that obeys
saturation kinetics and, therefore, can be blocked by competing
anions, e.g., probenicid.   These substances cross the cerebral
capillaries only slowly and can exit at a much faster rate via the
choroid plexus anion transport system.

The cation system transports inorganic cations such as K^+ out
of the CSF across the epithelial cells of the choroid plexus. It
also transports organic cations and the cationic species of weak
bases. Such cations as morphine, TEA, and N-methyl nicotinamide
leave the CSF by this route.

As a result of the rapid exit of substances from the brain and
CSF by bulk flow through the arachnoid villi and/or by active transport across the choroid plexus and their slow entrance into the
brain and CSF via the cerebral capillaries (site of blood-brain
barrier) there results a low steady-state concentration of these
types of substances in the brain and CSF. This has given rise to
concept of the "sink effect" which is due to the low permeability
of the cerebral capillaries to substances coupled with their rapid
exit from the CSF by bulk flow and/or active transport across the
choroid plexus. If CSF secretion is inhibited or active transport

of ions out of the CSF blocked, the steady-state levels of substances in the brain and CSF increase because the sink effect is negated.

CHANGES WHICH OCCUR IN THE BLOOD-BRAIN AND BLOOD-CSF BARRIER SYSTEMS DURING MATURATION

Capillary permeability

The histological changes in cerebral capillaries with age have been described by Donahue and Pappas (1961) and Caley and Maxwell, (1970). The basement membrane progresses from a thin band of variable thickness and density to a thicker structure of more or less uniform width and density above any given capillary. The endothelial cells in the immature animals are relatively thick. These cells become attenuated in the adult. The rather complete glial investment of the cerebral capillaries in the adult is absent in the immature animals. Cell bodies, rather than cell processes which occur in the adult brain, are in close proximity to the capillaries in the mature brain. Whether the decreased ability of various substances to enter the brain from the plasma in the mature animal is related to these anatomical changes in the cerebral capillaries has not been ascertained as yet.

The permeability of the cerebral capillaries to large molecules such as albumin and trypan blue is absent in the immature as well as the adult animal. However, molecules such as inulin, sucrose, sodium, potassium chloride, iodide, perchlorate, ouabain and other drugs, glutamic acid, lysine and other amino acids, phosphate, and cholesterol have been shown to enter brain and CSF more rapidly or have higher steady-state concentrations relative to plasma in fetal neonatal animals than in adults (Bakay, 1953; Katzman and Leiderman, 1953; Himwich and Himwich, 1955;Lajtha, 1958; Dobbing and Sands, 1963; Vernadakis and Woodbury, 1965; Woodbury, 1967; Luciano, 1968; Ferguson and Woodbury, 1969; Brøndsted and Woodbury, 1973).

The rate of uptake of these materials might be even faster, but there are fewer arterioles/cm^2 of brain surface in young as compared with older animals. The number of vessels/cm^2 increases sharply with age in both man and rats and then levels out. In the rat this plateau occurs at 21 days (Caley and Maxwell, 1970; Rhodes and Hyde, 1965). Thus the rate of uptake of substances in young animals may be blood-flow limited.

An example of the change in rate of entrance of substances into the brain with age is the observation of Luciano (1968) that the $t\frac{1}{2}$ for the uptake of Na^{22} by newborn rat brain is 40 minutes whereas it is 75 minutes in the adult. Even correcting for the larger volume of distribution of Na in the younger animals, the

rate constant was faster than that of adult rats. The same is true
for Cl^{36} uptake in neonatal as compared with adult rats (Vernadakis
and Woodbury, 1965) and for ^{14}C-inulin in which the rate of entry
into the brain was 7 times faster in -4-day-old (17 days of gestation)
rats than in 16-day-old rats and about 25 times faster than the uptake into the brain of adult rats (Ferguson and Woodbury, 1969).

Extracellular Volume

In Figure 2 are summarized the changes in the K concentration,
Na and Cl spaces and extracellular and intracellular volume of brain
during development of the rat. The extracellular fluid volume was
measured by the brain/CSF ratio of ^{14}C-inulin in rats of different
ages (-6 days old to adult) (Ferguson and Woodbury, 1969). In -6 days
old animals the CSF-plasma ratio of inulin was about 1.0 and in the
adult it was 0.01. The corresponding brain spaces of inulin
measured simultaneously with the CSF values are 50% and 1%. The
brain/CSF ratio measures the ECF volume up to 16 days of age in rats
since CSF and brain interstitial fluid appear to be in rapid
equilibrium during this period of time.

It is evident, therefore, that the volume of the extracellular
space of the brain, as measured by the marker technique decreases
with age. A decrease in ECF volume with age has also been noted
with anatomical studies of the brain utilizing the electronmicroscope (see, for example, Pysh, 1969; Caley and Maxwell, 1970).

It is also seen from Figure 2 that the Na and Cl spaces of
brain decrease with age, the intracellular water increases (despite
a decrease in total water, because the ECF volume decreases to a
greater extent than total water decreases), and the K concentration
increases with age (Vernadakis and Woodbury, 1962, 1965). The increase in K concentration and decrease in Na and Cl concentrations
with age are indicative of the increase in number of neuronal cell
processes and glial cells and decrease in the extracellular space
with age, as indicated by electron microscopis studies.

Glial Cell Numbers and Volume

In Figure 3 are shown the changes in the weight, carbonic
anhydrase activity and total CO_2 of the brain with age. The brain
weight has reached about half of its maximal value by 10 days but
the carbonic anhydrase activity, which is very low in the first 10
days of life, has not changed during this period, and the total
CO_2, which is very high, also has not changed during the first 10
postnatal days. However, from 10 to 21 days the brain carbonic
anhydrase activity increases rapidly to 21 days and then levels out
somewhat although it continues to increase more gradually for the
rest of the life of the rats. The total CO_2 decreases rapidly from

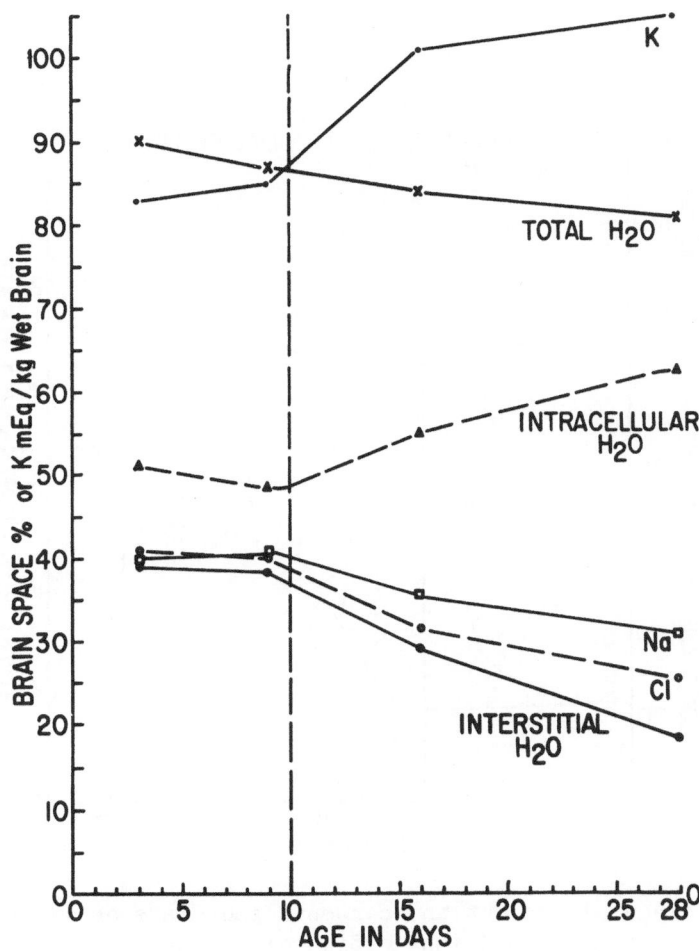

Fig. 2. Changes in K concentration, Na and Cl spaces, and extracellular and intracellular volume of brain during maturation in the
rat.

    Ordinate: Changes in brain concentration or space of the
various parameters. Abscissa: Age in days after birth. See
text for discussion.

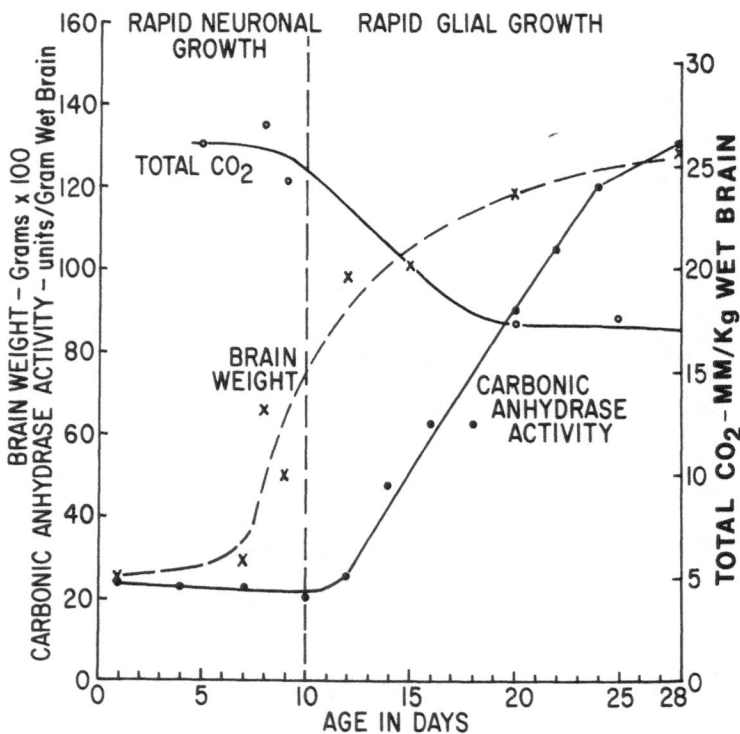

Fig. 3. Changes in weight and carbonic anhydrase activity (left
ordinate) and total CO_2 (right ordinate) of the brain with age in
days (abscissa). The period of rapid neuronal growth is separated
from the period of rapid glial growth bv a vertical dashed line at
10 days of age. See text for further discussion. (From Woodbury,
1971).

10 to 21 days, then levels out and tends to decrease more slowly
thereafter. Since carbonic anhydrase is localized to glial cells
(Giacobini, 1962)and it is assumed that the activity per cell does
not change, the increase in carbonic anhydrase activity during
development indicates increased glial cell growth with age. This
is consistent with electron microscopic observations of Brizzee and
Jacobs (1959) that the glial-neuron index (number of glial cells
per number of neurons per unit area) increases with age (see for
example, Caley and Maxwell, 1968, and Vaughn and Peters, 1967).
Tissue fractionation studies in which glial cells and neurons are
separated also demonstrate increased number and volume of glial
cells with maturation of the brain. In fetal and neonatal animals
the glial cells are immature and seem to be freely permeable to
Cl^- and possibly other substances, including drugs. At the onset
of rapid proliferation of glial cells, which begins at 10 days,
glial cell permeability to Cl appears to decrease (cf. Vernadakis
and Woodbury, 1965) and this may account in part for the decreased
volume of distribution and rate of uptake of Cl that occurs during
this period of time in maturing rats. The decreased rate of uptake
of drugs that occurs at this time also may be due in part to decreased permeability of glial cells as they mature.

Neuronal Cell Volume and Synapses

There is both electron microscopic and neurophysiologic evidence
that marked proliferation of neuronal processes (axons and dendrites)
and synapses occurs during maturation of the brain. The proliferat-
ing neuronal processes and glial cells encroach upon the large
extracellular space of the neonatal animals and account for its
decrease with age. This is evident from the increase in brain K
concentration and decrease in Na and Cl concentration in the brain
that occurs with age (see Figure 2). Very few data are available
on the changes in the permeability of neuronal membranes to drugs
and other substances with age.

Permeability of the Ependymal Lining

As maturation proceeds the ability of drugs or other substances
to cross the ependymal lining decreases. This layer of cells possesses gap junctions and small molecules can freely cross. However,
larger molecules such as albumin and, to some extent inulin, are
restricted in their movements. The increase in the brain/CSF ratio
for inulin that occurs after 16 days in the study of Ferguson and
Woodbury (1969) can be explained by a decrease in the ability of
inulin to cross the ependymal border as the animal matures.

Rate of CSF Production and Flow With Age

This aspect is discussed in the paper by Johanson and Woodbury elsewhere in this monograph. The data of Ferguson and Woodbury (1969) demonstrate a decrease in CSF/plasma ratio of inulin with age. Since inulin is not actively transported out of the CSF and exits only by bulk flow through the arachnoid villi it may be employed to measure CSF flow rate. The results thus suggest that immature animals have lower rates of CSF formation than do adult animals. Others have also demonstrated low rates of CSF flow in immature animals (e.g., Shaywitz et al., 1969).

That immature animals have lower CSF formation rates than adults is also suggested by the data shown in Figure 4 which depicts changes in CSF to aplasma electrolyte ratios with age (Ferguson and Woodbury, 1969). The ratios of Na and Cl in CSF to that in the plasma increase with age whereas that of K decreases. At 9 days after birth the electrolyte ratios have leveled out and reached the adult value. These data suggest that at 9 days the Na-K transport system in the choroid plexus is mature.

The reduced CSF flow rate in immature animals coupled with increased permeability of the cerebral capillaries to various substances and a larger extracellular volume as compared with adult animals all contribute to faster rates of entrance and higher concentrations of drugs and other molecules in brain and CSF. As the animal matures, CSF flow increases, cerebral capillary permeability decreases and the extracellular volume decreases. Thus, the rate of entrance of substances into brain CSF and their concentrations there are reduced.

Transport of Substances Across the Choroid Plexus

a. Cation transport. As indicated from the data presented in Figure 4 and discussed above, the K-Na choroid plexus transport system does not appear to mature until about 9 days after birth in rats. Magnesium ion is also transported actively from blood to CSF against an electrochemical gradient. This system also appears to be immature in fetal animals (but is the first cation system to mature). According to Saunders and Bradbury (1973) the specific transport systems for ions mature in the order: magnesium (fetal stage), sodium and chloride, and potassium (postnatal). Calcium levels in the CSF reach adult values after birth but there is no convincing evidence as yet that Ca^{++} is actively transported across the choroid plexus. Thus the transport systems are established at adult values at very different ages for different ions.

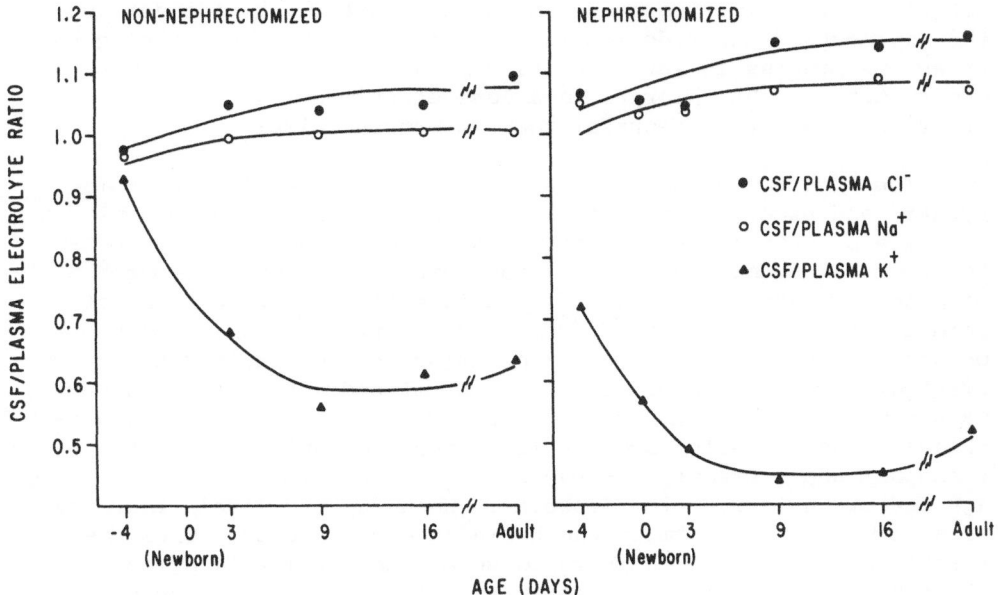

Fig. 4. Plot of CSF/plasma electrolyte concentration ratios for
rats of various ages. Graph on left represents changes with age
in normal rats and that on right the changes occurring in
nephrectomized rats of various ages. See text for discussion
(from Ferguson and Woodbury, 1969).

Organic cation transport across the choroid plexus also occurs
but the changes with age have not been well documented. However,
the accumulation of morphine in the choroid plexus in vitro appears to be lower in neonatal than in adult rats.

b. Anion transport. Mediated transport of chloride from blood
into cerebrospinal fluid has been described by Bourke et al. (1960)
and inhibitors of anion transport systems in other tissues have
been shown to inhibit chloride transport into CSF (Woodbury, 1968).
But changes with age have been little studied. As already
described and as shown in Figure 4, chloride levels in the CSF
increase with age and reach adult values at about 9 days of age.
Whether these changes are a result of development of an active

transport system cannot be decided because measurements of the potential difference between CSF and blood at the different age periods studied were not made. However, perchlorate ion competitively inhibits inorganic anion transport (e.g., iodide) and the movement of chloride ion from blood to the CSF, suggesting that an active process is involved (Barham and Woodbury, unpublished observations). Perchlorate is a less effective inhibitor of chloride movement in neonatal than in mature animals.

The monovalent inorganic anions, perchlorate, iodide, thiocyanate and bromide are also transported across the choroid plexus but in a direction opposite from that of chloride, i.e., from CSF to blood. The changes of this transport system for ^{36}Cl-perchlorate with age are shown in Figure 5. It is evident that in neonatal animals little transport of ^{36}Cl-perchlorate from CSF to blood occurs and that a large load of perchlorate has little effect. The transport system, therefore has not developed. As the animals mature the CSF to plasma ratio decreases and a large load of perchlorate has a greater and greater effect to inhibit perchlorate transport and increase CSF-levels. As the CSF levels decrease with age the brain levels also decrease. When the CSF levels increase with perchlorate treatment the brain levels increase. Thus the perchlorate in the CSF appears to determine the levels of perchlorate in the brain. Iodide transport out of the CSF across the choroid plexus also changes with age (Woodbury, 1968) as does that of sulfate (Robinson et al., 1968) but at a slower rate. Thus the two systems seem to be independent.

The changes in organic anion transport with age have been little studied. The available evidence suggests that this system is also incompletely developed in fetal and neonatal animals.

It is apparent from this discussion that the entrance of drugs into brain and CSF with age and their exit therefrom depends upon a number of properties of the blood-brain-CSF system: permeability of the brain capillaries, rate of flow of CSF, active transport across the choroid plexus, and volume of the extracellular fluid. Other factors, are also of importance, such as protein binding of the drug, lipid solubility and pKa. Some of these factors change with age and, therefore, in order to define the changes in distribution of drugs with age each of these properties has to be identified. The dose of a drug is also important in affecting its own distribution, as is the presence of other similar drugs. For example, probenecid competes with many organic anions for transport across choroid plexus cells. Thus it blocks the exit of penicillin, 5HIAA, and homovanillic acid. But if given in large doses, probenecid can also block its own transport out of the CSF. Many drugs may act on the brain by inhibiting transport of other drugs or endogenous metabolites out of the CSF. This would result in

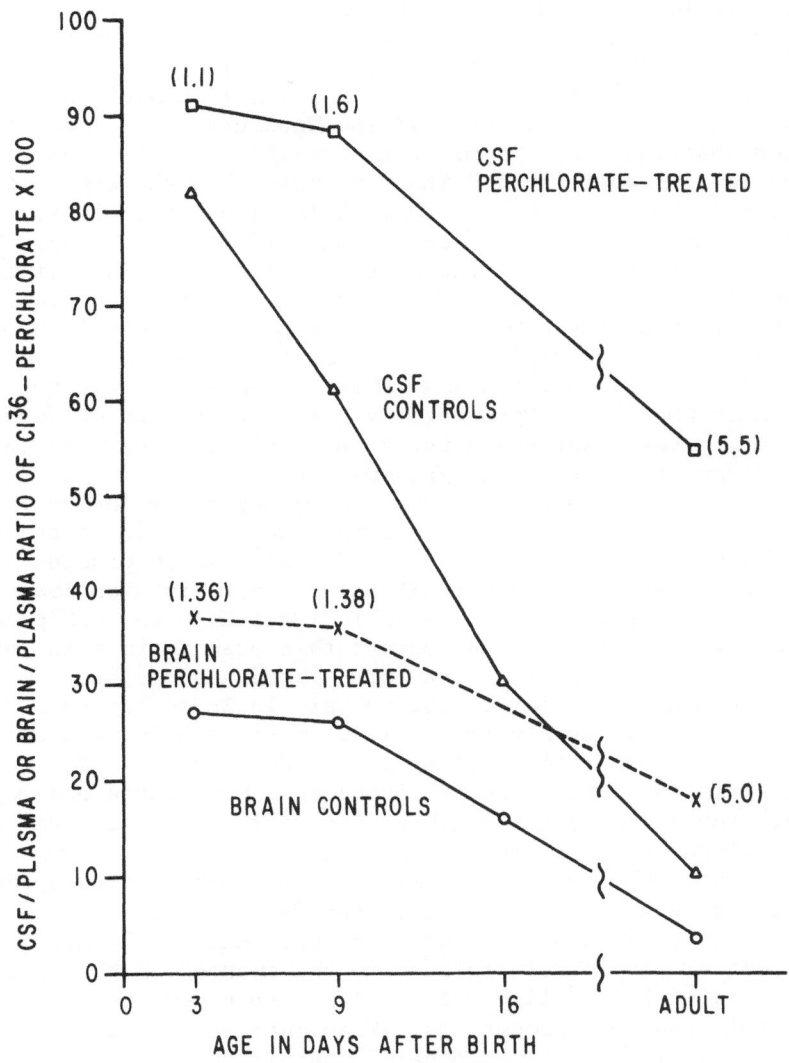

Fig. 5. Changes in CSF/plasma and brain/plasma ratio of ^{36}Cl-perchlorate with age in untreated and perchlorate-treated rats. See text for discussion.

an increase in their level of CSF and in brain and, if this level is sufficiently elevated, may cause pharmacological effects on the brain.

Fetal and neonatal animals are particularly vulnerable to the effects of centrally acting drugs because the various factors which maintain low levels of drugs in the brain of adult animals are not developed. The concentrations in fetal brain and CSF can reach high levels and thereby exert damaging effects. An example of this is the study on the distribution of ^{3}H-ouabain in brain and CSF in animals at various ages (Brøndsted and Woodbury, 1973, and unpublished observations). Some of the results of this study are depicted in Figures 6 and 7. These figures show the uptake of ^{3}H-ouabain into plasma, brain, CSF, skeletal muscle, liver, and heart of 3-day-old (Figure 6) and 35-day-old (Figure 7) rats. The ordinate in both figures is the amount of _free_ ouabain activity per gram of tissue or fluid and the abscissa is time in hours after injection of ^{3}H-ouabain. It is evident that the liver/plasma, heart/plasma and muscle/plasma ratios of free ouabain are very low in the 3-day-old animals and that they increase with age to values much greater than 1.0. Consequently active transport of ouabain occurs into these tissues and the transport increases with age. In the 3-day-old rats the CSF/plasma ratio is very low (< 1.0) and is less than the corresponding CSF/plasma ratio for inulin at this age period. This is suggestive evidence that ouabain is transported out of the CSF even at this age period. As seen in Figure 7, the CSF/plasma ratio for ouabain in 35-day-old rats is even lower than in the 3-day-old rats and considerably lower than the CSF/plasma ratio for inulin. These data suggest that ouabain is transported out of the CSF and that the transport system also develops with age. The brain/CSF ratio of free ouabain in 3-day-old rats is less than 1.0 and in 35-day-old rats > 1.0. Thus ouabain is transported into brain cells and this ability increases with age. The transport in brain and other tissues, is blocked by a large dose of ouabain. Hence the system exhibits saturation kinetics and it is also inhibited by increasing the plasma K concentration. The permeability of the cerebral capillaries to ouabain also appears to decrease with age. It is evident, therefore that the concentration of ouabain in brain and CSF and its effects thereon at different age periods are intimately related to the changes in the blood brain-CSF epithelial cell barriers with respect to their permeability and transport properties. That this is important is indicated by the fact that the dose of ouabain for producing seizures in 50% of animals in 3-day-old rats is about 2 mg/kg whereas in 35-day-old rats a dose of about 70 mg/kg which is the LD50, does not produce seizures. Thus, sufficient levels of drug to cause convulsions cannot be reached in adults but in newborn animals a dose 1/35 as large can readily reach sufficinetly high levels in the brain to cause seizures.

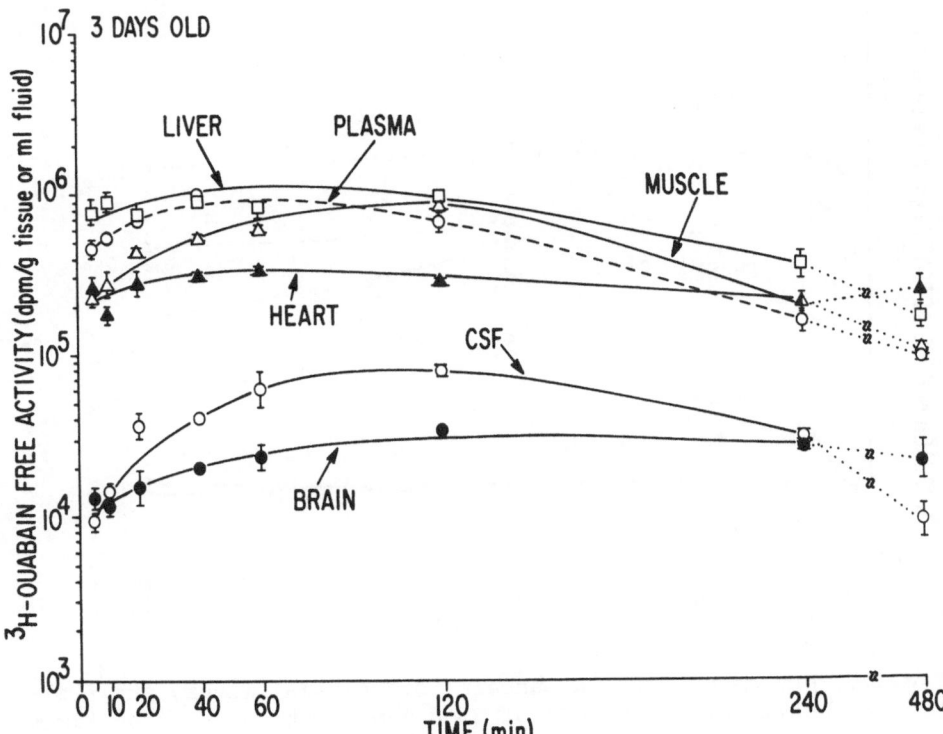

Fig. 6. Uptake of free ³H-ouabain into plasma, liver, skeletal muscle, heart, brain and CSF of 3-day-old rats at various times after i.p. injection. Note that levels of activity in muscle, liver and heart are about the same as in plasma and that the CSF activity is higher than that in brain. See text for discussion (from Brøndsted and Woodbury, unpublished observations).

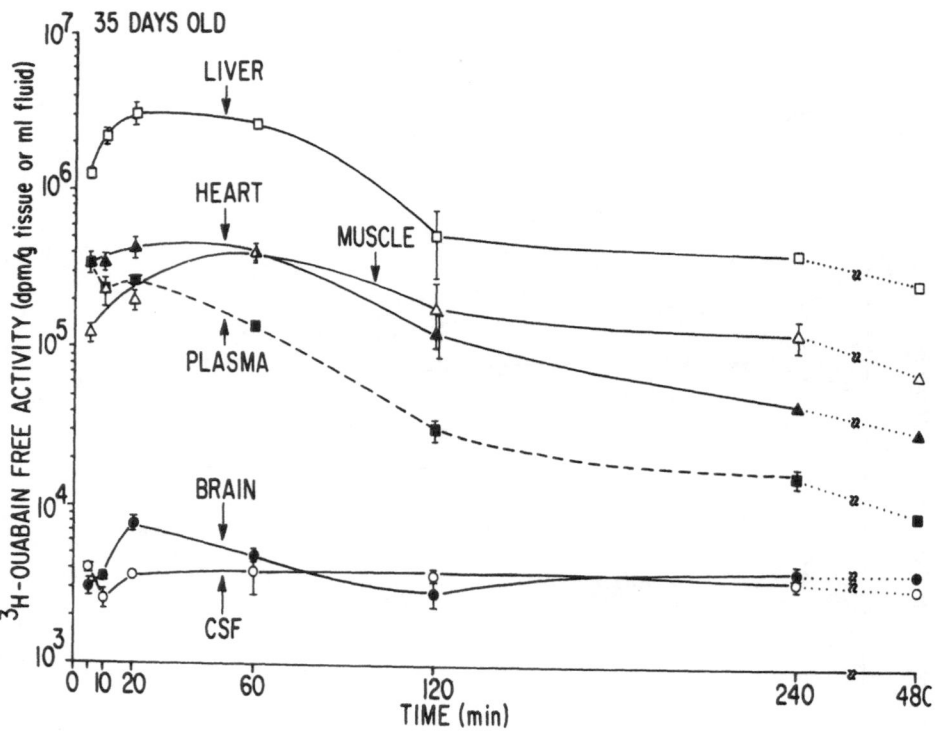

Fig. 7. Uptake of _free_ ³H-ouabain into plasma, liver, skeletal muscle, heart, brain and CSF of 35-day-old rats at various times after i.p. injection. Note that levels of activity in liver, muscle and heart are considerably higher than in plasma and that the brain activity is higher than that in CSF. This suggests that there is active transport of ouabain into these tissues from plasma or CSF. Note also that the CSF/plasma ratio in the 35-day-old rats is lower than that in the 3-day-old rats shown in Figure 6. This suggests that the transport of ouabain out of the CSF which is present in 3-day-old rats is even greater in 35-day-old rats. See text for further discussion (from Brøndsted, Woodbury, unpublished observations).

ACKNOWLEDGMENTS

Unpublished data presented in this paper were supported by a grant (5-P01-NS-04553) from the National Institute of Neurological Diseases and Stroke. Dr. Dixon M. Woodbury is the recipient of U.S. Public Health Service Research Career Award 5-K6-NB-13,838 from the National Institute of Neurological Diseases and Blindness, National Institutes of Health.

REFERENCES

Bakay, L., 1953, Studies on BBB with radioactive phosphorus. III. Embryonic development of the barrier, Arch. Neurol. Psychiat. (Chic.) 70: 30-39.

Bourke, R. S., Gabelnick, H. L. and Young, O., 1970, Mediated transport of chloride from blood into cerebrospinal fluid. Exp. Brain Res. 10: 17-38.

Brightman, M. W. and Reese, T. S., 1969, Junctions between intimately apposed cell membranes in the vertebrate brain, J. Cell. Biol. 40: 648-677.

Brizzee, K. R. and Jacobs, L. A., 1959, The glial-neuron index in the submolecular layers of the motor cortex in the cat, Anat. Rec. 134: 97-105.

Brøndsted, H. E. and Woodbury, D. M., 1973, Uptake and distribution of ^{3}H-ouabain in brain and other tissues of developing rats, in "Fetal Pharmacology", (L. O. Boreus, ed.), pp. 89-92, Raven Press, New York.

Caley, D. W. and Maxwell, D. S., 1968, An electron microscopic study of the neuroglia during postnatal development of the rat cerebrum, J. Comp. Neur. 133: 45-70.

Caley, D. W. and Maxwell, D. S., 1970, Development of the blood vessels and extracellular spaces during postnatal maturation of rat cerebral cortex, J. Comp. Neurol. 138: 31-48.

Chrone, C., 1971, The blood-brain barrier facts and questions, in "Ion Homeostasis of the Brain", Alfred Benzon Symposium III, (B. K. Siesjo and S. C. Sorensen, eds.), pp. 52-66, Munksgaard, Copenhagen.

Davson, H., 1973, Ontogeny of the blood-brain barrier, in "Fetal Pharmacology", (L. O. Boreus, ed.), pp. 75-88, Raven Press, New York.

Dobbing, J. and Sands, J. A., 1963, The entry of cholesterol into rat brain during development, J. Physiol. (Lond.), 166: 45P.

Donahue, Sheila and Pappas, G. D., 1961, The fine structure of capillaries in the cerebral cortex of the rat at various stages of development, Am. J. Anat. 108: 331-347.

Ferguson, R. K. and Woodbury, D. M., 1969, Penetration of ^{14}C-inulin and ^{14}C-sucrose into brain, cerebrospinal fluid, and skeletal muscle of developing rats, Exp. Brain Res. 7: 181-194.

Giacobini, E., 1962, A cytochemical study of the localization of carbonic anhydrase in the nervous system, J. Neurochem., 9: 169-177.

Grazer, F. M. and Clemente, C. D., 1957, Developing blood brain barrier to trypan blue, Proc. Soc. exp. Biol. Med. 94: 758-760.

Henn, F. A., Haljamäe, H. and Hamberger, A., 1972, Glial cell function: active control of extracellular K^+ concentration, Brain Res. 43: 437-443.

Himwich, H. E. and Himwich, W. A., 1955, The permeability of the blood-brain barrier to glutamic acid in the developing rat, in "Biochemistry of the Developing Nervous System", (H. Waelsch, ed.), p. 202, Academic Press, New York.

Katzman, R. and Leiderman, P. H., 1953, Brain potassium exchange in normal adult and immature rats, Am. J. Physiol. 174: 263-270.

Kuffler, S. W. and Nicholls, J. G., 1966, The physiology of Neuro-glial cells, Ergebn. Physiol. 57: 1-90.

Lajtha, A., 1958, Amino acid and protein metabolism of the brain II. The uptake of L-lysine by brain and other organs of the mouse at different ages, J. Neurochem. 2: 209-215.

Luciano, Dorothy S., 1968, Sodium movement across the blood-brain barrier in newborn and adult rats and autoradiographic-local-ization, Brain Res. 9: 334-350.

Olsson, Y., 1968, Blood-brain barrier to albumin in embryonic, new born and adult rats, Acta Neuropath. 10: 117-122.

Orkand, R. K., 1969, Neuroglial-neuronal interactions, in "Basic Mechanisms of the Epilepsies", (H. H. Jasper, A. A. Ward and A. Pope, eds.), pp. 737-746, Little, Brown & Co., Boston.

Pappenheimer, J. R., 1970, On the location of the blood-brain barrier, in "Proceedings of a Symposium on the Blood-Brain Barrier", (R. V. Coxon, ed.), pp. 66-84, Truex Press, Oxford. (Also see discussion by Brightman, M. R. on page 237-238 of this same Symposium and Figure opposite page 240).

Pollen, D. A. and Trachenberg, M. D., 1970, Neuroglia: gliosis and focal epilepsy, Science 167: 1252-1253.

Pysh, J. J., 1969, The development of the extracellular space in neonatal rat inferior colliculus: an electron microscopic study. Am. J. Anat. 124: 411-430.

Reed, D. J. and Woodbury, D. M., 1963, Kinetics of movement of iodide, sucrose, inulin and radioiodinated serum albumin in central nervous system and cerebrospinal fluid of rat, J. Physiol. (Lond.) 169: 816-850.

Rhodes, A. J. and Hyde, J. B., 1965, Postnatal growth of arterioles in the human cerebral cortex, Growth 29: 173-182.

Robinson, R. J., Cutler, R. W. P., Lorenzo, A. V. and Barlow, C. F., 1968, Development of transport mechanisms for sulphate and iodide in immature choroid plexus, J. Neurochem. 15: 455-458.

Saunders, N. R. and Bradbury, M. W. B., 1973, The development of the internal environment of the brain, in "Fetal Pharmacology", (Boreus, ed.) pp. 93-109, Raven Press, New York.

Shaywitz, B. A., Katzman, R. and Escriva, A., 1969, CSF formation and ^{24}Na clearance in normal and hydrocephalic kittens during ventriculocisternal perfusion, Neurology 19: 1159-1168.

Trachtenberg, M. C. and Pollen, D. A., 1970, Neuroglia: biophysical properties and physiologic function, Science 167: 1248-1252.

Vaughn, J. E. and Peters, A., 1967, Electron microscopy of the early postnatal development of fibrous astrocytes, Am. J. Anat. 121: 131-152.

Vernadakis, Antonia and Woodbury, D. M., 1962, Electrolyte and amino acid changes in rat brain during maturation, Am. J. Physiol. 203: 748-752.

Vernadakis, Antonia and Woodbury, D. M., 1965, Cellular and extra-cellular spaces in developing rat brain, Arch. Neurol. 12: 284-293.

Woodbury, D. M., 1968, Distribution of nonelectrolytes and
    electrolytes in the brain as affected by alterations in
    cerebrospinal fluid secretion, in "Progress in Brain Research",
    29, (A. Lajtha and D. Ford, eds.), pp. 297-313, Elsevier
    Publishing Co., Amsterdam.

Woodbury, D. M., 1971, Discussion, in "Ion Homeostasis of the Brain",
    Alfred Benzon Symposium III, (B. K. Siesjo and S. C. Sorensen,
    eds.), pp. 337-339, Munksgaard, Copenhagen.

CHANGES IN CSF FLOW AND EXTRACELLULAR SPACE IN THE DEVELOPING RAT

Conrad E. Johanson and Dixon M. Woodbury

Department of Pharmacology, University of Utah College

of Medicine, Salt Lake City, Utah

The effect of bulk flow of cerebrospinal fluid on the distribution of substances in the central nervous system has been a problem appreciated especially by those who have attempted to quantify the interstitial volume of the brain. The implications of this so-called "CSF sink" effect, particularly with regard to the measurement of brain extracellular space, have been treated thoroughly in reviews by Davson (1965) and by Woodbury (1967).

Results obtained from developmental studies by Ferguson and Woodbury (1969) indicate that the brain/CSF concentration ratio for inulin apparently reflects the brain extracellular space in young rats, but not in older animals. These authors have suggested that during the third postnatal week there are changes in the permeability of the ependymal membrane and/or CSF flow rate, the result being that this extracellular marker does not equilibrate between the interstitial fluid and the CSF; thus, when inulin is administered intraperitoneally to rats 3 weeks of age or older, the brain extracellular space is overestimated when the CSF is used as the reference fluid.

In order to shed more light on this particular problem, we have investigated patterns of CSF flow in neonatal rats of various ages. Previously, changes in CSF flow during development have been inferred from changes in electrolyte concentration ratios of CSF and plasma. However, in this study we have perfused the ventricular systems of young rats in order to evaluate changes in CSF flow more directly by the method of indicator dilution.

METHODS

Ventriculo-cisternal perfusions were carried out in rats, the ages of which ranged from 8 to 23 days. Results of preliminary experiments had indicated that one of the main problems associated with small animal perfusion involved the fixation of the head so that the needle cannulae could be properly positioned and maintained as such. This problem was solved by casting body molds (with acrylic resin) to accomodate animals approximately 1, 2 and 3 weeks old. Each of the molds was made to fit snugly into a lucite block, the latter mountable on an adjustable platform.

Each infant rat was anesthetized with sodium pentobarbital (30 mg/kg) and prepared for perfusion as subsequently described. The skull bone overlying parietal cortex was exposed, scraped clean and burred with a small bit at a point 2-3 mm caudal to the coronal suture and 2-3 mm to the left of the midline. After cannulation of the trachea, artificial ventilation was accomplished with a rodent respirator. The rat was then placed in the appropriate mold and lucite block and mounted on the platform of the perfusion apparatus. With the aid of a dissection microscope the atlanto-occipital membrane over the cisterna magna was exposed. The ventricular and cisternal cannulae (no. 27 and no. 26 gauge needles, respectively) were lined up normal to their respective puncture sites. Prior to the puncturings, the head was further secured in the mold by means of tightly drawn thread. The cisternal catheter (affixed to the hub of the needle) was filled with saline so that successful puncture would be manifested by fluid movement in the catheter. The left lateral ventricle was punctured and a unilateral ventriculo-cisternal perfusion slowly begun. Throughout the perfusion the ambient temperature was kept at 30°C by a heat lamp.

All animals were perfused with a synthetic CSF containing ^{14}C-inulin (1 μc/ml). The end of the outflow catheter was lowered 5 to 6 cm below the level of the cisterna magna to encourage maximal drainage. Effluent samples from the cistern were collected in shell vials (capped with parafilm) over several 20-min-intervals during the course of the 2 to 3 hour perfusions.

Calculations

The production rate of CSF, $\dot{V}_f$, has been calculated by the common formula

$$\dot{V}_f = \dot{V}_i \times (C_i - C_o) / C_o$$

where C_i and C_o represent the activities of ^{14}C-inulin in the perfusion fluid and perfusate, respectively, and $\dot{V}_i$ is the rate of inflow determined gravimetrically by pre- and post-experimental calibration of fluid delivery by the infusion pump.

TABLE I

ATTAINMENT OF STEADY-STATE CONDITIONS DURING
VENTRICULO-CISTERNAL PERFUSION OF A 13-DAY-OLD RAT

Inflow Rate = 13.8 µl/min
Inflow Activity = 80,412 CPM of ^{14}C-Inulin/50 µl Perfusion Fluid

Sample #	Collection Interval (min)	Cisternal Outflow Rate (µl/min)	Effluent Activity (CPM/50 µl)
3	40–60	13.8	75,056
4	60–80	13.2	76,422
5	80–100	13.4	76,598
6	100–120	13.7	77,558
7	120–140	13.0	77,378

RESULTS

Data obtained from a typical perfusion are listed in Table I
to illustrate the attainment of steady-state conditions. After about
an hour of perfusion, a steady state with respect to outflow rate and
indicator activity is achieved. In the majority of perfusions the
average rate of outflow is approximately 90-95% of the rate of perfusion when the cisternal samples are collected under a negative
perfusion pressure.

Inulin activity data obtained from radioisotopic counting of
each steady-state outflow sample can be used to calculate a production rate of CSF for each steady-state period during perfusion.
Each of the points plotted in Figure 1 is an experimental mean value
for $\dot{V}_f$ and thus represents the average of several such steady-state
values for $\dot{V}_f$ obtained from one rat. When CSF production ($\dot{V}_f$) is
plotted as a function of the age of the animal for which $\dot{V}_f$ was determined, a correlation coefficient of 0.8 is obtained, suggesting
that there is a progressive increase in CSF flow with age. The equation of the regression line in Figure 1 can be used to calculate a
value of -4 days (i.e., 4 days prenatal) for the x-intercept which
is the predicted age for which the CSF flow is essentially zero. This
extrapolated value is consistent with the findings of Ferguson and
Woodbury (1969) that CSF secretion, as inferred from CSF and plasma
electrolyte data, commences in the rat between the ages of 6 and 4
days before birth. At the other extreme, the rate of CSF secretion

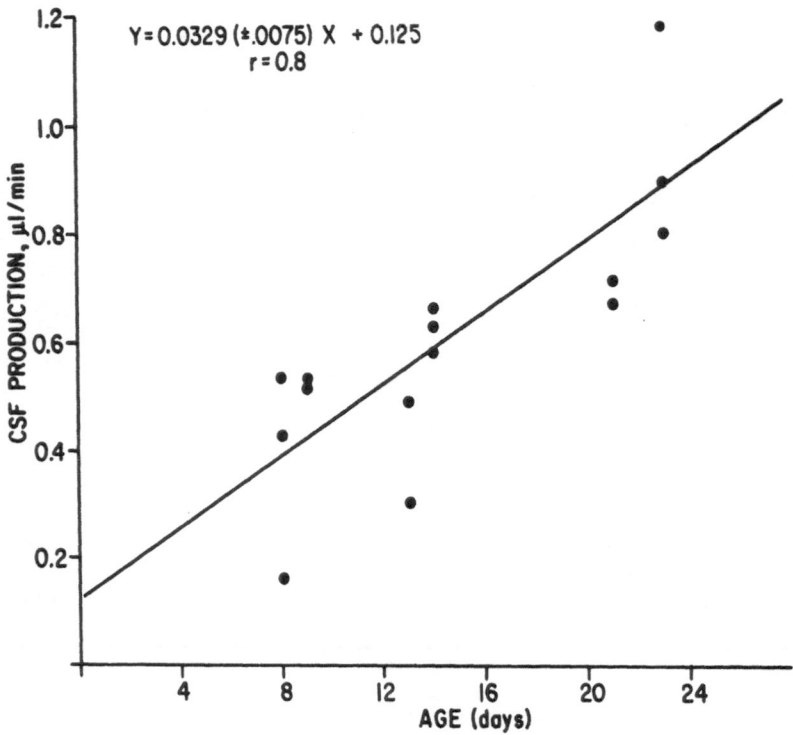

Fig. 1.   Rates of CSF Production in Neonatal Rats.   Each filled circle
represents a control value of $\dot{V}_f$ for one rat and is the average of
3 to 6 steady-state values for $\dot{V}_f$ obtained from one perfusion.   The
regression line was obtained by the method of least squares.   The
correlation coefficient is 0.8.

---

in the adult rat is approximately 2 µl/min.   If there is an essentially
linear progression of CSF flow rate with age during development, such
as is described by the equation in Figure 1, a flow rate of 2 µl/min
can be predicted to occur at approximately 60 days of age.   However,
until flow data are obtained from animals 4 to 8 weeks old, no conclusion can be made as to when the CSF system achieves maturity.

Since the choroidal epithelium is thought to be the primary
source of the cerebrospinal fluid, it seems desirable to relate the
CSF production to plexus tissue weight for each of the age groups
studied in order to ascertain if the capacity of the tissue for
volume secretion changes with age.   Choroid plexus tissues were excised from lateral ventricles and weighed on an electrobalance.
Since these tissues are very small (0.4 to 0.9 mg) and lose a sub-

TABLE II

CHANGES IN CSF PRODUCTION AND INULIN SPACE IN DEVELOPING RATS

Age Group	Rate of CSF Production (µl/min)	Weight of Ch. Plexus (mg)	CSF Flow/ Wt. Ch. Pl. (µl/min/mg)	Inulin Space (ml ECF/g Cortex) x 100
8-9 Days N=5	0.44 ±.06	1.14 ±.15	0.39	10.9 ±.8
13-14 Days N=5	0.53 ±.06	1.36 ±.10	0.39	7.9 ±1.2
21-23 Days N=5	0.86 ±.10	1.52 ±.11	0.57	4.6 ±.5

stantial amount of water before a weight can be recorded, it is
necessary to determine the rate of water loss for each tissue and
then, by graphical analysis, to extrapolate to time zero (i.e., the
time of tissue removal from the ventricular cavity) in order to estimate the fresh weight of the tissue. Average weights of plexus
tissues (from both lateral ventricles) for each of the 3 groups of
animals are listed in Table II. Not unexpectedly, there is a tendency for the weight of the plexus tissue to increase with age. Comparison of the data (8-9 days vs. 21-23 days) reveals a significant
increase in both CSF production and choroid plexus weight with increasing age. Moreover, the plexus tissue in the 3-week-old rats
may be more mature than in the 1-week-old animals since there is a
greater volume secretion per unit weight of tissue in the 21-23 day
rats than in the 8-9 day animals (See column 4 in Table II). The
ratio of CSF production to choroid plexus weight eventually reaches
a value of 0.8 µl/min/mg tissue in the adult rat (250-350 g). That
the choroid plexus is still in the process of maturing three weeks
after birth is suggested by the figure of about 0.6 µl/min/mg that
we have found for the 21- to 23-day-old rats.

Another objective of this study was to determine the extracellular space of each developing brain by allowing inulin to equilibrate between perfusion fluid and brain tissue. Listed in Table II
are activity ratios for ^{14}C-inulin (cortex/perfusion fluid) that were
determined for rats perfused for 2 to 3 hours. The finding that there
is a significant decrease ($P<.05$) in the inulin space with age agrees
with previous reports that the extracellular space of the CNS undergoes a progressive decrease in size at the expense of the expanding
cellular compartment. However, the inulin spaces of the brain for

the respective age groups are considerably lower than corresponding
measurements that have been previously obtained by different techniques (Vernadakis and Woodbury, 1965; Ferguson and Woodbury, 1969).
One possibility for this discrepancy is that our perfusion time is
not of long enough duration to permit the indicator to equilibrate
between interstitial fluid and ventricular fluid. Thus, longer perfusions are indicated to determine if these inulin spaces that we
have found increase with perfusion time.

DISCUSSION

In experiments in which inulin has been injected into plasma,
the inulin space (on the basis of brain/CSF ratio) has been found to
decrease until 16 days of age; between the 16th and 26th day the
ratio reverses itself and then increases steadily to an adult value
of 55% (Ferguson and Woodbury, 1969). It is unlikely that the extracellular space actually increases after 16 days and so a previous
explanation attributed this phenomenon to the development of an ependymal barrier in the maturing animal. The results of the present
study suggest another explanation, namely that the CSF sink effect
must increase with age since it has been shown that the CSF flow
approximately doubles between the ages of 2 and 3 weeks.

There is evidence that the active mechanisms that produce CSF
in neonatal rats are still maturing as late as three weeks after birth.
At approximately 1 week and 3 weeks of age the CSF formation per unit
weight of plexus is about one-half and three-fourths, respectively,
of the value for adult rats. However, this kind of evidence for an
immature plexus in the neonatal rat is not unequivocal since there
may be an extrachoroidal tissue which elaborates CSF. The latter
possibility has also been considered by Holloway and Cassin (1972)
who have established that the rate of CSF formation per unit weight
of choroid plexus in the 2- to 4-day-old pup is approximately one-
fifth the value for the adult dog.

Finally, an attempt has been made to gain an accurate measurement of cortical extracellular space in the developing rat. Inulin,
which has been used as the extracellular marker, has been presented
to the CSF side of the brain tissue in order to eliminate the CSF
sink effect. Further experiments are necessary to ascertain if the
2 to 3 hour inulin spaces that we have determined actually represent
steady-state values.

ACKNOWLEDGMENTS

This study was supported by U.S. Public Health Service Pharmacology Training Grant No. GM00153 and U.S. Public Health Service Pro-
gram-Project Grant 5-P01-NS-04553 from the National Institute of Neurological Diseases and Stroke.

REFERENCES

Davson, H., 1965, The extracellular space of the brain, in "Progress in Brain Research," Vol 12, (E.D.P. De Robertis and R. Carrea, eds.), pp. 124-134, Elsevier Publishing Co., Amsterdam, London and New York.

Ferguson, R.K., and Woodbury, D.M., 1969, Penetration of ^{14}C-inulin and ^{14}C-sucrose into brain, cerebrospinal fluid, and skeletal muscle of developing rats, Exp. Brain Res. 7: 181.

Holloway, L.S., and Cassin, S., 1972, Cerebrospinal fluid dynamics in the newborn dog during normoxia and hypoxia, Am. J. Physiol. 223: 499.

Vernadakis, A., and Woodbury, D.M., 1965, Cellular and extracellular spaces in developing rat brain, Arch. Neurol. 12: 284.

Woodbury, D.M., 1967, Distribution of nonelectrolytes and electrolytes in the brain as affected by alterations in cerebrospinal fluid secretion, in "Progress in Brain Research," Vol. 29, (A. Lajtha and D. Ford, eds.), pp. 297-313, Elsevier Publishing Co., Amsterdam.

DEVELOPMENTAL CHANGES IN IONIC COMPOSITION OF THE BRAIN IN HYPO

AND HYPERTHYROIDISM

Theony Valcana

Department of Physiology-Anatomy, University of

California, Berkeley, California

Disturbances in the levels of thyroid hormones are known to affect the normal function of the central nervous system (CNS), manifested most dramatically when they occur during development. Lack of thyroid hormones at critical stages of CNS maturation can result in an irreversible condition, which, when not diagnosed and treated early, leads to severe mental retardation. With specific reference to the developing CNS, not only is the basic mode of action of thyroid hormones not known, but the particular alteration(s) that characterizes the cretinoid condition also remains to be established, despite reported findings from many laboratories that numerous biochemical parameters important to brain growth and differentiation are altered in hypothyroidism (see Geel and Timiras, 1970; Balázs et al., 1971; Hamburgh et al., 1971). One parameter of special significance to normal CNS growth and function is that of its ionic composition; maturational disturbances in the levels of various ions would be expected to have their repercussions on the development of specialized CNS functions. In the present study, the ionic composition of the "hypothyroid brain" is described and, in order to distinguish those alterations that are specific to neural tissue, ionic changes in other body tissues are presented in parallel and related to corresponding observations reported by others. The effects of exogenous thyroxine administration also are presented in order to ascertain the influence of the hormone on normal brain development and on the alterations induced by hypothyroidism.

The effects of thyroid hormone deficiency on the ionic metabolism of the brain has been less well studied than its corresponding effects on the whole organism. One of the well-known symptoms of myxedematous patients, for example, is the retention of excessive Na and water in tissues and the loss of Na and water from the plasma

(Aikawa, 1956). Other clinical studies of hypothyroid patients, conducted by Byrom (1933), indicated that thyroxine treatment leads to diuresis, followed by a decrease in total body Na and K, the loss of Na being greater than the loss of K. The effect was dependent on the dose of thyroxine administered.

A relationship also has been drawn between thyroid function and Mg metabolism (Dine and Lavietes, 1942). Soffer and associates have reported almost no bound Mg in the serum of myxedmatous patients, yet total serum Mg was not changed. Conversely in most patients with hyperthyroidism, a greater than normal percentage of bound serum Mg was observed (Soffer et al., 1941). Experimental research in animals also shows a relationship between thyroid function and Mg metabolism; for example, Vitale and his associates (1957) have demonstrated a relationship between thyroxine and Mg requirements in rats. Furthermore, a decrease occurs in total plasma Mg after treatment with L-thyroxine (Liu and Overman, 1964), and, correspondingly, an increase in plasma Mg following thyroidectomy (Szelenyi et al., 1968). Thyroid hormones also appear to influence the metabolism of Ca. In hyperthyroidism, greater than normal excretion of Ca occurs whereas in hypothyroidism, excretion levels are subnormal (Pitt-Rivers and Tata, 1959a; Geschwind, 1961; Care, 1968).

With specific respect to the interdependence of thyroid function and ionic metabolism in the brain, Timiras and Woodbury (1956) have found that thyroidectomy of adult rats leads to an increase in plasma Na concentration with no change in plasma K or Cl concentrations. Furthermore, these investigators observed a decrease in the intracellular Na concentration in the brain, when using the Cl space as a measure of cerebral extracellular space, whereas brain K and Cl concentrations were not changed. On the other hand, thyroxine and triiodothyronine treatment of normal adult rats significantly decreased Na and increased K of plasma. Again using Cl space for evaluating intracellular Na concentration, it was found that total brain Na content, intracellular Na concentration and Na space were increased by hormonal treatment whereas brain Cl space and Cl concentration in plasma and brain were not modified.

From the literature summarized above, it emerges that thyroid hormones play an important role in the metabolism of inorganic ions, and one which warrants more intensive investigation in the developing organism, and, in particular, the brain. Accordingly, the specific aim of the present research is to clarify the developmental changes that occur in ionic composition in the rat brain under various conditions of thyroid function. The ionic composition of any tissue, as well as of the CNS, is maintained by many intricately interrelated processes. In our studies, we have selected to relate any such changes either to changes in the extracellular milieu - as reflected by changes in plasma composition, or to changes at cell membrane level - as may be reflected by changes in the activity of Na-K-ATPase, an enzyme implicated in active sodium and potassium transport. We also have examined the ionic composition of the red blood cell (RBC), not only for comparative purposes but because changes in nerve tissue-plasma, unlike those in RBC-plasma, may also reflect alterations occuring in the extracellular space.

The data presented is based on separate findings from a number of experiments we have conducted in this area, some of which already have appeared in published form (Valcana and Timiras, 1969; Valcana and Timiras, 1971).

The experimental groups consisted of normal control rats, hypothyroid rats, hypothyroid rats receiving thyroxine and normal controls receiving thyroxine. In all cases, hypothyroidism was induced at one day of age by intraperitoneal administration of 100 μC of ^{131}I, according to the method of Goldberg and Chaikoff (1949).

Replacement therapy, initiated to determine whether restoration of thyroxine is capable of returning the parameters studied to normal control values, consisted of daily subcutaneous injections of 10 μg/100 g body weight L-thyroxine from the 6th postnatal day until sacrifice. Hyperthyroidism, initiated to test the effects of excess thyroxine both in the developing and adult CNS, was induced as follows: for developing rats, two experimental groups were employed, one receiving daily injections of L-thyroxine 10 μg/100 g body weight from day 6 until sacrifice and one receiving graded doses of thyroxine - 2.5 μg/100 g body weight from day 1 to day 5 and 10 μg/100 g body weight from day 6 until sacrifice. Thyroxine treatment of adult animals consists of daily subcutaneous injection of 40 μg/100 g body weight for a period of 4 consecutive days.

Animals were sacrificed by decapitation and cerebral cortical tissue was rapidly removed and assayed for electrolytes and/or ATPase activity (see Valcana and Timiras, 1969, for methods). The details of the exact conditions of enzyme preparation and incubation for the ATPase assay are included in the legends to the pertinent tables.

IONIC CHANGES

During normal maturation, Cl, Na and Ca concentrations in plasma increased whereas K concentration decreased. No change occurred in Mg concentration, in agreement with the findings of Silverman and Gardner (1954), who found no differences in total plasma Mg between children and adults. The changes in Na, Cl and K content in plasma correspond to those previously observed by Vernadakis and Woodbury (1962).

TABLE I

EFFECT OF NEONATAL HYPOTHYROIDISM AND THYROXINE ON WATER AND ELECTROLYTE
CONCENTRATIONS OF PLASMA IN THE DEVELOPING RAT

Experimental Groups	meq/kg wet tissue				
	Cl	Na	K	Mg	Ca
Control (10)[a]	96.25 ± 2.48	138.50 ± 2.79	6.39 ± 0.48	1.67 ± 0.05	4.29 ± 0.05
Hypothyroid (10)[b]	96.06 ± 1.35	134.54 ± 4.88	6.72 ± 0.77	1.80 ± 0.06	4.34 ± 0.10
Control (16)	102.00 ± 0.39	140.47 ± 2.65	5.49 ± 0.15	1.69 ± 0.02	4.86 ± 0.12
Hypothyroid (16)	103.51 ± 1.29	139.81 ± 0.75	5.45 ± 0.17	1.61 ± 0.06	4.93 ± 0.13
Control (22)	107.89 ± 0.78	143.03 ± 0.20	5.85 ± 0.19	1.63 ± 0.05	5.00 ± 0.11
Hypothyroid (22)	106.95 ± 1.02	142.25 ± 0.67	5.02 ± 0.33	1.38 ± 0.03	4.55 ± 0.01
			$P<0.05$	$P<0.001$	$P<0.01$
Thyroxine-treated[c] (Hypothyroid) (22)	106.75 ± 0.82	142.54 ± 0.62	6.00 ± 0.31	1.71 ± 0.09	5.05 ± 0.18
Thyroxine-treated[c] (Control) (22)	100.23 ± 1.25	136.00 ± 1.91	6.55 ± 0.35	1.41 ± 0.03	4.25 ± 0.13
	$P<0.05$	$P<0.01$	$P<0.01$	$P<0.01$	$P<0.01$
Control (32)	106.17 ± 1.32	145.34 ± 1.08	5.71 ± 0.18	1.76 ± 0.06	5.49 ± 0.08
Hypothyroid (32)	105.35 ± 1.27	143.19 ± 2.13	4.50 ± 0.20	1.46 ± 0.04	4.93 ± 0.08
		$P<0.001$	$P<0.001$	$P<0.001$	$P<0.001$

[a]Numbers in parentheses represent age of animals in days.

[b]Hypothyroidism was induced at 1 day of age according to the method of Goldberg and Chaikoff (1949).

[c]Animals received daily subcutaneous injections of L-thyroxine at a dose of 10 μg/100g body weight.

Values are means ± S.E. from 8 or more animals; one sample per animal, 2 determinations per sample. P values refer to significance of difference between experimental and control groups.

Data taken from Valcana and Timiras (1971).

TABLE II

EFFECT OF NEONATAL HYPOTHYROIDISM AND THYROXINE ON WATER AND ELECTROLYTE
CONCENTRATIONS IN THE CEREBRAL CORTEX OF THE DEVELOPING RAT

Experimental Groups	%H$_2$O	meq/kg wet tissue				
		Cl	Na	K	Mg	Ca
Control (10)[a]	85.37 ± 0.20	40.40 ± 0.61	59.87 ± 2.32	82.18 ± 0.81	13.05 ± 0.25	3.06 ± 0.19
Hypothyroid[b] (10)	86.17 ± 0.18	42.95 ± 0.73	63.95 ± 1.59	77.05 ± 0.56	12.00 ± 0.23	2.96 ± 0.18
	$P<0.05$	$P<0.05$	$P=0.05$	$P<0.001$	$P<0.01$	
Control (16)	82.24 ± 0.49	38.15 ± 1.96	51.13 ± 0.49	103.92 ± 1.21	13.78 ± 0.11	3.51 ± 0.19
Hypothyroid (16)	83.35 ± 0.38	45.39 ± 1.25	56.84 ± 1.08	92.83 ± 2.87	12.67 ± 0.37	3.66 ± 0.29
	$P<0.05$	$P<0.01$	$P<0.001$	$P<0.02$	$P<0.01$	
Control (22)	81.90 ± 0.06	32.42 ± 0.48	49.33 ± 0.68	108.82 ± 2.39	14.75 ± 0.23	2.87 ± 0.11
Hypothyroid (22)	82.80 ± 0.09	34.28 ± 0.99	54.37 ± 0.75	100.71 ± 1.89	13.78 ± 0.22	2.67 ± 0.08
	$P<0.001$	$P<0.05$	$P<0.001$	$P<0.01$	$P<0.02$	
Thyroxine-[c] treated (Hypothyroid) (22)	81.90 ± 0.09	32.00 ± 0.69	48.11 ± 1.45	109.41 ± 1.25	14.88 ± 0.19	2.85 ± 0.13
Thyroxine-[c] treated (Control) (22)	81.78 ± 0.25	31.37 ± 1.46	48.83 ± 0.73	110.81 ± 0.84	14.65 ± 0.45	2.56 ± 0.11
Control (32)	82.75 ± 0.96	28.02 ± 0.81	42.15 ± 0.35	102.23 ± 0.81	13.31 ± 0.12	3.25 ± 0.45
Hypothyroid (32)	82.90 ± 0.60	34.44 ± 0.94	48.39 ± 0.70	97.93 ± 0.26	12.89 ± 0.06	3.11 ± 0.32
	$P<0.001$	$P<0.001$	$P<0.001$	$P<0.001$	$P<0.01$	

a,b,cAs in Table I. Values as in Table I. Data taken from Valcana and Timiras (1969).

Neonatal hypothyroidism induced a decrease in plasma K, Mg and Ca concentrations which first became evident in 22 day-old animals. In contrast, no significant changes were observed in plasma Na and Cl concentrations at any age interval studied. Thyroxine treatment of hypothyroid rats (10 μg/100 g body weight) from day 6 until sacrifice at day 22, returned all observed changes to control values.

Control animals receiving thyroxine from day 6 until sacrifice at day 22 showed an increase in plasma water content and a decrease in Na, Cl, Mg and Ca concentrations. Plasma K increased in this group (Table I).

The ionic changes that occur in cerebral cortical tissue with development and under various thyroid conditions are shown in Table II and in Figure 1. In both control and hypothyroid animals, K and Mg content increases and Na and Cl content decreases with development, changes which are more marked from 10 to 22 days of age. Ca levels in cerebral cortex, however, show no definite developmental pattern in either group (Table II). When compared with control rats, hypothyroid animals demonstrated significantly higher water, Na and Cl content and lower K and Mg content (Table II and Figure 1). These differences were evident as early as 10 days of age and except for water, were sustained throughout the experimental period. Ca levels showed no significant differences between control and hypothyroid animals in the cerebral cortex at any age interval studied.

When hypothyroid animals were treated with thyroxine from day 6 until sacrifice at day 22, changes observed in brain electrolytes returned to control values (Table II). Control animals similarly treated with thyroxine, however, showed no significant differences from non-treated controls. Although changes in Na, K and Mg content reported here are similar to those found in muscle tissue of adult

---

Fig. 1. Effects of neonatal hypothyroidism on Na and K contents, Mg-ATPase and Na-K ATPase activity in the DOC-extractable fraction (pH 6.5) from the cerebral cortex of the rat brain during development. Na-K ATPase activity is the difference between the total ATPase activity determined in the presence of Na, K and Mg ions and that of Mg-ATPase determined in the presence of Mg ions only. The Mg-ATPase activity was determined in a 2 cc. volume of incubation mixture of the following composition: 100 mM-histidine, pH 7.2, 3 mM-tris-ATP, and 3 mM-Mg; the incubation mixture for determination of total ATPase activity contained in addition 100 mM-Na and 20 mM-K. Incubation 30 min. at 37°. For ATPase activity, each point represents mean ± S.E. of duplicate determinations from 16 enzyme preparations and for Na and K contents, each point represents mean ± S.E. of 8 or more samples. The squares in all parameters at day 22 represent mean values obtained from hypothyroid animals treated daily with thyroxine (day 6 to day 22, 10 μg/100 g body weight). From Valcana and Timiras (1969).

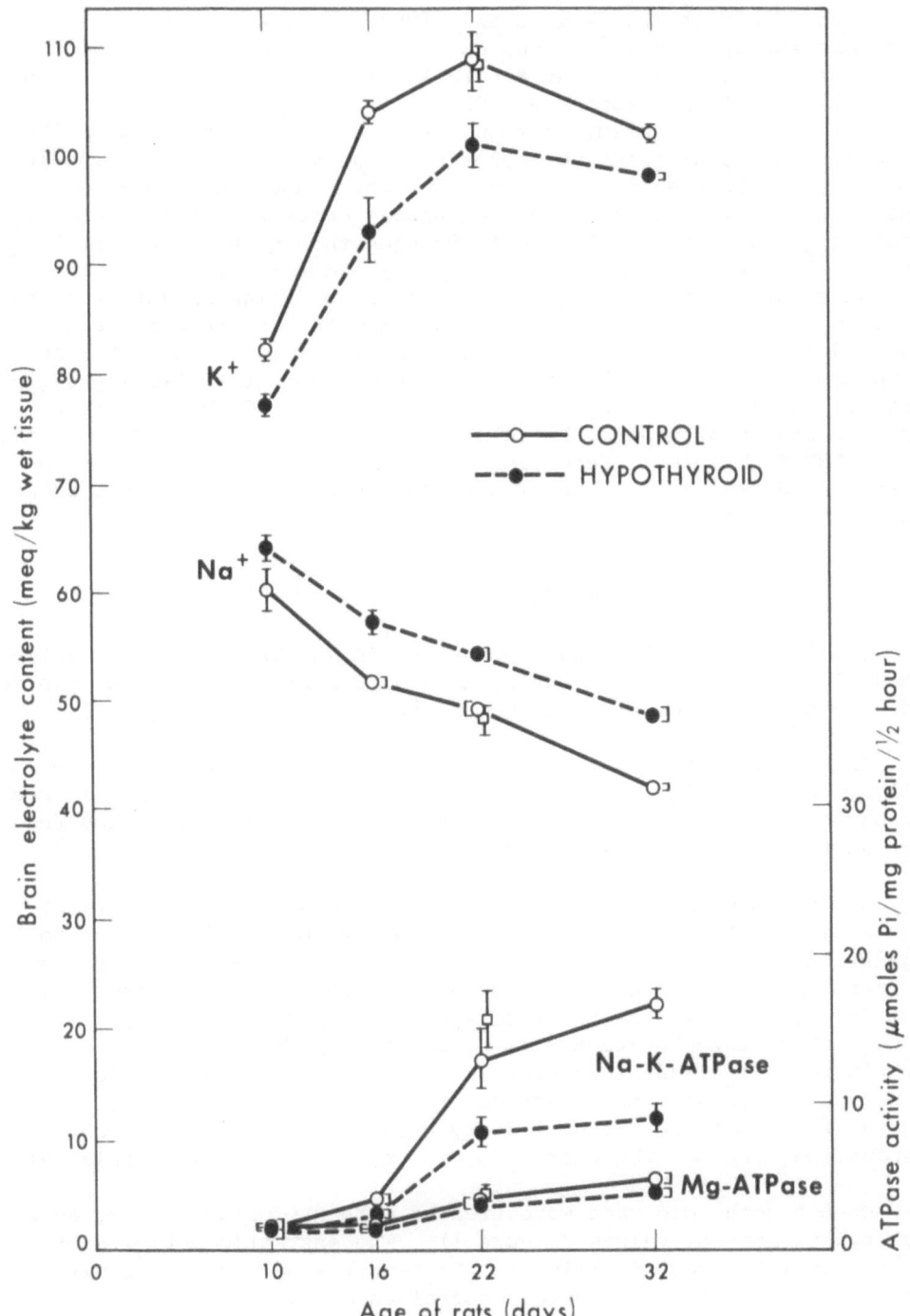

hypothyroid animals (Pandazi et al., 1959), they are in contrast to
those previously observed in the CNS of adult thyroidectomized animals, where a decrease in intracellular Na with no changes in K and
Cl content was found (Woodbury, 1958; Timiras and Woodbury, 1956).
Similarly, while no effect is found on the ionic composition of the
developing CNS consequent to thyroxine treatment (Table II), studies
in adult animals treated with thyroxine have shown that total Na content in the brain increases but no changes occur in total K content
(Timiras et al., 1955). The ionic changes that occur in cerebral
cortical tissue in the developing hypothyroid rat are similar to
changes occurring in the red blood cell where a significant increase
in Na content and a decrease in K, Mg and water contents are also
observed (Table III). The Cl content was lower in the hypothyroid
group than in controls, but the decrease was not statistically significant. The lack of change in ionic composition of the cerebral
cortical tissue of control animals is in contrast to what was observed
in the RBC from animals receiving thyroxine, where Na and water increased, K decreased, and no significant changes were observed in Mg
and Cl concentrations.

                         ATPase CHANGES

     The developmental changes occurring in Mg-ATPase and Na-K-acti-
vated ATPase extracted with deoxycholate from brain tissues of control
and hypothyroid animals are shown in the lower part of Figure 1.

     The specific activity of Mg-ATPase and Na-K-activated ATPase nor-
mally increased with age, and the latter showed a significant increase
during that period of brain development characterized by marked redistribution of Na and K content (Figure 1).

     Hypothyroidism induced a decrease in the specific activity of
Na-K-activated ATPase in the cerebral cortex but did not appear to
significantly affect the specific activity of Mg-ATPase. Inasmuch
as it is important to establish whether thyroxine really shows such
a differential action on these related enzymes and inasmuch as it is
thought that deoxycholate treatment may inhibit the Mg-ATPase or convert it to Na-K-ATPase (Järnefelt, 1964), we reexamined this effect
in tissue homogenates that were not treated with deoxycholate. These
studies show that when we omit deoxycholate treatment of the enzyme
preparation, the Mg-ATPase is also affected considerably (Table IV).

     When hypothyroid rats were treated with thyroxine, enzyme activity
reverted to control values (Figure 1). The enzymatic activity of
control animals treated daily with Na-L-thyroxine was not significantly different from untreated control animals, regardless of whether
the treatment was initiated at birth or at 6 days of age, and regardless of the age interval examined (Tables IV and V). Thyroxine

TABLE III

EFFECT OF NEONATAL HYPOTHYROIDISM AND OF THYROXINE ON H_2O, Cl, Na, K AND Mg
CONTENT OF RED BLOOD CELLS IN 22 DAY-OLD RATS

Experimental Groups	$\%H_2O$	meq per liter of cells			
		Cl	Na	K	Mg
Control	69.16 ± 0.37	64.41 ± 2.36	10.58 ± 0.37	118.44 ± 1.83	9.50 ± 0.24
Hypothyroid[b]	67.39 ± 0.39 P<0.02	62.87 ± 2.70	13.29 ± 0.97 P<0.01	112.28 ± 1.80 P<0.02	8.58 ± 0.21 P<0.01
Thyroxine-treated[c] (Control)	71.05 ± 0.32 P<0.05	64.21 ± 2.55	13.48 ± 0.73 P<0.01	113.05 ± 1.83 P<0.05	9.86 ± 0.48

[b],[c]As in Table I.

Values are means ± S.E. from 8 or more samples; P values refer to significance of differences between control and experimental groups.

TABLE IV

EFFECTS OF NEONATAL HYPOTHYROIDISM AND TREATMENT[a] WITH L-THYROXINE ON THE
ATPase ACTIVITY OF RAT CEREBRAL CORTICAL TISSUE

(μmoles Pi/hr/mg wet tissue)

	13-days old			22-days old		
	Control	Thyroxine Treated	Hypothyroid	Control	Thyroxine Treated	Hypothyroid
Na-K-Mg-ATPase	2.37 ± 0.09	2.44 ± 0.05	1.77[b] ± 0.18	3.97 ± 0.16	4.13 ± 0.26	3.46[b] ± 0.11
Mg-ATPase	1.04 ± 0.05	1.16 ± 0.04	0.69[b] ± 0.04	1.39 ± 0.10	1.72 ± 0.16	1.14[b] ± 0.05
Na-K-ATPase	1.32 ± 0.08	1.28 ± 0.04	1.08[b] ± 0.15	2.58 ± 0.12	2.41 ± 0.14	2.29[b] ± 0.11

[a] Animals were treated with 2.5μg/100g body weight from day 1 to day 5 and 10 μg/100g body weight from day 6 to sacrifice. Numbers represent means ± S.E. from tissues isolated from 4-6 animals. ATPase activity of each tissue homogenate was assayed in duplicate under the following incubation conditions: 2cc volume of incubation mixture composed of 50 mM Tris pH 7.4 3 mM Tris-ATP 3 mM Mg^{++} and, when present, 100 mM Na^+ and 20 mM K^+; incubation time 10 min at 37°C. Cerebral cortex was homogenized in 0.32 M sucrose, and 50λ of 2.5% homogenate was utilized for each assay.

[b] significantly different from control $p < 0.05$.

TABLE V

EFFECTS OF L-THYROXINE TREATMENT[b] OF ADULT RATS ON
THE ATPase ACTIVITY OF CEREBRAL CORTICAL TISSUE

	(μmoles Pi/hr/mg wet tissue)		
	Na-K-Mg-ATPase	Mg-ATPase	Na-K-ATPase
Control	3.74 ± 0.15[a]	1.95 ± 0.04	1.79 ± 0.13
Thyroxine Treated	4.07 ± 0.10	2.01 ± 0.11	2.05 ± 0.05

[a]Values represent means ± S.E. from 6 animals assayed in duplicate; homogenization and incubation conditions as described
in Table IV.

[b]Animals were injected subcutaneously with 40 μg/100 g body
weight per day for 4 consecutive days.

treatment of adult animals (65 days old) similarly showed no significant change in either Na-K-ATPase or Mg-ATPase activity (Table V),
findings which are in agreement with those reported by Raskin and
Fishman (1966) and Ismail-Beizi and Edelman (1971). However, in view
of the tendency toward higher values noted in these animals, sub-
fractionation studies should be conducted to determine whether this
finding reflects a change of this enzyme in a small subcellular compartment.

The decrease in Na concentration and the increase in K concentration between the 10th and 22nd postnatal days implies an exchange
of these ions during neonatal development (Figure 1). This ionic
redistribution in the cerebral cortex has been previously ascribed
to acid-base changes that may occur during maturation; according to
Woodbury and his co-workers (1958), for example, K concentration is
regulated by total anion content of the cell, which may vary considerably, being dependent on cellular pH as well as on the metabolic processes affecting the concentrations of free acidic and basic
amino acids and on the cellular concentration of bicarbonate. In
addition, however, K concentration depends on the coupling of potassium movement to active sodium transport. The results of the present study suggest that Na and K redistribution may be consequent
to the onset of active transport, inasmuch as it occurs concomitantly
with a marked increase in the Na-K-activated ATPase activity in this
tissue. This interpretation is consistent with the role ascribed

to ATPase in brain and other tissues in which it is found (Deul and McIlwain, 1961; Skou, 1962; Skou, 1965; Bonting et al., 1962). The increase in Na and the decrease in K content in the developing brain consequent to neonatal hypothyroidism may involve intracellular changes resulting from a depression in the Na-K pump, particularly since they occur in association with a decrease in the activity of Na-K-ATPase, an enzyme considered to be either the pump itself or, at least, intimately involved in the transport. That the ionic changes observed in the hypothyroid brain represent intracellular changes is further substantiated by their similarity to the ionic changes observed in the red blood cell (Table III). The lack of ATPase changes in the CNS of adult animals treated with thyroxine, known to lead to an increase in intracellular Na (Timiras et al., 1955) is in agreement with the studies of Gallagher and Glaser (1968) who have shown that ATPase activity in the CNS is not affected in adrenalectomy, an experimental situation which, like thyroxine treatment, has been shown to induce a shift of Na into the brain intracellular compartment (Woodbury, 1958).

That thyroxine may affect ionic levels through interactions at the membrane level is supported by the findings of Matty and Green (1962) and Green and Matty (1964) which indicate that thyroxine accelerates active sodium transport across isolated toad skin and bladder membranes, and by many studies showing that thyroxine alters mitochondrial membrane properties (see Pitt-Rivers and Tata, 1959b; Peachey and Greif, 1965). More recently, support has come from the work of Ismail-Beigi and Edelman (1970, 1971) who have shown that thyroid hormones activate Na extrusion and K accumulation by stimulating the Na pump in all tissues in which thyroxine is found to have a stimulatory effect on O_2 consumption.

It is of interest that this relationship holds in these tissues but that in the brain it holds only during development and only in thyroid deficiency. It is possible that the ATPase system in the CNS operates at maximum efficiency, and, therefore, further stimulation by thyroxine is not possible. In general, the lack of response of the adult and the developing CNS to excess thyroxine indicates that the brain maintains a tight regulatory control with respect to the stability of its electrolyte composition and the activity of ATPase. It would be of interest, however, to determine whether this control could be maintained in situations of extreme CNS activity; it is possible that one might detect differences in ionic composition and ATPase activity between adult and developing CNS tissue excised from animals treated with thyroxine, if examined in vitro at various time intervals after electrical stimulation.

Thus far, we have considered changes in ionic composition in the brain in relation to changes in ATPase activity. It should be recalled, however, that ionic changes in plasma were also investigated, and, as noted, no changes in plasma Na and Cl were evident in the hypothyroid animals, suggesting that the extracellular compartment may not be affected by neonatal hypothyroidism, and that plasma changes do not directly contribute to the alterations observed in the brain. In addition, changes in the brain are detected as early as the 10th postnatal day, whereas changes that occur in plasma are not evident until day 22. This hypothesis is strengthened by our observation that Na and Cl in the brain of control animals treated with thyroxine is not affected, whereas in plasma the levels of these ions do change following thyroxine treatment.

Of particular importance, both with respect to the subnormal growth characteristic of hypothyroid animals as well as to a proper interpretation of the mechanisms of action of thyroid hormones on the brain is the consistent observation that hypothyroidism is associated with a decrease in Mg. Mg deficiency, alone, could explain almost all of the changes observed in this study, not only underlying the abnormal growth patterns of hypothyroidism, but also the specific alterations occurring in Na and K content (see MacIntyre and Davidsson, 1958), and ATPase activity, inasmuch as Mg is implicated in normal monovalent cation permeability and the stability of the internal molecular arrangement of the cellular membrane. The decrease in Mg in hypothyroid animals may reflect alterations in the permeability of the membrane to the passive diffusion of Na and K down their electrochemical gradients, thus producing a "leakier" cell.

While it is true that numerous and complex changes occur in the hypothyroid brain of which those reported here represent but another example, alterations at the membrane level, as reflected in disturbances of ionic composition and associated enzymatic activity are of fundamental significance to other brain processes and may well underlie some of the abnormalities observed in hypothyroidism, generally.

ACKNOWLEDGMENTS

This work was partially supported by U.S.A.E.C. HT(04-3)-34, project 82. The technical assistance of Mrs. Carole Miller and the editorial advice of Mrs. Laurel Cook is gratefully acknowledged.

REFERENCES

Aikawa, J.K., 1956, The nature of myxoedema: alterations in the serum electrolyte concentrations and radiosodium space and in the exchangeable sodium and potassium contents, Ann. Intern. Med. 44: 30.

Balázs, R., Cocks, W.A., Eayrs, J.T. and Kovács, S., 1971, Biochemical effects of thyroid hormones on the developing brain, In: "Hormones in Development", (M. Hamburgh and E.J.W. Barrington, eds.), p. 357, Appleton-Century-Crofts, New York.

Bonting, S.L., Caravaggio, L.L. and Hawkins, N.M., 1962, Studies on sodium-potassium-activated adenosine triphosphatase. IV. Correlation with cation transport sensitive to cardiac glycosides, Arch. Biochem. Biophys. 98: 413.

Byrom, F.B., 1933, The nature of myxoedema, Clin. Sci. 1: 273.

Care, A.D., 1968, Significance of the thyroid hormones in calcium homeostasis, Federation Proc. 27: 153.

Deul, D.H. and McIlwain, H., 1961, Activation and inhibition of adenosine triphosphatases of subcellular particles from the brain, J. Neurochem. 8: 246.

Dine, R.F. and Lavietes, P.H., 1942, Serum magnesium in thyroid disease, J. Clin. Invest. 21: 781.

Gallagher, B.B. and Glaser, G.H., 1968, Seizure threshold, adrenalectomy and sodium-potassium stimulated ATPase in rat brain, J. Neurochem. 15: 525.

Geel, S.E. and Timiras, P.S., 1970, The role of hormones in cerebral protein metabolism, In: "Protein Metabolism of the Nervous System", (A. Lajtha, ed.), p. 335, Plenum Press, New York.

Geschwind, I.I., 1961, Hormonal control of calcium, phosphorus, iodine, iron, sulfur and magnesium metabolism, In: "Mineral Metabolism", (C.L. Comar and F. Bronner, eds.), p. 387, Vol. 1, Part B, Academic Press, New York.

Goldberg, R.C. and Chaikoff, I.L., 1949, A simplified procedure for thyroidectomy, Endocrinology 45: 64.

Green, K. and Matty, A.J., 1964, The effects of thyroid hormones on water permeability of the isolated bladder of the toad Bufo bufo, J. Endocr. 28: 205.

Hamburgh, M., Mendoza, L.A., Burkart, J.F. and Weil, F., 1971, Thyroid dependent processes in the developing nervous system, In: "Hormones in Development", (M. Hamburgh and E.J.W. Barrington, eds.), p. 403, Appleton-Century-Crofts, New York.

Ismail-Beigi, F. and Edelman, I.S., 1970, Mechanism of thyroid calorigenesis: role of active sodium transport, Proc. Nat. Acad. Sci. 67: 1071.

Ismail-Beigi, F. and Edelman, I.S., 1971, The mechanism of the calorigenic action of thyroid hormone, J. Gen. Physiol. 57: 710.

Järnefelt, J., 1964, Conversion of the Na^+ and K^+ independent part of the brain microsomal ATPase to a form requiring added Na^+ and K^+, Biochem. Biophys. Res. Comm. 17: 330.

Liu, C.T. and Overman, R.R., 1964, Effects of toxic doses of L-thyroxine on tissue H_2O electrolytes and plasma proteins, Proc. Soc. Exp. Biol. Med. 117: 232.

MacIntyre, J. and Davidsson, O., 1958, The production of secondary potassium depletion, sodium retention, nephrocalsinosis and hypercalcaemea by magnesium deficiency, Biochem. J. 70: 456.

Matty, A.J. and Green, K., 1962, Active sodium transport in response to thyroxine, Life Sci. No. 9, 487.

Pandazi, A.A., Herrington, J.K. and Schlueter, D.P., 1959, Sodium, potassium and magnesium distribution after thyroidectomy, Federation Proc. 18: 117.

Peachey, C.D. and Greif, R.L., 1965, Alterations of mitochondrial structure induced by thyroid hormones in vivo and in vitro, Endocrinology 77: 61.

Pitt-Rivers, R. and Tata, J.R., 1959a, Physiological actions of thyroid hormones, In: "The Thyroid Hormones", p. 75, Pergamon Press, London.

Pitt-Rivers, R. and Tata, J.R., 1959b, Some current concepts of the mechanism of action of thyroid hormones, In: "The Thyroid Hormones", p. 99, Pergamon Press, London.

Raskin, N.H. and Fishman, R.A., 1966, Effects of thyroid on permeability, composition and electrolyte metabolism of brain and other tissue, Arch. Neurol. 14: 21.

Silverman, S.H. and Gardner, L.I., 1954, Ultrafiltration studies on serum magnesium, New Eng. J. Med. 250: 938.

Skou, J.C., 1962, Preparation from mammalian brain and kidney of the enzyme system involved in active transport of Na^+ and K^+, Biochim. Biophys. Acta 58: 314.

Skou, J.C., 1965, Enzymatic basis for active transport of Na^+ and K^+ across cell membrane, Physiol. Rev. 45: 596.

Soffer, L.J., Cohn, C., Grossman, E.B., Jacobs, M. and Sobotka, H., 1941, Magnesium partition studies in Graves' disease and in clinical and experimental hypothyroidism, J. Clin. Invest. 20: 429.

Szelényi, I., Nam, L.B., Rigó, J., Nemesánszky, E., Simon, G. and Pósch, E., 1968, Magnesium metabolism and thyroid function, Acta Physiol. Acad. Sci. Hung. 33: 83.

Timiras, P.S. and Woodbury, D.M., 1956, Effect of thyroid activity on brain function and brain electrolyte distribution in rats, Endocrinology 58: 181.

Timiras, P.S., Woodbury, D.M. and Agarwall, S.L., 1955, Effect of thyroxine and triiodothyronine on brain function and electrolyte distribution in intact and adrenalectomized rats, J. Pharmac. Exp. Ther. 115: 154.

Valcana, T. and Timiras, P.S., 1969, Effect of hypothyroidism on ionic metabolism and Na-K-activated ATP phosphohydrolase activity in the developing rat brain, J. Neurochem. 16: 935.

Valcana, T. and Timiras, P.S., 1971, Effect of thyroid hormones on ionic metabolism of the developing rat brain, In: "Hormones in Development", (M. Hamburgh and E.J.W. Barrington, eds.), p. 453, Appleton-Century-Crofts, New York.

Vernadakis, A. and Woodbury, D.M., 1962, Electrolyte and amino acid changes in rat brain during maturation, Am. J. Physiol. 203: 748.

Vitale, J.J., Hegsted, D.M., Nakamura, M. and Connors, P., 1957, The effect of thyroxine on Mg^{++} requirement, J. Biol. Chem. 226: 597.

Woodbury, D.M., 1958, Effect of hormones on brain excitability and electrolytes, Recent Prog. Horm. Res. 10: 65.

Woodbury, D.M., Koch, A. and Vernadakis, A., 1958, Relation between excitability and metabolism in brain as elucidated by anticonvulsant drugs, Neurology 8: 113.

SOME ASPECTS OF ACID-BASE METABOLISM IN THE IMMATURE CENTRAL

NERVOUS SYSTEM

C.D. Withrow

Department of Pharmacology, College of Medicine

University of Utah, Salt Lake City, Utah

INTRODUCTION

Tissue acid-base metabolism is an important, but often neglected, area of investigation for several reasons. In the first place, the millieu in which cellular enzymatic reactions occur and in which many drug effects are exerted is intracellular fluid rather than extracellular fluid or blood. Second, tissue pH affects drug distribution, particularly if the drugs are weak electrolytes and non-ionic diffusion is an important determinant of their tissue-plasma ratios. Third, the processes, both active and passive, that are responsible for cellular hydrogen ion homeostasis are perhaps closely linked with other cellular activities of demonstrated significance, e.g., sodium transport. Finally, in the central nervous system (CNS), tissue acid-base balance is intimately related to cerebrospinal fluid (CSF) acid-base parameters and their regulation. Thus, it is appropriate to include a discussion of CNS and CSF acid-base metabolism in a symposium concerned with drug effects and distribution in the developing nervous system. There are, however, few data available concerned with acid-base regulation in the immature CNS and CSF. The purpose of this report is to summarize this information, and, more importantly, to point out what is not known about CNS acid-base balance in the immature animal. It is hoped that the questions not answered, and, in some cases not even directly proposed, will serve as a stimulus for more inquiry in this special research area.

REGULATION OF TISSUE pH

Adult Animals

Values for total acid-labile CO_2 in brain have been reported
that range from approximately 11 to 17 μmoles/g wet weight (Brodie
and Woodbury, 1958; Nichols, 1958; Koch and Woodbury, 1960; Thompson
and Brown, 1960; Pontén and Siesjö, 1964a; Weyne et al., 1968).
Since CO_2 is a labile tissue metabolite, care must be taken to prevent its production or loss when the tissue is taken from the animal.
Although placement in an enzyme inhibitor or immediate freezing of
the tissue sample in liquid nitrogen after removal from the animal
does arrest CO_2 production to some degree, freezing of the tissue
in situ appears to give the most consistent results (Pontén and
Siesjö, 1964b). Thus, the tissue CO_2 levels of 13-14 mmoles/kg wet
weight reported by Siesjö's group are probably good normal values
for total CO_2 in the cerebral cortex, at least in the rat. Maklari
and Kovach (1968) have reported tissue total CO_2 values (in mmoles/
kg wet weight) for different parts of dog brain as follows: frontal
cortex, 18.8; occipital cortex, 19.1; thalamus, 17.3; hypothalamus,
14.9; pons, 15.9; and medulla oblongata, 14.9. The significance of
these results is not apparent at present because they have not been
confirmed and they were obtained with a tissue CO_2 method not widely
used. Of course, there could be still other species and strain differences and differences in experimental design that could yield
other "normal" control values in any given experiment.

The total CO_2 content of brain has been fractionated into extracellular and intracellular HCO_3^-. After assumptions and calculations
have been made of intracellular pCO_2 values in this tissue, it has
been possible to calculate brain intracellular pH. Calculations of
tissue pH from CO_2 data show that the value in normal rats is approximately 7.1 with some scatter in values ranging upward to about 7.3
(Waddell and Bates, 1969).

Supplementary information about pH in brain cells has been obtained by study of the distribution of the weak acid, 5,5'-dimethyl-
oxazolidine-2,4-dione (DMO). Two values determined for rat cerebral
cortex cell pH were 6.93 and 7.13 (Rollins et al., 1970; Roos, 1971).
Intracellular pH has been shown to be 7.10 in dog cortex (Kibler
et al., 1964), 7.13 in the cortex of the cat (Roos, 1965), and 6.95
in the entire brain of the elasmobranch (Robin et al., 1964). In
vitro measurements of cell pH in whole brains of frogs disclosed
that pH was 7.29 when the bathing media had a pH=7.26 (Grayman et al.,
1968). DMO distribution determined in various parts of the rat brain
(Hertz et al., 1970) and in different anatomical sites in cat brain
(Roos, 1965) have not revealed any regional differences in cell pH
in these species.

It should be mentioned at this point that intracellular pH in brain is a derived value. The concentration of an indicator substance in cells is arrived at by subtraction of the amount in extracellular fluid from the total amount of indicator substance in the tissue. Hence, correct measurements of extracellular space are crucial to cell pH derivations. Since brain is a multicompartment tissue, extracellular space determinations are difficult to interpret. Further, cell pH values are presented as if intracellular water were a homogeneous fluid insofar as hydrogen ion concentrations are concerned. This is certainly not true if brain subcellular particles, e.g., mitochondria, have the same "intracellular pH" as do beef heart mitochondria (Addanki and Sotos, 1969). The lack of homogeneity in cells has been discussed in detail by Siesjö and Pontén (1966a) and by Waddell (1972).

Brain intracellular HCO_3^- is not changed when blood HCO_3^- levels are altered by acid excesses and deficits, except when these changes are a result of variation in blood carbonic acid concentrations (Kibler et al., 1964; Siesjö and Pontén, 1966b; Weyne et al., 1970; numerous references in Siesjö and Sørenson, 1971). In terms of cell pH considerations, this means that intracellular pH is rigidly controlled in metabolic acidosis and alkalosis if compensatory changes in respiration are prevented. When blood carbonic acid levels are altered, intracellular HCO_3^- levels and intracellular pH values change in brain but some regulation of pH occurs (Brodie and Woodbury, 1958; Kibler et al., 1964; Roos, 1965, 1971; Weyne et al., 1968; Granholm and Pontén, 1969; Rollins et al., 1970). Exposure of animals to prolonged changes in CO_2 concentrations results in a less drastic alteration of intracellular pH than is observed in acute CO_2 changes (Nichols, 1958; Weyne et al., 1968; Messeter and Siesjö, 1970). Thus, brain can regulate its internal H^+ levels and continue to function despite acid-base insults of all types.

Since it is known that gaseous CO_2 (numerous references in Siesjö and Sørensen, 1971) and that H^+ and HCO_3^- ions (Woodbury, 1971) penetrate cells, the question arises as to how intracellular pH is regulated. It has been proposed that the intracellular pH of slightly over 7 in cerebral cortex is indicative of active transport of H^+ from cells (or HCO_3^- into cells) since a pH nearer 6 would be predicted if H^+ were passively distributed across cell membranes (Grayman et al., 1968; Kjällquist et al., 1970; Siesjö and Messeter, 1971). Friede and Hu (1971) have presented somewhat direct evidence for H^+ transport out of bowfin brain. In other tissues in which better extracellular space measurements are possible and in which the cell population is homogeneous, there is good evidence that H^+ in tissues is distributed against an electrochemical gradient (Withrow et al., 1971). Further, this distribution is maintained in the face of serious acid-base insults as pointed out above. Therefore, it is reasonable to accept tentatively the proposition that H^+ transport is one means by

TABLE I

TOTAL ACID-LABILE CO_2 CONTENT OF CEREBRAL CORTEX
RAT AND GUINEA PIG[a]

Age	mmoles/kg wet weight	
	Rat	Guinea Pig
Infant	27.1 ± 0.6[b] (26)	13.7 ± 0.5[c] (7)
Adult	17.7 ± 0.6[b] (20)	13.5 ± 0.8[c] (8)

[a]All values are means ± S.E. Values in parentheses are number
of brain samples from separate animals analyzed.

[b]Values for 8-day old and adult male rats taken from Withrow
et al., 1964.

[c]Infants were 4-day-olds; adults were the mothers of the infants.

which cells maintain H^+ homeostasis. Siesjö and Messeter (1971) have
quantitated H^+ transport and have shown clearly that physicochemical
buffering and organic acid, particularly lactate, production or consumption also control intracellular pH in brain. Therefore, there
are multiple ways by which intracellular pH may be maintained at
tolerable levels. There are perhaps other mechanisms still undefined
that might be important such as the possible effects of parathyroid
hormone on acid-base homeostasis (Wills, 1970).

Immature Animals

Millichap et al.(1958) found that the total CO_2 content of rat
cerebrum was about 25 mmoles/kg wet weight in rats less than 5 days
old, and that brain total CO_2 levels fell rapidly to about 15 mmoles/kg
during the first month afterbirth. Withrow and coworkers (1964) confirmed these observations by use of a different tissue CO_2 method,
and further showed that brain cell HCO_3^- was elevated in the immature
rat. Cell pH calculations by the CO_2 method (Withrow et al., 1964)
suggested that brain cell pH in 8-day-old rats was above that seen
in adult animals. Later work by Withrow and Woodbury (1964), in which
cell pH measurements were made by the DMO method, did not support the

TABLE II

TOTAL CO_2 CONTENT OF INFANT RATS EXPOSED TO 40% CO_2[a]

Age In Days	mmoles/kg wet weight		
	Room Air Control	40% CO_2	Increase in Tissue Total CO_2
5	26.2 ± 1.0[b] (4)	36.7 ± 1.2 (4)	10.5
9	24.3 ± 1.4 (4)	35.0 ± 2.0 (4)	10.7
20	17.4 ± 0.3 (4)	27.3 ± 0.7 (4)	9.9

[a]Brain taken from animals decapitated immediately without exsanguination after 8 minutes exposure to 40% CO_2, 20% CO_2, and 40% N_2 gas mixture.

[b]Values are means ± S.E. Numbers in parentheses are numbers of animals used for CO_2 analysis.

earlier observations that cell pH changes during maturation. At present the entire concept of cell pH in the maturing animals is being reinvestigated in our laboratory with better techniques and additional experience in handling the infant rat.

The total CO_2 content of the cerebral cortex of infant and adult rats and guinea pigs is given in Table I. The most striking difference between the rat and the guinea pig is that guinea pig brain CO_2 content is not elevated in infants but rather exhibits adult values near birth. Millichap and coworkers (1958) showed that rat brain CO_2 content is inversely related to tissue carbonic anhydrase acitivity, and that the immature guinea pig has high levels of carbonic anhydrase activity (Millichap, 1957). It is thus possible that the "low" CO_2 content in brain of new-born guinea pigs is a consequence of carbonic anhydrase activity. It remains, however, to be shown exactly how tissue carbonic anhydrase activity results in lower tissue levels of CO_2.

The response of the immature brain to metabolic acid-base challenges has not been studied. It is not known whether the cells in immature brain with a more permeable blood brain barrier can be affected by changes in blood HCO_3^- levels. Further, the role of lactate in tissue pH regulation has not been determined in the immature brain.

Similarly, the response of the immature brain to CO_2 variations has not been measured in detail. The data in Table II represent some preliminary results of changes in tissue total CO_2 when small rats were exposed to 40% CO_2. The increase in total CO_2 amounts above that of controls is about the same in all groups. Because the exposure time to CO_2 is so short in the experiments summarized in Table II, the changes in tissue CO_2 content almost certainly represent physicochemical buffering in blood and in brain cells. However, there are important differences among the three age groups which complicate interpretation of these data. First, brain extracellular space is very large, about 40%, in the 5-day-old rat, and the size of this space decreases during the first month of life to the adult value of 13.5% (Ferguson and Woodbury, 1969). Second, the hematocrit of 8-day-old rats is about 30 as compared to a normal of 45 in adult rats in our laboratory. Since considerable buffering of CO_2 occurs in red blood cells when the CO_2 tension of blood is increased, it would be predicted that 5-day-old rats would buffer less CO_2 extracellularly because of the reduced amount of hemoglobin present. Third, there is no difference between plasma HCO_3^- levels in 8- and 28-day-old rats (Withrow et al., 1964). It is therefore obvious that until tissue CO_2 content is measured concurrently with blood acid-base parameters, it is not possible to compare physicochemical buffering in the cells of very immature rats with that of older rats. Further, longer exposure times to CO_2 are also necessary if the importance of active transport in tissue buffering of CO_2 in infants is to be quantitated.

REGULATION OF CSF pH

Adult Animals

The regulation of CSF pH in the mature animal has been extensively studied and recently has been reviewed in detail by several authors (Siesjö, 1972; Leusen, 1972; various authors in Siesjö and Sørenson, 1971). The following summary is taken liberally from these reviews and references in these papers should be consulted for more detail.

In a normal adult rat, typical acid-base parameters in cisternal CSF are pH=7.34, pCO_2=48 mm Hg, and HCO_3^-=24 mM. Values vary slightly in other species but most workers agree that cisternal CSF compared to arterial blood is more acid (about 0.04 pH units) and has a higher

pCO_2 (4-10 mm Hg). The usual ratio of HCO_3^- concentrations between cisternal CSF and plasma H_2O is 0.90 (Fencl, 1971; Siesjö, 1972).

There is a net electrical potential difference between cisternal CSF and jugular vein blood. At a normal blood pH of 7.4, CSF is approximately 4 mV positive with respect to blood. In the rat, dog and goat, cisternal CSF becomes more positive as plasma pH decreases, and becomes less positive as blood pH increases. In the cat, however, a fall in blood pH results in the CSF becoming more negative with respect to blood (Pannier et al., 1971). Metabolic acid-base distortions cause about 43 mV/pH unit change. Carbonic acid acidosis and alkalosis cause less change in CSF-blood potentials, approximately 30 mV/pH unit change in blood pH (Seisjö, 1972).

It has been calculated that HCO_3^- and H^+ are not in electrochemical equilibrium between blood and CSF. CSF is more acid and contains less HCO_3^- than it should if H^+ and HCO_3^- were passively distributed between plasma and CSF. Most authors agree that the electrochemical potential, $\Delta \mu$, is about two to ten mV for both H^+ and HCO_3^-. Or, phrased in another way, CSF pH would be about 7.45 and CSF HCO_3^- levels would be approximately 33 mM if these ions were in electrochemical equilibrium. The disequilibrium of H^+ and HCO_3^- between blood and CSF has been interpreted as evidence for either HCO_3^- transport out of CSF or H^+ transport into CSF (see Siesjö, 1972).

In non-respiratory acid-base disturbances, CSF pH is generally well-defended despite striking alterations in blood pH. CSF pH, however, does tend to follow slightly changes in blood pH. When carbonic acid concentrations are altered and blood pH varies greatly, CSF pH eventually returns to near normal values despite the fact that CO_2 rapidly penetrates body membranes. If, however, hypoxia accompanies hypercapnia, pH compensation in CSF is not complete and is much less than that observed in well-oxygenated patients or animals (Siesjö, 1972).

The regulation of CSF pH is complex and is different for metabolic and respiratory acid-base changes. In non-respiratory acid-base distortions, CSF HCO_3^- levels do not change as rapidly as do HCO_3^- concentrations in blood. Thus, some maintenance of CSF pH is due to the slow penetration of HCO_3^- (or H^+) into CSF (Leusen, 1972). Further, changes in the DC potential between CSF and blood appropriately, at least in several species, attract (in acidosis) or repel (in alkalosis) HCO_3^- to or from CSF. Finally, respiration is stimulated in systemic acidosis and depressed somewhat in systemic alkalosis. These changes in pCO_2 are immediately reflected in CSF and mitigate CSF HCO_3^- changes that passively occur because of changes in blood HCO_3^- levels. Thus, CSF pH is regulated by changes in both CSF HCO_3^- and pCO_2.

In respiratory acid-base disturbances, the systemic changes in pCO_2 are immediately reflected in the CSF and its pH changes rapidly in acute respiratory acidosis or alkalosis. When blood pCO_2 remains altered for several hours or days, HCO_3^- levels in CSF change so that near normal HCO_3^- - H_2CO_3 ratios are observed. Renal compensation for the respiratory acidosis or alkalosis increases or decreases blood HCO_3^- levels respecitvely, and these changes are passively reflected in CSF and contribute to normalization of CSF pH. Again, appropriate changes in the DC potential between CSF and blood also help regulate CSF HCO_3^- levels. Finally, the addition of lactic acid to CSF is a very important regulatory mechanism for CSF pH in hyperventilation, and the comsumption of lactate may help regulate CSF pH when pCO_2 is elevated (Siesjö and Kjällquist, 1969).

It is not clear whether the passive and non-CSF mechanisms already discussed are solely responsible for the modifications of CSF HCO_3^- described above when systemic acidosis or alkalosis is produced. On the one hand, the lack of change of electrochemical gradients during acidosis is cited as evidence against active HCO_3^- (or H^+), transport being important as a regulatory process for CSF pH maintenance (Messeter and Siesjö, 1971; Siesjö, 1972). Others, however, have presented evidence that active transport of HCO_3^- is necessary for pH regulation in CSF (Mines and Sørensen, 1971; Mines et al., 1971; Pannier et al., 1971). A complete argument of this point is beyond the scope of this paper, and the interested reader is referred to the reviews of Siesjö (1972) and Leusen (1972) for additional information. Suffice it to say that if active HCO_3^- transport does indeed contribute to CSF pH stability, it is a potential site of drug effects and is thus important to keep in mind.

Two final points concerning CSF acid-base homeostasis merit mention. The first is that changes in cerebral blood flow can contribute to CSF pH regulation in acute hypercapnia and hypocapnia. Blood flow is probably of little importance in most chronic acid-base disorders (Siesjö, 1972). The second point is that the CSF HCO_3^- level, even in normal animals, is probably altered as CSF flows from its site of formation, the choroid plexus, to its usual site of sampling in experimental animals, the cisterna magna. It has been speculated on the basis of charge balance that cisternal CSF has about 7 mEq/l less HCO_3^- than does freshly secreted CSF sampled from the surface of choroid plexus (Ames et al., 1960). The recent data of Miner and Reed (1972) calculated in the same way support the earlier findings. There does not appear to be further modification of CSF between the cisterna magna and the lumbar region, although the CSF pH is slightly lower in lumbar CSF (Siesjö, 1972). Thus, it appears that the rate of CSF formation and flow are possible determinants of CSF acid-base balance.

Immature Animals

There is a paucity of data on CSF composition in immature animals. Mann et al. (1972) have reported the following CSF acid-base data for fetal sheep: pH=7.18, pCO_2=58.5 mm Hg, and HCO_3^-=18.8 mEq/kg H_2O. Blood data in the same animals were: pH=7.29, pCO_2=48.3 mm Hg and HCO_3^-=27.2 mEq/kg H_2O. Qualitatively similar data, i.e., CSF more acid than blood because of lower HCO_3^- levels and higher pCO_2, were reported for fetal lambs by Hodson et al.(1968). Herrington and coworkers (1971), however, found that fetal lambs had a pH equal to that of blood, and that HCO_3^- levels were higher in CSF than in blood, so that their results differ from those of Hodson et al. and Mann et al. Neonatal lamb CSF was found by Hodson et al. to be more acid and to have a lower HCO_3^- than did blood.

Careful studies of the regulation of CSF pH in fetal lambs exposed to metabolic insults have been done by Hodson et al. (1968). These workers found that acute elevation of blood HCO_3^- causes a significant increase in CSF HCO_3^- levels. However, severe metabolic acidosis does not appear to decrease CSF HCO_3^- levels. Unpublished data from our laboratory show that metabolic acidosis in neonatal rats decreases CSF HCO_3^- levels and hence do not confirm these data. CSF pH was well regulated despite marked changes in blood pH in both cases.

Mann et al. (1972) measured the effects of acute respiratory acidosis and alkalosis in fetal lambs. Systemic hypocarbia and hypercarbia caused immediate changes in CSF pH and pCO_2. HCO_3^- levels in CSF were not correlated with blood HCO_3^- concentrations. These experiments, however, were so acute that no information concerning CSF pH regulation in immature animals could be gleaned from these data.

With the exception of these few experiments, nothing else is known about pH regulation in the CSF of immature animals. What is the DC potential? How does it change with metabolic and respiratory pH disturbances? What about the effects of reduced CSF flow in the neonate (see Johanson, this proceedings)? What effect does the development of the blood brain barrier have on HCO_3^- and H^+ permeabilities? What is the importance of organic acid production and consumption in the immature animal with incomplete biochemical systems? If and when we can answer some of these questions, this topic can be discussed more completely.

SUMMARY

The information above is a brief discussion of tissue and CSF
pH regulation in mature and immature animals. With regard to mature
animals, there are numerous data and several working hypotheses to
test with additional experiments. When immature animals are considered, there is not enough information even to speculate about
control mechanisms. Therefore, there is much work to be done. There
is enough information, however, to suggest that normal acid-base
balance and the response to acid-base challenges in the immature
animal could be different from those in the mature animal. It is
imperative that interpretation of drug effects or speculation about
drug distribution in the immature animal be tempered with this
thought.

The immature animal offers much as a model for acid-base studies
in the CNS. The possible absence of some transport systems may allow
us to quantitate their importance. Differences in enzyme activity
levels and blood-brain permeabilities may permit more definitive
studies. Finally, study of the immature nervous system and its development may help elucidate the intriguing problem of the possible
role of glia in tissue pH regulation (Friede and Hu, 1971).

ACKNOWLEDGMENTS

The work described in this paper was supported by National
Institutes of Health Grants NS0455309 and GM00153-14. The author
is grateful to Ms. Jill Jones for typing the manuscript and for
assistance with the references.

REFERENCES

Addanki, S. and Sotos, J.F., 1969, Observations on intramitochondrial
     pH and ion transport by the 5, 5-dimethyl 2, 4-oxazolidinedione
     (DMO) method, Ann. N.Y. Acad. Sci. 147: 756.

Ames, A., III, Sakanoue, M. and Shinichiro, E., 1964, Na, K, Ca, Mg,
     and Cl concentrations in chroid plexus fluid and cisternal fluid
     compared with plasma ultrafiltrate, J. Neurophysiol. 27: 672.

Brodie, D.A. and Woodbury, D.M., 1958, Acid-base changes in brain and
     blood of rats exposed to high concentrations of carbon dioxide,
     Am. J. Physiol. 192: 91.

Fencl, V., 1971, Distribution of H^+ and HCO_3^- in cerebral fluids. In:
     "Ion Homeostasis of the Brain", (Siesjö and Sørensen, eds.),
     Academic Press, New York.

Ferguson, R.K. and Woodbury, D.M., 1969, Penetration of ^{14}C-inulin and ^{14}C-sucrose into brain, cerebrospinal fluid, and skeletal muscle of developing rats, Exp. Brain Res. 7: 181.

Friede, R.L. and Hu, K., 1971, Hydrogen ion transfer and pH control in bowfin brain in vitro, Brain Res. 25: 161.

Granholm, L. and Pontén, U., 1969, The in vitro CO_2 buffer curve of the intracellular space of cat cerebral cortex, Acta Neurol. Scand. 45: 493.

Grayman, G., Bradbury, M.W.B. and Kleeman, C.R., 1968, Intracellular pH of the amphibian brain incubated in vitro, Life Sci. 7: 499.

Herrington, R.T., Harned, H.S., Ferreiro, J.I. and Griffin, C.A., 1971, The role of the central nervous system in perinatal respiration studies of chemoregulatory mechanisms in the term lamb, Pediatrics 47: 857.

Hertz, L., Schousboe, A. and Weiss, G.B., 1970, Estimation of ionic concentrations and intracellular pH in slices from different areas of rat brain, Acta Physiol. Scand. 79: 506.

Hodson, W.A., Fenner, A., Brumley, G., Chernick, V. and Avery, M.E., 1968, Cerebrospinal fluid and blood acid-base relationships in fetal and neonatal lambs and pregnant ewes, Res. Physiol. 4: 322.

Kibler, R.F., O'Neill, R.P. and Robin, E.D., 1964, Intracellular acid-base relations of dog brain with reference to the brain extracellular volume, J. Clin. Invest. 43: 431.

Kjällquist, A., Messeter, K. and Siesjö, B.K, 1970, the in vivo CO_2 buffer capacity of rat brain tissue under carbonic anhydrase inhibition, Acta Physiol. Scand. 78: 94.

Koch, A. and Woodbury, D.M., 1960, Carbonic anhydrase inhibition and brain electrolyte composition, Am. J. Physiol. 198: 434.

Leusen, I., 1972, Regulation of cerebrospinal fluid composition with reference to breathing, Physiol. Rev. 52: 1.

Maklári, E. and Kovách, A.G.B., 1968, Carbon dioxide content of brain tissue and acid-base balance in haemorrhagic shock after pretreatment with dibenzyline, Acta Medica Academiae Scientiarum Ungaricae 25: 13.

Mann, L.I., Carmichael, A. and Duchin, S., 1972, Fetal cerebrospinal fluid acid-base regulation, Amer. J. Obstet. Gynec. 114: 546.

Messeter, K. and Siesjö, B.K., 1971, Electrochemical gradients for H+ and HCO$_3^-$ between blood and CSF during sustained acid-base changes. In: "Ion Homeostasis of the Brain," (Siesjö and Sørenson, eds.), Academic Press, New York.

Messeter, K. and Siesjö, B.K.,1970, Regulation of intracellular pH in the rat brain in chronic hypercapnia, Acta Physiol. Scand. 79: 136.

Millichap, J.G., 1957, Development of seizure patterns in newborn animals. Significance of brain carbonic anhydrase, Proc. Soc. Exp. Biol. Med. 97: 125.

Millichap, J.G., Balter, M. and Hernandez, P., 1958, Development of susceptibility to seizures in young animals III. Brain water, electrolyte and acid-base metabolism, Proc. Soc. Exp. Biol. Med. 99: 6.

Miner, L.C. and Reed, D.J., 1972, Composition of fluid obtained from choroid plexus tissue isolated in a chamber in situ, J. Physiol. 227: 127.

Mines, A.H. and Sørensen, S.C., 1971, Changes in the electrochemical potential difference for HCO$_3^-$ between blood and cerebrospinal fluid and in cerebrospinal fluid lactate concentration during isocarbic hypoxia, Acta Physiol. Scand. 81: 225.

Mines, A.H., Morril, C.G. and Sørensen, S.C., 1971, The effect of isocarbic metabolic acidosis in blood on (H+) and HCO$_3^-$) in CSF with deductions about the regulation of an active transport of H+/HCO$_3^-$ between blood and CSF, Acta Physiol. Scand. 81: 234.

Nichols, G., Jr., 1958, Serial changes in tissue carbon dioxide content during acute respiratory acidosis, J. Clin. Invest. 37:1111

Pannier, J.L., Weyne, J. and Leusen, I., 1971, The CSF blood potential and the regulation of the bicarbonate concentration of CSF during acidosis in the cat, Life Sci. 10: 287.

Pontén, U. and Siesjö, B.K., 1964a, A method for the determination of total carbon dioxide content of frozen tissues, Acta Physiol. Scand. 60: 297.

Pontén, U. and Siesjö, B.D., 1964b, Acid-labile carbon dioxide of rat brain after freezing the tissue in situ, Acta Physiol. Scand. 60: 309.

Robin, E.D., Murdaugh, H.V., Jr., and Weiss, E., 1964, Acid-base, fluid and electrolyte metabolism in the elasmonbranch, I. Ionic composition of erythrocytes, muscle and brain, J. Cell Comp. Physiol. 64: 409.

Rollins, D.E., Withrow, C.D. and Woodbury, D.M., 1970, Tissue acid-base balance in acetazolamide-treated rats, J. Pharmac. Exp. Ther. 174: 535.

Roos, A., 1971, Intracellular pH and buffering power of rat brain, Am. J. Physiol. 221: 176.

Roos, A., 1965, Intracellular pH and intracellular buffering power of the cat brain, Am. J. Physiol. 209: 1233.

Siesjö, B.K., 1972, The regulation of cerebrospinal fluid pH, Kidney International 1: 360.

Siesjö, B.K. and Kjällquist, A., 1969, A new theory for the regulation of the extracellular pH in the brain, Scand. J. Clin. Lab. Invest. 24: 1.

Siesjö, B.K. and Messeter, K., 1971, Factors determining intracellular pH. In: "Ion Homeostasis of the Brain," (Siesjö and Sørensen, eds.), Academic Press, New York.

Siesjö, B.K. and Pontén, U., 1966a, Intracellular pH - True parameter or misnomer?, Ann. N.Y. Acad. Sci. 133: 78.

Siesjö, B.K. and Pontén, U., 1966b, Acid-base changes in the brain in nonrespiratory acidosis and alkalosis, Exp. Br. Res. 2: 176.

Siesjö, B.K. and Sørensen, S.C., eds., 1971, "Ion Homeostasis of the Brain," Academic Press, New York.

Thompson, A.M. and Brown, E.B., Jr., 1960, Tissue carbon dioxide concentrations in rats during acute respiratory acidosis, J. Appl. Physiol. 15: 49.

Waddell, W.J., 1972, Subcellar and molecular aspects of intracellular pH, Chest 61: 56S.

Waddell, W.J. and Bates, R.G., 1969, Intracellular pH, Physiol. Rev. 49: 285.

Weyne, J., Demeester, G. and Leusen, I., 1968, Bicarbonate and chloride shifts in rat brain during acute and prolonged respiratory acid-base changes, Arch. Int. Physiol. et de Biochimie 76: 415.

Weyne, J., Pannier, J.L., Demeester, G. and Leusen, I., 1970, Bicarbonate and chloride of rat brain during infusion-induced changes in bicarbonate concentration of blood, Pflugers Arch. 320: 45.

Wills, M.R., 1970, Fundamental physiological role of parathyroid
    hormone in acid-base homeostasis, Lancet 2: 802.

Withrow, C.D. and Woodbury, D.M., 1964, Tissue acid-base changes
    during maturation. In: "Progress in Brain Research," (Himwich
    and Himwich, eds.), Vol. 9, Elsevier Publishing Company,
    Amsterdam.

Withrow, C.D., Woodbury, D.M. and Wilcox, W.D., 1964, Acid-base
    changes in brain and skeletal muscle of maturing rats, Am. J.
    Physiol. 206: 521.

Withrow, C.D., Elsmore, T., Williams, J.A. and Woodbury, D.M., 1971,
    Hydrogen ion distribution and regulation in various rat tissues.
    In: "Ion Homeostasis of the Brain," (Siesjö and Sørensen, eds.),
    Academic Press, New York.

Woodbury, J.W., 1971, Fluxes of H^+ and HCO_3^- across frog skeletal
    muscle cell membrane. In: "Ion Homeostasis of the Brain,"
    (Siesjö and Sørensen, eds.), Academic Press, New York.

DEVELOPMENTAL ASPECTS OF LEARNING AND MEMORY
Samuel Barondes, Chairman

THE DEVELOPMENT OF BEHAVIOR IN NORMAL AND BRAIN-DAMAGED INFANT RATS,

STUDIED WITH HOMING (NEST-SEEKING) AS MOTIVATION

Joseph Altman, Robert L. Brunner, Fatma G. Bulut and

Kiran Sudarshan

Laboratory of Developmental Neurobiology, Department of

Biological Sciences, Purdue University, West Lafayette,

Indiana

INTRODUCTION

The behavioral, especially learning, capabilities of normal and treated preweaning rats has received only limited experimental atten- tion due mainly to the shortage of testing procedures that can be profitably administered to them. In addition to their limited sen- sory and motor capacities, serious difficulties arise when motivation- al conditions appropriate for adults are applied to nursling rats. What is needed in this field of investigation is reward and punish- ment situations which are relevant to the needs of infants. In al- tricial species an obvious such situation is the disturbance of filial-maternal interrelationship. A drastic example of this is the removal of the infant from the nest or home cage where it is provided by the mother with food, shelter and the various other necessities of survival. Perhaps another, related situation is the removal of a pup from its siblings who contribute to the comforts that the grow- ing infant needs and seeks.

An instance of filial-maternal interrelationship that has been extensively utilized in behavioral studies is the following-response of newly-hatched precocial birds, such as the chick or duckling. These studies provided a considerable amount of information about the nature of a type of early learning, i.e., imprinting (Lorenz, 1935; Hess, 1959, Sluckin, 1965). Another, less extensively used example is the food-begging response of newly-hatched herring gull chicks, which was exploited to study the nature of visual "releasers"

321

responsible for this response (Tinbergen and Perdeck, 1950; Tinbergen, 1963). The tendency of altricial (mammalian) infants to
return when removed from the nest was recently examined in kittens
(Rosenblatt et al., 1969) and rats (Rosenblatt and Lehrman, 1963),
and some beginnings have been made in using this "homing" response
to examine the development of sensory abilities, especially olfaction (Tobach et al., 1967; Salas et al., 1970; Schapiro and Salas,
1970; Gregory and Pfaff, 1971, in the rat; Rosenblatt et al., 1969;
Rosenblatt, 1971, in kittens; Devor and Schneider, unpublished,
in hamsters).

HOMING (NEST-SEEKING) BEHAVIOR

Rosenblatt and Lehrman (1963) divided the nursing-suckling relation between mother and young in cats and rats into three phases:
(a) the neonatal phase, when the mother plays a major role in initiat-
int suckling in the nest by arousing the young and facilitating their
suckling; (b) the second phase, when the young begin to follow their
mother and initiate suckling, sometimes outside the nest region, with
the cooperation of the mother; and (c) the last phase, which ante-
dates weaning, when the mother cooperates less and less and eventually
rejects the suckling attempts of the young. While this schema suggests
passivity on the part of the very young in suckling, quite early
during the assumption of filial-maternal relationship the infants
assume a more and more active role, as indicated by their behavior
when removed from the nest area. Kittens as young as 1-4 days
(Rosenblatt et al., 1969; Rosenblatt, 1971) distinguish between their
home cage and an alien environment and vocalize when placed in the
latter, which then is relieved when returned to their home cage.
When 5 day old kittens were placed in the home cage 18 inches from
the nest, they oriented toward it and then crawled home; when the
separation was increased to 28 inches, there was intense vocalization
but they could not return. The ability to orient and locomote from
greater distances developed gradually. An examination of the question
whether airborne odors or materials deposited on the floor guided
the kittens to the nest suggested that cues from the latter source
were primarily utilized.

Schapiro and Salas (1970) investigated the effects of mother
odor on the behavior of rats aged 2 to 12 days by noting the inhibition of motor activity (restlessness) in the field when the
mother was interposed in the air stream. Rats 6 days and younger
showed a slight trend to slow their motor activity; this inhibition
was more pronounced in rats 8 days or older. In a complementary
study, Salas et al. (1970) could detect only minimal, nonspecific
effects by the odor of food or mother on the electrical activity of
the olfactory bulb of rats before the age of day 6, but thereafter
there was a progressive discrimination of the two odors, as indicated
by differential effects on several electrophysiological parameters.

These studies suggest minimal or no olfactory responses in rats to odors related to the nest during the first week; it may be noted, however, that responsiveness to noxious (nonphysiological) odors, such as ammonia vapor, is already manifest in neonates (Small, 1899; Bolles and Woods, 1964; unpublished observations). In the hamster, preference for home cage bedding over fresh bedding was first seen at 7-8 days of age, although other odor preferences were noted as early as 4 days (Devor and Schneider, unpublished).

Clear olfactory responses related to filial-maternal interaction have been noted in rats during the second and third week after birth. Nyakas and Endröczi (1970) reported that 10-day old rats select that arm of the maze where the mother (or a lactating female) is located in preference to a male; this choice is abolished when olfaction is inhibited by tetracaine. Gregory and Pfaff (1971) found that 12-day old rats displayed a preference for shavings from the home cage over clean wood shavings or shavings from the cage of a nonpregnant female; such a discrimination could not be obtained in rats younger than 7 days. Some of the other relevant studies were carried out in older rats. Hofer (1970) noted in 14-day old rats a decline in heart and respiratory rate when they were separated from their mothers, and Leon and Moltz (1971) found in 16-day old rats a strong attraction exerted by the mother's odor which they could distinguish in preference tests from the odor of a nulliparous female, though not from another lactating female. When the choice was between two soiled goal boxes, they chose the box previously occupied by a lactating female.

The nature of this homing response of infant rats, its dependence on the development of sensory and motor capacities, and on the needs that are satisfied in the nest, have yet to be established in detail. However, the studies that were described do document the existence of such a tendency which is presumably complementary to the retrieval response displayed by the lactating female (Wiesner and Sheard, 1933). Perhaps in agreement with the stages proposed by Rosenblatt and Lehrman (1963) that were previously described, there is a reciprocal relationship between maternal retrieval and infant homing, and as retrieval begins to decline by the middle of the second week (Moltz and Robbins, 1965) homing increases. The present series of studies were concerned less with the clarification of the nature of the homing response as with its exploitation as a source of motivation in infants and thus as a means of controlling their behavior for the purposes of experimental studies of behavioral development.

HOMING IN NORMAL AND UNDERNOURISHED RATS: PILOT STUDIES

The first study in which we attempted to use "homing" as motivation was concerned with the assessment of behavioral development in undernourished infant rats (Altman, Sudarshan, Das, McCormick and

Barnes, 1971). Constant-size litters were raised by Purdue-Wistar albino mothers that received during lactation 40 percent or 20 percent ad lib diet consumed by control mothers; these litters constituted the severely and mildly undernourished groups. In this first study, instead of true homing, single rats were placed in a test chamber and their latency of reaching the chamber where their littermates were located was determined (Fig. 1B). The animals were tested between days 6 and 21, each being given a 180 second trial per day. None of the normal animals reached the chamber containing the siblings before day 8, and none of the severely undernourished rats before day 14. In a related test, specifically involving homing (Fig. 1A), the animals had a choice of approaching the home cage or a similar empty cage on the opposite side of the test box. The majority of the normal animals moved toward the home cage on days 6-7, but the performance of the undernourished animals was much poorer. In both tests a rapid decline was noted in the time taken to reach the target region, and asymtotic levels were reached by the end of the third week. The improvement with age could be attributed to the increase in the number of successful animals and to an increase in the speed of locomotion, but few clues were offered as to what variables (sensory, motor, emotional, etc.) were specifically affected.

              HOMING USED TO STUDY THE DEVELOPMENT OF LOCOMOTION

     We have recently undertaken an extensive survey of the post-natal development of motor skills in the rat (Altman and Sudarshan, in preparation). This investigation, as earlier ones (Bolles and Woods, 1964; Altman et al., 1971a) has relied heavily on the quantification of naturally emitted responses in the open field. For instance, it was established that rats do not locomote during the first week, as measured by crossing "squares" in the open field, and this failure could be attributed to the circumstance that during this period overt activity takes the form of "pivoting", that is, rotatory movements produced by the forelimbs with little assistance from the hindlimbs to produce effective forward progression. Pivoting declines rapidly during the second week to be replaced by crawling but effective locomotion remains low. It became evident in the course of this study that in order to survey the development of various motor skills and analyze the maturation of underlying mechanisms it is necessary to induce the animals to perform various emerging skills such as balancing, jumping, climbing, etc., which they do not display spontaneously in the open field. Removal from the home cage or separation from siblings were among the motivational situations that were utilized to induce animals to display such skills.

     Because successful homing is dependent on at least two variables, i.e., the ability and disposition to orient towards the home cage (or mother or siblings) and the capacity to ambulate, the first task

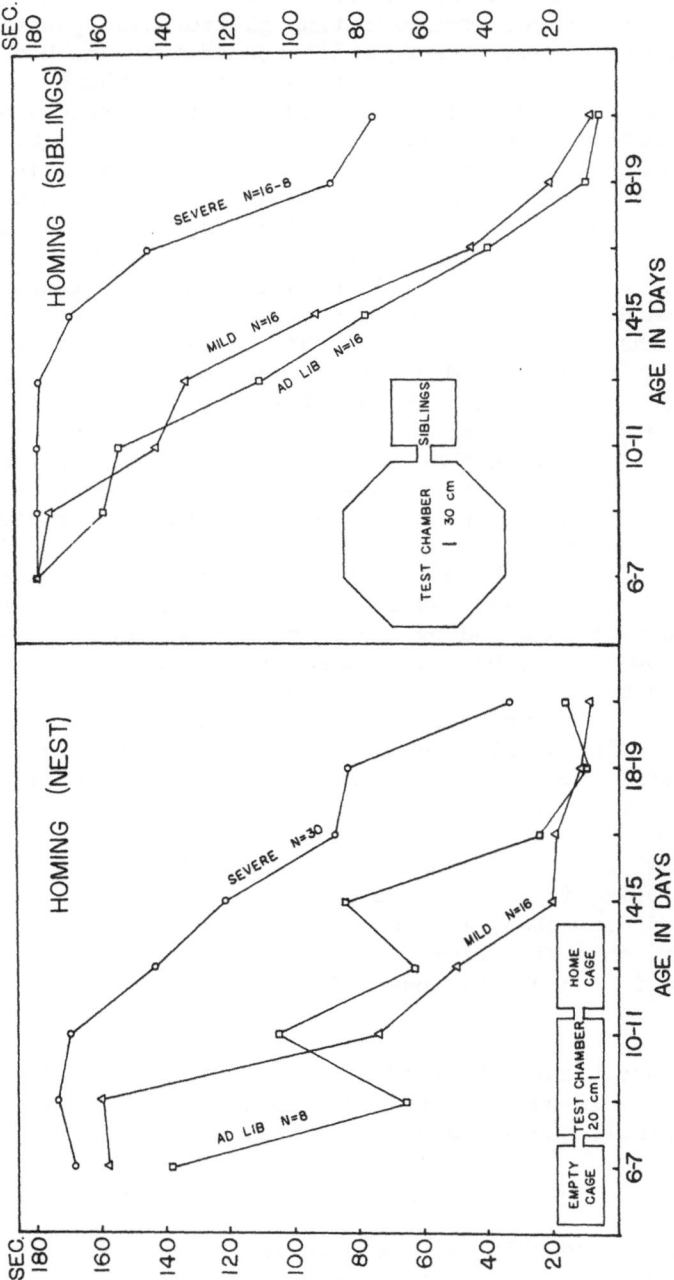

Fig. 1. A: Latency of reaching home cage in a choice situation as a function of age in normal, severely undernourished and mildly undernourished rats. B: Siblings used as the incentive instead of the home cage. (From Altman et al., 1971b).

was to separate the two and examine nonambulatory orientation by letting the animal utilize its early-developing pivoting skill. The apparatus consisted of a central circular area 4-1/2" in diameter and surrounded by a wire fence. The orienting platform was positioned between two enclosed alleys 3" long which opened into the home cage on one side and an empty cage on the opposite side. The size of the fenced-in area limited locomotion. In order to facilitate scoring the animal's orientation, the circular area was demarcated by octagonally oriented lines. The animal was placed randomly facing the right or left line at a right angle to the entrances; these were the null points. Turning toward the home cage or empty cage was scored as +1 or -1, and turning half-way to the two entrances was scored as +1/2 or -1/2. Each animal was placed daily into the fenced circle for 180 seconds and its orientation was recorded every 10 seconds. For each animal the scores were summed for the day and the grand means of all animals for that day were calculated. (Maximum individual daily score was +18, if the animal was oriented at all observation periods toward the opening of the home cage.) The results are summarized in Fig. 2. Although some infants were oriented partially or completely away from the home cage during some of the observation periods, the positive tendency of orienting towards the home cage began to emerge by day 3 with 50% of the animals orienting at least partially toward the home cage at least half of the observation periods. By days 5-6, 8-9 out of 14 animals were oriented fully toward the home cage and by day 8 most of the animals were fully oriented towards the home cage most of the time. Many of the animals displayed by then a tendency to ambulate towards the home cage by rearing and pushing against the fence facing the entrance to home and attempting to climb over it. It is interesting that positive orientation toward the home cage was evident several days before that obtained in tests which required ambulation (Nyakas and Endröczi, 1970; Gregory and Pfaff, 1971). Moreover, the successful orientation of all animals emerged several days before active head pointing and sniffing is seen in the open field (beginning on days 10-11, Altman and Sudarshan, in preparation), and so did rearing, which was seen in this situation by day 8 and not until day 13-14 where the homing incentive was absent (Altman and Sudarshan, in preparation).

Whereas orientation without locomotion is evident by day 7 in all of the animals, if homing involved actual locomotion towards the home cage few animals succeeded until several days later and the

_____

Fig. 2. Orientation toward the home cage in a circular platform surrounded by a wire fence. Orientation of the animal was scored, as indicated in the inset, every 10 seconds during a 180 second daily observation period.

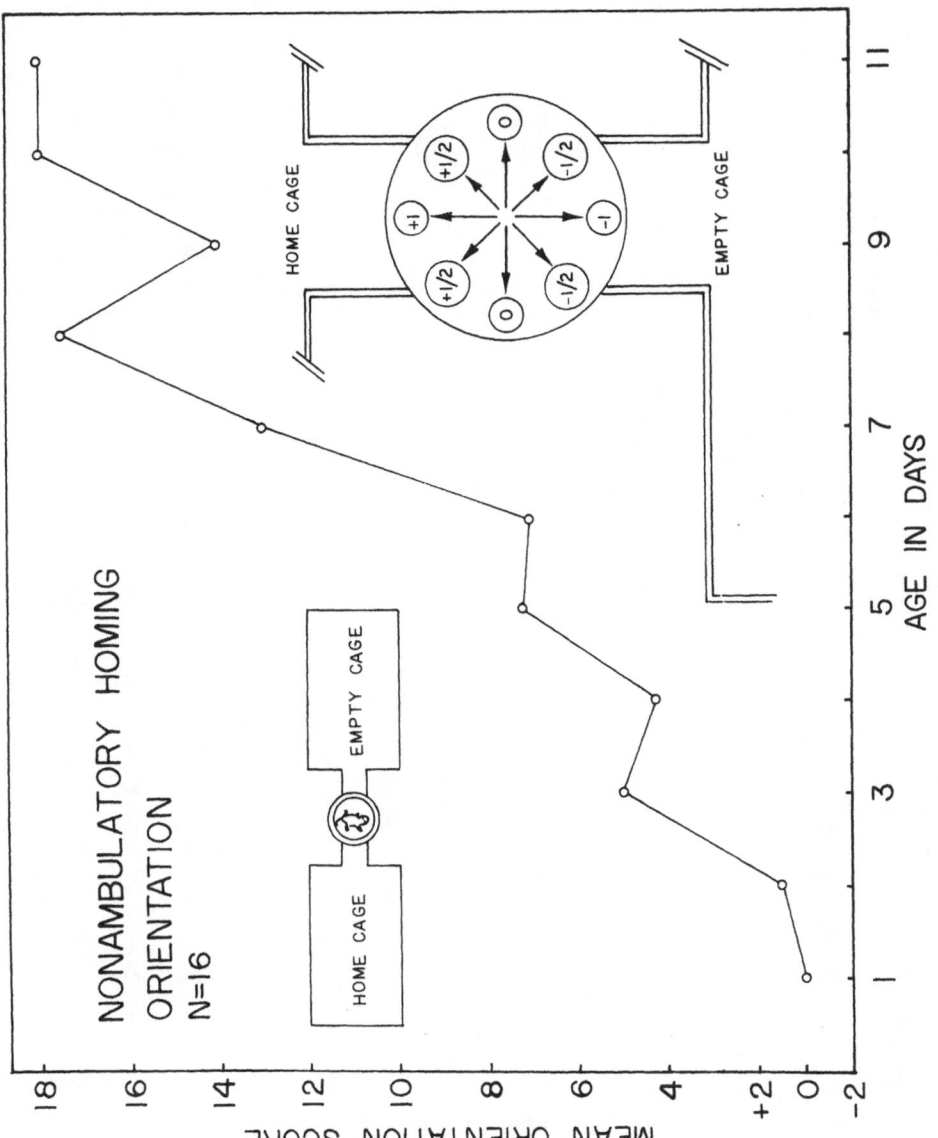

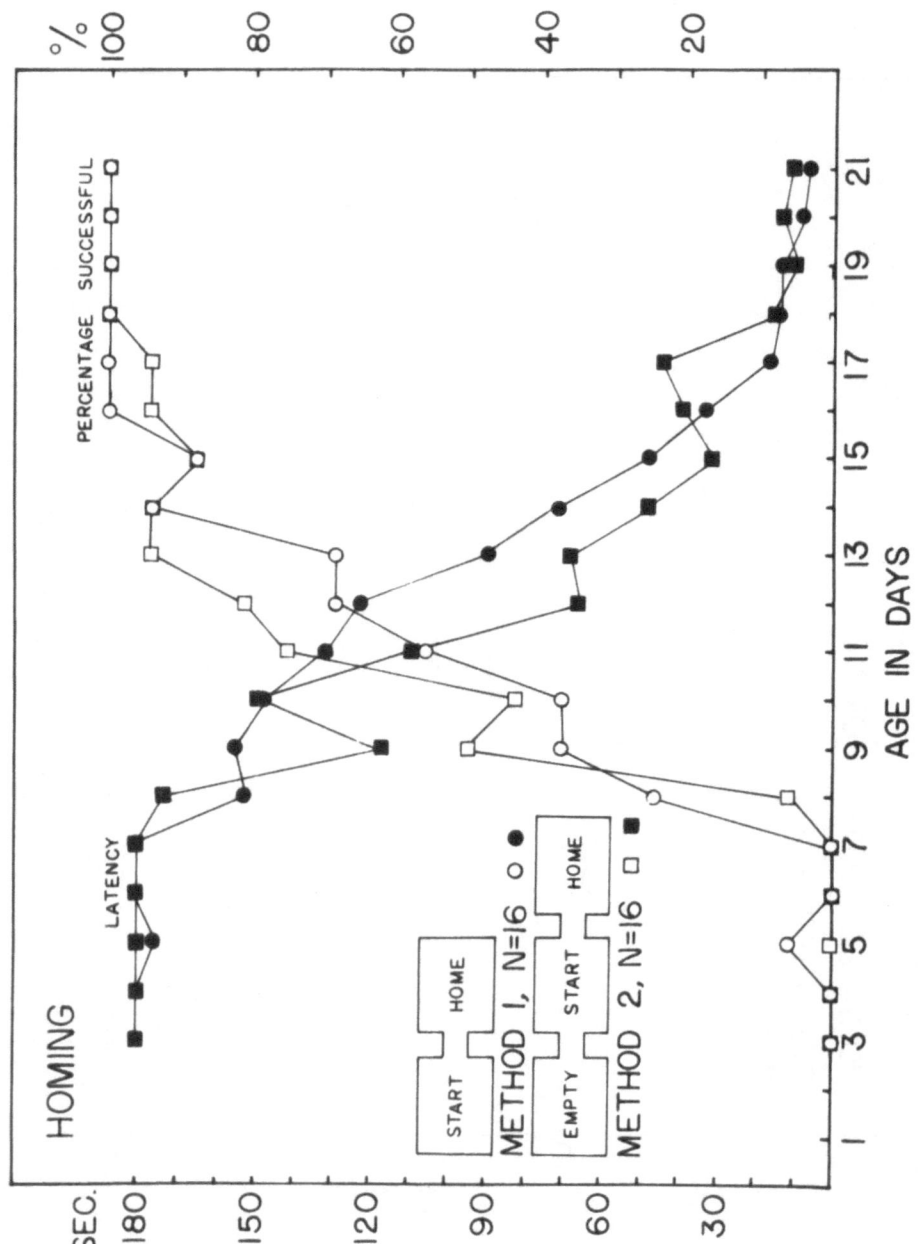

majority did not until days 13-14. Two methods were used (Fig. 3).
The first apparatus consisted of a start chamber and a modified home
cage. The home cage had an opening which allowed the isolated pup
to rejoin its mother and siblings; a wire fence inside the cage prevented the mother from leaving the cage to retrieve the young. In
the second method the start box had two openings, one leading to the
home cage, the other to an empty cage, providing the animal with a
choice. There were little differences with the two methods. Some
animals homed successfully by day 8, which required traversing a
minimal distance of 8 inches, more than half of them by day 11, and
the majority of animals (about 90%) homed by day 13. While in the
open field, as it was mentioned before, there is minimal locomotion
during the second week, when homing is introduced as a motivation,
the animals traverse an appreciable distance speedily.

Homing used as a motivation made it also possible to study the
development of motor skills that are more complex than ambulation
on a flat surface with adequate traction. In some of these tests
true homing was employed, in others a litter was placed in a goal
compartment and isolated pups had to negotiate different obstacle
courses to rejoin their siblings. The skills tested included the
ability to traverse elevated paths of different lengths and widths;
climbing up or descending on ropes and rods of different textures
and widths; ascending or descending on a wire mesh surface or ladder;
jumping down from different heights or across gaps of different
widths (Altman and Sudarshan, in preparation).

Two experiments will be described here. In one test an elevated
platform held a litter and attached there was a "bridge" 24" long
and either 1-1/4" or 1/4" wide. Isolated pups were placed at the
end of these bridges and their ability and speed of rejoining the
litter was determined (a sawdust-filled box at the base served as a
protection for the falling infants). Daily tests of 3-minute duration were administered, and animals that rejoined their siblings in
that period were scored successful. On the wide bridge falls decreased and distances covered increased from day 13, but on the
narrow bridge all animals fell off up to day 15, evidencing their
inability to balance themselves (Fig. 4). In general, successful
ambulation emerged later on the wide bridge than on solid surface
(more than half of the animals were successful on the ground by
day 11, and only by day 15 on the wide bridge) and still later (by
about a 2 day delay) on the narrow bridge, indicating the slow maturation of balancing skill. A slower maturation of hindlimb coordination than coordination of the forelimbs was indicated by the

-----

Fig. 3. Latency of homing and percentage of animals succeeding in
reaching the home cage in a choice and nonchoice situation.

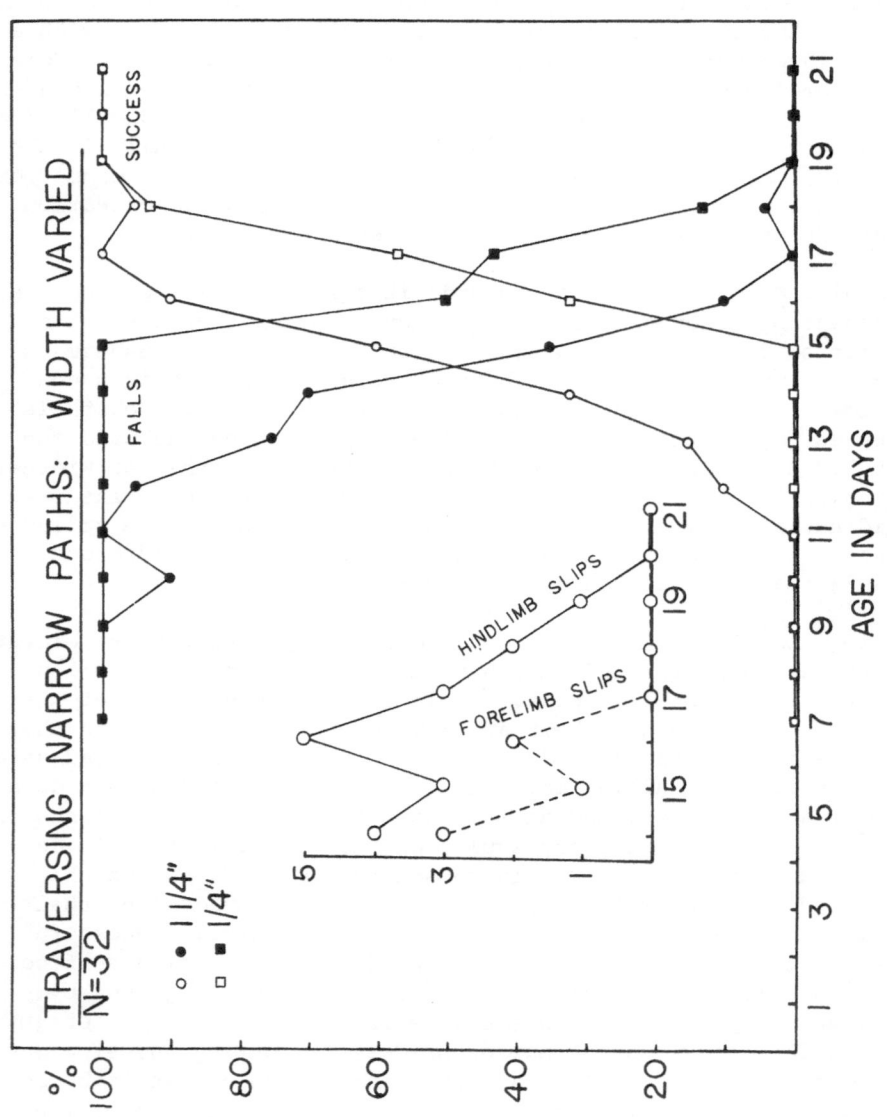

longer persistence of hindlimb slips, even after the animals stopped falling (Fig. 4, inset).

In the other experiment, a surface consisting of 1/4" wire mesh attached to a wooden frame 18" high and 6" wide was placed at an angle of 70 degrees with its top in contact with a platform and its base in water. A litter of rats was placed on the platform and individual rats were placed at the bottom of the wire mesh. In a complementary experiment the isolated pup was placed on the top platform and its littermates at the base of the wire mesh. As is shown in Fig. 5, all animals were successful in climbing up and rejoining their siblings by day 14, but it was not until day 20 that nearly all succeeded in descending. Although this points to a differential rate of maturation of these two skills, it must be mentioned that there is a multiple motivation in the case of ascending, as the animal is placed on the incline and falling into the water is aversive, whereas staying on the platform does not involve these additional motive forces. Indeed, it may be seen that in the ascending situation there are many falls, while descending is not attempted by most animals until the skill has matured (Fig. 5). Other studies (Altman et al.,1971a; Altman and Sudarshan, in preparation) do indicate the later maturation of descending skills in other situations.

The use of homing has enabled us to study the maturation of motor skills in normal rats during the suckling period, before most of those skills have been acquired which allow the animal to fend for itself and be weaned. With the normative data that are being gathered it has become possible to assess objectively the retardation of motor development produced by such agents as low-level irradiation of various brain structures (Altman et al., 1971a), undernutrition (Altman, et al., 1971b) and other treatments (work in preparation).

HOMING USED TO STUDY THE DEVELOPMENT
OF DISCRIMINATION LEARNING

While successful classical and instrumental conditioning has been reported in neonates and young infants of various species (rat: Caldwell and Werbogg, 1962; dog: Fuller et al., 1950; Cornwell and Fuller, 1961; Stanley et al., 1963; monkey: Mason and Harlow, 1958; man: Lipsitt, 1963, 1969; Kaye, 1965; Papoušek, 1969; Siqueland, 1968) the study of the development of discrimination and other complex learning tasks has been hindered for the same reasons as has

---

Fig. 4. Percentage of falls and successful crossing over bridges 1-1/4" and 1/4" wide leading to the platform holding the siblings. Number of forelimb and hindlimb slips on the wide bridge, after the animals acquired the ability to balance themselves, is shown in inset.

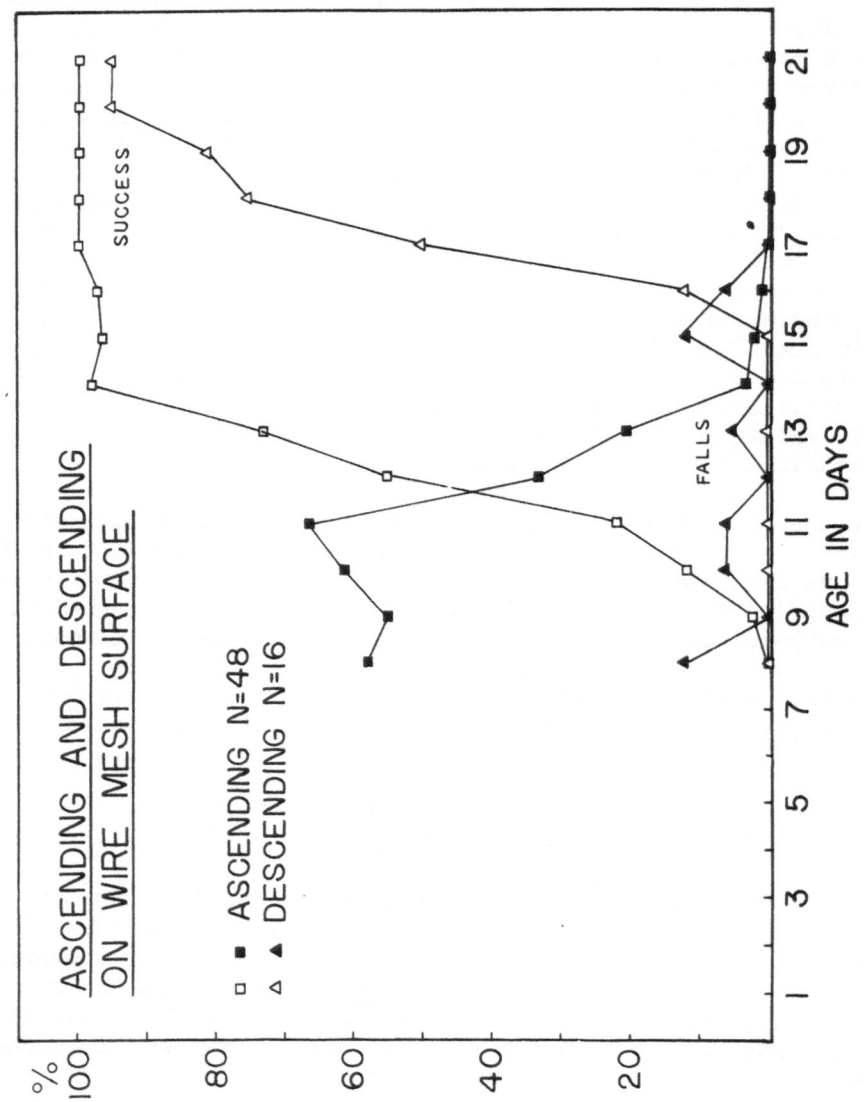

been the assessment of other behavioral capacities, namely, the difficulty of creating appropriate reward and punishment situations and of circumventing their sensory and motor handicaps. For such practical reasons, past studies of the development of learning have mainly been carried out in rats during the "juvenile" rather than "infantile" stage of development. For example, in maze learning, the youngest age studied has been 16 days old, involving a water escape task, and performance improved up to 29 days of age (Biel, 1938, 1940). The other studies employed rats or mice 30 days or older (Yerkes, 1909; Hubbert, 1915; Liu, 1928; Stone, 1929a,b).

More recently, punishment has been used successfully in training infant rats in escape and avoidance paradigms. Goldman and Tobach (1967) found evidence for one-way avoidance learning in 10 and 13 day old rats. However, this experiment was designed in such a way that maturation of motility and learning could not be separated. Misanin et al. (1970) were able to demonstrate in rats as young as 5 days old a within-session decrease of a non-goal directed competing response (turning in the wrong direction) in an escape situation; the ability to retain the improved performance level for a 24-hour period was not evident until 9 days of age in rats (Misanin et al., 1971) and mice (Nagy et al., 1972). Unfortunately escape behavior is not readily adaptable to more complex forms of discrimination learning. Another approach has been the study of the development of passive avoidance learning which utilizes the natural tendency of the rat to step down from a slightly elevated platform or from a large lighted to a small darkened compartment. Rats as young as 10 days old learn to withold their stepdown tendency (Riccio and Schulenburg, 1969); however, the speed of acquisition of this response is much longer in infants than in juveniles and in juveniles than in adults (Brunner, 1969; Riccio et al., 1968; Riccio and Schulenburg, 1969; Feigley and Spear, 1970; Schulenburg et al., 1971; Riccio and Marazzo, 1972). However, since weanling rats are comparable to adults in one-way active avoidance learning (Kirby, 1963; Klein and Spear, 1969; Feigley and Spear, 1970; Riccio and Marazzo, 1972) it is conceivable that poor performance on passive avoidance is due to an inability of young animals to withold a prepotent response (Altman et al., 1973).

As important as these learning paradigms may be, it seemed desirable to introduce other procedures which might allow the study of more complex discrimination learning tasks in infant rats. In this paper we report an attempt to utilize return to the nest area as a reward to motivate the acquisition and reversal of simultaneous

---

Fig. 5. Ascending or descending on an inclined (70 degrees) wire mesh surface to rejoin siblings with percentage of falls and success as a function of age.

discrimination problems in normal and retarded preweaning rats. The apparatus employed was a two-choice discrimination box (Fig. 6). It had a small start chamber and a choice compartment in which a T-shaped divided provided two routes to the goal box. The goal box was a modified nursing cage with a large opening on one side, and a wire screen behind the opening which prevented the mother from leaving the cage to retrieve the removed young. The discrimination box could be hooked onto the home cage in such a way that its choice routes were aligned with the opening on the home cage. A movable wire screen allowed closing the exit through one of the openings, without substantial interference with air currents that carry the home odor to the choice point in the discrimination box.

Position Discrimination: The subjects were Purdue-Wistar albino rats. On the day of birth each litter was culled to 8 pups (4 males and 4 females) and 1 day before the experiment was started the litters with their mothers were transferred from their standard breeding cages to the experimental nursing cages. Three groups were used, with training started on 6, 10 and 15 days of age. Each rat was given 20 trials a day, trial duration was 60 seconds, intertrial interval 5 minutes, and half an hour elapsed between two sessions of 10 trials. Half of the litter (2 males and 2 females) was required to select the right alley to gain entrance to the home cage, the other half had to choose the left alley. If an animal made an error or failed to respond within 60 seconds, it was placed in an isolation box for 60 seconds as a punishment. The criterion of learning was 34 correct choices in 40 consecutive trials over 2 days. Individual animals upon reaching criterion were put on reversal training; criterion for reversal learning was 17 correct responses out of 20. The measures recorded were latency in responding, number of responses, number of errors, and number of trials (or days) to criterion.

No differences were observed within the three groups between males and females or the subgroups that had to turn to the right or the left; all the data were therefore pooled. Fig. 7a shows that in 12 days of training all the 6-day group animals acquired the position habit and the mean to criterion was 9.3 days. All the animals of the 10-day group reached criterion level of performance in 10 days with a mean of 8.0; while all the 15-day group animals took 5.0 days, with the mean of 4.0 days. It was observed that animals in the 6-day group were greatly handicapped in learning the discrimination task because few of them left the start chamber during the trials administered on the first day, as suggested by their below chance level of performance (Fig. 7a), and many opportunities were missed on the subsequent days. Accordingly, the error scores were separated into true choice errors and non-responding errors (Fig. 8b). It is evident that the 6-day group differed appreciably from the 10-day group in nonresponding scores. Computation of choice errors to criterion indicated no difference (t-test; $p = <.01$) between the

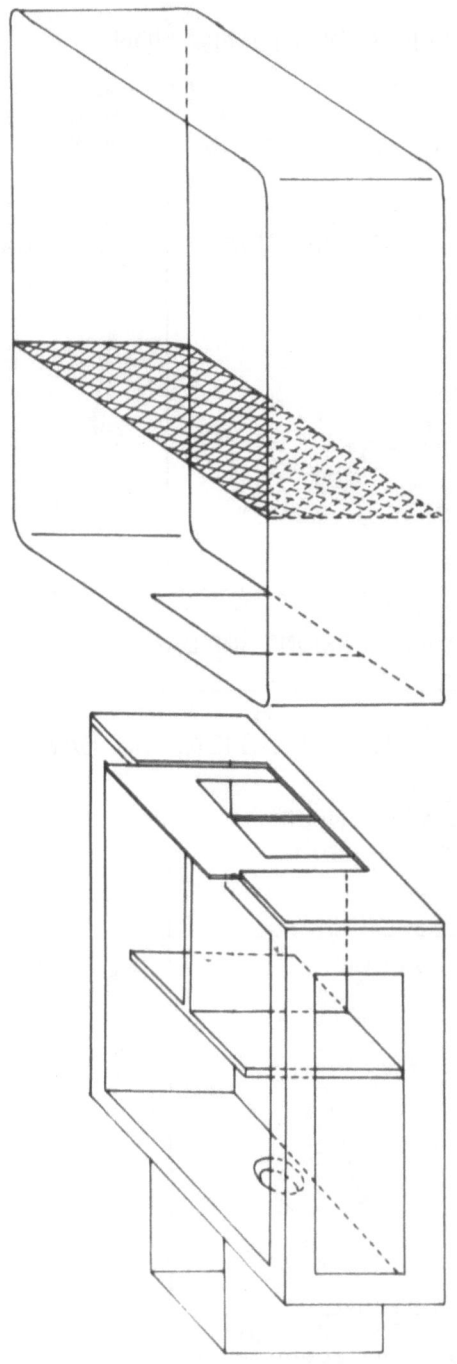

Fig. 6. Apparatus used to study discrimination learning. The two-alley choice box had two exits, one of which could be closed by means of a movable screen which did not interfere with penetration of odor from the home cage. The choice box was attached to the modified home cage (right) in which a wire screen prevented the mother from leaving the cage to retrieve the isolated pup.

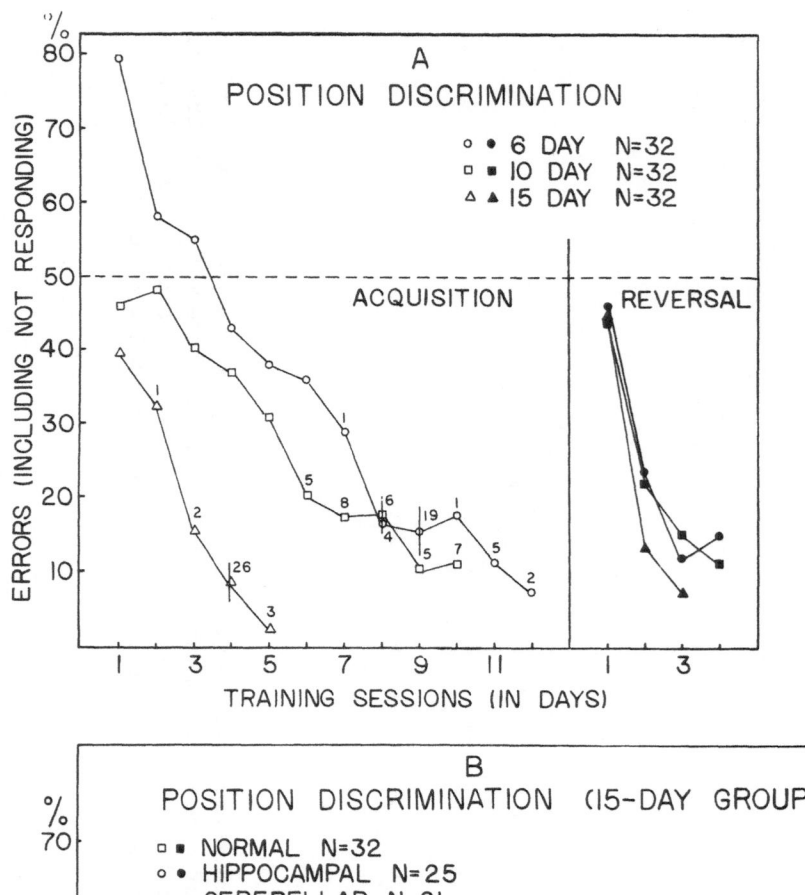

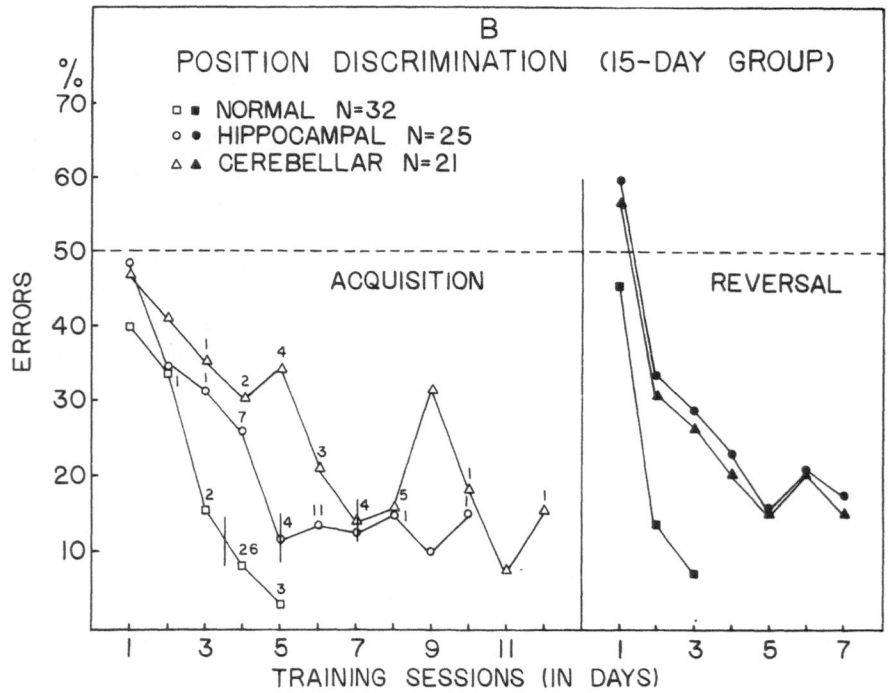

6-day and 10-day groups, but the differences between the 6-day and 15-day groups, and between the 10-day and 15-day groups were significant.

These results suggested that if the non-responding trials of the 6-day old animals are disregarded, which could be attributed to locomotor immaturity and during which no experience could be gained, that then the younger group was not significantly inferior to the intermediate group in the number of actual trials utilized. However, the 15-day animals were greatly superior to the younger groups and required half the number of trials. It is too early to speculate why there was little difference in learning ability following 6 and 10 days of age and the sudden improvement after 15 days. Among the possibilities are maturation of added afferent channels that provide information about spatial position; the reorganization of some of the central nervous structures being utilized; or the mediation of learning in the maturing animals by different brain mechanisms than those utilized during early infancy. However, this is not to be construed that the early training was of no utility to the animal. If age at the start of training is summed with the mean number of days required to reach criterion level of performance, the position habit was acquired by the early-starters by day 15, by the next group by day 18, and the late-starters acquired the habit by day 19, indicating a slight advantage offered by training started at an early age.

Tactile Discrimination: As in the previous experiment, 3 groups were used, with training started at the ages of 6, 10 and 15 days. For tactile discrimination the floor of the choice compartment was rough on one side (Garnet paper #40) and smooth on the other (backside of the sand paper). Half of each litter (2 males and 2 females) was required to choose the rough side as the correct alley, the other half the smooth side. Position of the correct surface was changed from trial to trial following a table of random numbers. The number of trials per day and all the other variables were the same as in the previous experiment.

Within the three groups there were no significant differences between sexes and the data were pooled. However, there was pronounced

---

Fig. 7. A: Mean percentage of errors (including failure to move and make a choice) on a side discrimination task, and its reversal, in animals that began training on days 6, 10 and 15. Numerals above scores indicate the number of animals that reached criterion on the day indicated; vertical bar is the mean for the group. B: Acquisition and reversal of the position habit in 15-day old normal animals, and animals in which the development of the cerebellum or hippocampus was retarded with x-irradiation, as described in the text.

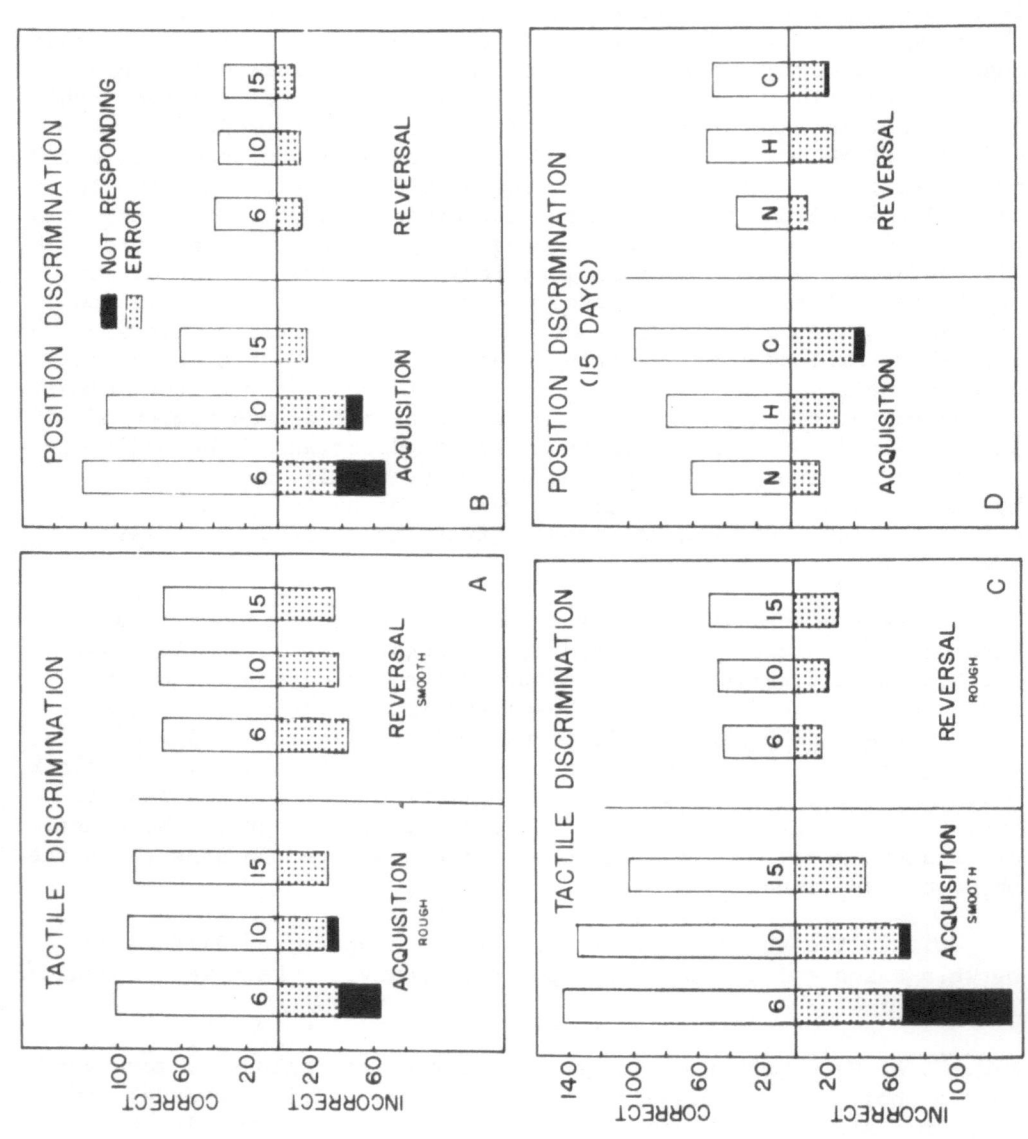

preference for the rough side (with better traction) over the smooth
side and this affected both acquisition and reversal. Therefore,
data for these two types of tactile discrimination learning were
plotted separately. Fig. 9a shows that with the rough-floored alley
being correct, criterion level of performance (not disregarding
errors due to nonresponding) was reached by all animals of the 6-,
10- and 15-day groups in 11, 10 and 7 days, respectively. The corresponding mean number of days were 9.0, 6.6 and 6.0 days. Disregarding nonresponding errors (Fig. 8a) computation of choice errors
to criterion indicated that only the difference between the 6-day
and 15-day groups was significant. In reversal training which required shifting to the nonpreferred smooth side, training was protracted (Figs. 8a, 9a) but there was no difference between the three
groups.

Acquisition of the tactile discrimination task with the smooth
side correct was a more protracted process (Fig. 9b) than with the
preferred rough side the correct choice and it took 15, 12 and 9 days,
respectively, for all the animals of the 6-, 10- and 15-day groups
to reach criterion level of performance. The corresponding mean
days to criterion were 13.1, 10.3 and 7.4 days. Actual choice errors
to criterion were not different between the 6- and 10-day groups
(Fig. 8c) but were significantly different between the 6- and 15-day
and the 10- and 15-day groups. That is, in this task, as in the
acquisition of the position habit, there was a discontinuous improvement in learning ability around 15 days. The absence of such a
sudden improvement in the discrimination task with the preferred side
correct may indicate that with the inadvertent "baiting" used this
did not represent a pure learning situation. The latter task was
acquired by the 6-day group in fewer trials than the position discrimination. It is difficult to say why the 15-day group was not
facilitated on this task, unless their preference for the rough side
was less pronounced. This is supported by several considerations.
First in the 15-day group the difference in acquisition scores between rough and smooth sides was the smallest. In reversal training,
which required shifting to the rough side the 6-day group, indeed,
performed significantly better than either the 10-day or 15-day

---

Fig. 8. Number of trials to criterion in acquisition and reversal.
A: Tactile discrimination with preferred rough-floor the cue to the
correct alley. B: Tactile discrimination with the nonpreferred
smooth-floor as the cue. C: Position discrimination in normal animals started at three ages (6, 10 and 15). D: Position discrimination in three groups of animals (N=normal; H=hippocampus-irradiated;
C=cerebellum-irradiated) that started training on day 15. The total
number of trials were divided in each case into correct and incorrect
responses; the latter were subdivided into errors of commission and
omission (not responding).

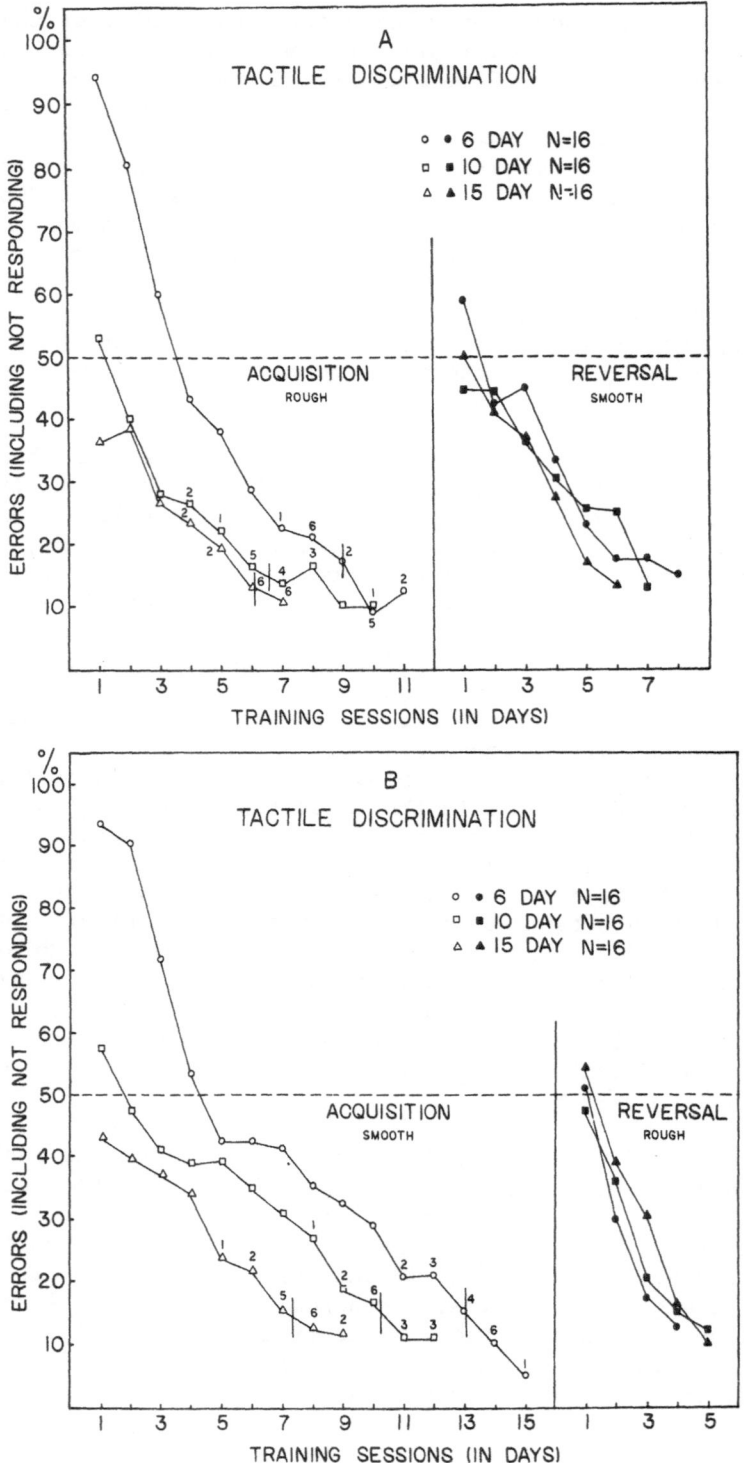

groups, supporting the idea that the preference confounding factor was strongest in this group in which the smooth surface may have added to the locomotor handicap. Finally, a previous study has shown (Finger and Frommer, 1968) no differences in adult rats in tactile discrimination in a T-maze between the rough or smooth surface being the correct arm.

HOMING USED TO STUDY EXPERIMENTAL RETARDATION OF REGIONAL BRAIN DEVELOPMENT

Spaced, low-level x-irradiation of the area of the cerebellum leads to depopulation of the postnatally-forming microneurons of the cerebellar cortex (Altman and Anderson, 1971, 1972). Similar effects may be obtained with irradiation of the forebrain region containing the hippocampus, which leads to selective depopulation of the granule cells of the dentate gyrus (Bayer et al., 1973). The behavioral consequences of experimental retardation of cerebellar growth were examined to some extent in infants (Wallace and Altman, 1969a) and adults (Wallace and Altman, 1969b; Altman et al., 1971a; Anderson and Altman, 1971) with special emphasis on deficits produced in postural and locomotor functions. Infantile retardation of hippocampal development was found to lead in adults to syndromes similar to those obtained after surgical lesions of the hippocampus de toto, such as deficits in spontaneous alternation and in passive avoidance learning, augmented open field motility, and facilitation of two-way avoidance learning (Bayer et al., 1973).

In the experiment to be described in this section, the original intent was to study the time course of alterations in the acquisition and reversal of a discrimination task following hippocampal irradiation. Because the cerebellum is not usually implicated in learning, animals with cerebellar irradiation were included in this study to serve as irradiated controls. The results, however, pointed to the importance of the cerebellum as well as the hippocampus in maze learning; a conclusion which is supported by recent experiments in adults (Brunner and Altman, in preparation).

Male, Purdue-Wistar rat pups were irradiated, following a procedure described in detail elsewhere (Altman et al., 1971a). Twenty-five pups were x-rayed with a beam limited to the forebrain containing the hippocampus on postnatal days 2,3 (200r), 3,5,7,9,11,13 and 15 (150r), resulting in a reduction of approximately 85% of the

---

Fig. 9. Mean percentage of errors (including failure to move) on a texture discrimination task. A: Preferred rough surface correct in acquisition, nonpreferred smooth side on reversal. B: Nonpreferred smooth side correct in acquisition, preferred side on reversal. Numbers and bars, as in Fig. 7.

granule cells of dentate gyrus but sparing all pyramidal cells of
Ammon's horn. A similar schedule of irradiation limited to the region of the cerebellum was delivered to 21 animals. This produced
a cerebellar cortex essentially devoid of stellate, basket and granule
cells but sparing Purkinje cells. Beginning on day 15 both groups
of irradiated animals were trained on the same position discrimination task that was described in the previous section and were compared with normal animals of the same age group (Figs. 7b, 8d). The
results indicate that the hippocampal-retarded animals were handicapped with respect to controls both in acquisition and reversal of
a position habit (t=<.01). Unexpectedly, cerebellar irradiation had
an even greater effect on acquisition (though not on reversal) than
did irradiation of the hippocampal region though the two irradiated
groups did not differ significantly from each other.

The poor performance of hippocampal animals in reversal learning is in agreement with several studies in adults which showed reversal deficits in a T or Y maze following hippocampal lesions
(Thompson and Langer, 1963; Teitelbaum, 1964; Kimble and Kimble,
1965; Niki, 1966; Douglas and Pribram, 1966). However, no such deficits were reported in the acquisition of a black and white Y-maze
discrimination (Kimble, 1963). Even more surprising was the severe
deficit seen in the cerebellar group. Whether cerebellar retardation
selectively affects position discrimination learning or has the same
effect on other forms of discriminations, remains to be determined.
The possibility also remains that the locomotor deficits produced
in these animals has an adverse effect on performance.

                                    SUMMARY

Infant rats begin to display a positive tendency to orient
towards the home cage by 3 days of age, before they can successfully
return to it, and this tendency is fully mature by the end of the
first week. We made use of this nest-seeking proclivity, and the
inclination of infant rats to re-join their siblings, to study the
maturation of simple locomotor skills, such as returning to the home
cage on a solid substrate, and the emergence of more complex motor
skills, such a traversing narrow bridges, climbing up or down on inclines, ropes or rods. Homing was also used as an incentive to motivate normally developing and retarded infant rats to master various
discrimination learning tasks.

Over 90% of 13-day old normal rats returned in about 1 minute
to the home cage when placed into an adjacent chamber, but virtually
all animals fell off a relatively wide bridge (1-1/4") leading to
siblings at that age. Comparable level of success was not seen on
the wide bridge until day 16 and on a narrower (1/4") bridge until
day 19, indicating the late maturation of balancing skills. Tests

on inclines suggested that ascending skills matured earlier than descending skills. Little has been done so far to use such norms of motor development to study the effects of such treatments as drug administration, hormonal imbalance, undernutrition or experimental retardation of brain development.

In a two-alley discrimination apparatus with side or floor-texture as the cue to the correct alley, rats as young as 6 days of age can begin to profit from training. The 6-day old rats often failed to respond initially due to their motor immaturity but if the missed opportunities are disregarded, they mastered the position habit in about the same number of actual trials as another group of animals started on day 10. However, the animals that began training on day 15 were greatly superior to the two younger groups and required only half as many trials. Fifteen-day old rats in which the growth of the cerebellum or hippocampus was retarded by a schedule of low-level x-irradiation, were handicapped both in the acquisition and reversal of the position habit.

Little difference was found in the three age groups in a tactile discrimination task in which the correct alley had a rough surface, presumably because the younger animals had a preference for this texture which provides better traction. In the experiment in which the alley with smooth floor was correct the younger animals profited from the training but, again, there was clear evidence of discontinuous improvement in learning ability in the animals older than 2 weeks. The mechanisms underlying this change in learning ability remain to be identified.

ACKNOWLEDGMENTS

This research is supported by the National Institute of Mental Health and the U.S. Atomic Energy Commission. We would like to thank Deborah Duncavage and Zeynep Kurgun for their assistance.

REFERENCES

Altman, J., and Anderson, W.J., 1971, Irradiation of the cerebellum in infant rats with low level x-ray: Histological and cytological effects during infancy and adulthood, Exp. Neurol. 30: 492.

Altman, J., and Anderson, W.J., 1972, Experimental reorganization of the cerebellar cortex: I. Morphological effects of elimination of all microneurons with prolonged x-irradiation started at birth, J. Comp. Neurol. 146: 355.

Altman, J., Anderson, W.J., and Strop, M., 1971a, Retardation of cerebellar and motor development by focal x-irradiation during infancy, Physiol. Behav. 7: 143.

Altman, J., Brunner, R.L., and Bayer, S.A., 1973, The hippocampus and behavioral maturation, Behav. Biol. in press.

Altman, J., Sudarshan, K., Das, G.D., McCormick, N., and Barnes, D., 1971b, The influence of nutrition on neural and behavioral development: III. Development of some motor, particularly locomotor patterns during infancy, Devel. Psychobiol. 4: 97.

Anderson, W.J., and Altman, J., 1971, Retardation of cerebellar and motor development in rats by focal x-irradiation beginning at four days, Physiol. Behav. 8: 57.

Bayer, S.A., Brunner, R.L., Hine, R., and Altman, J., 1973, Behavioral effects of interference with the postnatal acquisition of hippocampal granule cells, Nature, in press.

Biel, W.C., 1938, The effect of early inanition upon maze learning in the albino rat, Comp. Psychol. Monogr. 15: 1.

Biel, W.C., 1940, Early age differences in maze performance in the albino rat, J. Genet. Psychol. 56: 439.

Bolles, R.C., and Woods, P.J., 1964, The ontogeny of behavior in the albino rat, Anim. Behav. 12: 427.

Brunner, R.L., 1969, Age differences in one-trial passive avoidance learning, Psychon. Sci. 14: 134.

Caldwell, D.F., and Werboff, J., 1962, Classical conditioning in newborn rats, Science 136: 1118.

Cornwell, A.C., and Fuller, J.L., 1961, Conditioned responses in young puppies, J. Comp. Physiol. Psychol. 54: 13.

Douglas, R.J., and Pribram, K.H., 1966, Learning and limbic lesions, Neuropsychol. 4: 197.

Feigley, D.A., and Spear, N.E., 1970, Effect of age and punishment condition on long-term retention by the rat of active- and passive-avoidance learning, J. Comp. Physiol. Psychol. 73: 515.

Finger, S., and Frommer, G.P., 1968, Effects of cortical lesions on tactile discriminations graded in difficulty, Life Sci. 7: 897.

Fuller, J.L., Easler, C.A., and Banks, E.M., 1950, Formation of conditioned avoidance responses in young puppies, Amer. J. Physiol. 160: 462.

Goldman, P.S., and Tobach, E., 1967, Behavior modification in infant rats, Anim. Behav. 14: 559.

Gregory, E.H., and Pfaff, D.W., 1971, Development of olfactory-guided behavior in infant rats, Physiol. Behav. 6: 573.

Hess, E.H., 1959, Imprinting: an effect of early experience, Science 130: 133.

Hofer, M.A., 1970, Physiological responses of infant rats to separation from their mothers, Science 168: 871.

Hubbert, H.B., 1915, The effect of age on habit formation in the albino rat, Behav. Monogr. 2: 1.

Kaye, H., 1965, The conditioned Babkin reflex in human newborns, Psychonom. Sci. 2: 287.

Kimble, D.P., 1963, The effects of bilateral hippocampal lesions in rats, J. Comp. Physiol. Psychol. 56: 273.

Kimble, D.P., and Kimble, R.J., 1965, Hippocampectomy and response perseveration in the rat, J. Comp. Physiol. Psychol. 60: 474.

Kirby, R.H., 1963, Acquisition, extinction, and retention of an avoidance response in rats as a function of age, J. Comp. Physiol. Psychol. 56: 158.

Klein, S.B., and Spear, N.E., 1969, Influence of age on short-term retention of active-avoidance learning in rats, J. Comp. Physiol. Psychol. 69: 583.

Leon, M., and Moltz, H., 1971, Maternal pheromone: discrimination by preweanling albino rats, Physiol. Behav. 7: 265.

Lipsitt, L.P., 1963, Learning in the first year of life, in "Advances in Child Development and Behavior," (L.P. Lipsitt and C.C. Spiker, eds.), pp. 147-195, Vol. 1, Academic Press, New York.

Lipsitt, L.P., 1969, Learning capacities of the human infant, in "Brain and Behavious," (R.J. Robinson, ed.), pp. 227-245, Academic Press, London.

Liu, S.Y., 1928, The relation of age to the learning ability of the white rat, J. Comp. Psychol. 8: 75.

Lorenz, K., 1935, Der Kumpan in der Umwelt des Vogels, J. Ornithol. 83: 137.

Mason, W.A.,and Harlow, H.F., 1958, Formation of conditioned responses in infant monkeys, J. Comp. Physiol. Psychol. 51: 68.

Misanin, J.R., Nagy, Z.M., Keiser, E.F. and Bowen, W., 1971, Emergence of long-term memory in the neonatal rat, J. Comp. Physiol. Psychol. 77: 188.

Misanin, J.R., Nagy, Z.M., and Weiss, E.M., 1970, Escape behavior in neonatal rats, Psychon. Sci. 18: 191.

Moltz, H., and Robbins, D., 1965, Maternal behavior of primiparous and multiparous rats, J. Comp. Physiol. Psychol. 60: 417.

Nagy, Z.M., Misanin, J.R., and Olsen, P.L., 1972, Development of 24 hour retention of escape learning in neonatal C3H mice, Devel. Psychobiol. 5: 259.

Niki, H., 1966, Response preservation following the hippocampal ablation in the rat, Jap. Psychol. Res. 8: 1.

Nyakas, C., and Endröczi, E., 1970, Olfaction guided approaching behaviour in infantile rats to the mother in maze box, Acta Physiol. Acad. Sci. Hung. 38: 59.

Papoušek, H., 1969, Individual variability in learned responses in human infants, in "Brain and Early Behaviour," (R.J. Robinson, ed.), pp. 251-263, Academic Press, London.

Riccio, D.C., and Marazzo, M.J., 1972, Effects of punishing active avoidance in young and adult rats, J. Comp. Physiol. Psychol. 79: 453.

Riccio, D.C., Rohbaugh, M., and Hodges, L.A., 1968, Developmental aspects of passive and active avoidance learning in rats, Devel. Psychobiol. 1: 108.

Riccio, D.C., and Schulenburg, C.J., 1969, Age related deficits in the acquisition of a passive avoidance response, Canad. J. Psychol. 23: 429.

Rosenblatt, J.S., 1971, Suckling and home orientation in the kitten: A comparative developmental study, in "The Biopsychology of Development," (E. Tobach et al., eds.), pp. 345-410, Academic Press, New York.

Rosenblatt, J.S., and Lehrman, D.S., 1963, Maternal behavior of the laboratory rat, in "Maternal Behavior in Mammals," (H.L. Rheingold, ed.), pp. 8-57, Wiley, New York.

Rosenblatt, J.S., Turkewitz, G., and Schneirla, T.C., 1969, Development of home orientation in newly born kittens, Trans. N.Y. Acad. Sci. 31: 231.

Salas, M., Schapiro, S., and Guzman-Flores, C., 1970, Development of olfactory bulb discrimination between maternal and food odors, Physiol. Behav. 5: 1261.

Schapiro, S., and Salas, M., 1970, Behavioral response of infant rats to maternal odors, Physiol. Behav. 5: 815.

Schulenburg, C.J., Riccio, D.C., and Stikes, E.R., 1971, Acquisition and retention of passive-avoidance response as a function of age in rats, J. Comp. Physiol. Psychol. 74: 75.

Siqueland, E.R., 1968, Reinforcement patterns and extinction in human newborns, J. Exp. Child Psychol. 6: 431.

Sluckin, W., 1965, "Imprinting and Early Learning," Aldine, Chicago.

Small, W.S., 1899, Notes on the psychic development of the young white rat, Amer. J. Psychol. 11: 80.

Stanley, W.C., Cornwell, A.C., Poggiani, C., and Trattner, A., 1963, Conditioning in the neonate puppy, J. Comp. Physiol, Psychol. 56: 211.

Stone, C.P., 1929a, The age factor in animal learning. I. Rats in the problem box and the maze, Genet. Psychol. Monogr. 5: 1.

Stone, C.P., 1929b, The age factor in animal learning. II. Rats on a multiple light discrimination box and a difficult maze, Genet. Psychol. Monogr. 6: 125.

Teitelbaum, H., 1964, A comparison of effects of orbitofrontal and hippocampal lesions upon discrimination learning and reversal in the cat, Exp. Neurol. 9: 452.

Thompson, R., and Langer, S.K., 1963, Deficits in position reversal learning following lesions of the limbic system, J. Comp. Physiol. Psychol. 56: 987.

Tinbergen, N., 1963, "The Herring Gull's World," Collins, London.

Tinbergen, N., and Perdeck, A.C., 1950, On the stimulus situation releasing the begging response in the newly-hatched herring gull chick (Larus argentatus), Behaviour 3: 1.

Tobach, E., Rouger, Y., and Schneirla, T.C., 1967, Development of olfactory function in the rat pup, Amer. Zool. 7: 792.

Wallace, R.B., and Altman, J., 1969a, Behavioral effects of neonatal irradiation of the cerebellum. I. Qualitative observations in infant and adolescent rats, Devel. Psychobiol. 2: 257.

Wallace, R.B., and Altman, J., 1969b, Behavioral effects of neonatal irradiation of the cerebellum. II. Quantitative studies in young-adult rats, Devel. Psychobiol. 2: 266.

Wiesner, B.P., and Sheard, N.M., 1933, "Maternal Behavior in the Rat," Oliver and Boyd, Edinburgh.

Yerkes, R.M., 1909, Modifiability of behavior in its relations to the age and sex of the dancing mouse, J. Comp. Neurol. Psychol. 19: 237.

DRUG ACTIONS: MYELINOGENESIS
J. Folch-Pi, Chairman

PROTEOLIPIDS

J. Folch-Pi

Harvard Medical School, Boston, Massachusetts and

McLean Hospital, Belmont, Massachusetts

INTRODUCTION

During the development of a method for the extraction and purification of lipids from central nervous system (Folch et al., 1951),
it was observed that a chloroform: methanol 2:1 mixture, v/v, (CM) extracted from central nervous system some protein material (Folch and
Lees, 1951). This material was not removed from the extract upon repeated washing with water. Its presence in the extract was revealed
by the fact that when the extract was taken to dryness by evaporation
of the solvents, the resulting residue proved to be only partly soluble in the chloroform: methanol mixture that had been used in the
original extraction of the tissue. The portion of the residue that
was insoluble in CM, was found also to be insoluble in water, and in
all of a large number of aqueous solutions and organic solvents that
were tested. The insoluble material contained 14% N, 1.76% S and
between 0.2% and 0.4% P. Upon adequate acid hydrolysis, over 91% of
its N could be recovered chromatographically as free amino acids,
i.e., the insoluble material was mainly protein in nature.

It was assumed that this protein material was extracted from the
tissue as a protein-lipid complex, and that the latter moiety con-
ferred to the complex characteristic lipid-like solubility in chloroform: methanol mixtures and its insolubility in water. The only
protein-lipid complexes described up to that time had been blood
plasma lipoproteins, which were soluble in water, and destroyed, or
dissociated by organic solvents. To emphasize the marked difference
in solubility properties between plasma lipoproteins and the recently
discovered brain protein-lipid complexes, the latter were designated
as proteolipids.

351

TABLE I

AMINO ACID COMPOSITION OF PROTEOLIPID APOPROTEIN (PLA) FROM DIFFERENT TISSUES

Tissue and PLA Preparation

(Moles per 100 moles recovered in hydrolysate)

Amino Acid	Central White Matter	Central Gray Matter		Heart		Liver		Kidney
		71-VII	72-VI	72-III	72-VII	72-V	72-IX	72-IV
Arginine	2.6	2.39	2.62	2.41	3.26	3.34	3.15	2.99
Histidine	1.8	1.65	1.90	1.91	1.61	1.73	1.48	1.82
Lysine	3.8	3.86	3.70	3.31	3.26	3.90	3.08	3.80
Aspartic	4.0	4.78	4.84	6.29	6.78	6.12	6.57	5.98
Glutamic	5.8	6.07	5.76	5.22	5.69	6.03	5.70	5.69
Half Cystine	4.0	2.39	1.74	--	0.36	0.27	0.80	--
Methionine	1.9	2.39	2.78	5.35	4.65	3.90	3.68	3.94
Serine	8.5	5.61	5.70	6.03	6.29	6.03	6.76	6.21
Threonine	8.5	7.54	7.36	6.69	6.67	5.85	6.30	5.98
Proline	2.8	3.86	4.52	5.29	4.96	5.48	5.43	5.25
Glycine	10.3	10.58	10.23	8.90	9.11	9.09	9.44	9.71
Alanine	12.5	12.06	12.04	10.05	10.28	10.02	10.38	10.80
Valine	6.9	7.27	7.15	5.82	6.11	6.87	6.69	6.58
Leucine	11.1	11.60	11.88	14.59	13.09	14.20	13.60	14.09
Isoleucine	4.9	5.71	5.60	7.50	6.60	6.40	6.43	6.86
Tyrosine	4.6	4.69	4.58	3.41	3.67	3.53	3.47	3.43
Phenylalanine	7.9	7.54	7.55	7.23	7.15	7.24	7.03	6.86

The amino acid composition of proteolipids is rather unusual, with a high content of sulphur and non-polar amino acids, and a comparatively low content of acidic and basic amino acids (Table I). Proteolipids are resistant to the usual animal proteolytic enzymes. Proteolipids are extracted from tissues by chloroform:methanol 2:1, v/v. A subsequent extraction with the same solven mixture fails to yield additional amounts of proteolipids, i.e., the extraction appears to be quantitative in the first extraction. Alternatively, the absence of additional proteolipids in second and subsequent extracts might indicate an "insolubilization" of any possible unextracted proteolipids by the changes brought about by the first extaction:dehydration, removal of lipids, of many small molecule solutes, etc.

The amount of proteolipids in extracts may be estimated in a number of ways: 1)by determining the amount of solutes that become insoluble in chloroform:methanol upon removal of the solvents by vacuum distillation; this procedure must be repeated three times, if a quantitative result is sought; 2)by estimating total protein by the method of Lowry et al. (1951), or by one of its modifications; 3)by estimating the amount of amino acids released by acid hydrolysis, and computing from it the amount of protein by the use of an empirical factor (Folch and Lees, 1951); 4)for the purposes of monitoring the presence of proteolipids, the extinction coefficient at 278 nm provides an indicator which is quite quantitative, especially for comparative purposes, and which has the advantage of simplicity and sensitivity.

PROTEOLIPIDS

Distribution of Proteolipids

Although especially abundant in central nervous tissue, proteolipids are present in a wide variety of animal and vegetable tissues: bovine tissues contain the following amounts of proteolipid protein (mg/g fresh tissue weight): heart, 3.5; kidney, 2.0; lung, 0.95; skeletal muscle (biceps), 0.4; smooth muscle (uterus), 0.6. In spinach chloroplasts proteolipids represent 2-4% of dry weight (Zill and Harmon, 1961). All the values reported are only indicative, because often the yields obtained may have been incomplete.

In the central nervous system, they are especially abundant in brain white matter, where they have been shown to be mainly myelin components (Autilio, 1966). They are absent or present in very small amounts in fetal brain (Folch, 1955) and their appearance and progressive accumulation is concurrent with myelination.

In a study of 28 different anatomical areas of the human nervous system Amaducci (1962) observed marked and consistent differences from

one anatomical area to another (Amaducci, 1962). The highest concentration is found in corpus callosum and centrum ovale, where they
constitute 2.5 to 2.8% of fresh tissue weight. In cerebral gray
matter they are present at 1/5 to 1/10 of their concentration in brain
white matter. They exhibit a rostro-caudal decrease in concentration,
and they are present at very small concentrations in peripheral nerve.
Hence, although in central white matter they are mainly myelin components, their concentration does not parallel exactly the concentration of myelin, an observation that suggests that the protein composition of myelin shows quantitative differences among anatomical
areas.

Proteolipids in central nervous system are found in structures
other than myelin (Lees et al., 1968). In heart muscle, they are
mainly components of mitochondria (Joel et al., 1958; Murakami et al.,
1962). In general, proteolipids have been found in relation to membranous structures. Hence it is justifiable to think of them prin-
cipally as membrane components.

Study of Central White Matter Proteolipids

In brain white matter, proteolipids represent almost exclusively
myelin protein. Indeed, it was found that myelin was soluble in
chloroform:methanol (Laatsch, 1963; Autilio et al., 1964) and it was
inferred that all central myelin protein was proteolipid. A number
of observations, however, soon indicated that the solubility of myelin
in chloroform:methanol was misleading and that proteins other than
proteolipids were present in myelin. Thus, Lees (1968) demonstrated
that when brain tissue homogenates are freed of diffusable electrolytes, chloroform:methanol will dissolve proteins other than proteolipids. Also, it was known that isolated myelin produced allergic
encephalomyelitis when injected into animals with the necessary ad-
juvants, indicating that myelin contained the antigenic protein
(Laatsch, 1963). Since this was known to be a basic protein quite
different from proteolipids, it was clear that myelin contained at
least the antigenic basic protein, in addition to classical proteolipids. These and other observations have shown that myelin contains
at least three different types of protein; namely, the classical
proteolipids of Folch and Lees (1951), the antigenic basic protein
responsible for the experimental allergic encephalomyelitis and the
so-called proteolipid of Wolfgram (1966) which is quite different
from the classical proteolipid of Folch and Lees.

These three proteins can be separated from isolated myelin by
a very simple method that has been developed in our laboratory by
Gonzalez-Sastre (1970). The method is based on the observations that
Wolfgram's proteolipid is insoluble in neutral chloroform:methanol
mixtures, and that the encephalitogenic basic protein is insoluble
in chloroform:methanol in presence of electrolytes. In this method

myelin, isolated by one of the standard methods of subcellular fractionation, is dissolved in chloroform:methanol. The solution is then
centrifuged at about 100 g for 10 minutes or until clear. A small
amount of insoluble residue is thus collected. It amounts to 2% or
3% of the dry weight of myelin, i.e., 10% to 15% of the total proteins
present. The supernatant is then diluted by addition of 1/20th its
volume of 0.5 M KCl. A precipitate is formed which is collected by
centrifugation. We thus have divided myelin into three different
fractions: the original chloroform:methanol fraction (I), the subsequent fraction insoluble in chloroform:methanol:KCl mixture (II),
and the final supernatant (III). These three fractions have been
analyzed chemically, and by polyacrylamide gel electrophoresis. It
has been found that (I) had the electrophoretic mobility and the amino
acid composition of the basic antigenic protein and that (III) has mobility and an amino acid composition of the basic antigenic protein
and that (III) has mobility and an amino acid composition undistinguish-
able from those of classical proteolipids. The respective amounts
of these three fractions as percent of total myelin protein are:
Wolfgram's proteolipid, 15-17%; basic protein, 30%; classical proteolipids, 50-55%. These values are consistent with results obtained
by other authors using different methods (Eng et al., 1968).

A large amount of work has gone not only into the purification
of proteolipids proper, i.e., the separation of the protein-lipid
complex from adventitious lipids, but also into the preparation of
the protein moiety free of lipids, i.e., the proteolipid apoprotein.
It has been found that proteolipids can be concentrated by solvent
fractionation, by differential centrifugation, by dialysis in organic
solvents, by gel permeation, or by a combination of these procedures.
The specific procedures that have been developed are: 1) the "fluff"
method of Folch and Lees (1951) which was the one first used for the
separation of proteolipid-enriched fractions from the tissue chloro-
form:methanol extract. The extract is overlaid with at least 5-fold
its volume of water. Eventually, a "fluff" accumulates at the interface, which can be collected by freezing. From this fluff, by solvent
fractionation, two preparations, proteolipids A and B are obtained.
From the chloroform:methanol solution underlying the fluff, a proteolipid C is obtained by solvent fractionation. 2) the emulsion-
centrifugation procedure (Folch et al., 1959) is based on the difference between the specific gravity of protein and that of lipids. The
lipid and proteolipid mixture recovered from a washed lipid extract
is emulsified in 30-fold its weight of water; by centrifugation, proteolipids are collected quantitatively at the bottom (crude proteolipid), leaving the majority of lipids in emulsion in the supernatant.
From the pellet, by solvent fractionation, a "concentrated proteolipid"
preparation is obtained. 3) By dialysis in organic solvents, free
lipids diffuse through the dialysis membrane, whereas the proteolipids are retained by it. At the completion of dialysis, the retentate contains proteolipids freed of the greater part of lipids.
4) In gel permeation, as in dialysis, the proteolipids are separated

from free lipids because of their larger molecular size. Using
polystyrene gel, Autilio (1966) was able to separate proteolipids
from isolated myelin. Later, Mokrasch (1967), by combining diethyl
ether precipitation with permeation of Sephadex LH20, obtained a
highly enriched preparation of proteolipids. Finally, Soto et al.,
(1969) also used Sephadex LH20 in the purification of proteolipids
from white matter and from gray matter. From the latter they were
able to separate a distinct fraction which exhibited many of the
properties postulated for an acetylcholine receptor, and for which
the function of physiological receptor is being claimed (de Robertis
and Soto, 1967).

Since these procedures were not always designed to yield proteolipids of the highest possible protein content, the different products obtained show a wide range of variation in lipid composition.
The preparations with the highest protein content, which are those
obtained by dialysis or by gel permeation, still contain about 15
percent lipids or more. These lipids, which are the most firmly
bound to the protein, are mainly, if not exclusively, phosphatidyl-
serine, sulfatides and polyphosphoinositides, i.e., they are acidic
lipids. They appear to be bound to the protein moiety by ionic
linkages. They can be removed in part by chromatography on silicic
acid (Matsumoto et al., 1964) or on a Dowex 1-X2 column (Mokrasch,
1967), both procedures yielding products with about 95 percent protein. To remove the lipids completely, however, it is necessary to
submit the proteolipid to dialysis in chloroform:methanol acidified
by addition of concentrated HCl to a final HCl concentration of 0.04 N.
A protein is then obtained which contains only traces of some lipids,
with the exception of 2 to 4 percent covalently bound fatty acids
(see below). This is termed the proteolipid apoprotein.

The chromatography of proteolipids on silicic acid has been
carried out by Matsaumoto and Folch-Pi (1964) with preparations obtained by the emulsion-centrifugation procedure. Typical conditions
are a 10 mm inner diameter column packed with 4 g silicic acid and
loaded with about 70 mg of a preparation containing 60 percent protein. The column is eluted with a discontinuous gradient of chloro-
form:methanol:water mixtures of increasing polarity starting at 85
percent chloroform and ending with chloroform:methanol (1:1, v/v)
containing 12 percent 0.05 N HCl. Free lipids appear at 85 and 75
percent chloroform, and three protein peaks appear at 75, 70 and 50
percent chloroform (acidified). No difference is found among the
three protein peaks in amino acid composition and in the nature of
the up to 5 percent lipids that each contains, which are mainly polyphosphoinositides.

The preparation of maximally delipidated apoprotein was first
carried out by Tenenbaum and Folch-Pi (1966). It consisted in dialy-
zing a washed lipid extract against chloroform:methanol (2:1, v/v)
(CM) for seven days with daily changes of the diffusate, followed by

dialysis for seven more days against chloroform:methanol:HCl, 2:1:0.04 N (CM, HCl), followed by dialysis against a series of outer phases in which water was replacing gradually the organic solvents, until the latter were completely eliminated. The final retentate contained a "water-soluble proteolipid protein".

Properties and Composition of Central White Matter Proteolipids

The different proteolipid preparations obtained by the fore-going procedures are freely soluble in chloroform:methanol mixtures, and insoluble in water and in aqueous solutions. In the biphasic system chloroform:methanol:water (8:4:3, v/v) they will concentrate quantitatively in the lower chloroform phase, and will be completely absent from the upper methanol:water phase (with the exception of the last protein peak eluted from silicic acid column: about 1/5 of the protein partitions into the upper phase). The retention of the ori-ginal solubility properties throughout the gradual removal of lipids forces the conclusion that the characteristic solubilities of pro-teolipids must be explained in terms of the conformation of the pro-tein moiety. Studies of some of these preparations by optical ro-tatory dispersion (ORD) show that proteolipids are characterized by a high content of α-helix which remains unchanged throughout the procedure of gradual delipidation (Shermand and Folch-Pi, 1970; Zand, 1968). Upon removal of the last traces of lipids, the result-ing apoprotein proves to be soluble in water, although still retain-ing its solubility in organic solvents. The newly acquired solubility in water is paralleled by a decrease of the α-helix content to below detectable limits (<10%), i.e., there is a conformational change which apparently makes available to the medium the hydrophilic groups of the protein which in the starting proteolipids must have been buried inside the molecular structure.

The solutions of proteolipids in chloroform:methanol (2:1, v/v) are very stable and they keep for years without developing turbidity or precipitates, even at room temperature. They can be taken to dry-ness by evaporation of the solvents without loss of solubility of the proteolipids in the residue, provided the evaporation takes place at 40° or lower, and provided no biphasic system results in partial or total insolubilization of the proteolipid protein unless corrected immediately by addition of a proper solvent (usually methanol). A similar result is obtained by exposing the proteolipid solution in a biphasic system to slight alkalinity, in the presence of ions. For instance, at pH 8.8, in the biphasic system chloroform:methanol:water (8:4:3, v/v), proteolipids will become insoluble to an extent which is proportional to the logarithm of the ionic strength, between 0.001 and 1.0 M NaCl. The same result is obtained with Na_3 or K_3 citrate solution (Webster and Folch, 1961).

All the proteolipid preparations have been found to be resistant
to the action of pepsin, trypsin, papain and erepsin. This resistance
is not due to the presence of lipids because it persists in the apoprotein. The only enzyme that attacks proteolipids is pronase, although the extent of this susceptibility has not been thoroughly explored (Messinger et al., 1967). Lees et al. (1969) have reported that trypsin attacks proteolipids in the presence of Triton
X-100.

The amino acid composition, the protein moiety of the various
proteolipids appears to be the same in all preparations; the lipid
"moiety" varies according to the procedure of preparation. Fractionation by solvents, emulsion-centrifugation, permeation of Sephadex
LH20, and dialysis in CM separate from the protein, cholesterol and
the bulk of cerebrosides, sulfatides and phospholipids; hence these
lipids are bound to the protein, if at all, by labile bonds that are
easily disrupted. Most remaining phospholipids are removed by chroma-
trogrphy on silicic acid leaving only polyphosphoinositides and small
amounts of sulfatides. With Dowex 1X2 a similar removal of lipids is
attained, although no information is available on the exact nature
of the lipids still remaining. Finally, with dialysis in CM HCl, the
highest degree of delipidation is obtained, which proves that the
most tightly bound lipids must be bound through ionic linkages.

The amino acid composition of the different preparations up to
and including the apoprotein, shows that the amino acid pattern of
proteolipids is not affected by the previous procedures of purification. The amino acid pattern has the following characteristics:
a) a relatively scarcity of basic and acidic amino acids; arginine,
lysine and histidine account jointly for less than 10 percent of
amino acids in the hydrolysate, and aspartic and glutamic amount
jointly to about 10 percent. b) There is a relative abundance of
the so-called non-polar amino acids, i.e., amino acids that, when
combined in a peptide chain, offer only non-polar groups to the medium; leucine, isoleucine, valine, glycine, proline, phenylalanine,
and alanine amount to 57-58 percent of amino acids. If tryptophan
is added, about 60 percent of amino acids are non-polar. The relatively high concentration of tryptophan is indicated by the high absorption at 280 nm. c) There is a relative abundance of methionine
and half-cystine, as is to be expected from the high concentration
of sulfur in proteolipid protein (1.76 percent). Lees et al. (1967)
in a study of the conditions necessary for the preparation of the
carboxymethylcysteine derivatives of proteolipids, have shown that
the protein contains both sulfhydryl and disulfide groups, but the
sulfhydryl groups are difficult to demonstrate. They are available
for reaction with alkylating agents only in the presence of sodium
dodecyl sulfate, and a portion of them react slowly. Approximately
one-third of the half-cystine residues exist in the sulfhydryl form
when exposed to SDS; the remainder occurs in disulfide linkages which
must be reduced before alkylation can occur.

PROTEOLIPID APOPROTEIN

Preparation of a Stable Central White Matter Proteolipid Apoprotein

The apoprotein prepared by Tenenbaum and Folch-Pi (1967) proved too unstable for careful chemical and physical studies. It was obtained in the form of an aqueous solution containing only 0.1% protein. The protein precipitated at neutral pH, and when recovered by lyophilization, it proved either insoluble in water or soluble only below pH 5. On standing, either the original solution or the reconstituted solution developed precipitates. The protein remained soluble in chloroform:methanol. As already stated, ORD measurements showed it to have no measurable α-helix content, compared to the high helicity of the starting proteolipid.

In an attempt to obtain more stable apoprotein preparations, the procedure followed was reinvestigated. The result of this study is a new procedure which yields a consistent and stable preparation of proteolipid apoprotein, upon which extensive studies have been carried out. The details of the development of this procedure have been discussed in some detail elsewhere (Folch-Pi, 1972). In outline, central white matter is homogenized with five-fold its volume of chloroform:methanol, 1:1, v/v, and one-half its volume of aqueous 2M KCl. In the resulting biphasic system, the lower phase contains essentially all of the tissue lipids and proteolipids, including the polyphosphoinositides. The upper phase contains gangliosides, non-proteolipid protein, and low molecular weight tissue components.

The system is resolved by centrifugation, and the lower phase collected, placed in dialysis bags, and dialyzed against several changes of 10-fold its volume of CM 2:1, preferably in the dark and at 4°C. When 2/3 of the starting total solutes have dialyzed out, dialysis is continued against CM HCl 800:100:3, v/v until at least 85 percent of the solutes in the starting lower phase have been removed. Then dialysis is continued further for at least 5 changes of neutral CM, or until the solutes in the outer fluid amount to 0.05 percent or less of the starting solutes, whichever is longer. The length of time required to reach these levels of dialysis varies from sample to sample of dialysis tubing and it can be as little as 2 days to reach diffusion of 2/3 of starting solutes, and 4 days to reach more than 85 percent, to two-fold or three-fold these lengths of time.

The reason for the prolongation of the dialysis in acid medium until at least 85 percent of the solutes in the original lower phase have been removed by dialysis is that after removal of the acidic lipids, the proteolipid protein may form complexes with sphingo-myelin, upon return to a neutral medium. These sphingomyelin-protein complexes are not dissociated by additional dialysis either in acidified or neutral CM. Empirically, it has been found that if the removal of lipids is continued to the point at which 85 percent at least of the original solutes have been removed, these complexes are not formed.

The final retentate is usually clear and contains about 5 mg apoprotein per ml. Upon evaporation, it yields the apoprotein as a residue which has a characteristic glass-like appearance. By comparison, apoprotein samples that have not been maximally delipidated appear whitish.

Preparation of the Water-Soluble Apoprotein

The apoprotein recovered from the retentate is freely soluble in CM and in many other organic solvents, and it is completely insoluble in water. To render it water-soluble it is necessary to make it pass from solution into chloroform:methanol into solution in water by placing the CM solution in, or under, a stream of nitrogen, which removes chloroform preferentially (Folch-Pi and Stoffyn, 1972). When about 4/5 of the weight of the solution has thus been removed, water is added to the concentrate until cloudiness develops, or until a volume of water equal to the concentrate has been added. Passage of nitrogen is continued until the weight of the solution has again been reduced by half. At this stage, the solution is essentially free of chloroform and methanol, and can be kept for further study as an aqueous solution of apoprotein. Alternatively, it can be taken to dryness in a vacuum desiccator. The residue, glass-like in appearance, will prove freely soluble in water and also in chloroform:methanol, although some time of contact between residue and solvent may be required and, in the case of chloroform:methanol, addition of 1 or 2 percent water to the mixture may be necessary to bring about complete solution. The residue retains these solubilities for as long as we have kept it, which is several weeks. Aqueous solutions up to 3 or 4% can be easily prepared. Above 4 percent concentration, the aqueous solutions show increasing viscosity, and at 5 or 6 percent they become essentially gels.

It must be emphasized that only the maximally delipidated apoprotein is soluble in water. The presence of very small amounts of residual lipids results in incomplete insolubility in water. For instance, the sphingomyelin-protein de novo complexes are quite insoluble in water.

The aqueous solutions of apoprotein are indefinitely stable at neutral or slightly acid pH's. They appear to be markedly, if not totally, resistant to bacterial contamination. In our experience, solutions stored at 4°, but with frequent periods at room temperature, and also frequently opened for the taking of samples, have remained sterile for as long as they have been kept, which in some cases has been as long as eighteen months.

At pH 7.5 and above, aqueous solutions of apoprotein develop a
turbidity which disappears at higher pH's but persists upon acidification. Aqueous solutions brought rapidly to 0.1 N NaOH or higher
alkali concentrations, develop a transient turbidity followed by
complete clarification. This turbidity is so transient as to go
unnoticed unless special attention is paid to its appearance and disappearance. The solutions in 0.1 N NaOH or higher remain clear for
several days at least but, upon acidification, there is formation of
a massive precipitate which collects readily, leaving a supernatant
that shows only negligible absorption at 280 nm, i.e., the apoprotein
appears to have precipitated out quantitatively. This insolubilization of the apoprotein, exposed to 0.1 N NaOH, in aqueous acid develops over a period of about 2 hours.

The apoprotein is insolubilized, just as proteolipids are, by
taking to dryness from biphasic solutions, and by exposure to low
alkalinity in presence of ions. Thus, when a solution of apoprotein
in chloroform:methanol (2:1, v/v) is diluted with one-fifth its volume of 0.1 M Na_3 citrate, the bulk, if not all, of the protein is
precipitated out of solution, and collects as an insoluble residue
at the interface. This residue is completely insoluble in all aqueous
solutions and organic solvents that have been used, including 5 percent SDS (Na-dodecyl-sulfate). It has the same chemical composition
as that of the apoprotein, including the amount of covalently bound
fatty acids (see below). Treatment of the residue with CM HCl fails
to extract any of the bound fatty acids. Hence, it appears that exposure to alkali may render the apoprotein completely insoluble without any release of its bound fatty acids.

Although no systematic study has been made of the influence of
salts on the solubility of the apoprotein in water, it has been observed that the apoprotein is precipitated out of solution by NaCl
at about 0.27 M concentration. The precipitation is reversible, and
upon elimination of NaCl, or lowering of its concentration, the apoprotein goes back into solution.

Physical Properties of the Apoprotein

Apoprotein in aqueous solution exhibits one main peak and a much
smaller second peak, both in the ultracentrifuge and by moving boundary
electrophoresis at both pH 7.0 and 5.0. In both analyses, the main
peak accounts for 90 percent or more of the material in solution
(Folch-Pi and Stoffyn, 1972).

Under various conditions of polyacrylamide gel electrophoresis,
several authors have reported single bands for proteolipid apoprotein,
using either isolated myelin (Gonzalez-Sastre, 1970), partly purified
proteolipids (Thorun and Mehl, 1968), or apoprotein preparations
(Braun and Radin, 1969). In our experience, gel electrophoresis has

given far from satisfactory results. Penetration of the apoprotein
in the gel was only obtained originally by using gel concentrations
below 5 percent or by increasing cross-linking. Better penetration
has been obtained later by using phenol-formic acid, water and SDS,
but the extent of the penetration does not permit drawing any final
conclusions as to the physical homogeneity or heterogeneity of the
preparation.

In summary, although from past physical evidence proteolipid
apoprotein has been judged by many to be homogeneous, we have recently
concluded tentatively that the evidence available does not permit
any statement beyond saying that proteolipid apoprotein shows a high
tendency to aggregate, and that more work is necessary, especially
with gel electrophoresis, before the question of its homogeneity or
heterogeneity is settled.

The apoprotein shows an absorption peak at 278 nm. Its $E_{1\%}^{1cm}$
at 278 nm is 13.6. This is lower than the values reported in other
studies (Tanenbaum and Folch-Pi, 1966). The higher values may reflect contamination and, in some cases, the lack of correction for
turbidity.

Relationship Between the Solubilities of the Proteolipid Apoprotein and its Conformation

The apoprotein occurs in two different forms, a lipophilic form
soluble in organic solvents, and a hydrophilic form soluble in aqueous
media. It can pass from one form to the other reversibly under the
proper conditions of operation. To pass from the lipophilic to the
hydrophilic form, it is necessary to follow the procedure described
under "Preparation of water-soluble apoprotein". The reverse passage
is much easier, and the apoprotein dried from aqueous solutions can
be dissolved directly into CM, although the addition of a small
amount of water may be necessary.

It is not known what exact changes occur with these reversible
changes in solubility, but it is fair to assume that, in the lipophilic apoprotein, the lipophilic groups predominate at the surface
of the molecule, whereas in the hydrophilic apoprotein, it is the
hydrophilic groups that predominate at the molecular surface. Optical
rotatory dispersion and circular dichroism measurements on solutions
of apoprotein in different solvents (see Table IV) (Folch-Pi and
Stoffyn, 1972) bear out that conformational changes occur, without
defining their nature. Zand (1968) reported originally that proteolipid was characterized by a high content of α-helix, whereas the
"water-soluble" protein of Tenenbaum and Folch-Pi (1966) showed no
measurable α-helix. Sherman and Folch-Pi (1970) confirmed Zand's observations on proteolipids and extended them to show that the α-helix
content did not change in the course of the gradual delipidation of

the proteolipid to the apoprotein stage. They found, however, that
in sharp contrast with the absence of measurable α-helix of the
"water-soluble" apoprotein of Tenenbaum and Folch-Pi, the present
apoprotein retained about one-half of the α-helix content of the CM
soluble apoprotein, and that this change in conformation was reversible. Upon being placed back into solution in CM, the apoprotein
regained its former α-helix content. This change appeared to be repeatedly reversible and a given sample of apoprotein could be changed
back and forth repeatedly from its CM soluble form into its water
soluble form with the corresponding changes in α-helix content.

Sherman and Folch-Pi (1970) found that the reversibility of this
change in conformation can only be preserved if exposure to water-
methanol mixtures, or to pure methanol, is kept to a minimum. Apparently methanol changes the conformation of the apoprotein irrever-
sibly. The result is an apoprotein with a reduced α-helix content
which is soluble in methanol and which, if it goes into solution
into CM at all, will do so without regaining its former α-helix content. In water, this apoprotein will form only very dilute solutions
which gradually yield a precipitate which is insoluble in all the
solvents that have been used. Presumably, it is this effect of methanol that is responsible for the instability and the low α-helix
content of the water soluble apoprotein of Tenenbaum and Folch-Pi.

The contrast between the stability of solutions of apoprotein in
organic solvents and in water, and the ease with which the apoprotein
can be obtained as an almost universally insoluble residue (short of
chemical breakdown) by such simple means as drying from biphasic solutions, exposing to low alkaline pH's in presence of ions or exposure to methanol, suggests that the apoprotein is apt to undergo
a number of changes in conformation, some reversible and some irreversible. None of these changes appears to change the chemical composition of the apoprotein.

Chemical Composition of the Proteolipid Apoprotein

The apoprotein does not show any spots on thin-layer chromatography for lipids even when samples as large as 5 to 10 mg are taken.
It contains traces of P (0.01 to 0.04%), and of carbohydrate (<0.1%
as galactose). Its P is released by treatment with 0.1 N NaOH at
room temperature for 16 hrs as water soluble organic P, i.e., it is
not phosphoprotein P; the water solution shows no absorption at 260nm,
which indicates that the P is not a nucleic acid derivative. As discussed below, this P most likely represents traces of phospholipids.
The carbohydrate present is mainly galactose, and most likely corresponds to residual sulfatides and cerebrosides. In summary, the
apoprotein is neither a phosphoprotein, a glycoprotein, nor a nucleo-
protein.

The most striking feature of the chemistry of the apoprotein is
the presence of from 2.0 to 3.2 percent fatty acids. These fatty
acids (Sherman and Folch-Pi, 1970) show a consistent pattern of about
60 percent palmitic, 25 percent oleic and 10 percent stearic acids
with 5 percent other acids (Table II). Stoffyn and Folch-Pi (1971)
have established conclusively that these fatty acids are esterified
since they do not react with diazomethane and they react with Na
borohydride, with production of the corresponding alcohols.

These fatty acid residues do not belong to any recognizable lipid.
An exhaustive analysis of the apoprotein for possible lipid moieties,
with which these fatty acids might be bound, shows that the amounts
of P, ethanolamine, choline, sphingosine, inositol, galactose and other
sugars, sialic acid, and glycerol present in the apoprotein are individually and jointly unable to account for from less than one-tenth
to no more than one-fourth, of the fatty acids present. In summary,
it is necessary to conclude that these fatty acids esterified in the
apoprotein, must be esterified on the polypeptide chain itself, except for the remote possibility that they are constituents of an as
yet unidentified lipid. Such a hypothetical lipid would be singularly
devoid of the most common moieties of lipids known at the present time.

The apoprotein exhibits an amino acid composition indistinguishable from that of the crude, and of the partly purified proteolipids.

The apoprotein preserves intact the resistance to most proteolytic enzymes, that is characteristic of the proteolipids. On the
basis of the least abundant residue being 2 methionines per mole of
protein, the apoprotein appears to have 125 residues, giving a possible molecular weight of about 12,000 daltons.

The apoprotein dried to constant weight, in high vacuum, in
presence of NaOH, gives aqueous solutions with pH's around 3.5.
Apparently by the method described, the apoprotein is obtained as
a fully, or almost fully, protonated anion. Titration of two different apoprotein preparations between pH 3.5 and 7.17 requires one
μmole of NaOH for each 3.58 mg of apoprotein. Braun and Radin (1969)
report the use of one μmole of HCl for each 2 mg of apoprotein between pH's 6.0 and 3.0. Although the two sets of values are not
strictly comparable, it is obvious that the apoprotein of Braun
and Radin exhibited a larger number of titratable acid groups than
do our preparations. A possible explanation for this discrepancy is
that the procedure followed by Braun and Radin involved a much more
prolonged exposure to acid than our own procedure, with the result
that some glutamine residues may have been deaminated to glutamic
acid.

TABLE II

FATTY ACIDS COMBINED IN PROTEOLIPID APOPROTEIN (PLA)

PLA Preparation[a]	Total Fatty Acids as % of Weight of PLA	Composition of Fatty Acid Mixture as % of Values in Column (a)						P in PLA
	(a)	14:0	16:0	16:1	18:0	18:1	20:0	%
White Matter PLA								
69-XVII	2.0	--	56.0	--	9.7	27.0	n.d.[c]	0.01-0.04
69-XIX	3.2	--	62.0	--	9.1	23.0	n.d.	"
69-XXI	3.2	--	62.0	--	8.6	26.0	n.d.	"
70-III-2	3.0	--	58.5	--	10.6	25.4	n.d.	"
70-XII	2.45	--	60.0	--	9.1	26.0	n.d.	"
Gray Matter PLA								
72-VII	3.88	15.1	49.2	3.1	14.1	18.5	n.d.	0.077
72-VI	3.30	4.4	54.0	5.3	11.1	25.2	n.d.	0.042
Heart PLA[b]								
72-III	0.40							0.033
72-VII	0.52							0.042
Kidney PLA[b]								
72-IV	0.56							0.017
Liver PLA								
72-V	2.45	6.7	26.2	--	37.3	26.6	n.d.	0.015
72-IX	2.17	6.6	32.9	5.9	20.2	24.6	n.d.	--

[a]All these preparations contained about 0.1% carbohydrate, as galactose. As galactolipids, this would account for about 0.15% fatty acids but this is unlikely because of the absence of fatty acids 20:0 or longer.

[b]The amounts of fatty acids present in Heart and in Kidney PLA can readily be attributed to phospholipids, since in a diacylphosphoglyceride, fatty acids amount to 18-fold the concentration of P, on a weight basis.

[c]n.d. = not detectable.

The Question of the Homogeneity of the White Matter
Proteolipid Apoprotein and its Molecular Size(s)

As already stated, under certain conditions of operation, proteolipid protein exhibits a single band on polyacrylamide gels, indicating a physical homogeneity in each particular case. However,
and especially by the use of SDS and various denaturing agents, the
same preparations of PLA will exhibit more than one band, although
usually there is a main band present. In summary, thus the question
of the homogeneity of PLA remains to be proven. In view of the marked
tendency of PLA to aggregate, the physical heterogeneity indicated
by various bands might well represent different degrees of aggrega-
tion of a single monomer. This brings up the problem of the molecular size of PLA. In 1969, Thorun and Mehl, using gel electrophoresis on a polyacrylamide density gradient, obtained a value of 34-
36,000 for the molecular weight of their proteolipid preparation.
In 1971, Eng, using a 10% acrylamide gel and phosphate buffer in
0.1% SDS, reported a molecular weight of 22,000-23,000 for his preparation. This molecular size has also been observed by Waenheldt
and Mandel (1972) and by Agrawal et al. (1972). The latter group
has, of course, shown the presence of a different protein of the
proteolipid type in the range of 20,500.

Speculating on the size of a possible monomer, Folch-Pi in 1959
computed from the amino acid composition of proteolipids a possible
monomeric molecular size of about 12,500, based on two methionines
as the least abundant constituent amino acid. In 1971, Folch-Pi reported that a portion of the proteolipid is dialyzable through cello-
phane membranes, presumably impermeable to molecules above a size
of 12,000. This dialyzable fraction accounts for a greater or smaller fraction according to the relative permeability of the cellulose
membrane used. Paradoxically, the more permeable the membrane, the
smaller the fraction of proteolipid protein that diffuses through it.
In addition, this diffusion of proteolipid protein occurs only at the
very beginning of the dialysis process, and it ceases completely, so
that a second dialysate does not contain any protein. This behavior
suggests that in the original tissue extract, a major or minor fraction of the total proteolipid may be maintained in a diffusable monomeric form of dispersion by a factor or factors. This factor or
factors is changed or eliminated during the dialysis process, and,
with its removal, the proteolipid changes to an aggregate, undialyzable form.

The following recent observations appear to support this sequence of events. A CM extract is submitted to dialysis until diffusion of protein through the membrane ceases. At this moment the
retentate is collected and replaced in the dialysis bag by a fresh
portion of the same CM extract. The diffusion of protein starts
again in a manner comparable to the course observed with the original
portion of extract, i.e., the permeability of the membrane to protein

does not appear to have changed. At the same time, the original
retentate is placed in a fresh dialysis bag, cut from the same roll
as the first one. No diffusion of protein is observed, i.e., the
protein remaining in the retentate after diffusion of protein ceases
to occur, is truly undialyzable. Finally, if a diffusate containing
protein is submitted to dialysis, it is observed that little or none
of the protein proves dialyzable, i.e., the protein that had originally diffused out has become undialyzable.

If, indeed, proteolipid protein possesses a monomer size of
12,500, the values obtained by Eng (1971) and by Thorun and Mehl
(1968) would represent a dimer and a trimer respectively.

In another approach to the problem of molecular size of PLA,
Whikehart and Lees (1973) have determined the amino and carboxyl end
groups of various preparations of central white matter proteolipids.
The results show that bovine PLA exhibits two N-terminal end groups,
glycine and glutamic acid in the approximate molar proportions of
3:1 (Table III). The corresponding C-terminal amino acids are phenylalanine and glycine. The yields obtained are low for the molecular
sizes indicated by polyacrylamide gel electrophoresis. However, the
presence of two N-terminal amino acids and two C-terminal amino acids
indicates heterogeneity.

Study of PLA from central gray matter and from Non-neural Sources

By the same procedure used with central white matter, Folch-Pi
and Sakura (1973) have obtained PLA from central gray matter, heart,
kidney and liver. The study of their chemical and physical properties show interesting differences among the different PLA, within a
framework of common properties. Thus the amino acid compositions
show for all PLA the same abundance of non-polar amino acids and S-
amino acids, and the relative poverty in polar amino acids. However,
non-neural PLA show little or no half-cystine, with a proportionate
increase in methionine. They show less glycine, alanine and tyrosine,
and more aspartic acid, proline, leucine and isoleucine than white
matter PLA. Gray matter PLA shows a composition intermediate between that of white matter and of non-neural tissues. PLA from non-
neural tissues show only aspartic acid as N-terminal, and lysine as
C-terminal amino acids. The most marked chemical difference among
the different PLA is the presence of covalently bound fatty acids
in which matter, gray matter and liver PLA, and their absence from
heart and kidney PLA (Table III). Physically all PLA share the
ability to change conformation reversibly according to the polarity
of the solvent medium (Table IV). In addition, in the course of the
preparation, the CM extracts from the different tissues showed the
same diffusion of protein during the first stage of dialysis in CM,
that had been first observed with central white matter CM extracts.

TABLE III

N-TERMINAL AMINO ACIDS OF PROTEOLIPID APOPROTEIN (PLA)
FROM DIFFERENT BOVINE TISSUES

PLA Sample	N-Terminal Amino Acid Expressed as Nanomoles per mg of Protein		
	Aspartic Acid (or Asparagine)[a]	Glutamic Acid (or Glutamine)[a]	Glycine
70-IX White Matter PLA	trace[b]	5.8	16.8
	trace	6.9	16.5
70-XII White Matter PLA (dialyzable)	trace	6.9	21.2
	trace	6.8	19.0
71-VII Gray Matter PLA[c]	3.2	1.8	8.3
72-III Heart PLA[c]	34.2	n.d.[d]	n.d.
72-IV Kidney PLA[c]	15.8	n.d.	n.d.
72-V Liver PLA[c]	14.5	n.d.	n.d.

[a]The procedure followed does not differentiate between the acids and the corresponding amides.

[b]Trace indicates amounts below 1 nanomole per mg of protein.

[c]Average of two determinations.

[d]n.d. = not detectable.

(From Whikehart and Lees, 1973.)

TABLE IV

CHANGES IN α-HELIX CONTENT OF PROTEOLIPID APOPROTEIN (PLA) FROM DIFFERENT BOVINE TISSUES ACCORDING TO THE POLARITY OF THE SOLVENT MEDIUM. REVERSIBILITY OF SUCH CHANGES

ORD/CD No.	Source of PLA	α-helix Content of PLA		
		In CM 2:1 (original dialysis retentate)[a]	In water (prepared from the retentate)[b]	In CM (by dilution of the aqueous solution)
	White Matter			
108	71-VI-1	67%	22%	69%
116	71-VI-2	67%	41%	–
–		66%	37%	66%
131	Gray Matter	58%	37%	(80%)
129	Heart	68%	26%	60%
130	Kidney	58%	22%	54%
127	Liver	61%	22%	–

[a]From ORD measurements (m') 233 nm

[b]From CD measurements (θ) 208 nm

Finally, in polyacrylamide gels, the various PLA have exhibited single bands or several bands according to the conditions of the operation.

Since the presentation of this symposium, Folch-Pi and Sakura (1973) have shown that the heterogeneity shown on polyacrylamide gels by the different PLA increases with the addition of SDS and of denaturing, and of reducing agents during the electrophoresis. The effect is especially marked with non-neural PLA, which exhibit as many as 10 bands in presence of SDS and 8M urea. The molecular size of these bands ranges from 6000 upwards, with main components at 30,000. Central white matter PLA shows a main band at 24,000, and minor bands at 12,000 and 20,000, the latter presumably corresponding to the protein described by Agrawal et al. (1971). The presence in all PLA of protein bands at 12,000 lends support to the dialyzability of varying proportions of proteolipid protein, and to their change to a polyaggregated state during dialysis.

REFERENCES

Agrawal, H.C., Burton, R.M., Fishman, M.A., Mitchell, R.F., and Prensky, A.L., 1972, Partial characterization of a new myelin protein component, J. Neurochem. 19: 2083.

Amaducci, L., 1962, The distribution of proteolipids in the human nervous system, J. Neurochem. 9: 153.

Autilio, L., 1966, Fractionation of myelin proteins, Fed. Proc. 25: 764.

Autilio, L., Norton, W.T. and Terry, R.D., 1964, The preparation and some properties of purified myelin from the central nervous system, J. Neurochem. 11: 17.

Braun, P.E. and Radin, N.S., 1969, Interaction of lipids with a membrane structural protein from myelin, Biochemistry 8: 4310.

Eng, L.F., 1971, Molecular weights of the major myelin proteins, Fed. Proc. 30: 1248.

Eng, L.F., Chao, F.C., Gerstl, B., Pratt, D. and Tavaststjerna, M.G., 1968, The maturation of human white matter myelin. Fractionation of the myelin membrane proteins, Biochemistry 7: 4455.

Folch, J., 1955, Composition of the brain in relation to maturation, in "Biochemistry of the Developing Nervous System, (Waelsch, ed.), Academic Press, New York.

Folch, J., Ascoli, I., Lees, M., Meath, J.A., and LeBaron, F.N., 1951, Preparation of lipide extracts from brain tissue, J. Biol. Chem. 191: 833.

Folch, J. and Lees, M., 1951, Proteolipids, a new type of tissue lipoproteins. Their isolation from brain, J. Biol. Chem. 191: 807.

Folch, J., Webster, G.R. and Lees, M., 1959, The preparation of proteolipids, Fed. Proc. 18: 228.

Folch-Pi, J. and Stoffyn, P.J., 1972, Proteolipids from membrane systems, Ann. N.Y. Acad. Sci. 195: 86.

Folch-Pi, J., 1959, Études récentes sur la chimie du cerveau et leur rapport avec la structure de la gaine myelinique, Exp. Ann. Biochim. Med. 21: 81.

Folch-Pi, J., 1971, Nature of the dialyzable brain white matter proteolipid, Third Intern. Meet. Intern. Soc. Neurochem., Abstract 239.

Folch-Pi, J., Sakura, J.D., 1973, Proteolipid apoprotein (PA) from bovine non-neural tissues, Fed. Proc. 32: 624.

Gonzalez-Sastre, F., 1970, The protein composition of isolated myelin, J. Neurochem. 17: 1049.

Joel, C.D., Karnovsky, M.L., Ball, E.G. and Cooper, O., 1958, Lipide composition of the succinate and reduced diphosphopyridine nuceotide oxidase system, J. Biol. Chem. 233: 1565.

Laatsch, R.H., 1963, Fractionation of myelin constitutents by a two-phase system, Fed. Proc. 22: 316.

Lapetina, E.G., Soto, E.F. and DeRobertis, E., 1968, Lipids and proteolipids in isolated subcellular membranes of rat brain cortex, J. Neurochem. 15: 437.

Lees, M.B., 1966, Influence of sucrose on the extraction of proteo-lipids from brain and other tissues, J. Neurochem. 13: 1407.

Lees, M.B., 1968, Effect of ion removal on the solubility of rat brain proteins in chloroform-methanol mixtures, J. Neurochem. 15: 153.

Lees, M.B., Leston, J.A. and Marfey, P., 1969, Carboxymethylation of sulphidryl groups in proteolipids, J. Neurochem. 16: 1025.

Lowry, O., Rosebrough, N.J., Farr, A.L. and Randall, R.L., 1951, Protein measurement with the Folin phenol reagent, J. Biol. Chem. 193: 265.

Matsumoto, M., Matsumoto, R. and Folch-Pi, J., 1964, The chromatographic fractionation of brain white matter proteolipids, J. Neurochem. 11: 829.

Messinger, B.F., Lees, M.B. and Burnham, J.D., 1967, Tryptic hydrolysis of brain proteolipid, Biochem. Biophys. Res. Comm. 28: 185.

Mokrasch, L.C., 1967, A rapid purification of proteolipid protein adaptable to large quantities, Life Sci. 6: 1905.

Murakami, M., Sekine, H. and Funahashi, S., 1962, Proteolipid from beef heart muscle. Application of organic dialysis to preparation of proteolipid, J. Biochem. 51: 431.

deRobertis, E., Fiszer, S. and Soto, E.F., 1967, Cholinergic binding capacity of proteolipids from isolated nerve-ending membranes, Science 158: 928.

Sherman, G. and Folch-Pi, J., 1970, Rotatory dispersion and circular dichroism of brain proteolipid protein, J. Neurochem. 17: 597.

Soto, E.F., Pasquini, J.M., Placido, R. and LaTorre, J.L., 1969, Fractionation of lipids and proteolipids from cat grey and white matter by chromatography on an organophilic dextran gel, J. Chromatog. 41: 400.

Stoffyn, P.J. and Folch-Pi, J., 1971, On the type of linkage binding fatty acids present in brain white matter proteolipid apoprotein, Biochem. Biophys. Res. Com. 44: 157.

Tenenbaum, D. and Folch-Pi, J., 1966, The preparation and characterization of water-soluble proteolipid protein from bovine white matter, Biochem. Biophys. Acta. 115: 141.

Thorun, W. and Mehl, E., 1968, Determination of molecular weights of microgram quantities of protein components from biological membranes and other complex mixtures. Gel electrophoresis across linear gradients of acrylamide, Biochim. Biophys. Acta. 160: 132.

Waehneldt, T.V. and Mandel, P., 1972, Isolation of rat brain myelin, monitored by polyacrylamide gel electrophoresis of dodecyl sulfate-extracted proteins, Brain Res. 40: 419.

Webster, G.R. and Folch, J., 1961, Some studies of the properties of proteolipids, Biochim. Biophys. Acta. 49: 399.

Wikehart, D.R. and Lees, M.B., 1973, Amino and carboxyl-terminal amino acids of proteolipids proteins, J. Neurochem. 20: 1303.

Wolfgram, F., 1966, A new proteolipid fraction of the nervous system, J. Neurochem. 13: 461.

Zand, R., 1968, Solution properties and structure of brain proteo-lipids, Biopolymers. 6: 939.

Zill, L.P. and Harmon, E.A., 1961, Chloroplast proteolipid, Biochim. Biophys. Acta. 53: 579.

PROTEIN AND ENZYME CHANGES WITH BRAIN DEVELOPMENT

Elizabeth R. Einstein

Department of Physiology-Anatomy and Institute of

Human Development, University of California, Berkeley,

California

INTRODUCTION AND BACKGROUND

Recent studies have focused on the biochemical changes occurring in the process of myelination, an important measure of brain maturation. Although documented earlier by light and electron-microscopic techniques that the most pronounced alteration to occur during brain development is in the myelin, not until recently were attempts made to relate these findings to biochemical aspects of the myelin (for review, see Davison and Peters, 1970; Mokrasch, 1971; Norton 1972).

Of the two main myelin constituents, proteins and lipids, the latter have been well studied in the normal animal (Smith and Eng, 1965; Smith, 1967, 1969; Cuzner and Davison, 1968; Horrocks, 1968; Dalal and Einstein, 1969; Davison, 1971, 1972; Dalal et al., 1971); and significant data have been accumulated from this research. It has been concluded that those lipids characteristic of myelin are present in low concentration during early stages of brain development; specifically, the concentration of cerebroside and cholesterol is very low before the 10th postnatal day in the rat (Eng and Noble, 1968; Cuzner and Davison, 1968; Dalal et al., 1971) and in the rabbit (Dalal and Einstein, 1969). The pronounced difference between early and mature myelin is in the ratio of cerebrosides to phospholipids. In the case of the rabbit, our values on cerebroside and phospholipid ratio in the immature animal (Dalal and Einstein, 1969) corresponded to those reported by Davison et al. (1966) for the glial-rich fraction of the adult rat brain. If the composition of immature myelin is close to that of the glial membrane, this would support the thesis of

375

Bunge et al., (1962) that myelin is formed by a wrapping process of the oligodendroglial membrane around the nerve fibers, and that of Hirano (1968) that myelin is of oligodendroglial origin; however, according to Mokrasch (1971), no definitive biochemical evidence has yet been presented to prove this hypothesis. The biochemical studies that have been carried out to determine the process of myelinogenesis have been based largely on lipid analysis; but because myelin, like other biological membranes, is formed of lipid and protein complexes, it is of prime importance that the sequential development of myelin proteins also be investigated before drawing final conclusions.

The two proteins which together constitute over 80% of the total myelin proteins are the proteolipids and basic protein(s). The chairman of this session, Dr. Folch-Pi, has discussed the proteolipids in detail; in order to make the report complete on the myelin proteins, a brief account of the properties of the basic protein is included here.

The basic protein has been localized in the myelin by techniques using fluorescent antibodies with the polarizing microscope (Rauch and Raffel, 1964) and by immuno-electronmicroscopy (Herndon et al., 1973). It has been prepared directly from myelin (Laatsch et al., 1962; Autilio et al., 1964). At present myelin is prepared routinely in many laboratories. For reviews on the chemistry of the myelin see Davison and Peters, 1970; Norton, 1971, 1972; and the basic protein see Eylar, 1971; Einstein, 1972.

A unique property of the basic myelin protein is that when injected into experimental animals it induces paralysis with infiltration of lymphocytes into the brain. The resultant neuroallergic disease, called experimental allergic encephalomyelities (EAE) is comparable in certain of its manifestations to multiple sclerosis, and, for this reason, the basic protein has been the object of intensive studies in recent years. The relationship of this protein to human and experimental neurological diseases, however, is not pertinent to our present report and the interested reader is referred to the reviews and conference reports of Kies and Alvord, 1959; Scheinberg et al., 1965; Paterson, 1966; Alvord, 1970; Field et al., 1972; Einstein and Chao, 1970; Einstein, 1972; Adams and Leibowitz, 1971).

Although the mode of preparation for the homogenous basic myelin protein has been worked out as early as 1962 (Einstein et al., 1962) only recently has its correct molecular weight (17000-18000) been determined by sedimentation equilibrium and gel filtration techniques (Eylar and Thompson, 1969; Chao and Einstein, 1969, 1970; Deibler et al., 1970). Optical rotary measurements (ORD) indicate that this protein lacks helical structure and this finding, viewed together with its high intrinsic viscosity, suggests an extended conformation (Eylar and Thompson, 1969; Chao and Einstein, 1970). Its characteristic lack of secondary structure explains its easy degradation by neural acid proteinase (Einstein et al., 1968). The basic myelin protein has 170 amino acid residues (Eylar, 1970) and of these over 25% are basic (Nakao et al., 1966; Eylar and Thompson, 1969).

An important contribution has been made toward elucidating its structure by three groups of investigators (Eylar, 1970; Carnegie, 1971; Shapira et al., 1971) who have determined its complete amino acid sequence.

The basic protein is closely associated with brain maturational processes because in some species which have been studied (human, rabbit, rat, mouse), it progressively increases postnatally but cannot be demonstrated at birth (Einstein and Csejtey, 1966; Gaitonde and Martenson, 1970; Einstein et al., 1970; Morell, 1972). The basic protein appears in the later stages of myelinogenesis, and accordingly the emphasis in this report will be placed on three important stages of postnatal brain development in the rat at 10, 24 and 37 days.

We have extended our investigations on the developmental changes also to the enzyme 2'3'-cyclic nucleotide 3'-phosphohydrolase in the myelin. This particular enzyme was reported to exhibit high activity in the myelin (Kurihara and Tsukada, 1967, 1968). It is of interest that the period of active myelination in the rat brain is also the period recognized as critical in terms of the influence of thyroid hormones (ref. Valcana and Timiras, 1969; Balazs et al., 1969; Geel and Timiras, 1970; Eayrs, 1971).

The myelin protein and enzyme studies presented here summarize changes occurring with normal development and in the thyroid deficient state, and the analytical data will be interpreted in terms of brain development. The results on lipid changes under the same experimental conditions have been reported by Dalal et al., 1971.

The problem of the regulatory role of thyroid hormones during CNS maturation is being presented at this symposium by Drs. Timiras, Valcana and Ford (see this proceedings).

MATERIALS AND METHODS

Animals. Long-Evans female rats born to mothers fed on a low-iodine diet were used. Each group, representing 6-8 animals, were divided into the following experimental groups: normal (not treated) as control; hypothyroid; hypothyroid receiving replacement thyroxine therapy.

Experimental Hypothyroidism. Hypothyroidism was induced at one day of age by administration of 100 μC ^{131}I, according to the method of Goldberg and Chaikoff (1949) as described by Dalal et al. (1971).

Thyroxine Replacement Therapy. One group of hypothyroid rats received daily subcutaneous injections of Na L-thyroxine (Smith, Kline and French Laboratories) as a dose of 10 μg/100 g body weight given in a volume of 0.05 ml from the 6th postnatal day until sacrifice (Valcana and Timiras, 1969).

Preparation of Brain Tissue. Rats were killed by decapitation on the 10th, 24th, and 37th postnatal days. The brain was removed, stripped of grossly-visible blood vessels and blotted free of moisture. The brain was stored at -70°C for myelin preparations and for enzyme determinations.

The Preparation of Myelin. Myelin was prepared according to the methods of Suzuki et al. (1967) and Norton (1971), with the time for centrifugation extended for one hour.

Protein Determination. Total protein of the brain and myelin was determined by the procedure of Lowry et al. (1951), using bovine serum albumin as a standard.

Acrylamide Gel Electrophoresis. Recently, methods have been devised to separate, identify and quantitate proteins on a microscale. The method of Mehl (1968) has been modified and used by us as follows: 2-2.5 mg of lyophilized myelin was dissolved in phenol-formic acid-water (14:3:3) and 10 μl of this applied to the gel pretreated in the following manner: 10% acrylamide gel of 3mm thickness is cut into 10x8 cm slabs and soaked in phenol-formic acid-water (14:3:3) for 48 hours. The protein sample was applied to the gel, and the electrophoresis performed by using a current of 50 Volt (5 V/cm) for 24 hours. The plates were stained with 0.5% amido black dissolved in acetic acid-methanol-water (1:4:5) and the excess dye removed by destaining the plates with 7.5% acetic acid. The pattern was traced in a densitometer at 560 nm and the peaks measured. From the values thus obtained and from the total protein content, the distribution of the various proteins was estimated.

Determination of 2'3'-cyclic Nucleotide 3'-phosphohydrolase. The method is based on hydrolysis of adenosine 2'3'-cyclic phosphate by the enzyme 2'3'-cyclic nucleotide 3'phosphohydrolase resulting in 2'-cyclic phosphate. (Drummond et al., 1962; Drummond et al., 1971; Kurihara and Tsukada, 1967; Olafson et al., 1969). The method (see footnote * for detailed procedure) we used in these studies however represents a combination of the techniques of Kurihara et al. (1969), Zanetta et al. (1972), and G. Gombos (personal communication). One unit of enzyme activity is defined here as producing from adenosine 2'3'-cyclic phosphate one μmole adenosine 2'-cyclic phosphate

per minute. The specific enzyme activity is expressed in units per
mg of protein.

RESULTS AND DISCUSSION

Brain Weight and Myelin Yield. Data obtained on brain weight,
dry matter and total protein are presented in Table I. Brain weights
among experimental animals were quite uniform in each group studied.
Brain weight and percent dry matter increased with age and percent
total protein decreased. Under the same conditions, the total lipids
were found to increase as reported earlier (Dalal et al., 1971).
Generally, the age related pattern observed in the rat corresponded
to that previously reported in the rabbit (Dalal and Einstein, 1969).

In the ultracentrifugal technique of myelin preparation, the
brain tissue is homogenized with subsequent centrifugation for the
purpose of removing the nuclei and mitochondrial fraction (including
the lysomes, synaptosomes and microsomes). Because these fractions
are in great excess in the immature brain in comparison with the
myelin, the loose floating myelin layer which has to be collected
at the interface of 0.32M and 0.85M sucrose is difficult to separate
and, as a consequence, results in low yield, as shown in Table II
(the myelin yields are calculated per fresh brain and as percentage
on dry basis). When our experiments were terminated at 37 days, we
still obtained a low myelin yield. Myelin accumulation in this
species is known to continue as long as 425 days (Davison, 1971).

---

*Assay of 2'3'-cyclic Nucleotide 3'-phosphohydrolase

2 mg tissue homogenized with 3 ml 0.018M phosphate buffer, pH 7.4
Centrifuged at 16,000 RPM for 80 min
Pellet extracted with 0.4 ml of 0.2M Tris HCl, pH 7.5, + 1.4 ml
    1% Na-deoxycholate
0.2 ml of enzyme extract added to the incubation medium of 0.1 ml
    buffer (0.2M Na_2HPO_4 - 0.1M citric acid, pH 6.2, + 0.1 ml
    substrate of 30 mM 2'3'-cyclic AMP) at 37°C
The reaction stopped at 20 min with 0.04 ml glac. acet. acid
Aliquots chromatog. on silica-gel G plate, with methyl acetate +
    isopropanol + 25% ammonia + water (9:6:4:3) (70 min)
Plates dried for 5 min at 100°C
Spots revealed under U.V. light and eluted with 2 ml of 0.01N HCl
    and read at 254 nm against standard of 30 mM adenosine
    2'-phosphate
Unit of enzyme = the amount that produces 1 μmole of adenosine-
    2'-phosphate from adenosine-2'3'-cyclic phosphate/min
Specific activity: units/mg protein/min

TABLE I

CHANGES IN WEIGHT AND TOTAL PROTEIN IN
BRAINS OF RATS DURING DEVELOPMENT

Age	10 days	22-24 days	35-37 days
Average Weight of Brain (g)	0.83 ± 0.06[a]	1.32 ± 0.10	1.50 ± 0.08
Dry Matter % of Total Weight	13.70 ± 0.12	19.25 ± 0.08	20.50 ± 0.10
Total Protein[b]	51.25 ± 0.10	45.72 ± 0.04	41.88 ± 0.06

[a]Values represent mean ± S.E. of 4 samples
[b]Total protein expressed as percent of dry matter

Few data are available in the literature on myelin yield from
immature brain. In comparison with the myelin values reported by
Suzuki et al. (1967) - 4.2 mg - in the 10-day-old rat brain, our
yield was 5.6 mg and at 24 days Suzuki et al. reported a value of
24.0 mg whereas ours was 27.0 mg. Norton (1972) reports that he
obtained from one 15-day-old brain 4 mg myelin, which increases
sixfold during the next 15 days.

Even with the difficulty encountered in obtaining sufficient
myelin from immature brain it is to be noted from our data that
during the period when brain weight increases 1.8 fold, myelin
accumulation is ninefold.

Electrophoresis and Distribution of Myelin Proteins. The electrophoretic pattern of the proteins in the myelin at different ages
is presented in Figure 1. In contrast to the myelin of human, rabbit,
bovine and monkey which has one basic protein, the rat myelin has
two basic proteins as reported by several investigators (Mehl, 1968;
Martenson et al., 1970) as does the mouse (Morell, 1972). (In the
electrophoretic pattern presented here, Figure 1, bovine basic myelin
protein has been used for comparison.)

It is of interest that the same techniques used for preparation
of myelin and for electrophoresis of the myelin proteins from human
brain or from bovine cord result in a comparatively small number of
high molecular weight proteins close to the origin, in contrast to

TABLE II

CHANGES IN YIELD OF MYELIN IN CONTROL (C) AND THYROIDECTOMIZED (T)
RATS DURING POSTNATAL DEVELOPMENT

Age	10 days		22-24 days		35-37 days	
Treatment	C	T	C	T	C	T
mg Dry Myelin/ One Wet Brain	5.70	4.15	26.77	20.20	50.60	32.03
Myelin Yield on Dry Basis (%)	4.96	3.77	10.39	10.31	16.58	14.71

the large number of these proteins in the electrophoretic pattern
of rabbit (Einstein et al., 1970), mouse (Morell et al., 1972) and
rat brains (Mehl and Halaris, 1970) and the present study. The question is whether the disparity arises from technical difficulty (or
problems) involved in preparing myelin from the brain of small animals, that is, whether the multiple bands observed in the electrophoretic pattern represent contamination from other subcellular elements such as microsomes, or are these true myelin constituents.
Using electron microscopic and biochemical procedures for testing the
purity of the myelin preparation, Mehl and Halaris (1970) and Morrell et
al. (1972) concluded that very little contamination was present. Nevertheless a group of proteins close to the origin could be observed.
These protein bands are present in high concentration in myelin from
10-day-olds. At the same age the basic proteins are represented by
slightly fading weak bands, indicating a very low concentration or
absence of these proteins. This segment of the electrophoretic
pattern is similar to that of Agrawal et al. (1970) who describes it
as a myelin like fraction. In our electrophoretic pattern of the two
basic proteins, the faster moving one shows a more pronounced increase at 37 days.

Using the electrophoretic pattern to group the various proteins
into the conventionally named proteolipids, acidic and basic proteins,
presents certain difficulties. One of the proteins classified as
proteolipid has been demonstrated recently to differ in its properties
from the classical proteolipids (Csejtey et al., 1972; Agrawal et al.,
1972). We have divided the myelin protein into conventional groups,
and their distribution is presented in Table III. The total protein
content is low (9.5%) at 10 days of age and increases to 18.4% at
24 days. These results are in substantial agreement with those of

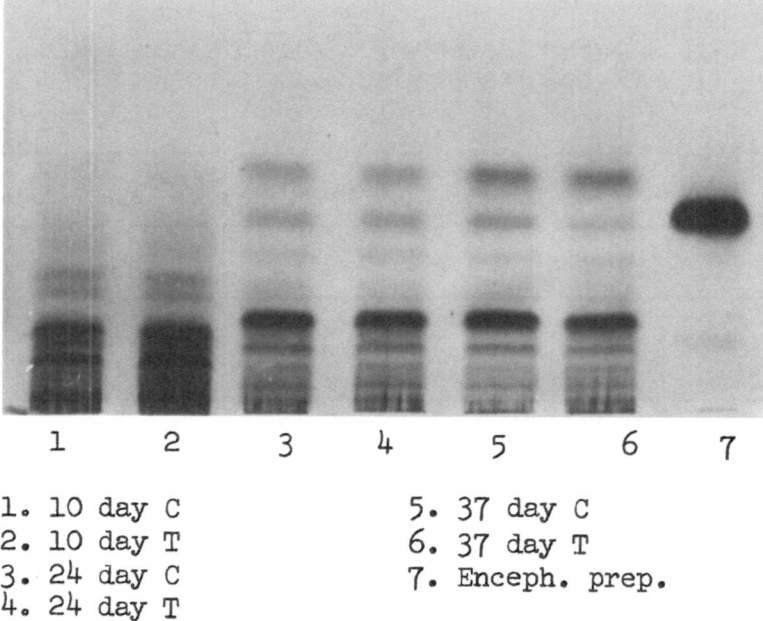

1. 10 day C   5. 37 day C
2. 10 day T   6. 37 day T
3. 24 day C   7. Enceph. prep.
4. 24 day T

Fig. 1. Acrylamide gel electrophoresis of control (C) and thyroidectomized (T) brain myelin in rats at various stages of postnatal development.

Eng and Noble (1968). Quantitative measurements of proteolipids and
basic proteins based on electrophoresis, do indicate a general increase with development as reported also by Morrell et al. (1972) in
the mouse.

The Enzyme 2'3'-cyclic Nucleotide 3'-phosphohydrolase in the
Developing Brain. The results of our determinations on the activity
of the enzyme 2'3'-cyclic nucleotide 3'-phosphohydrolase in the brain
and myelin are presented in Table IV. As noted previously, this
enzyme may serve as a criterion of myelin formation (Kurihara and
Tsukada, 1967, 1968) and therefore may be useful for investigating
the influence of the thyroid hormones on myelination.

The increase in this enzyme in the brain was fivefold between
the 10th and 24th day and an increase in the myelin was sixfold
during this period which is associated in the rat with accelerated
myelinogenesis. The only comparative data in the literature are that
of Zanetta et al. (1972) who reported a fivefold increase in the
brain. The cerebroside level recognized as an index for estimating
the degree of myelination also was found to rise sharply between

TABLE III

CHANGES IN MYELIN PROTEINS IN CONTROL (C) AND THYROIDECTOMIZED (T) RATS DURING POSTNATAL DEVELOPMENT

Age (days)	Total Protein	Acidic Protein	Proteolipid Protein	Minor Protein	Basic Proteins	
					Slow Moving	Fast Moving
10 C	9.53 ± 0.08[a]	3.87 ± 1.60[b] (40)[c]	2.77 ± 1.50 (29)	1.47 ± 0.20 (16)	0.83 ± 0.24 (9)	0.60 ± 0.17 (6)
10 T	8.93 ± 0.14	3.50 ± 0.43 (39)	2.30 ± 1.38 (26)	1.50 ± 0.45 (17)	0.80 ± 0.40 (9)	0.83 ± 0.22 (9)
24 C	18.42 ± 0.06	4.57 ± 0.60 (25)	7.05 ± 1.07 (38)	1.70 ± 0.44 (9)	2.57 ± 0.33 (14)	2.52 ± 0.71 (14)
24 T	17.77 ± 0.10	4.52 ± 0.42 (25)	7.15 ± 0.92 (40)	1.62 ± 0.43 (9)	1.95 ± 0.50 (11)	2.52 ± 0.38 (14)
35 C	20.55 ± 0.05	3.55 ± 0.73 (17)	9.18 ± 0.74 (44)	1.12 ± 0.42 (5)	2.65 ± 0.29 (13)	4.25 ± 0.74 (21)
35 T	18.50 ± 0.12	3.80 ± 0.50 (20)	7.02 ± 0.81 (38)	1.35 ± 0.59 (7)	1.95 ± 0.24 (10)	4.38 ± 0.71 (24)

[a] Values represent mean ± S.E.

[b] Expressed as percent of dry weight

[c] Expressed as percent total protein in parentheses

TABLE IV

CHANGES IN 2',3'-CYCLIC NUCLEOTIDE 3'-PHOSPHOHYDROLASE ACTIVITY
IN BRAIN AND MYELIN OF RATS DURING DEVELOPMENT

Effect of Thyroid Ablation by ^{131}I and Thyroxine

Treatment	10 days Brain	10 days Myelin	24 days Brain	24 days Myelin	37 days Brain	37 days Myelin
Control	0.40[a] ± 0.04	1.87[a] ± 0.08	2.00 ± 0.13	11.55 ± 0.37	2.10 ± 0.15	12.06 ± 0.27
Hypothyroid	0.36 ± 0.04	1.70 ± 0.04	1.70 ± 0.11	9.67 ± 0.27	1.80 ± 0.13	10.60 ± 0.19
Hypothyroid Injected With Thyroxine	0.39 ± 0.03	1.82 ± 0.04	1.80 ± 0.12	11.49 ± 0.25	2.00 ± 0.11	11.91 ± 0.28

[a]Values represent mean ± S.E. of 4 myelin preparations, each made from 1-3 brains; expressed: micromoles/mg protein/min.

the 10th and 24 th day and an increase in the myelin was sixfold during this period which is associated in the rat with accelerated myelinogenesis. The only comparative data in the literature are that of Zanetta et al. (1972) who reported a fivefold increase in the brain. The cerebroside level recognized as an index for estimating the degree of myelination also was found to rise sharply between 10 and 20 days. We used the figures obtained on cerebroside content in this species from a previous study (Dalal et al., 1971) and compared them with the present data on 2'3'-cyclic phosphohydrolase activity (Figure 2). An age related increase in these two compounds is shown.

Influence of the Thyroid Hormone. The results obtained in the thyroid experiments are included in the same tables where the influence on the myelin composition is presented.

Thyroidectomy retards myelin formation (see Table II); at 37 days, 22% reduction was found. A decrease at this age parallels the reduction in cerebroside and cholesterol levels as reported earlier

by Dalal et al. (1971) and Ghittoni and de Raveglia (1972). The influence of the thyroid hormone on several biochemical constituents
of the brain has been reviewed by Balazs (1970, 1971), and Timiras
(1972).

The electrophoretic pattern as illustrated by a representative
pattern (Figure 1) indicates that the slower-moving basic protein is
reduced in hypothyroid conditions in comparison with normal control
at 37 days. A reduction was noted in the slow moving basic protein
23% at 24 days and 26% in the 35-day-old rat myelin. Thyroidectomy
has an effect also on the proteolipids with 24% reduction in the
35-day-old animal (Table III).

The results of our determination on the activity of the enzyme
2'3'-cyclic nucleotide 3'-phosphohydrolase in the brain and myelin
are presented in Table IV. As noted previously, this particular
enzyme serves as criterion of myelin formation (Kurihara and Tsukada,
1967, 1968) and is useful also for investigating the influence of
the thyroid hormones on myelination.

At 24 days the hypothyroid rats showed a significant reduction
in the specific activity of 2'3'-cyclic nucleotide 3'-phosphohydrolase
in the myelin as compared to the corresponding controls. After thyroxine treatment the activity of 2'3'-cyclic nucleotide 3'-phospho-
hydrolase was restored to normal level already at 24 days (Table IV).

While our experiments were in progress, Wysocki and Segal (1972)
published their findings on the influence of the thyroid on this
enzyme in the brain and spinal cord. Our values are comparable to
theirs with respect to control animals. (The enzyme levels determined as activity/mg protein in the brain of the 12-day-old control
in their experimental series was 0.51 and in our series at 10 days,
the value was 0.40. The value for the hypothyroid was 0.35, ours
was 0.36.)

On the other hand, although the values in hypothyroid animals
were similar in the 10-day-old animal, the reduction of this enzyme
in the brain at 23 days was 25% in their study compared to our figure
of 15%. This disparity may be due to a difference in the respective
technique used for inducing hypothyroidism: Wysocki and Segal administered n-propylthiouracil in the drinking water to the mothers
from the 13th day of pregnancy, and subsequently to offspring by
intraperitoneal injection; in our experiment ^{131}I was injected intraperitoneally at one day of age. Despite the difference in the methods used to induce hypothyroidism, it was shown by both groups of
investigators that the enzyme activity could be restored to normal
level by daily injections with thyroxine.

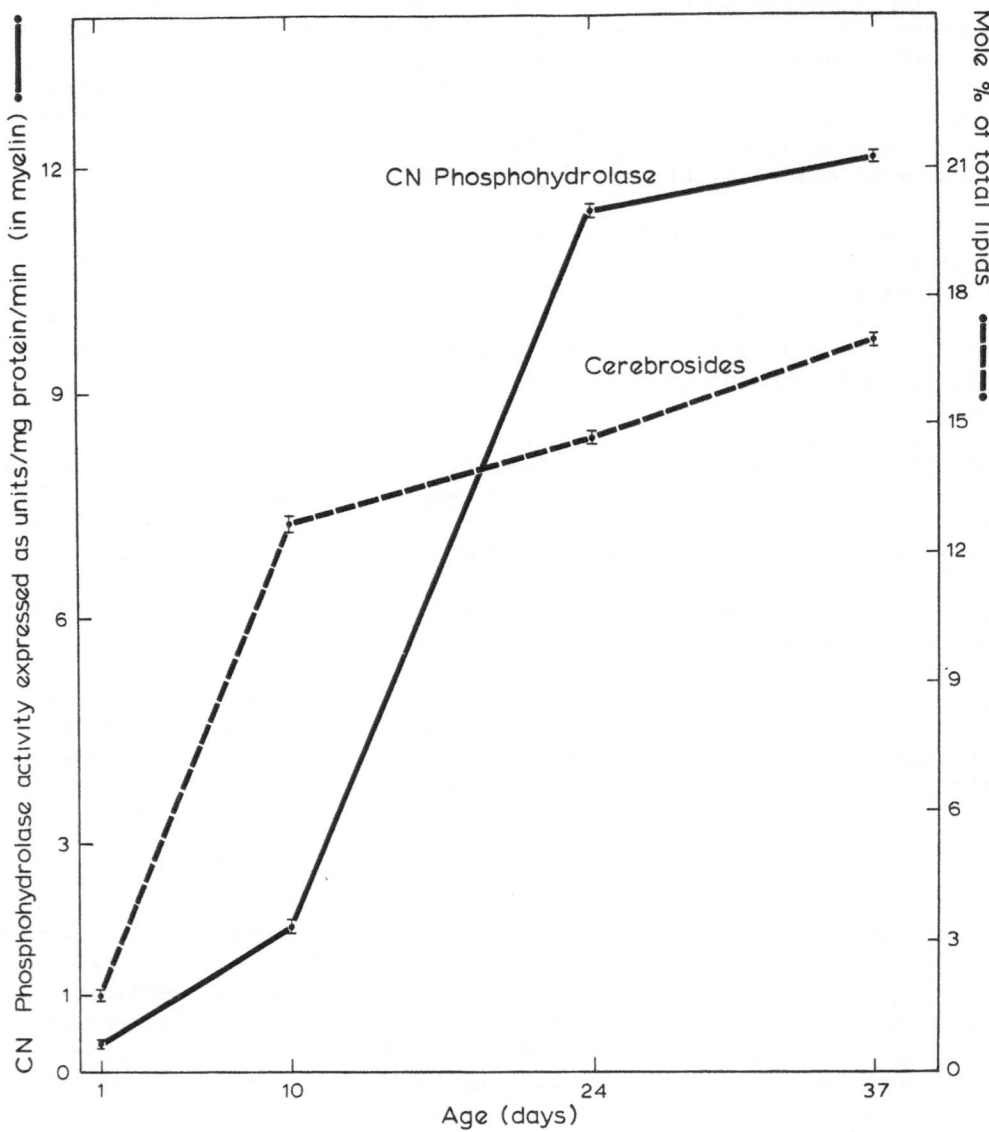

CONCLUDING REMARKS

In our efforts to study myelin formation during development and under conditions of thyroid hormone deprivation and excess, we have conducted systematic studies on the lipids (Dalal et al., 1971), and have now investigated the other major component of the myelin, the proteins. The emphasis in the present study was placed on the basic protein which was described in terms of physicochemical properties and its ability to form a tight bond with acidic lipids such as phosphatidyl inositides, thereby resulting in compact myelin in the mature brain. We also noted that this protein is low in the early stages of brain development, and the myelin changes in consistency. The quantity of the protein increases in parallel with the myelin formation. Since this protein has been demonstrated exclusively in the myelin, it can serve as a marker for the development of the myelin membrane. Furthermore, because thyroid hormones are known to stimulate protein synthesis, it is reasonable to hypothesize that hypothyroidism would have an effect on the myelin proteins and thus on the process of myelination, as demonstrated in this study.

The enzyme, 2'3-cyclic nucleotide 3'-phosphohydrolase, although not exclusive to the myelin, also has been shown to be a sensitive index for myelin formation. A marked reduction of this enzyme was noted in the myelin of hypothyroid animals, in agreement with the work of Tsukada and Nomura (1971) who reported suppression of this enzyme in the cerebrum and that of Wysocki and Segal (1972) in the rat brain. The effects of altered thyroid hormone levels do not necessarily reflect a specific action on this particular enzyme. It is known, for example, that thyroid disease is associated with metabolic disturbances in general (Sokoloff, 1967) and that changes occur in the activity of a number of enzymes (Hoch, 1962). Although the mode of action of this enzyme and its substrate in the nervous system is not known, we can conclude from the present study that the reduction observed in the levels of this enzyme in the hypothyroid brain represent an impairment of myelination.

ACKNOWLEDGMENTS

Some of the work reported here results from the collaborative effort of the author with several members of the laboratory, primarily Dr. K.B. Dalal, Dr. T. Valcana and J. Csejtey, and was supported by NSF Grant #GB-28202.

Fig. 2. Changes in the activity of 2'3'-cyclic phosphohydrolase in myelin expressed as units/mg protein/min and in cerebroside content expressed as mole percent of total lipids in rats during postnatal development.

REFERENCES

Adams, C.W.M. and Leibowitz, S., 1971, "Research on Multiple Scle-
    rosis", Charles C Thomas Publishers, Springfield, p. 182.

Agrawal, H.C., Banik, N.L., Bove, A.H., Davison, A.N., Mitchell,
    R.F. and Spohn, M., 1970, The identity of a myelin-like fraction
    isolated from developing brain, Biochem. J. 120: 635.

Agrawal, H.C., Burton, R.M., Fishman, M.A., Mitchell, R.F. and Pren-
    sky, A.L., 1972, Partial characterization of a new myelin pro-
    tein component, J. Neurochem. 19: 203.

Alvord, E., 1970, Acute disseminated and allergic neuroencephalopaths,
    in: "Multiple Sclerosis and Other Demyelinating Diseases",
    pp. 500-571, American Elsevier Publishing Co., New York.

Autilio, L.H., Norton, W.T. and Terry, R., 1964, The preparation and
    some properties of purified myelin from central nervous system,
    J. Neurochem. 11: 17.

Balazs, R., 1970, Effects of hormones on the biochemical maturation
    of the brain, in: "The Influence of Hormones on the Nervous
    System", Proc. of Int. Soc. Psychoneuroendocrinology, p. 150,
    S. Karger, Basel.

Balazs, R., 1971, Biochemical effects of the thyroid hormone in the
    developing brain, in: "Cellular Aspects of Neural Growth and
    Differentiation", UCLA Forum Medical Sci., No. 14 (D.C. Pease,
    ed.), pp. 273-311, University of California Press, Los Angeles.

Balazs, R., Brooksbank, B.W.L., Davison, A.N., Eayrs, J.R. and
    Wilson, D.A., 1969, The effects of neonatal thyroidectomy on
    myelination in the rat brain, Brain Res. 15: 219.

Bunge, M.B., Bunge, R.P. and Pappas, G.D., 1962, Electron microscopic
    demonstrations of connections between glia and myelin sheaths
    in the developing mammalian central nervous system, J. Cell
    Biol. 12: 448.

Carnegie, P.R., 1971, Properties, structure and possible neuroreceptor
    role of the encephalitogenic protein of human brain, Nature
    229: 25.

Chao, L-P and Einstein, E.R., 1969, Estimation of the molecular
    weight of flexible disordered proteins by exclusion chromato-
    graphy, J. Chromat. 42: 485.

Chao, L-P and Einstein, E.R., 1970, Physical properties of the ence-
    phalitogenic protein: Molecular weight and conformation,
    J. Neurochem. 17: 1121.

Csejtey, J., Hallpike, J.F., Adams, C.W.M. and Bayliss, O.B., 1972, Histochemistry of myelin XIV peripheral nerve myelin proteins electrophoretic and biochemical correlations, J. Neurochem. 19: 1931.

Cuzner, M. and Davison, A.N., 1968, The lipid composition of rat brain myelin and subcellular fractions during development, Biochem. J. 106: 29.

Dalal, K.B. and Einstein, E.R., 1969, Biochemical maturation of the central nervous system. I. Lipid changes, Brain Res. 16: 441.

Dalal, K.B., Valcana, T., Timiras, P.S. and Einstein, E.R., 1971, Regulatory role of thyroxine on myelinogenesis in the developing rat, Neurobiology 1: 211.

Davison, A.N., 1971, Lipids and brain development, in: "Cellular Aspects of Neural Growth and Differentiation", UCLA Forum in Medical Sciences, pp. 365-384, University of California Press, Berkeley.

Davison, A.N., 1972, Biosynthesis of the myelin sheath, in: "Lipids, Malnutrition and the Developing Brain", Ciba Foundation Symposium, pp. 73-83, Elsevier, Amsterdam.

Davison, A.N. and Peters, A., 1970, "Myelination", Charles C Thomas Publisher, Springfield, p. 238.

Davison, A.N., Cuzner, M.L., Banik, N.L. and Oxberry, J., 1966, Myelinogenesis in the rat brain, Nature 212: 1373.

Deibler, G.E., Martenson, R.E. and Kies, M.W., 1970, Gel filtration of proteins at acid pH, application to molecular weight estimation of myelin basic proteins, Biochem. Biophys. Acta 200: 342.

Drummond, G.I., Iyer, N.T. and Keith, J., 1962, Hydrolysis of ribonucleoside 2'3'-cyclic phosphates by diesterase from brain, J. Biol. Chem. 237: 3535.

Drummond, G.I., Eng, D.Y. and McIntosh, C.A., 1971, Ribonucleoside 2'3'-cyclic phosphate diesterase activity and cerebroside levels in vertebrate and invertebrate nerve, Brain Res. 28: 157.

Eayrs, J.T., 1971, Thyroid and developing brain, in: "Hormones in Development", (M. Hamburgh and E.J.W. Barrington, eds.), Appleton-Century-Crofts, New York.

Einstein, E.R., 1972, Basic protein of myelin and its role in experi-
    mental allergic encephalomyelitis and multiple sclerosis, in:
    "Handbook of Neurochemistry", Vol. 7, (A. Lajtha, ed.), pp. 107-
    129, Plenum Press, New York.

Einstein, E.R. and Chao, L-P, 1970, Problems related to the protein-
    eliciting experimental allergic encephalomyelitis, in: "Protein
    Metabolism of the Nervous System", (A. Lajtha, ed.), pp. 643-657,
    Plenum Press, New York.

Einstein, E.R. and Csejtey, J., 1966, Proteins in the developing
    human brain, Trans. Amer. Neurol. Assoc. 91: 212.

Einstein, E.R., Robertson, D.M., DiCaprio, J.M. and Moore, W., 1962,
    The isolation from bovine spinal cord of a homogeneous protein
    with encephalitogenic activity, J. Neurochem. 9: 353.

Einstein, E.R., Csejtey, J. and Marks, N., 1968, Degradation of en-
    cephalitogen by purified brain acid proteinase, FEBSOL 1: 191.

Einstein, E.R., Dalal, K.B. and Csejtey, J., 1970, Biochemical matu-
    ration of the central nervous system. II. Protein and proteo-
    lytic enzyme changes, Brain Res. 18: 35.

Eng, L.F. and Noble, E.P., 1968, Maturation of rat brain myelin,
    Lipids 3: 157.

Eylar, E.H., 1970, Amino acid sequence of the basic protein of the
    myelin membrane, Proc. Nat. Acad. Sciences, USA 68: 1425.

Eylar, E.H., 1971, Encephalitogenic basic protein, in: "Neurosciences
    Res. Prog. Bull." Vol. 9, (L.C. Mokrasch, R.S. Bear and F.O.
    Schmitt, eds.), p. 545, Brookline, Mass.

Eylar, E.H. and Thompson, M., 1969, Allergic encephalomyelitis, the
    physico-chemical properties of the basic protein encephalitogen
    from bovine spinal cord, Arch. Biochem. Biophys. 129: 468.

Field, E.J., Bell, T.M. and Carnegie, P.R., eds., 1972, "Multiple
    Sclerosis: Progress in Research", North-Holland Publishing Co.,
    Amsterdam, p. 273.

Gaitonde, M.K. and Martenson, R.E., 1970, Metabolism of highly basic
    proteins of rat brain during postnatal development, J. Neurochem.
    17: 551.

Geel, S.E. and Timiras, P.S., 1970, The role of hormones in cerebral
    protein metabolism, in: "Protein Metabolism of the Nervous Sys-
    tem", p. 335, Plenum Press, New York.

Ghittoni, N.H. and de Raveglia, I.F., 1972, Influence of neonatal undernutrition on the lipid composition of cerebral cortex and cerebellum of the rat, Neurobiology 2: 41.

Goldberg, R.C. and Chaikoff, I.L., 1949, A simplified procedure for thyroidectomy of the newborn rat without concomitant parathyroidectomy, Endocrinology 45: 64.

Herndon, R.M., Rauch, H.C. and Einstein, E.R., 1973, Immunoelectron microscopic localization of the encephalitogenic basic protein in myelin, J. Immunol. Comm. (in press).

Hirano, A., 1968, A confirmation of the oligodendroglial origin of the myelin in the adult rat, J. Cell Biol. 38: 637.

Hoch, F.L., 1962, Biochemical actions of thyroid hormones, Physiol. Rev. 49: 605.

Horrocks, L.A., 1968, Composition of mouse brain myelin during development, J. Neurochem. 15: 483.

Kies, M.W. and Alvord, E.C., eds., 1959, "Allergic Encephalomyelitis", Charles C Thomas, Springfield.

Kurihara, T. and Tsukada, Y., 1967, The regional and subcellular distribution of 2'3'-cyclic nucleotide 3'-phosphohydrolase in the central nervous system, J. Neurochem. 14: 1167.

Kurihara, T. and Tsukada, Y., 1968, 2'3'-cyclic nucleotide 3'-phosphohydrolase in the developing chick brain and spinal cord, J. Neurochem. 15: 827.

Kurihara, T., Nussbaum, J.L. and Mandel, P., 1969, 2'3'-cyclic nucleotide 3'-phosphohydrolase in the brain of the jimpy mouse, a mutant with deficient myelination, Brain Res. 13: 401.

Laatsch, R.H., Kies, M.W., Gordon, S. and Alvord, E.C., 1962, The encephalomyelitic acitivity of myelin isolated by ultracentrifugation, J. Exp. Med. 115: 777.

Lowry, O.H., Rosebrough, N.J., Farr, A.L. and Randall, R.J., 1951, Protein measurement with the Folin phenol reagent, J. Biol. Chem. 193: 265.

Martenson, R.E., Deibler, G.E. and Kies, M.W., 1970, Myelin basic proteins of the rat central nervous system. Purification, encephalitogenic properties and amino acid compositions, Biochim. Biophys. Acta 200: 353.

Mehl, E., 1968, Electrophoresis of membrane proteins from brain, in: "Macromolecules and the Function of the Neuron", (Z. Lodin and S.P.R. Rose, eds.), p. 22, Wiley Interscience.

Mehl, E. and Halaris, A., 1970, Stoichiometric relation of protein components in cerebral myelin from different species, J. Neurochem. 17: 659.

Mokrasch, L.C., 1971, Biological chemistry and dynamics of myelin, Neurosciences Res. Prog. Bull. 9: 452.

Morell, P., Greenfield, S., Constantino-Ceccarini, E. and Wisniewski, H., 1972, Changes in the protein composition of mouse brain myelin during development, J. Neurochem. 19: 2545.

Nakao, A., Davis, W.J. and Einstein, E.R., 1966, Basic proteins from acidic extract of bovine spinal cord. Isolation and characterization, Biochem. Biophys. Acta 130: 163.

Norton, W.T., 1971, Recent developments in the investigation of purified myelin, in: "Advances in Experimental Medicine and Biology", Bol. 13: Chemistry of Brain Development, (R. Paoletti and A.N. Davison, eds.), pp. 327-337, Plenum Press, New York.

Norton, W.T., 1972, The myelin sheath, in: "The Cellular and Molecular Bases of Neurologic Disease", (S.M. Sky, E.S. Goldenson and S.M. Appel, eds.), Lea and Febiger, Philadelphia.

Olafson, R.W., Drummond, G.T. and Lee, J.F., 1969, Studies on 2'3'-cyclic nucleotide 3'-phosphohydrolase from brain, Can. J. Biochem. 47: 961.

Paterson, P.Y., 1966, Experimental allergic encephalomyelitis and autoimmune disease, Adv. in Immunol. 5: 131.

Rauch, H.C. and Raffel, S., 1964, Immunofluorescent localization of encephalitogenic protein in myelin, J. Immunol. 92: 452.

Scheinberg, L.C., Kies, M.W. and Alvord, E.C. (conference co-chairmen), 1965, Research in demyelinating diseases, Ann. N.Y. Acad. Sci. Vol. 122, pp. 570.

Shapira, R., Chou, F.C.H., McKneally, S., Cerban, E. and Kibler, R.F., 1971, Biological activity and synthesis of an encephalitogenic determinant, Science 173: 736.

Smith, M.E., 1967, Metabolism of myelin lipids, Adv. Lipids Res. 5:241.

Smith, M.E., 1969, An in vitro system for the study of myelin synthesis, J. Neurochem. 16: 83.

Smith, M.E. and Eng, L.F., 1965, The turnover of the lipid components
of myelin, J. Amer. Oil Chem. Soc. 42: 1013.

Sokoloff, L., 1967, Action of thyroid hormones and cerebral development, Am. J. Diseases of Children 114: 498.

Suzuki, K., Poduslo, S.E. and Norton, W.T., 1967, Gangliosides in
the myelin fraction of developing rats, Biochem. Biophys. Acta
144: 375.

Timiras, P.S., 1972, "Developmental Physiology and Aging", The
Macmillan Co., New York, p. 692.

Tsukada, Y. and Nomura, M., 1971, Neurochemical studies on the developing rat brain after neonatal thyroidectomy, in: Third
International Meeting of Soc. for Neurochemistry, Budapest,
p. 194 (abstract).

Valcana, T. and Timiras, P.S., 1969, Effects of hypothyroidism on
ionic metabolism and Na-K activated ATP phosphohydrolase activity
in the developing rat brain, J. Neurochem. 16: 935.

Wysocki, S.J. and Segal, W., 1972, Influence of thyroid hormones on
enzyme activities of myelinating rat central nervous tissues,
Eur. J. Biochem. 28: 183.

Zanetta, J.P., Benda, P., Gombos, G. and Morgan, I.S., 1972, The
presence of 2'3'-cyclic AMP 3'phosphohydrolase in glial cells
in tissue culture, J. Neurochem. 19: 881.

THE MORPHOLOGY OF THE DEVELOPING MYELIN SHEATH

Alan Peters

Department of Anatomy, Boston University School of

Medicine, Boston, Massachusetts

Myelinated axons are present in the peripheral and central nervous systems, and in both, the myelin sheaths have the form of segmented cylindrical tubes. The segments of the sheaths are the internodes and the intervals between them are the nodes of Ranvier.

The earlier electron microscopic studies on the structure and formation of myelin sheaths are considered in reviews such as those presented by Causey (1960), Peters (1968), Elfvin (1968), Bunge (1968), Peters and Vaughn (1970) and Peters, Palay and Webster (1970). In the present article, it is not intended to consider the earlier literature in any detail, but to direct attention to the recent studies on myelin sheath development. However, to put these studies in perspective, a brief account will first be given of the form of mature myelin sheaths.

MATURE MYELIN SHEATHS

In the peripheral nervous system, a myelin sheath is derived from the plasma membrane of the Schwann cell, an individual Schwann cell being responsible for the formation of a single internodal length of myelin. In transverse sections of internodes viewed with the electron microscope, Schwann cell cytoplasm is usually present as complete layers on both the inside of the myelin, adjacent to the axon, and on the outside (Fig. 1). It is in the outer layer of cytoplasm that the elongated nucleus of the Schwann cell is located, generally in a position midway along an internodal length. Sandwiched between the outer and inner cytoplasmic layers is the myelin, which is composed of a series of regularly repeating lamellae that are the turns of a spirally wrapped pair of plasma membranes. The

395

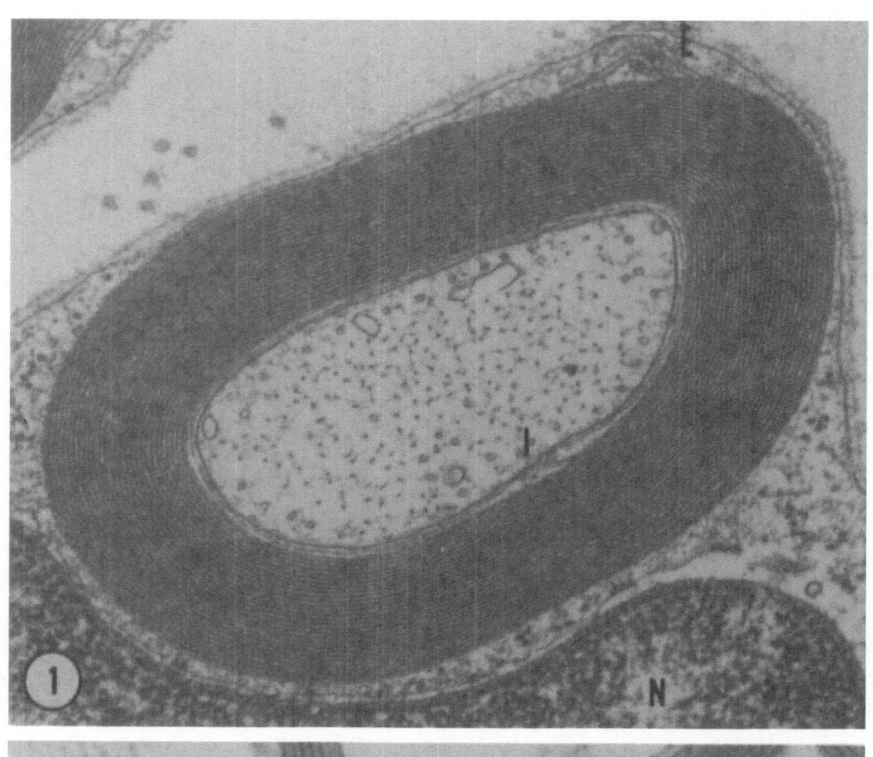

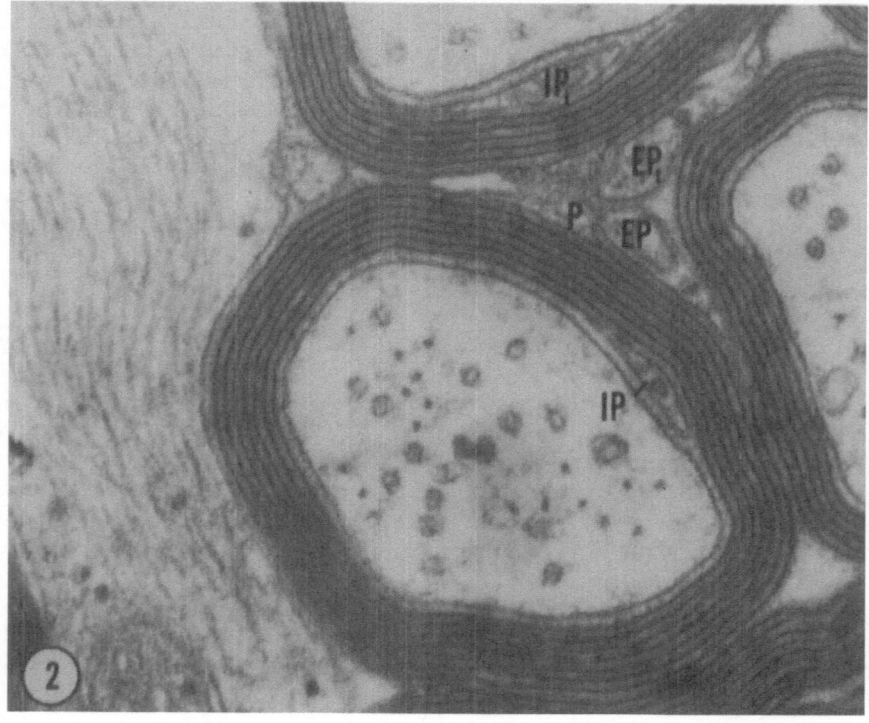

spiral of lamellae terminates on the outer surface of the sheath as
the external mesaxon and at the inner side as the internal mesaxon
(Fig. 1).

At the mesaxons, two areas of the plasma membrane of a Schwann
cell come together so that their outer surfaces are apposed and as
a result of this apposition the intraperiod line of the myelin sheath
is formed. The intraperiod line is evident in most electron micrographs of compact myelin as a relatively dense and thin line. Throughout the width of the sheath, it alternates with the thicker and more
prominent major dense line, which results from apposition of the
cytoplasmic surfaces of the same pair of membranes.

Fundamentally, the electron microscopic appearance of central
myelin sheaths in transverse sections (Fig. 2) is like that of peripheral myelin. Differences exist, however, and the most obvious of
these are perhaps a consequence of the difference in the location of
the perikarya of the myelin forming cells in the two systems. In
the central nervous system, there are no nuclei present in the cytoplasm on the outsides of the myelin sheaths, for the myelin forming
cells, the oligodendrocytes, are situated some distance away from
the sheaths and are attached to them by means of cytoplasmic processes.
While one Schwann cell forms each internodal length in the peripheral
nervous system, in the central nervous system an oligodendrocyte
forms a number of internodal lengths of myelin. Calculations have
shown that in the optic nerve of the rat for example, each oligodendrocyte could form between 20 and 40 separate internodal lengths
(Peters and Proskauer, 1969). In the spinal cord of the cat, the
number seems to be between 18 and 60 (Matthews and Duncan, 1971),
but in the cranial nerves of the cat, only 2 to 3 (McFarland and
Friede, 1971). A process of an oligodendroglial cell is connected
to the cytoplasm on the outside of the myelin lamellae and in the

---

Fig. 1. Transverse section of a myelinated axon from the trigeminal
nerve of a rat. The section is at the level of the Schwann cell
nucleus (N). The spiral of lamellae starts at the internal mesaxon
(I) and ends at the external mesaxon (E). At this magnification only
the major dense line of the myelin is apparent. X 44,000.

Fig. 2. Transverse section of a myelinated axon from rat optic nerve.
Cytoplasm on the inside of the sheath is confined to an internal
tongue process (IP). This sheath is somewhat unusual in that an external mesaxon is present, for the cytoplasm on the outside of the
sheath is contained in an external tongue process (EP) and an adjacent
pocket (P). The external (EP$_1$) and internal (IP$_1$) tongue processes
of an adjacent sheath are also included in the micrograph. Note that
adjacent sheaths come into contact. X 100,000.

majority of sheaths, this cytoplasm does not form a complete cylinder around the myelin, but is confined to a long ridge that extends along the whole internodal length and appears in cross sections of a sheath as a small tongue process. Consequently, except in some instances (Fig. 2) an external mesaxon is not present. A similar situation usually exists on the inside of the central sheath.

An additional difference is that central and peripheral myelin lamellae are not of the same width. X-ray diffraction studies show peripheral lamellae to be 10 per cent thicker than central ones and this same difference exists in electron micrographs. Also as a consequence of the absence of basal laminae on the outsides of central sheaths, the outer surfaces of adjacent sheaths may come into apposition. Then a junction resembling an intraperiod line is formed between the apposed sheaths and a complete sequence of alternating intraperiod and major dense lines extends across the full thickness of two sheaths (Fig. 2).

In both central (Hirano, Zimmerman and Levine, 1966) and peripheral (Revel and Hamilton, 1969; Napolitano and Scallen, 1969; Peterson and Pease, 1972) myelin, it is now apparent that the intraperiod line is not a closed or tight junction as has previously been supposed. Instead it is open to penetration by lanthanum salts and the outer faces of the apposed plasma membranes are separated by an interval of about 20 $\AA$ (Fig. 4). Although the situation is less clear-cut, a recent study by Peterson and Pease (1972) strongly suggests that the major dense line may also contain a gap.

At a node of Ranvier the peripheral (see Robertson, 1959; Elfvin, 1968) and central (see Metuzals, 1965; Peters, 1966; Bunge, 1968) axons are not covered by myelin. The myelin lamellae end in the paranodal region, where the innermost lamella terminates first with the successively more external lamellae overlapping and extending beyond the one lying beneath. Thus, the myelin becomes progressively thinner as the node is approached. As the myelin lamellae terminate, the major dense line opens and accomodates cytoplasm.

Fig. 3. Sciatic nerve from a nine day postnatal rat. In the middle of the field is a group of axons (AA) bounded by a Schwann cell process. Below is an axon (A_1) that is individually enclosed. Note the interdigitating lips of the Schwann cell. At the right is an axon (A_2) around which the enveloping lips have completed one turn. The top axon (A_3) is surrounded by a process that has completed two turns. X 28,000.

Fig. 4. Portion of the myelin sheath from the trigeminal nerve of a mature rat to show the double nature of the intraperiod line (I), which alternates with the major dense line (M). X 250,000.

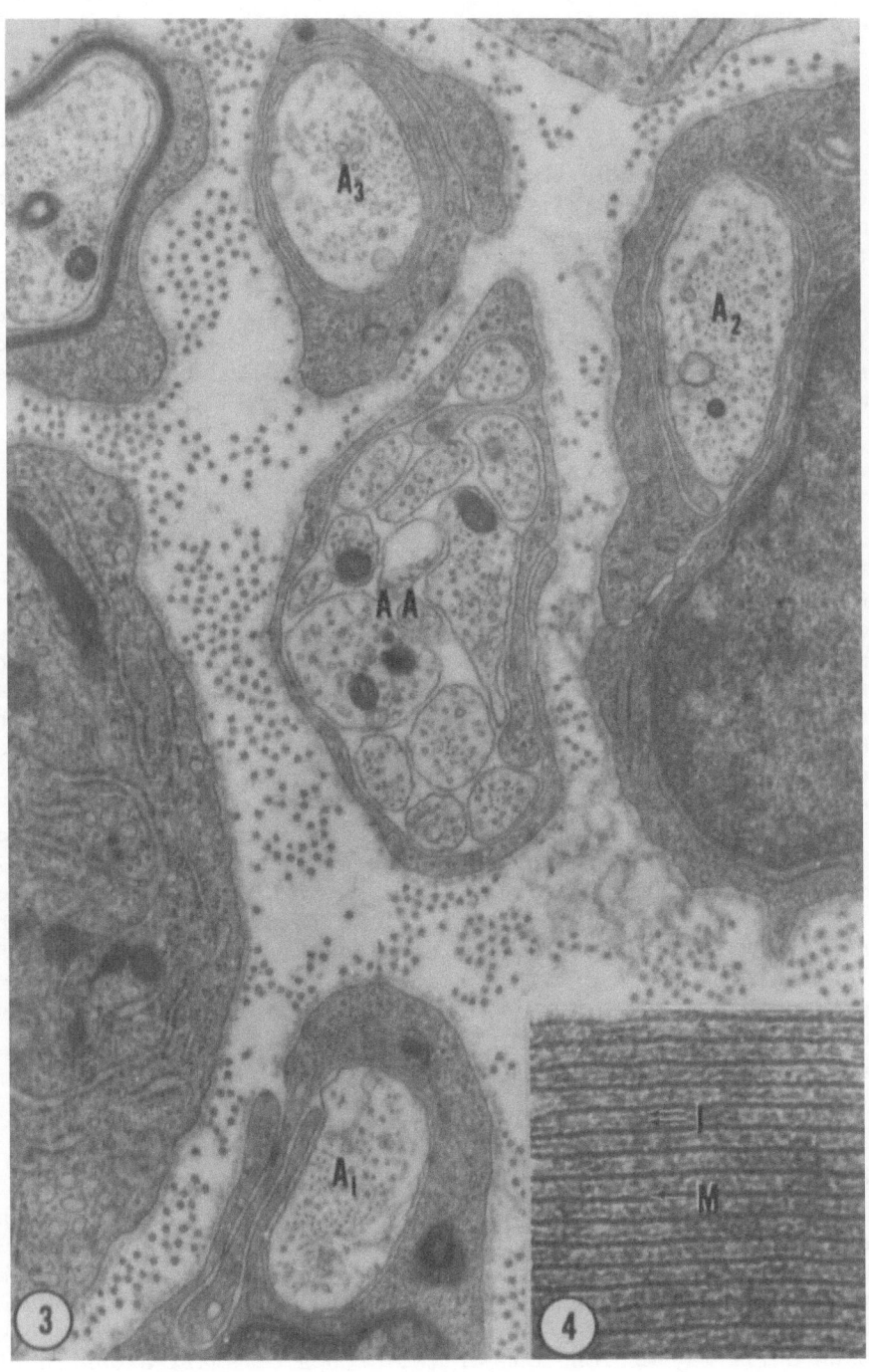

This paranodal cytoplasm, which appears in longitudinal sections as
a series of pockets lying along each side of the axon, has the form
of a helical spiral that is continuous with the cytoplasm on both
the inside and outside of the internodal sheath.

From the above description, it is apparent that if a myelin
sheath could be unwound and pulled out into a flat sheet, it would
have a trapezoidal shape, with cytoplasm contained in a pocket extending along all margins. In the peripheral sheath, the nucleus
of the Schwann cell would lie in the cytoplasm along the longer of
the parallel margins and in the central sheath this same side would
have a process of cytoplasm leading from it and extending to the
perikaryon of an oligodendroglial cell. Additional pockets of cytoplasm extending between the parallel edges would account for the
Schmidt-Lantermann clefts.

THE FORMATION OF PERIPHERAL MYELIN

As shown by Speidel (1964) in the tails of living tadpoles,
peripheral nerve fibers develop in the following manner. A pioneer
axon extends from a neuron and advances by means of an ameoboid
growth cone. Other axons then follow the path of the pioneer and
these are closely followed by Schwann cells that migrate into the
incipient peripheral nerves from the neural crest. At the distal
ends of growing nerves Webster and Billings (1972) have shown that
although Schwann cell processes envelop some axons either partially
or completely, they do not form a sheath around the bundle as a whole.
More proximally, however, where development is more advanced, the
migratory Schwann cells increase their number by mitotic division
and come to form a complete layer around the outside of the entire
bundle of immature nerve fibers, thus separating them from surrounding tissues (see Peters and Vaughn, 1970; Ochoa, 1971). When this
outer layer of Schwann cells has been formed, Schwann cells invade
the central core of axons, which at this stage have diameters of
between only 0.2 and 0.5 μ. In human peripheral nerves this invasion
occurs at about 11 weeks of intrauterine life (Cravioto, 1965;
Gamble, 1966).

The invading Schwann cells then partition off the axons by partially surrounding groups of them with thin processes (Fig. 3; AA).
As Schwann cells continue to proliferate, the numbers of axons in
the encircled groups become fewer and some of the larger axons become individually, although often partially, segregated. Indeed, the
process of maturation within a nerve at this time seems to be devoted
to the individual segregation of each axon, although the exact manner
in which it is achieved is not clear. But during the sequence some
Schwann cells may enclose one or two groups of small axons in addition
to one or two individually separated axons, and the processes of more
than one Schwann cell may contribute to the enclosure of the same

group of axons. At the same time, some individual Schwann cells
are involved with only a single larger diameter axon and since no
axons are free of envelopment, it must be assumed that this one-to-
one relationship is brought about by Schwann cell proliferation.
The acquisition of a length of one axon by a single Schwann cell
seems to be the relationship that must exist before myelination can
take place, since neither axons nor Schwann cells alone are capable
of forming myelin. This process of individual acquisition takes
place along the whole length of a nerve and the result is that an
axon destined to myelinate acquires a string of its own Schwann cells.

   An axon destined to myelinate lies in a furrow or groove that
indents the long axis of a Schwann cell. The furrow then deepens
so that the axon is more completely enveloped and the free edges of
the furrow approximate to form a mesaxon by apposition of the outer
faces of the two areas of the Schwann cell plasma membrane. At this
stage an axon is about 1 μ in diameter (Matthews, 1968; Friede and
Samorajski, 1968; Webster, 1971). Axons below this size do not seem
to myelinate and, indeed, later in development the circumferences of
axons which initiate myelination seem to be somewhat larger (Fraher,
1972).

   The mesaxon elongates next and essentially this elongation proceeds in a spiral manner around the enclosed axon. However, the
spiral formed by a mesaxon may not be simple, but tortuous (Fig. 3)
so that it is looped or turns back upon itself (e.g. see Peters and
Vaughn, 1970; Webster, 1971). In addition, as shown in a recent
three-dimensional study of the process of myelination in the sciatic
nerve of the rat (Webster, 1971), the elongation does not take place
at the same rate along an internode, for at this time the number of
turns is usually greater in the paranuclear region than at the ends
of the Schwann cell where the nodes of Ranvier will form. Webster
has also demonstrated that even the direction taken by the spiral,
that is clockwise or anticlockwise, can vary within the same internode.

   As the mesaxon continues to elongate and more turns of the spiral
are produced, fewer irregularities are observed in the configuration
of the mesaxon (Fig. 3 A_3) and once a few, but varying number of turns
of the mesaxon have been produced, cytoplasm is lost from between
them and compact myelin results. According to Fraher (1972), who examined anterior roots in the rat, compaction takes place when three
or four turns of a mesaxon are present. The loss of cytoplasm may
occur throughout the length of the spiral, but more frequently compact myelin forms initially in only one area of the spiral. Elsewhere,
cytoplasm persists between the turns and, as pointed out by Webster
(1971), it usually persists in the vicinity of the external mesaxon.
In three dimensions, this retained cytoplasm has the form of a series
of long strips that, at the nodal region, are in continuity with the
cytoplasm which always remains in the paranodal helix.

The apposition of the outer surfaces of the Schwann cell plasma membrane in the mesaxon leads to the formation of the intraperiod line, while the later loss of cytoplasm from between the turns of the spiralled mesaxon brings the cytoplasmic surfaces of these same membranes into apposition, so that the major dense line is formed.

As additional turns of myelin are produced, the loss of cytoplasm from between the lamellae is more complete. However, small helical channels persist both in the internodal portions of mature sheaths, where they result in Schmidt-Lantermann clefts or incisures (see Peters and Vaughn, 1970; Webster, 1971) and at the paranodes.

THE FORMATION OF CENTRAL MYELIN

Myelination in the central nervous system is best studied in a tract of axons. Early in development such a tract consists of small axons between which pass thin processes of immature glial cells and the first sign of myelination seen in single transverse sections is that some of the axons, still each somewhat less than 1 μ in diameter, become partially encircled by rather thin processes. These encircling processes are now generally considered to be the ends of the cytoplasmic processes emanating from oligodendroglial cells (see Peters and Vaughn, 1970; Bunge, 1968; Hirano, 1968; Matthews and Duncan, 1971), whose perikarya are located some distance away from the site of myelin formation. It should be pointed out, however, that Blunt, Baldwin and Wendell-Smith (1971) believe that, at least in the kitten optic nerve, the myelin forming cells are astroglioblasts. A thin process then completely encircles an axon, so that the advancing lips of the process come together to form a mesaxon as in peripheral myelin (Fig. 5). In three-dimensional terms, the axon is now lying inside a tube formed by the oligodendroglial cell process. Next the mesaxon elongates so that it begins to form a spiral as one of the advancing lips grows over the other. A recent study by Stempak and Knobler (1972) has shown that at this early phase of myelination, the direction in which the mesaxon elongates, that is clockwise or anticlockwise, can change within the length of the same enveloping process.

Fig. 5. Transverse section of axons from the developing white matter in the cerebral cortex of a 15 day postnatal rat. Most of the axons are still without sheaths. Three axons (A_1, A_2, A_3) are surrounded by glial processes whose lips have just come together to form mesaxons (arrows). Another axon (A_4) is surrounded by 2½ turns of a spiralling process, which has formed compact myelin only beneath the external tongue process (EP). Around two other axons (A_5 and A_6) myelination is more advanced. X 30,000.

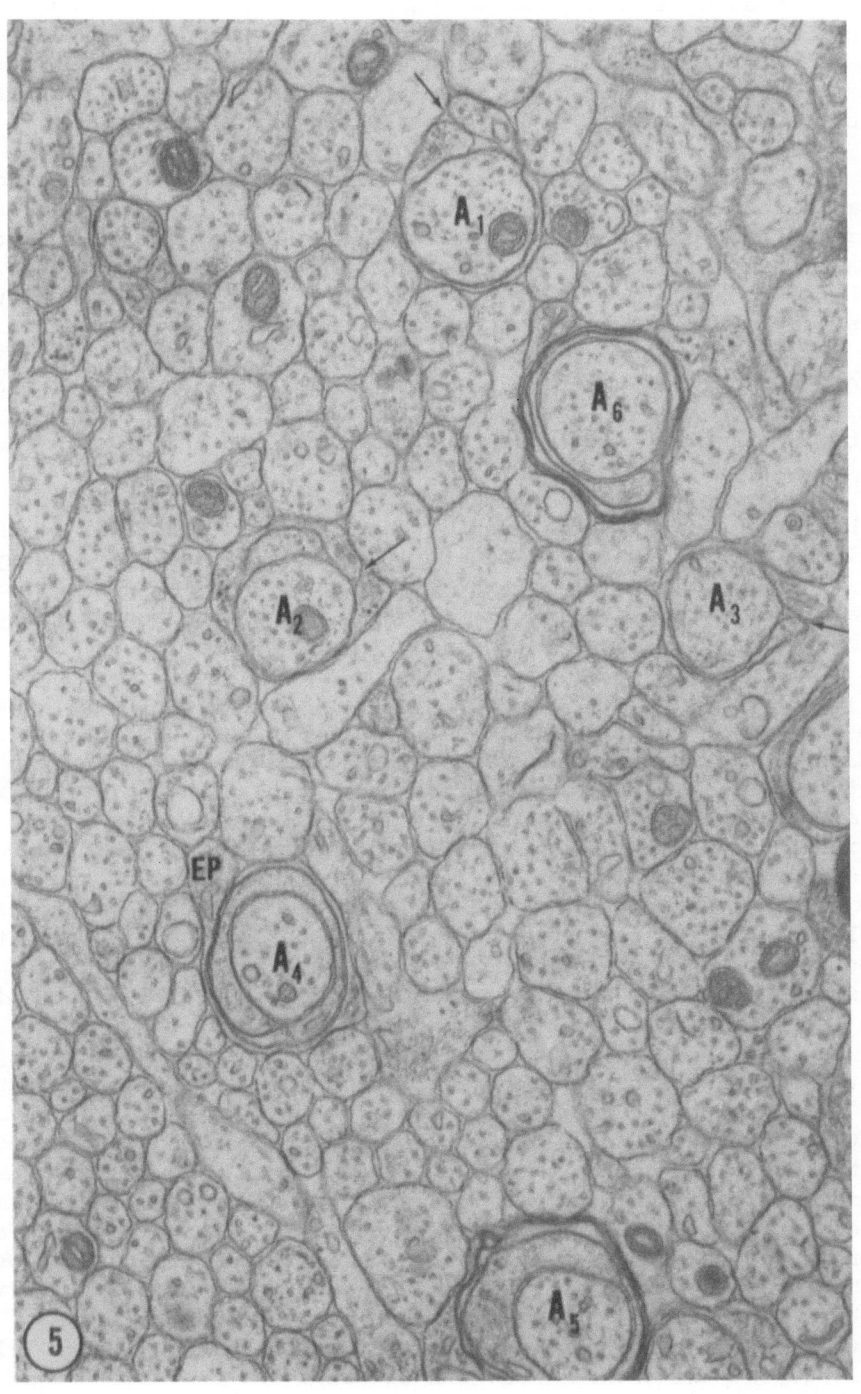

Thus, on each side of a location where the lips of the advancing
process meet to form the initial, short mesaxon, one of the advancing
lips occupies the outside position, while on the other side, they
reverse positions. Thus, the situation at this phase is reminiscent
of that in developing peripheral myelin (Webster, 1971).

Once the spiral of the mesaxon has formed a few turns, cytoplasm is lost from between the turns, so that the cytoplasmic or
inner leaflets of the plasma membrane forming the mesaxon come into
apposition. This results in the formation of the major dense line
and hence, compact myelin (Fig. 5). As in the peripheral nervous
system, myelination does not proceed in a uniform manner within the
same internodal length. Knobler and Stempak (1972) have shown that
along the length of a single axon, the myelinating process may not
completely encircle the axon at one site, whereas some distance away
one or two lamellae of compact myelin have formed.

During the formation of compact myelin, pockets of cytoplasm
may be retained within the spiral, but generally cytoplasm is only
retained to any extent in a single layer on the inside of the myelin
and in a terminal portion of the outer turn, where it forms the external tongue process (Fig. 5). These events have been described by
a number of authors (see Peters and Vaughn, 1970).

Caley (1967) has drawn attention to the fact that central myelin
does not always form in the manner described above and that it is
common for the major dense, rather than the intraperiod line to form
first. Thus, in transverse sections the process initially encircling
the axon may be seen to have a dumb-bell shape, with pockets of cytoplasm retained at the edges, but lost from the middle portion where
the cytoplasmic leaflets of the membrane on each face of the process
come into apposition. The mesaxon may form as the two ends of the
enveloping process meet, but examples can be observed in which the
apposition of the outer leaflets of the membrane to produce the
mesaxon is delayed until the enveloping process has begun to spiral.

As maturation of the central myelin continues, the axon expands
and the number of turns of compact myelin increases. Concomitant
with this growth the amount of cytoplasm both on the inside of the
sheath and in the external tongue process becomes reduced. Frequently, the cytoplasm on the inside no longer forms a complete layer, but
becomes confined to either a localized region on each side of an internal mesaxon, or to only the inner end of the spiral. Then, an
internal tongue process remains, but the internal mesaxon is lost.
It should again be emphasized that although the process of myelination
has been described as it would appear in transverse sections of nerve
fibers, the pockets of cytoplasm extend longitudinally, parallel to
the length of the axon. Thus, the external and internal tongue processes for example, have the form of ridges of cytoplasm that, as in
the peripheral sheath, are continuous with the cytoplasm present in

the helical channels at the paranodes.

THE MECHANISM OF MYELIN FORMATION

As far as peripheral myelin is concerned, it has been generally
supposed that the spiral of lamellae in each internode is produced
by a rotation of the Schwann cell around the enclosed axon. Movements of Schwann cells consistent with this hypothesis have been
observed in tissue cultures (e.g. see Pomerat et al., 1967), but
from observations on nerves growing in the tails of tadpoles, Speidel
(1964) states that he has failed to observe such a rotation. In any
case more than simple rotation of the Schwann cell must be involved,
for while the myelin sheath is growing in thickness, the axon is
increasing in diameter and the lengths of its internodes are increasing. Furthermore, rotation of the myelin-forming cell could almost
certainly not occur in the central nervous system, where each oligodendrocyte forms a number of separate internodal lengths on different axons.

An alternative to the addition of lamellae on the outside of
the sheath is growth at the inner end of the spiral. At first sight
this would appear to lead to constriction of the enclosed axon. But
increase in diameter of the sheath could be effected by slippage of
the lamellae over each other, as has been demonstrated to occur in
experimental edema of central axons (Hirano and Dembitzer, 1967),
and around the proximal portions of peripheral axons induced to swell
by placing a ligature around a nerve (Friede and Miyagishi, 1972).

Data indicating a linear growth in the length of the myelin
spiral has been published by Friede and Samorajski (1968) who studied
the sciatic nerve of the rat. They find a linear relationship between axon circumference and number of lamellae present during growth
and have calculated that the time taken for a complete turn of a
myelin lamella to form is 5 hrs between 4 to 10 days of age, 23 hrs
between 30 and 40 days and over 240 hrs beyond 70 days. In terms of
the average speed of advancement of the outer mesaxon, the maximum
rate occurs between 10 and 20 days. These authors (Samorajski and
Friede, 1968) also find a linear relationship between axon circumference and number of myelin lamellae present in the myelinating
pyramidal tracts of the rat.

In another study of the developing sciatic nerve of the rat,
Webster (1971) has quantified the growth of the Schwann cell membrane
and has arrived at a somewhat different conclusion. He finds that
while the membranes on the inner and outer surfaces of the sheath
grow in a linear fashion, the portion of the membrane involved in
the formation of myelin grows in an exponential manner with respect
to axon diameter. In terms of surface area changes, it seems that
the rate of increase in the area of myelin forming membranes is

proportional to the area already present. On this basis, it would
seem that the growth of the myelin spiral could not take place at
a localized site such as the external or internal mesaxon and that
the myelin membrane grows as a whole. This concept may be related
to the observation that in both central (Peters, 1966) and peripheral (Webster, 1971; Fraher, 1972) myelin, the external and internal
ends of the myelin spiral are not randomly disposed, but are most
frequently located opposite to each other, in the same cross-section-
al quadrant of the sheath. This would not be expected if either of
the two ends of the spiral is the site of myelin formation. In
addition, if growth occurs at one end of the spiral, in the central
nervous system it would have to progress at great speed in those
situations when excess myelin is formed, giving rise to sheaths many
times too large for the enclosed axon (see Peters and Vaughn, 1970)
or to sheaths surrounding oligodendrocytes or neurons (Blinzinger,
Anzil and Müller, 1972).

In experimental attempts to determine how myelin sheaths grow,
a number of authors have studied sheaths in which radioactive materials have been incorporated. For the most part, however, the
resolution of the radioautographs at the electronmicroscope level
is not good enough to provide unequivocal data. Hendelman and Bunge
(1969) have exposed myelinating cultures of peripheral nerves to
tritiated choline and report that the choline is incorporated along
the entire internodal lengths, with no preferential site of initial
incorporation. Hedley-Whyte et al., (1969) have injected labeled
cholesterol into mice and found it to be relatively concentrated
within the myelin, but not at a particular site (see Uzman and Smith,
1971). Hence, these two studies also suggest that the growth of
myelin is not localized at a specific site within the sheath.

Finally, reference should be made to the fact that myelination
may not be an entirely constructive process. Thus, Hildebrand (1971)
has shown that in the developing feline spinal cord, myelination
seems to be accompanied by myelin sheath disintegration, by demye-
lination of short internodes and by degeneration of some oligodendroglial cells.

FACTORS AFFECTING MYELINATION

In mature animals, the effects of a number of substances on the
structure of myelin sheaths have been considered and some of the
changes that can be induced have been recently reviewed by Lampert
(1968), Hirano (1972) and Adams and Liebowitz (1969). Unfortunately,
perhaps because of the difficulties in working with young animals,
few morphological studies of the effects of drugs on the formation
of myelin have been carried out with the exception of the effects
of cholesterol inhibitors and drugs producing hypothyroidism. The
structural effects produced by these substances will be considered

in the following brief discussion along with the changes that can be induced by mutations and by undernourishment.

Cholesterol Inhibitors

One of the major components of myelin is cholesterol. Biochemical studies have shown that certain drugs block cholesterol synthesis, so that the molecular composition of myelin is changed and the process of myelination retarded. The morphological effects of two of these inhibitors, triparanol (1-[p(β-diethylaminoethoxy) phenyl] -1-(p-tolyl)-2-(p-chlorophenyl)ethanol) and AY 9944 (trans-1,4-bis(2-chlorobenzylaminomethyl)cyclohexane dihydrochloride), on the process of myelination in the sciatic nerves of mice have been examined by Rawlins and Uzman (1970a). They find that when these drugs are injected together into either suckling mice or into their mother being fed on a cholesterol free diet, there is a reduction in both the number of lamellae around the myelinating axons and the number of axons being myelinated. Hence, Rawlins and Uzman (1970a) conclude that a decrease in endogenous cholesterol available to suckling mice can affect peripheral myelination by retarding the onset of myelination and by decreasing the rate of myelination already in progress. These cholesterol inhibitors also induce the formation of membranous and crystalline cytoplasmic inclusions in Schwann cells. In another study, these same authors (Rawlins and Uzman, 1970b) have tested the effects of AY 9944 alone, and find that myelination is again inhibited.

Undernutrition

It is well known that undernutrition during the early days of life affects the central nervous system. Thus, rats undernourished from birth have smaller brains (about 80 per cent of the control weight) and brains that contain less cholesterol, proteolipid and cerebroside than well-fed controls. In a study of myelination in rats underfed from birth, Benton et al., (1966) find that Loyez stained preparations show myelination to be retarded in all brain tracts. In another study, Bass, Netsky and Young (1970) find brains of neonatally malnourished animals, examined 40 to 50 days after birth in luxol-fast blue stained preparations, to show poorly stained myelinated fibers. Furthermore, they have discovered that the normal pattern of alignment of neuroglial cells in rows within myelinated tracts is absent, while many "spongioblasts", presumably destined to migrate through the white matter into the cerebral cortex, remain near the ependymal wall of the lateral ventricles. Hence, undernourishment seems to disrupt the normal pattern of development of the oligodendrocytes.

So far as could be determined, no detailed electron microscopic studies have been carried out on the brains of early postnatally undernourished animals, although Hedley-Whyte and Meuser (1971) report the optic nerves of such animals to have less myelin than controls. In a study of the sciatic nerves of undernourished rats Clos and Legrand (1970) find the number of myelin lamellae to be reduced in comparison with the number present around axons with similar diameters in controls and a similar conclusion has been reached by Hedley-Whyte and Meuser (1971). They find that after three days of postnatal deprivation there is no effect on the myelin sheaths in rat sciatic nerves, although the effect is apparent after 5, 8 and 12 days of partial starvation.

The study by Clos and Legrand (1970) also takes into account animals made hypothyroid with propylthiouracil, since experimental thyroidectomy reduces myelination in the rat (see Balazs et al., 1969). In the sciatic nerves, although there are fewer axons myelinated, the number of lamellae around fibers of similar diameter to those in controls seems to be the same, and there is a correlation between the number of lamellae present and the circumference of the enclosed axon. This is different from the situation in undernourished animals, where there is no correlation between these two parameters.

The indications from these studies are that while undernourishment retards and disrupts the normal pattern of myelination, perhaps due to a lack of myelin building blocks, hypothyroidism probably does not disturb myelination by inducing malnutrition.

Mutants

The two mice mutants most carefully studied are "quaking" and "jimpy", both of which have myelin deficiencies. An analysis of brain fatty acids and lipids reveals that they are deficient in cerebrosides and sulfatides and have a low cyclic AMP 3'-phosphohydrolase activity (see Mandel, 1971). Ultrastructural studies of portions of the peripheral and central nervous systems of the quaking mutant (Samorajski, Friede and Reimer, 1970) have shown that compared with nerve fibers of the same caliber from normal mice, only about half the number of lamellae are present in this mutant and that in the brain, more axons are unmyelinated. Similar results have been obtained by Wisniewski and Morell (1971), who point out that myelination appears to be arrested and the assembly of myelin is perhaps impaired because of the unavailability of a structural protein (Costantino-Ceccarini and Morell, 1971). In jimpy on the other hand, electron microscopic studies (Herschkowitz, Vassella and Bischoff, 1971) show almost no myelin in the cerebral cortex at any age when axons of normal mice are myelinated. In the sciatic nerve though, there is apparently no difference from normal mice. Another mutant that appears to have normal peripheral myelin and a deficiency in the CNS, is the msd mutant studied by Meier and MacPike (1970). Hence the indication from jimpy and msd is that myelination in central and peripheral nerves is under separate genetic control.

Another interesting finding is that of Hamburgh and Bornstein (1970) who studied tissue cultures of cerebella from two demyelinating mutants, "dilute lethal" and "wabbler". In these mutants myelin degeneration starts as early as two weeks after birth in vivo (Kelton and Rauch, 1962). In tissue cultures, however, the myelin is maintained normally and although the reason for this is not understood, Hamburgh and Bronstein (1970) interpret the result to mean that the block to myelin synthesis in these two mutants is probably external to the myelin-forming cells themselves.

SUMMARY

Although the form of the mature myelin sheath is quite well understood, it is not known how the spiral of lamellae is formed. However, the present indications are that the membranes grow interstitially by interposition of molecules into the myelin membrane, rather than grow at specific loci. Very little structural information is available about how different factors influence myelin development, but a deficiency in available myelin components, such as is brought about by undernutrition or by inhibition of cholesterol synthesis, inhibits myelin formation. The morphological changes affected by other drugs do not appear to have been studied. Central and peripheral myelin are under separate genetic control, but whether the two systems can be influenced independently in normal animals has not been studied.

ACKNOWLEDGMENTS

The work described in this paper has been supported by U.S. Public Health Service Research Grant NB-07016 from the National Institutes of Neurological Disease and Stroke.

REFERENCES

Adams, C.W.M., and Leibowitz, S., 1969, The general pathology of demyelinating disease, in "Structure and Function of Nervous Tissue", vol. 3 (G.H. Bourne, ed.), p. 309, Academic Press, New York and London.

Balázs, R., Brooksbank, B.W.L., Davison, A.N., Eayrs, J.T., and Wilson, D.A., 1969, The effect of neonatal thyroidectomy on myelination in the rat brain, Brain Res. 15: 219.

Bass. N.H., Netsky, M.G., and Young, E., 1970, Effect of neonatal malnutrition on developing cerebrum. II. Microchemical and histologic study of myelin formation in the rat, Arch. Neurol. 23: 303.

Benton, J.W., Moser, H.W., Dodge, P.R., and Carr. S., 1966, Modification of the schedule of myelination in the rat in early nutritional deprivation, Pediatrics 38: 801.

Blinzinger, K., Anzil, A.P., and Müller, W., 1972, Myelinated nerve cell perikaryon in mouse spinal cord, Z. Zellforsch. 128: 135.

Blunt, M.J., Baldwin, F., and Wendell-Smith, C.P., 1972, Gliogenesis and myelination in kitten optic nerve, Z. Zellforsch. 124: 293.

Bunge, R.P., 1968, Glial cells and the central myelin sheath, Physiol. Rev. 48: 197.

Caley, D.W., 1967, Ultrastructural differences between central and peripheral myelin sheath formation in the rat, Anat. Rec. 157: 223.

Causey, G., 1960, The Cell of Schwann, Livingston, Edinburgh.

Clos, J., and Legrand, J., 1970, Influence de la déficience thyroidienne et de la sous alimentation sur la croissance et la myelinisation des fibres nerveuses du nerf sciatic chez le jeune rat blanc. Étude au microscope electronique, Brain Res. 22: 285.

Constantino-Ceccarini, E., and Morell, P., 1971, Quaking mouse: In vitro studies of brain sphingolipid biosynthesis, Brain Res. 29: 75.

Cravioto, H., 1965, The role of Schwann cells in the development of human peripheral nerves. An electron microscopic study, J. Ultrastruct. Res. 12: 634.

Elfvin, L.G., 1968, The structure and composition of motor, sensory, and autonomic nerves and nerve fibers, in "Structure and Function of Nervous Tissue", vol. 1 (G.H. Bourne, ed.), p. 325, Academic Press, New York and London.

Fraher, J.P., 1972, A quantitative study of anterior root fibres during early myelination, J. Anat. 112: 99.

Friede, R.L., and Miyagishi, T., 1972, Adjustment of the myelin sheath to changes in axon caliber, Anat. Rec. 172: 1.

Friede, R.L., and Samorajski, T., 1968, Myelin formation in the sciatic nerve of the rat. A quantitative electron microscopic, histochemical and radioactive study, J. Neuropath. exp. Neurol. 27: 546.

Gamble, H.J., 1966, Further electron microscope studies of human foetal peripheral nerves, J. Anat. 100: 487.

Hamburgh, M., and Bornstein, M.R., 1970, Myelin synthesis in two demyelinating mutations in mice, Exp. Neurol. 28: 471.

Hedley-Whyte, E.T., and Meuser, C.S., 1971, The effect of under-nutrition on myelination of rat sciatic nerve, Lab. Invest. 24: 156.

Hedley-Whyte, E.T., Rawlins, F.A., Salpeter, M.M., and Uzman, B.G., 1969, Distribution of cholesterol-1,2-H^3 during maturation of mouse peripheral nerve, Lab. Invest. 21: 536.

Hendelman, W.T., and Bunge, R.P., 1969, Radioautographic studies of choline incorporation into peripheral nerve myelin, J. Cell Biol. 40: 190.

Herschkowitz, N., Vassella, F., and Bischoff, A., 1971, Myelin differences in the central and peripheral nervous systems in the "jimpy" mouse, J. Neurochem. 18: 1361.

Hildebrand, C., 1971, Ultrastructural and light-microscopic studies of the developing feline spinal cord white matter. II. Cell death and myelin sheath disintegration in the early postnatal period, Acta. physiol. scand. Suppl. 364: 109.

Hirano, A., 1968, A confirmation of the oligodendroglial origin of myelin in the adult rat, J. Cell Biol. 38: 637.

Hirano, A., 1972, The pathology of the central myelinated axon, in "The Structure and Function of Nervous Tissue", vol. 5 (G.H. Bourne, ed.), p. 73, Academic Press, New York and London.

Hirano, A., and Dembitzer, H.M., 1967, A structural analysis of the myelin sheath in the central nervous system, J. Cell Biol. 34: 555.

Hirano, A., Zimmerman, H.M., and Levine, S., 1966, Myelin in the central nervous system as observed in experimentally induced edema in the rat, J. Cell Biol. 31: 397.

Kelton, D., and Rauch, H., 1962, Myelination and myelin degeneration in the central nervous system of dilute lethal mice, Exp. Neurol. 6: 252.

Knobler, R.l., and Stempak, J.G., 1972, Serial section analysis of myelin development in the central nervous system of the albino rat: An electron microscopical study of early axonal ensheathment, in "Neurobiological Aspects of Maturation and Aging" (D.H. Ford, ed.), Progress in Brain Research, Elsevier Press.

Lampert, P.W., 1968, Fine structural changes of myelin sheaths in the central nervous system, in "Structure and Function of Nervous Tissue", vol. 1 (G.H. Bourne, ed.), p. 187, Academic Press, New York and London.

Mandel, P., 1971, Pathology: Mutants, in "Myelin" (L.C. Morasch, R.S. Bear and F.O. Schmitt, eds.), Neurosciences Res. Prog. Bull. 9: 486.

Matthews, M.A., 1968, An electron microscopic study of the relationship between axon diameter and the initiation of myelin production in the peripheral nervous system, Anat. Rec. 161: 337.

Matthews, M.A., and Duncan, D., 1971, A quantitative study of morphological changes accompanying the initiation and progress of myelin production in the dorsal funiculus of the rat spinal cord, J. comp. Neurol. 142: 1.

McFarland, D.E., and Friede, R.L., 1971, Number of fibres per sheath cell and internodal length in cat cranial nerves, J. Anat. 109: 169.

Meier, H., and MacPike, A.D., 1970, A neurological mutation (msd) of the mouse causing a deficiency of myelin synthesis, Exp. Brain Res. 10: 512.

Metuzals, J., 1965, Ultrastructure of the nodes of Ranvier and their surrounding structures in the central nervous system. Z. Zellforsch. 65: 719.

Napolitano, L.M., and Scallen, T.J., 1969, Observations on the fine structure of peripheral nerve myelin, Anat. Rec. 163: 1.

Ochoa, J., 1971, The sural nerve of the human foetus: Electron microscope observations and counts of axons, J. Anat. 108: 231.

Peters, A., 1966, The node of Ranvier in the central nervous system, Quart. J. exp. Physiol. 51: 229.

Peters, A., 1968, The morphology of axons of the central nervous system, in "Structure and Function of Nervous Tissue", vol. 1 (G.H. Bourne, ed.), p. 142, Academic Press, New York and London.

Peters, A., Palay, S.L., and Webster, H. de F., 1970, The Fine Structure of the Nervous System. The Cells and Their Processes, Harper and Row, New York, Evanston and London.

Peters, A., and Proskauer, C.C., 1969, The ratio between myelin segments and oligodendrocytes in the optic nerve of the adult rat, Anat. Rec. 163: 243.

Peters, A., and Vaughn, J.E., 1970, Morphology and development of they myelin sheath, in "Myelination" (A.N. Davison and A. Peters, eds.), p. 3, Charles C. Thomas, Springfield.

Peterson, R.G., and Pease, D.C., 1972, Myelin embedded in polymerized glutaraldehyde-urea, J. Ultrastruct. Res. 41: 115.

Pomerat, C.M., Hendelman, W.J., Raiborn, C.W., and Massey, J.F., 1967, Dynamic activities of nervous tissue in vitro, in "The Neuron" (H. Hydén, ed.), p. 119, Elsevier Pub. Co., Amsterdam, London, New York.

Rawlins, F.A. and Uzman, B.G., 1970a, Retardation of peripheral nerve myelination in mice treated with inhibitors of cholesterol biosynthesis. A quantitative electron microscopic study, J. Cell Biol. 47: 505.

Rawlins, F.A., and Uzman, B. G., 1970b, Effect of AY-9944. A cholesterol biosynthesis inhibitor, on peripheral nerve myelination, Lab. Invest. 23: 184.

Revel, J.P., and Hamilton, D.W., 1969, The double nature of the intermediate dense line in peripheral nerve myelin, Anat. Rec. 163: 7.

Robertson, J.D., 1959, Preliminary observations on the ultrastructure of nodes of Ranvier, Z. Zellforsch. 50: 553.

Samorajski, T., and Friede, R.L., 1968, A quantitative electron microscopic study of myelination in the pyramidal tract of rat, J. Comp. Neurol. 134: 323.

Samorajski, T., Friede, R.L., and Reimer, P.R., 1970, Hypomyelination in the quaking mouse. A model for the analysis of disturbed myelin formation, J. Neuropath. Exp. Neurol. 29: 507.

Speidel, C.C., 1964, In vitro studies of myelinated nerve fibers, in "International Review of Cytology", vol. 16 (G.H. Bourne and J.F. Danielli, eds.), p. 173, Academic Press, New York and London.

Stempak, J.G., and Knobler, R.L., 1972, Bidirectionality in the tongue processes of the oligodendroglial cell investment of axons in the albino rat, Am. J. Anat. 135: 287.

Uzman, B.G., and Smith, M.E., 1971, Myelin stability and turnover. Chemical aspects, in "Myelin" (L.C. Mokrasch, R.S. Bear and F.O. Schmitt, eds.), Neurosciences Res. Prog. Bull. 9: 477.

Webster, H. de F., 1971, The geometry of peripheral myelin sheaths during their formation and growth in rat sciatic nerves, J. Cell Biol. 48: 348.

Webster, H. de F., and Billings, S.M., 1972, Myelinated nerve fibers in Xenopus tadpoles: In vivo observations and fine structure, J. Neuropath. Exp. Neurol. 31: 102.

Wisniewski, H., and Morell, P., 1971, Quaking mouse: Ultrastructural evidence for arrest of myelinogenesis, Brain Res. 29: 63.

ENVIRONMENT, HORMONES: BRAIN DEVELOPMENT
Paola S. Timiras, Chairman

DEVELOPMENTAL CHANGES IN THE RESPONSIVITY OF THE BRAIN TO ENDOGENOUS

AND EXOGENOUS FACTORS

Paola S. Timiras

University of California, Department of Physiology-

Anatomy, Berkeley, California

Those of us working in the area of CNS development have become increasingly aware that the effects of drugs on this system, and especially on the brain, vary with age, the specific brain structure studied, and the selected neurologic parameter tested. The significance of such variables has been well demonstrated by the presentations delivered at this conference. Equally important in studies of the neurologic effects of drugs is the physiological state of the organism as a whole, and of the brain in particular at the time of drug administration, inasmuch as functional equilibrium is intrinsically related to neurologic competence. This consideration is crucial during development when the requirements for differentiation and growth impose an additional burden on the homeostatic capability of the organism (Timiras, 1972). Consequently, the role of internal factors (for example, the hormonal milieu) and external factors (represented by a variety of stressful environmental conditions) on the developing brain must be carefully evaluated in terms of possible synergisms or antagonisms with the effects of drugs. Additionally, it must be recognized that at no other time during the lifespan can drugs exert such dramatic effects as during development; indeed, the administration of drugs at selected critical periods in brain maturation, whether prenatally, neonatally or at puberty, is capable not only of immediately modifying the functional state of the brain but also of altering the normal timetable of development. In the latter case, irreversible deficits may be incurred that are only manifested at later ages when the respective functions affected reach maturity (Timiras et al., 1968; Vernadakis and Timiras, 1972).

The interrelationships among developmental processes, changes in hormonal state, physiological adjustments and drugs are little understood. Such multifactorial studies depend upon intensive research in each separate area. In this respect, many laboratories have first focused on elucidating the mode of action by which hormones and environmental factors regulate or influence brain development. The two communications presented by Drs. Petropoulos and Ford in this session are representative of these efforts.

The first communication (Petropoulos and Timiras, these proceedings) raises the question of the vulnerability of the fetal brain to environmental factors: for example, despite the protection afforded by the placenta, relatively minor disturbances such as a moderate degree of hypoxia in utero can induce alterations in brain maturation that are reflected in severe functional disturbances during postnatal life (Castillo and Timiras, 1964; Timiras, 1965; Williams et al., 1966; Wing et al., 1967; Woolley and Timiras, 1963, 1965; Woolley et al., 1963, 1966). These observations are significant for they may be extrapolated to the effects of pharmacological agents on the brain; that is, drugs inoffensive to the mother may be capable of inducing irreversible alterations in the developing brain of the fetus, without endangering survival. Data from Dr. Petropoulos' research further emphasize the susceptibility of the developing brain to a lack of oxygen (Atherton and Timiras, 1971; Heim and Timiras, 1964; Petropoulos et al., 1969, 1970, 1972; Timiras, 1963; Timiras and Woolley, 1966), the repercussions of which are often overlooked or minimized in the literature, particularly in studies using gross indices such as survival or body weight, as criteria of viability. Both experimental and clinical evidence clearly underscores the correlation between neurologic and mental disturbances in postnatal life and such unfavorable environmental conditions during fetal life as, for example, hypoxia, malnutrition, and hormonal deficiency or excess - each of which, even when moderate in degree, may not be adequately compensated by the placenta, or, in some cases, may result from placental dysfunction.

The second communication (Ford, these proceedings) is concerned with the distribution and action of thyroid hormones in the brain during the early stages of postnatal development: we know that normal thyroid function is prerequisite to the normal development of the brain and that hypothyroidism at birth leads to serious neurologic deficits which, in humans, culminate in cretinism, an extremely severe degree of mental retardation. Dr. Valcana and Dr. Einstein already have discussed (this proceedings) some of the alterations in electrolyte transport and myelin formation occurring in the brain of the hypothyroid rat. Other studies from our laboratory and elsewhere have demonstrated further that, in the cretinoid rat, protein synthesis (Geel and Timiras, 1970; Geel et al., 1967), selected enzymatic activities (Geel and Timiras, 1967a; Valcana, 1971; Valcana and Timiras, 1969), nucleic acid content and metabolism (Geel and Timiras, 1967b, 1970, 1971; Geel and Valcana, 1972) as well as dendritic and synaptic development (Eayrs, 1971; Legrand, 1971) are impaired and

that each of these parameters can be restored to normal by administration of appropriate doses of thyroxine at a circumscribed period
early in postnatal life.

My own interest in these introductory remarks is to call attention to yet another dimension of the research problem that confronts
us in assessing the effects of drugs on the developing brain; specifically, the necessity of taking into account the complexity of
homeostatic adjustments that occur in the CNS at critical growth
periods so that we may adjust our thinking in terms of the changing
interactions we may expect at any given age. Thus, my primary consideration here will be to select from the literature a few examples
that illustrate how hormonal and environmental factors can be expected to influence drug effects on the developing brain in a number
of ways - by accelerating or delaying the sequential patterns of brain
maturation, by acting competitively on receptor sites, by selectively
affecting specific cell types or cell function and metabolism or by
inducing alterations in blood brain barrier and brain circulation.

First, I would like to note that immediate and long-term effects
of hormonal and environmental factors on the developing brain have
been related to alterations in cell size, number or timetable of development; to changes in metabolism of brain cells; to interference
with the assembly of specific neuronal circuits or the development
of specific receptor sites; or, finally, to a combination of all
these effects. With respect to hormones, two types of action presumably might be involved: one action pleiotypic in nature, regulates
the existing machinery of the cell and is shared by most hormones.
The other type of action, "organizational" in nature, is exerted on
selected macromolecules, generating discrete responses specific for
each hormone (Tompkins and Gelehrter, 1972).

Similarly, external conditions also may act at several functional
levels: for example, insufficient or unbalanced nutrition, decreased
blood supply of oxygen, ionizing radiation, to mention but a few,
result in a wide spectrum of maturational deficits, ranging from
alterations in cell metabolism in the case of malnutrition, to chromosomal aberrations as a result of excessive radiation (Timiras and
Vernadakis, 1968). In addition, the possible interplay of internal
and external factors in brain development and function has raised
such questions as whether the characteristic impairment of myelin
formation in hypothyroid animals should be better attributed to
nutritional or hormonal deficiencies (Balázs et al., 1969; Dalal
et al., 1971; Davison, 1971; Legrand, 1971; Walrarens and Chase, 1969).
Although it is now clear that thyroid hormones per se influence myelin
formation, it cannot be excluded that the pathophysiology of severe
malnutrition, characteristically associated with faulty myelination,
may, in fact, involve hormonal insufficiencies induced by malnutrition.

When the internal and external environment are manipulated experimentally, we frequently find that the timetable of brain development is altered. Such an alteration can have profound repercussions, as perhaps best demonstrated by reference to the well-known organizational action of androgens in determining the sexual differentiation of the hypothalamus: Experiments, particularly in the rat, have shown that, irrespective of genetic sex, the hypothalamus and some areas of the limbic system are essentially feminine at birth, that is, in the absence of androgens, regulation of pituitary gonadotropin secretion and of sexual behavior, as well as patterns of electrical activity, will develop according to a pattern recognized as "feminine" (Flerkó, 1972; Timiras, 1971). Only, if androgens are secreted perinatally by the testis or administered in relatively small doses - whether these doses must be considered physiological or pharmacological remains undecided - the hypothalamus will differentiate in the male pattern of gonadotropin secretion and sexual behavior (Barraclough, 1961). The importance, for our purposes, of this effect of androgens is that it is age-specific: as early as the end of the first postnatal week, even pharmacological doses of androgens remain ineffective in determining hypothalamic differentiation of the male type (Gorski, 1968). If, however, the timetable of brain development is prolonged or accelerated, the period during which androgens are effective can be modified accordingly. The maturation of the rat brain may be delayed by inducing hypothyroidism before and after birth by administration of propylthiouracil to the mother; under these circumstances, the effectiveness of androgens with respect to neural differentiation is prolonged well beyond the first postnatal week; if, on the other hand, brain development is accelerated by thyroxine administration in relatively large doses, the organizing action of androgens is restricted to the first one or two days after birth (Kikuyama et al., 1972).

A second example of ways in which hormones and environmental influences can interact with drugs involves a competition for receptor sites. Evidence of the existence of hormone-binding proteins in various brain areas has been reported by several investigators. For example, it appears that estradiol forms complexes with a cytoplasmatic receptor protein, and this combination, or the translocation of the complex to the nucleus, represents the first step in the hormonal control of gene expression (Mueller, 1971). Indeed, on this basis, the perinatal action of androgens in the differentiation of the hypothalamus has been explained as acting on the estradiol-binding receptor or altering its affinity for estradiol in the hypothalamic estradiol-sensitive neurons, thus reducing the responsiveness of this area to estrogen (Flerkó, 1972). Because of its irreversibility, this action of androgen has been related to alterations in protein synthesis, a view that seems to be confirmed by experiments in which antibiotics were used to inhibit protein synthesis (Gorski and Shryne, 1972). The systemic administration or intrahypothalamic implantation of some, but not all, of a relatively large number of antibiotics prevented hypothalamic androgenization. Pentobarbital also has been shown to suppress the effects of androgen on the neo-natal hypothalamus, although its mechanism of action remains to be determined (Sunderland and Gorski, 1972).

Other evidence of competitive inhibition for receptor sites has been demonstrated with estradiol and several drugs of the phenothia-zine group (Widely used for drug therapy of psychoses) which, because they bear a steric resemblance to estradiol, can also bind strongly to the estradiol receptor and thereby modify its activity (Shani et al., 1971). For example, uptake of tritiated estradiol by the median eminence is significantly reduced when the hormone is injected after administration of perphenazine, whereas its uptake in the cere-bral cortex remains unaffected. (This observation, incidentally, confirms our consistent findings that dose effects of a number of exogenous agents vary depending upon the brain structure and its maturational stage - an important factor to consider in developmental neuropharmacology.) It is attractive to speculate that the psycho-tropic side effects of many steroids may be neutralized by pheno-thiazines via a common receptor. More importantly, the danger that such drugs administered to the mother during gestation might inter-fere with the normal development of the steroid receptors, and thereby prevent the organizational action of these hormones on the brain should be taken into account when we relate these findings to clinical situations.

Other examples are available to illustrate the ways in which changes in specific cell populations or cell function consequent to hormonal or environmental alterations might be implicated in the responses of the developing brain to drugs. Neonatal X-radiation is known to inflict the most severe damage to the cerebellum, and in particular, to the granule cells (Altman et al., 1967). Increased brain excitability also has been observed in animals subjected neo-natally to X-radiation (Vernadakis and Timiras, 1963), and inasmuch as the cerebellum is well known for its inhibitory properties, the altered electroconvulsive activity may reflect the damage incurred by this brain structure.

Experiments from our laboratory have shown that diphenylhydantoin, essentially an anticonvulsant drug, which acts upon both excitatory and inhibitory pathways, but particularly on the latter, when adminis-tered to the neonatally X-radiated animal has a convulsant effect (Valcana et al., 1971). It would seem that in the X-radiated animal, in which the development of inhibitory pathways has been delayed, the drug aggravates the immaturity of inhibition, and further enhances the increased excitation of the X-radiated brain (Vernadakis and Timiras, 1967). As the brain matures, the anticonvulsant effect of the drug is restored.

These observations are not only indicative of the interplay of environmental and pharmacological factors, but will recall the now established fact that the action of many drugs is frequently opposite in the young and in the mature animal. Also in this connection, in vivo and in vitro studies have shown that certain hormones act selectively on the development of glial cells, with consequent repercussions on overall function of the brain. For example, Dr. Vernadakis has suggested earlier in this conference that uptake of norepinephrine by the glial cells, that occurs when this catecholamine is in high concentration, can be decreased by administration of cortisol. The reciprocal relationship between hormones, environment and monoamines is currently a subject of intensive investigation.

The blood-brain barrier, which has been discussed in some detail by Dr. Woodbury (this proceedings) is also affected by hormonal states. Adrenocortical steroids, for example, by modifying the blood-brain barrier may alter the passage of drugs to the brain (Angel and Burkett, 1971; Eisenberg et al., 1970). Similarly, by effecting changes in the extracellular space and in the ionic composition of the brain, hormones can modify the distribution of drugs among the different brain compartments.

I know that you all appreciate the fact that time considerations necessarily confine the depth and scope of conference presentations - and perhaps happily so - I hope that this very brief commentary on certain aspects of developmental neurobiology that seem to me important, both from an experimental and a clinical standpoint, will provide an overview and an introduction for the speakers who follow.

ACKNOWLEDGMENTS

Among the studies cited here, those conducted in my laboratory were supported by NIH NS-08989 and NSF GB-28202 grants and by AEC contract AT (11-1) -34 Project #82.

REFERENCES

Altman, J., Anderson, W.J. and Wright, K.A., 1967, Selective destruction of precursors of microneurons of cerebellar cortex with fractionated low-dose x-rays, Exp. Neurol. 17: 481.

Angel, C. and Burkett, M.L., 1971, Effects of hydrocortisone and cycloheximide on blood-brain barrier function in the rat, Dis. Nerv. Syst. 32: 53.

Atherton, R.W. and Timiras, P.S., 1971, Effects of high altitude on selected biochemical aspects of brain maturation in the chick embryo, Environmental Physiology 1: 5.

Balázs, R., Brooksbank, B.W.L., Davison, A.N., Eayrs, J.T. and Wilson, D.A., 1969, The effect of neonatal thyroidectomy on myelination in the rat brain, Brain Res. 15: 219.

Barraclough, C.A., 1961, Production of anovulatory, sterile rats by single injections of testosterone propionate, Endocrinology 69: 62.

Castillo, L.S. and Timiras, P.S., 1964, Electroconvulsive responses of rats to convulsant and anticonvulsant drugs during high-altitude acclimatization, J. Pharmac. Exp. Ther. 146: 160.

Dalal, K.B., Valcana, T., Timiras, P.S. and Einstein, E.R., 1971, Regulatory role of thyroxine on myelinogenesis in the developing rat, Neurobiology 1: 211.

Davison, A.N., 1971, Lipids and brain development. In: "Cellular Aspects of Neural Growth and Differentiation", (D.C. Pease, ed.), (UCLA Forum in Medical Sciences No. 14), University of California Press, Berkeley, p. 365.

Eayrs, J.T., 1971, Thyroid and developing brain: anatomical and behavioral effects. In: "Hormones in Development", (M. Hamburgh and E.J.W. Barrington, eds.), Appleton-Century-Crofts, New York, p. 345.

Eisenberg, H.M., Barlow, C.F. and Lorenzo, A.V., 1970, Effect of dexamethasone on altered brain vascular permeability, Arch. Neurol. 23: 18.

Flerkó, B., 1972, Steroid hormones and the differentiation of the central nervous system. In: "Current Topics in Experimental Endocrinology", (V.H.T. James and L. Martini, eds.), Vol. 1, Academic Press, New York.

Geel, S.E. and Timiras, P.S., 1967a, Influence of neonatal hypothy-
    roidism and of thyroxine on the acetylcholinesterase activities
    in the developing central nervous system of the rat, Endocrinology
    80: 1069.

Geel, S.E. and Timiras, P.S., 1967b, The influence of neonatal hypo-
    thyroidism and of thyroxine on the ribonucleic acid and deoxy-
    ribonucleic acid concentrations of rat cerebral cortex,
    Brain Res. 4: 135.

Geel, S.E. and Timiras, P.S., 1970, The role of hormones in cerebral
    protein metabolism. In: "Protein Metabolism of the Nervous
    System", (A. Lajtha, ed.), Plenum Press, New York, p. 335.

Geel, S.E. and Timiras, P.S., 1971, The role of the thyroid and growth
    hormones on RNA metabolism in the immature brain. In: "Hormones
    in Development", (M. Hamburgh and E.J.W. Barrington, eds.),
    Appleton-Century-Crofts, New York, p. 391.

Geel, S.E. and Valcana, T., 1971, Cerebral RNA metabolism and thyroid
    function in early life. In: "Influence of Hormones on the
    Nervous System", (D.H. Ford, ed.), S. Karger, Basel, p. 165.

Geel, S.E. and Valcana, T., 1972, Synthesis of free and membrane-
    bound ribosomal RNA from cerebral cortex in hypothyroid rats
    during development, Neurobiology 2: 21.

Geel, S.E., Valcana, T. and Timiras, P.S., 1967, Effect of neonatal
    hypothyroidism and of thyroxine on L-(^{14}C) lysine incorporation
    in protein in vivo and the relationship to ionic levels in the
    developing brain of the rat, Brain Res. 4: 143.

Gorski, R.A., 1968, Influence of age on the response to perinatal
    administration of a low dose of androgen, Endocrinology 82: 1001.

Gorski, R.A. and Shryne, J., 1972, Intracerebral antibiotics and
    androgenization of the neonatal female rat, Neuroendocrinology
    10: 109.

Heim, L.M. and Timiras, P.S., 1964, Brain maturation measured by
    electroshock seizures in rats at high altitude (12,470 ft.,
    3,800 m.), Nature 204: 1157.

Kikuyama, S., Yamanouchi, K., Yanai, R. and Nagasawa, H., 1972,
    Effect of perinatal hypothyroidism on the synthesis and release
    of prolactin and growth hormone. Presented at: U.S.-Japan
    Cooperative Science Program: Seminar on Long-Term Effects of
    Perinatal Hormone Administration, Tokyo, September 18-22, p.11.

Legrand, J., 1971, Comparative effects of thyroid deficiency and undernutrition on maturation of the nervous system and particularly on myelination in the young rat. In: "Hormones in Development", (M. Hamburgh and E.J.W. Barrington, eds.), Appleton-Century-Crofts, New York, p. 381.

Mueller, G.C., 1971, Estrogen action: a study of the influence of steroid hormones on genetic expression. In: "The Biochemistry of Steroid Hormone Action", (R.M.S. Smellie, ed.), Biochemical Society Symposia: No. 32, p. 1.

Petropoulos, E.A., Vernadakis, A. and Timiras, P.S., 1969, Nucleic acid content in developing rat brain after prenatal and/or neonatal exposure to high altitude, Federation Proc. 28: 1001.

Petropoulos, E.A., Vernadakis, A. and Timiras, P.S., 1970, Neurochemical changes in rats subjected neonatally to high altitude and electroshock, Am. J. Physiol. 218: 1351.

Petropoulos, E.A., Dalal, K.B. and Timiras, P.S., 1972, Effects of high altitude on myelinogenesis in brain of the developing rat, Am. J. Physiol. 223: 951.

Shani, J., Givano, Y., Sulman, F.G., Eylath, U. and Eckstein, B., 1971, Competition of phenothiazines with oestradiol receptors in rat brain, Neuroendocrinology 8: 307.

Sunderland, S.D. and Gorski, R.A., 1972, An evaluation of the inhibition of androgenization of the neonatal female rat brain by barbiturate, Neuroendocrinology 10: 94.

Timiras, P.S., 1963, Comparison of growth and development of the rat at high altitude and at sea level. In: "Symposium on the Physiological Effects of High Altitude, Proceedings", (W.H. Weihe, ed.), Pergamon Press, New York, p. 21.

Timiras, P.S., 1965, High-altitude studies. In: "Methods of Animal Experimentation", (W. Gay, ed.), Vol. II, Academic Press, New York, p. 333.

Timiras, P.S., 1971, Estrogens as organizers of CNS function. In: "Influence of Hormones on the Nervous System" (D.H. Ford, ed.), S. Karger, Basel, p. 242.

Timiras, P.S., 1972, "Developmental Physiology and Aging", The Macmillan Co., New York.

Timiras, P.S. and Vernadakis, A., 1968, Brain plasticity: hormones and stress. In: "Endocrine Aspects of Disease Processes", (G. Jasmin, ed.), Warren H. Green, Inc., St. Louis, p. 151.

Timiras, P.S. and Woolley, D.E., 1966, Functional and morphologic
    development of brain and other organs of rats at high altitude,
    Federation Proc. 25: 1312.

Timiras, P.S., Vernadakis, A. and Sherwood, N., 1968, Development
    and plasticity of the nervous system. In: "Biology of Gestation",
    (N.S. Assali, ed.), Vol. II, Academic Press, New York, p. 261.

Tomkins, G.M. and Gelehrter, T.D., 1972, The present status of genetic
    regulation by hormones. In: "Biochemical Actions of Hormones",
    (G. Litwack, ed.), Vol. II, Academic Press, New York, p. 1.

Valcana, T., 1971, Effect of neonatal hypothyroidism on the develop-
    ment of acetylcholinesterase and choline acetyltransferase
    activities in the rat brain. In: "Influence of Hormones on the
    Nervous System", (D.H. Ford, ed.), S. Karger, Basel, p. 174.

Valcana, T. and Timiras, P.S., 1969, Effect of hypothyroidism on ionic
    metabolism and Na-K activated ATP phosphohydrolase activity in
    the developing rat brain, J. Neurochem. 16: 935.

Valcana, T., Vernadakis, A., Meisami, E. and Timiras, P.S., 1971,
    Interrelation between x-radiation and diphenylhydantoin in the
    central nervous system of developing rats, Neuropharmacology
    10: 359.

Vernadakis, A. and Timiras, P.S., 1963, Effects of whole-body
    x-irradiation on electroshock seizure responses in developing
    rats, Am. J. Physiol. 205: 177.

Vernadakis, A. and Timiras, P.S., 1967, Interrelation between con-
    vulsant drugs and x-radiation on the central nervous system of
    rats, Arch. Int. Pharmacodyn. 170: 146.

Vernadakis, A., and Timiras, P.S., 1972, Pathophysiology of nervous
    system disorders. In: "Pathology of Gestation", (N.S. Assali,
    ed.), Vol. III, Academic Press, New York, p. 233.

Walrarens, P. and Chase, H.P., 1969, Influence of thyroid on forma-
    tion of myelin lipids, J. Neurochem. 16: 1477.

Williams, B., Woolley, D.E. and Timiras, P.S., 1966, Synaptic delay
    and conduction time in brain during exposure to simulated high
    altitudes, Nature 211: 889.

Wing, M.E., Woolley, D.E. and Timiras, P.S., 1967, Electrical activity
    of the rhinencephalon during high altitude acclimatization,
    Am. J. Physiol. 212: 135.

Woolley, D.E. and Timiras, P.S., 1963, Changes in brain glycogen
    concentration in rats during high altitude (12,470 ft.) exposure,
    Proc. Soc. Exp. Biol. Med. 114: 571.

Woolley, D.E. and Timiras, P.S., 1965, Prepyriform electrical activity
    in the rat during high altitude exposure, Electroenceph. Clin.
    Neurophysiol. 18: 680.

Woolley, D.E., Herrero, S.M. and Timiras, P.S., 1963, CNS excitability
    changes during altitude acclimatization and deacclimatization
    in rats, Am. J. Physiol. 205: 727.

Woolley, D.E., Barron, B.A. and Timiras, P.S., 1966, Spectral com-
    ponents in prepyriform electrical activity and changes at high
    altitude, Electroenceph. Clin. Neurophysiol. 20: 175.

EFFECTS OF HYPOXIC ENVIRONMENT ON PRENATAL BRAIN DEVELOPMENT:

RECENT EVIDENCE VERSUS EARLIER DOGMA

Evangelos A. Petropoulos and Paola S. Timiras

Department of Physiology-Anatomy and White Mountain

Research Station, University of California, Berkeley,

California

The hypoxic environment of natural high altitude (HA) is both a challenge and a stress to man and to all living organisms. Survival, fitness and reproduction of the species in this environment depend on adaptive adjustments, which are not only species-specific but also age-specific within a given species, and system-specific within individual animals (Petropoulos and Timiras, 1973); that is to say, the rat responds differently from man, the developing animal from the mature and one body system from another (Petropoulos and Timiras, 1973). Studies from this and other laboratories have confirmed that exposure of rats to natural HA during critical periods of CNS organogenesis and development may alter both the structural and functional maturation of the CNS, and that the duration of exposure and the maturational stage of the CNS at the time of such exposure are significant determinants of the extent and severity of impairment (Heim, 1965; Heim and Timiras, 1964; Jilek et al., 1966; Petropoulos and Timiras, 1973; Petropoulos et al., 1969; Petropoulos et al., 1970; Petropoulos et al., 1972a; Timiras and Woolley, 1966).

For both practical and theoretical reasons, the studies noted above dealt with postnatal, but not prenatal, development at HA. The main theoretical rationale for this was the belief, widely held during the past decade, that the fetus, not only is protected in utero, provided the mother is already acclimatized to HA, but also it possesses metabolic advantages, such as ready access to anaerobic glycolysis; consequently - it was theorized - the fetus is not susceptible to the adverse effects of the hypoxic environment. These assertions stemmed, on the one hand, from experimental (Metcalfe et al., 1962a; Metcalfe et al., 1962b) and theoretical (Metcalfe et al., 1967)

evidence that the maternal organism is capable of securing proper
oxygen supply to the fetus at HA, and, on the other hand, from various
experiments showing that newborns (and, by extension, fetuses) can
successfully survive anoxic environments up to one hour without
"apparent damage" (Himwich, 1951; Windle, 1943). Yet, indirect evidence kept accumulating in subsequent years, to suggest that the fetus
was not entirely unaffected by the hypoxic environment at HA (Table I).

The present investigation was undertaken, therefore, to specifically study the effects of natural HA directly on the fetus, and
particularly, on the fetal CNS. We chose natural rather than simulated HA, in order to avoid elimination of the multifactorial influences to which native highlander populations are exposed (Petropoulos and Timiras, 1973) - influences that cannot be reproduced by
decompression chambers.

In view of our previous studies of postnatal CNS development
and function in the rat at HA, extending our research in this species
to the prenatal period, we hope to provide an integrated continuum
of information of rat brain maturation at HA. In this connection,
it is important that we also include data obtained in the newborn
animal, in which any developmental alterations induced by HA may be
most clearly related to changes occurring in utero, and further, may
provide the link between CNS alterations occurring prenatally and
their possible repercussions in postnatal life. Accordingly, consistent with our previous studies on postnatal brain maturation in
the rat at HA, nucleic-acid and protein content and their precursor
incorporation rates, as well as specific myelin lipids were the parameters investigated in the brain of both fetuses and newborns.

MATERIALS AND METHODS

Animals. The mothers of all progeny used in the experiment were
multiparous Long-Evans rats between 120 and 140 days of age. Two
groups of fetuses were studied: fetuses of parents native to sea level
(SL), and fetuses of parents acclimatized to HA; all fetuses were
studied at day 17 and day 21 of gestation. For each of these two
days of gestation, and for each environment (HA and SL), eight mothers
were used (a total of 32). Fetuses were distributed as follows:
52 for day 17 at HA, 53 for day 21 at HA, 61 for day 17 at SL, and
74 for day 21 at SL. The fetuses were obtained by casearean section,
performed under anesthesia. Newborns were divided into three groups:
sea level controls (SLC), males and females conceived and born at SL;
animals exposed perinatally to HA (Group A), males and females born
to mothers mated at SL and transported to the Barcroft Laboratory,
White Mountain Research Station (12,470 ft., 3,800 m.) on day 20 of
gestation, one day prior to normal delivery; first-generation HA
animals (F_1), male and female offspring conceived and born at the
Barcroft Laboratory from parent rats acclimatized to HA. Each group

TABLE I

SUMMARY OF REPORTED EFFECTS OF HIGH ALTITUDE ON FETUSES OF ACCLIMATIZED MOTHERS

FINDINGS	HIGH ALTITUDE	ANIMAL SPECIES	AUTHOR
Increased incidence of fetal resorptions and stillbirths; decreased litter size	simulated natural simulated	mice rats guinea pigs	Baird & Cook, 1962 Kelley & Pace, 1968; Nelson & Srebnik, 1970 Delaquerriere-Richardson and Valdivia, 1967
Decreased body weight at birth	natural	human	Lichty et al., 1957; Grahn & Kratchman, 1963; Baker 1969;Kruger & Arias-Stella,197
Decreased subcutaneous fat in newborns	natural	human	Frisancho, 1970
Decreased glycogen content in the liver at birth	natural	rat	Kelley & Pace, 1968
Increased red and white blood cell counts, heart and spleen weight, at birth	natural	rat	Timiras, 1964; Kelley & Pace, 1968
Increased hemoglobin concentration in fetal blood	natural	sheep	Metcalfe et al., 1967; Chabes et al., 1968; Frisancho, 1970
Increased brain, heart and peripheral muscle capillarity at birth	simulated	dog	Becker & Kreuzer, 1955

(SLC, A and F_1) consisted of ten male and ten female newborns, which were killed within 12 hours from the time of birth for brain sampling.

Brain Samples. After decapitation, the brains from fetuses and newborns were rapidly removed and stripped of grossly-visible blood vessels. The whole fetal brain was weighed and retained at $-70^{\circ}C$ for nucleic acid, protein and precursor-incorporation determinations, or for brain-lipid studies. In the case of newborns, a portion of somatosensory cortex of either cerebral hemisphere (sides were alternated from animal to animal), as well as the hypothalamus and half of the cerebellum (right or left alternately) were immediately removed, weighed and retained frozen for nucleic-acid, protein and precursor-incorporation determinations. The remainder of the brain was immediately stored at $-70^{\circ}C$ for later lipid determination and myelin preparation. The time between decapitation and freeze-storing of the brain was 2 min.

Lipid Determination. Extraction of brain lipids, preparation of myelin, extraction of myelin lipids, and quantitative thin-layer lipid chromatography were performed as described previously (Petropoulos et al., 1972a). Cyclic nucleotide phosphohydrolase activity was determined as described previously (Dalal et al., 1973).

Nucleic acid and Protein Determination. Nucleic acid extraction and analysis, as well as protein analysis were performed as previously described (Petropoulos, 1973).

Placenta Samples. Placentae obtained at the time of caesarean section were freed of fetal membranes, weighed, and frozen for subsequent nucleic acid and protein content determination, as well as precursor incorporation as described previously (Petropoulos, 1973).

Radioactive Precursors. ^{3}H-leucine (L-4, 5-^{3}H-leucine; specific activity 40 c/mmole; Schwartz), ^{3}H-uridine (5-^{3}H-uridine, specific activity 20 c/mmole; Schwartz) and ^{14}C-thymidine (2-^{14}C-thymidine, specific activity 30-50 mc/μmole) were used as precursors for protein, RNA and DNA, respectively, in both brain and placenta. For fetal and placental studies, 50 μc of ^{3}H-leucine, or 50 μc of ^{3}H-uridine and 10 μc ^{14}C-thymidine per animal were injected intravenously (under ether anesthesia) into the maternal external jugular vein; for neonatal studies, 25 μc of ^{3}H-leucine or 25 μc of ^{3}H-uridine and 5 μc ^{14}C-thymidine were injected intraperitoneally in each animal. Fetal brains, placentae, fetal and maternal plasma, as well as neonatal brains and plasma were obtained 15 min and 30 min after the injection of radioactive precursors, and their radioactivity was assessed by standard liquid scintillation counting in a Packard Tri-Carb Model 3310 scintillation counter, equipped with an external radioactive standard for quenching correction purposes.

TABLE II

NEUROCHEMICAL ABERRATIONS IN ONE-DAY-OLD RATS AT HIGH ALTITUDE:
BRAIN AND MYELIN LIPIDS AND ENZYMES

LIPIDS	SEA LEVEL CONTROLS C	HIGH ALTITUDE ANIMALS A	F_1
BRAIN			
Dry Matter	9.47 ± 0.04[a]	9.14 ± 0.07[b]	8.97 ± 0.03[cd]
Cholesterol	2.11 ± 0.04	1.98 ± 0.03[b]	1.62 ± 0.03[cd]
Serine & Inositol Phosphatides	6.37 ± 0.10	5.70 ± 0.04[b]	4.79 ± 0.08[cd]
Uncharacterized Lipids	5.50 ± 0.17	5.83 ± 0.11	6.22 ± 0.08[cd]
PREMYELIN			
Total Phospholipids	61.59 ± 0.16	60.38 ± 0.16[b]	58.18 ± 0.17[cd]
Ethanolamine Glycerophosphatide	14.81 ± 0.18	14.72 ± 0.09	14.31 ± 0.05[cd]
Uncharacterized Lipids	28.95 ± 0.44	30.12 ± 0.13[b]	32.50 ± 0.68[cd]
CN Phospho-hydrolase	0.28 ± 0.03	0.27 ± 0.03	0.24 ± 0.02

A = rats conceived at sea level and taken to high altitude
(12,470 ft.) the day before birth; F_1 = first-generation rats
conceived and born at high altitude from acclimatized parents.

a = Mean ± standard error. Dry matter is expressed as % of wet
weight. The individual lipids are expressed as % of dry
matter for brain, and as moles % of total lipids for myelin.
Cyclic nucleotide phosphohydrolase activity is expressed as
μmoles of 2'-AMP produced/min/mg of myelin protein at 37°C.

Statistically-significant differences at levels ranging from
$P<0.001$ to $P<0.05$ are cited for comparisons between A/C (b),
F_1/C (c) and F_1/A (d).

Other Fetal Parameters. Body weight, heart weight, and hematocrit (blood collected by heart puncture) were also recorded at the
time of autopsy.

Statistical Analysis. To determine whether the means of the
parameters measured in the various groups differed significantly,
the t test for nonpaired data was applied (Fisher, 1950).

RESULTS

Neonatal Changes. As shown in Table II, all lipids determined
in both brain and myelin, with the exception of uncharacterized lipids,
were significantly lower in HA neonates than in their SL counter-
parts; cyclic nucleotide phosphohydrolase activity also tended to be
lower at HA than at SL. Uncharacterized lipids were significantly
increased in both HA groups, an indication of brain dysmaturity
characteristic in adverse environments and/or conditions (Dalal et
al., 1971; Petropoulos et al., 1972a). F_1 rats were more severely
affected than A rats despite the fact that the mothers of A progeny
were not acclimatized to HA and thus presumably less suited than
mothers of F_1 progeny to protect their fetuses from hypoxia. It is
evident that the duration of exposure, and exposure during critical
organogenetic stages are more important factors in modulating the
response of the fetal brain to HA than previous acclimatization of
the mother. Table III indicates that DNA concentrations in the cerebral cortex were significantly decreased in both high altitude groups,
protein was significantly decreased in the A group, whereas RNA concentration was similar between HA and SL newborns; incorporation of
radioactive precursors into nucleic acids and protein was significantly
higher at HA than at SL. In A rats, ^{14}C-thymidine and ^{3}H-leucine
incorporation was higher, but ^{3}H-uridine incorporation was lower than
in F_1 rats.

Fetal Changes. In general, all brain lipids determined (with
the exception of uncharacterized lipids), showed a trend to be lower
in HA than in SL fetuses; this reduction was statistically significant
for total phospholipids, sphingomyelin, inositol and serine phospha-
tides (Table IV). As in newborns, HA fetuses demonstrated an increase
in uncharacterized-lipid content in their brain; in addition, dry
matter was significantly decreased at HA (Table IV). Nucleic acid
and protein concentration in the brain was lower in HA than in SL
fetuses; total DNA and protein content, however, was higher or normal in fetal brains at HA than at SL (Table V). This contrast between concentration and total content of DNA and protein as well as
the decreased dry matter and increased brain weight in HA fetal brains
(Table VIII) indicate not only a higher number of nuclei (and therefore of cells) but also a higher brain water content; these factors
in combination, would have the effect of "diluting" total DNA and
protein content and thus explaining the lower DNA, RNA, and protein

TABLE III

NEUROCHEMICAL ABERRATIONS IN ONE-DAY-OLD MALE AND FEMALE RATS AT HIGH ALTITUDE: NUCLEIC ACID AND PROTEIN METABOLISM IN CEREBRAL CORTEX

CONSTITUENTS	SEA LEVEL CONTROLS C	HIGH ALTITUDE A	ANIMALS F1
	Concentrations (μg/mg wet tissue)		
DNA	5.63 ± 0.21[a]	4.47 ± 0.24[b]	4.08 ± 0.24[c]
RNA	4.09 ± 0.13	4.48 ± 0.19	4.50 ± 0.22
PROTEIN	65.20 ± 1.88	53.11 ± 1.40[d]	60.96 ± 2.78[d]
	Incorporation of radioactive precursors (dpm/mg of DNA, or RNA, or protein) 15 min postinjection intraperitoneally		
THYMIDINE	746 ± 195	2838 ± 412[b]	981 ± 153[d]
URIDINE	3281 ± 654	4777 ± 1619	15985 ± 1247[d]
LEUCINE	6718 ± 1215	20456 ± 2297[b]	14616 ± 1244[c]

A = rats conceived at sea level and taken to high altitude (12,470 ft.) the day before birth; F1 = first-generation rats conceived and born at high altitude from acclimatized parents.

a = Mean ± standard error.

Statistically-significant differences at levels ranging from $P<0.001$ to $P<0.05$ are cited for comparisons between A/C (b), F1/C (c), and F1/A (d).

TABLE IV

DRY-MATTER AND LIPID CONTENT IN THE BRAIN OF RAT FETUSES AT SEA LEVEL AND AT HIGH ALTITUDE

LIPIDS	17th Day of Gestation		21st Day of Gestation	
	SL	HA	SL	HA
Dry Matter	7.73 ± 0.16^a	7.12 ± 0.09^b	8.34 ± 0.15	8.12 ± 0.10
Total Phospholipids	43.23 ± 0.18	42.49 ± 0.21^b	41.25 ± 0.23	40.13 ± 0.10^b
Uncharacterized Lipids	10.10 ± 0.09	10.85 ± 0.41	8.06 ± 0.08	10.00 ± 0.25^b
Sphingomyelin Inositol Phosphatides Serine Glycerophosphatide	7.33 ± 0.14	7.24 ± 0.12	6.49 ± 0.22	5.80 ± 0.07^b
Choline Glycerophosphatide	20.92 ± 0.13	20.55 ± 0.09	19.40 ± 0.18	18.94 ± 0.09
Ethanolamine Glycerophosphatide	14.97 ± 0.18	14.69 ± 0.09	15.60 ± 0.15	15.38 ± 0.07
Cholesterol	0.78 ± 0.04	0.76 ± 0.02	0.96 ± 0.10	0.90 ± 0.06
Cerebrosides Sulfatides	0.29 ± 0.04	0.25 ± 0.04	0.39 ± 0.04	0.37 ± 0.05

SL = sea level; HA = high altitude (12,470 ft.).

a = Mean ± standard error. Values for dry matter are expressed as % of wet weight; for lipids as % of dry matter.

b = Statistically-significant differences, at levels ranging from $P < 0.001$ to $P < 0.05$, for HA/SL comparison.

TABLE V

NUCLEIC-ACID AND PROTEIN CONCENTRATION AND TOTAL CONTENT IN FETAL BRAIN

| | 17th Day of Gestation | | | | 21st Day of Gestation | | | |
| | Sea Level | | High Altitude | | Sea Level | | High Altitude | |
CONSTITUENT	Concentration	Content	Concentration	Content	Concentration	Content	Concentration	Content
DNA	8.79^a ± 0.44	0.60 ± 0.02	8.46 ± 0.15	0.68^b ± 0.02	4.54 ± 0.15	0.91 ± 0.01	4.27 ± 0.06	0.97^b ± 0.01
RNA	8.52 ± 0.31	0.58 ± 0.01	6.02^b ± 0.10	0.49^b ± 0.02	5.64 ± 0.17	1.13 ± 0.01	4.84^b ± 0.06	1.10 ± 0.02
PROTEIN	69.82 ± 2.51	4.75 ± 0.11	61.11^b ± 0.57	5.12^b ± 0.10	52.81 ± 0.64	10.99 ± 1.00	48.48^b ± 0.53	11.23 ± 1.40

High Altitude = 12,470 ft

a = Mean ± standard error. b = Statistically-significant differences at levels ranging from $P<0.001$ to $P<0.05$, for HA/SL comparison.

Concentrations are expressed as μg/mg wet weight, total content as mg/brain

concentration recorded at HA. That the higher total DNA content
found at HA may reflect an acceleration of DNA synthesis is indicated
by the consistent findings of increased precursor (^{14}C-thymidine)
incorporation in HA fetuses (Table VI); only sporadic differences
between HA and SL were observed in the incorporation of RNA and protein precursors, ^{3}H-uridine and ^{3}H-leucine, respectively (Table VI).
It might be noted here that these alterations in precursor incorporation into fetal brain constituents at HA were not due to changes in
precursor kinetics in maternal or fetal circulation, as indicated
by the general similarity between HA and SL precursor levels in
maternal and fetal plasma (Table VII). All the changes described
above for fetuses as well as newborns, are summarized in Figure 1.

Fetal body weight at HA was similar to that at SL, whereas fetal
heart weight and hematocrit were significantly lower at HA as compared to SL control values (Table VIII).

Placental Changes (Figure 2). Total DNA content showed no differences between HA and SL, but total RNA and protein content were
higher at HA than at SL; ^{3}H-uridine and ^{3}H-leucine incorporation into
RNA and protein, respectively, was higher at HA than at SL, directly
correlating with the biochemical findings noted above. Placental
weight at 17 days was also higher at HA as compared to SL, indicating,
in conjunction with the above findings, that a true placental hypertrophy occurred at HA, perhaps as an adaptive response to the hypoxic
environment. In view of these placental findings as well as the increased brain weight and DNA content in HA fetuses, it should be noted
that Zamenhof et al. (1971a) presented statistical evidence that
fetuses with a heavier placenta are also likely to have a higher
brain weight and a higher cerebral DNA content.

                              DISCUSSION

The findings of the present study showing that fetal brain development is adversely affected by exposure of the mother to HA during
gestation indicate that despite the factor of maternal acclimatization
to hypoxia and the adaptive responses of the placenta, the mother rat
is not able to fully protect her progeny in utero. The increase over
control values in DNA content and in DNA-precursor incorporation, as
well as the increased brain weight in HA progeny represent direct and
indirect evidence of increased cellular proliferation in the brain of
these animals. Shivers and Roofe (1966) also have documented histo-
logically that subacute exposure of pregnant rats to simulated HA
induced a 20% increase in the cerebral cell population of their offspring, presumably because of glial cell proliferation. The increased
brain hydration attested by the decrease in dry matter content also
may account for the increased brain weight; yet it should be noted
that total RNA and protein content was virtually unchanged whereas
their concentrations were decreased, a fact which, when taken together

TABLE VI

INCORPORATION OF RADIOACTIVE PRECURSORS INTO NUCLEIC ACIDS AND PROTEIN OF FETAL-RAT BRAIN

| PRECURSOR | 17th Day of Gestation | | | | 21st Day of Gestation | | | |
| | 15 min | | 30 min | | 15 min | | 30 min | |
	SL	HA	SL	HA	SL	HA	SL	HA
^{14}C-Thymidine	4036[a] ± 73	4619 ± 291	4075 ± 281	6026[b] ± 372	1546 ± 69	1797[b] ± 68	1919 ± 160	2483[b] ± 180
^{3}H-Uridine	778 ± 117	1117 ± 105	1052 ± 128	999 ± 100	551 ± 43	436 ± 20	486 ± 55	430 ± 58
^{3}H-Leucine	3240 ± 76	3027 ± 173	3526 ± 47	2947[b] ± 243	2046 ± 117	2120 ± 132	2500 ± 116	2710 ± 118

SL = sea level; HA = high altitude (12,470 ft.).

a = Mean ± standard error. Incorporation, expressed in dpm/mg of DNA, or RNA, or protein, is given for 15 and 30 min after intravenous injection into the mother.

b = Statistically-significant differences at levels ranging from $P < 0.001$ to $P < 0.05$ for HA/SL comparison.

TABLE VII

LEVELS OF RADIOACTIVE PRECURSORS IN MATERNAL AND FETAL PLASMA 15 MIN AFTER INTRAVENOUS INJECTION INTO THE MATERNAL CIRCULATION

PRECURSOR	17th Day of Gestation		21st Day of Gestation	
	SL	HA	SL	HA
MATERNAL PLASMA				
^{14}C-Thymidine	46 ± 3[a]	34 ± 0.4[b]	38 ± 4	46 ± 0.2
^3H-Uridine	536 ± 20	497 ± 23	454 ± 33	557 ± 7
^3H-Leucine	346 ± 45	398 ± 31	324 ± 17	226 ± 51
FETAL PLASMA				
^{14}C-Thymidine	12 ± 2	13 ± 0.3	9 ± 0.6	7 ± 0.3[b]
^3H-Uridine	263 ± 17	251 ± 4	145 ± 9	170 ± 5[b]
^3H-Leucine	249 ± 54	556 ± 156	373 ± 31	313 ± 43

SL = sea level; HA = high altitude (12,470 ft.).

a = Mean ± standard error; Values represent dpm/μl of plasma. b = Statistically-significant differences, at levels ranging from $p < 0.001$ to $p < 0.05$, for HA/SL comparison.

TABLE VIII

SELECTED DEVELOPMENTAL PARAMETERS OF RAT FETUS AT HIGH ALTITUDE AND SEA LEVEL

PARAMETER	17th Day of Gestation		21st Day of Gestation	
	SL	HA	SL	HA
Body weight (mg)	840 ± 14^a	811 ± 15	5488 ± 62	5524 ± 100
Brain weight (mg)	69 ± 3	82 ± 2^b	209 ± 4	230 ± 4^b
Heart weight (mg)	---	---	31 ± 1	27 ± 1^b
Fetal Hematocrit	34 ± 1	30 ± 1^b	41 ± 1	37 ± 1^b

SL = sea level; HA - high altitude (12,470 ft.).

a = Mean ± standard error

b = Statistically-significant differences, at levels ranging from $P<0.001$ to $P<0.05$, for HA/SL comparison.

with the decrease in dry matter and the increased cellular population,
indicates that the size of brain cells was decreased in HA animals.
It would seem, therefore, that exposure to HA, although it stimulates
brain cell division, delays those cell processes necessary for attaining normal size and maturity. This postulate is further supported by
the deficiencies observed in brain lipids, constituents involved in
the formation of myelin, necessary to proper brain function. Moreover, while these deficiencies in lipids as well as in RNA and protein continue into the neonatal period, the increase in fetal brain
DNA content shows a marked reversal at this time - findings which
substantiate that brain maturational processes already have been
affected in the prenatal period. That precursor incorporation in
the neonatal brain was higher at HA than at SL also may indicate
that at the same chronological age, the HA brain is in an earlier
maturational stage than the SL brain. Although the possibility that
HA effects changes in the pool size of these precursors also should
be investigated as a causal factor in these differences, the interpretation given above is supported by other structural and functional
findings from our previous studies at HA (Dalal et al., 1973; Heim
and Timiras, 1964; Petropoulos et al., 1969; Petropoulos et al., 1970;
Petropoulos et al., 1972a; Timiras and Woolley, 1966).

Having established that the impairment consistently noted in
our previous investigations of postnatal brain maturation in rats
exposed to HA is initiated, at least partially, in utero, the present study, by comparing F_1 and A newborn rats, further indicates
that the duration of exposure to HA and the coincidence of such exposure with critical periods in brain organogenesis are more important factors in determining the ultimate extent and severity of brain
impairment than maternal acclimatization to hypoxia; for brain maturation in the offspring of mothers not acclimatized to HA (A rats) was
less adversely affected than F_1 rats whose mothers were acclimatized
to HA. Various other noxious factors and drugs also appear to differen-
tially affect the fetus depending on its maturational stage and the
duration of its exposure to these agents (cf. Petropoulos et al.,
1972b).

The contrast between the decreased fetal heart weight and hematocrit we observed at HA and the increased hemoglobin concentration
in the blood of the fetal Andean sheep recorded by Metcalfe et al.
(1967) is perhaps due to species specific differences, and to differences in the techniques employed and the stage of pregnancy studied;
yet, in a previous study Metcalfe et al. (1962b) reported no differences in fetal heart weight between HA and SL sheep.

In order to clarify the mechanisms involved in the effects of
HA on fetal brain, one must consider the adaptive responses of the
maternal organism, the placenta, and the fetus itself. Although
Metcalfe et al. (1962a, 1967) in the only such study thus far conducted, observed that the partial pressure of oxygen in the umbilical

		DNA	Thymidine incorp.	RNA	Uridine incorp.	Protein	Leucine incorp.	Dry matter	Cholesterol	Total phospholipids	Phosphatides	Uncharacterized lipids
DEVELOPMENTAL CHANGES IN ALL GROUPS	Fetus → Newborn	▽	▽	▽	Fetus ▽ / Newborn ▲	Fetus ▽ / Newborn ▲	Fetus ▽ / Newborn ▲	▲	▲	▽	▽	▽
COMPARISON BETWEEN HA AND SL GROUPS	Fetuses	conc. ~ / content ▲	▲	▽	~	conc. ▽ / content ▲	~	▽	~	▽	▽	▲
	Newborns HA$_A$/SL	▽	▲	~	~	▽	▲	▽	▽	▽	▽	~
	HA$_{F_1}$/SL	▽	~	~	▲	~	▲	▽	▽	▽	▽	▲
	HA$_{F_1}$/HA$_A$	~	▽	~	▲	▲	~	▽	▽	▽	▽	▲

Fig. 1. Developmental patterns of rat brain at high altitude (HA) and at sea level (SL). HA$_A$ = rats conceived at sea level and taken to high altitude (12,470 ft.) the day before birth; HA$_{F_1}$ = first-generation rats conceived and born at high altitude from acclimatized parents. ▽ indicates decrease; ▲ indicates increase; ~ indicates similarity.

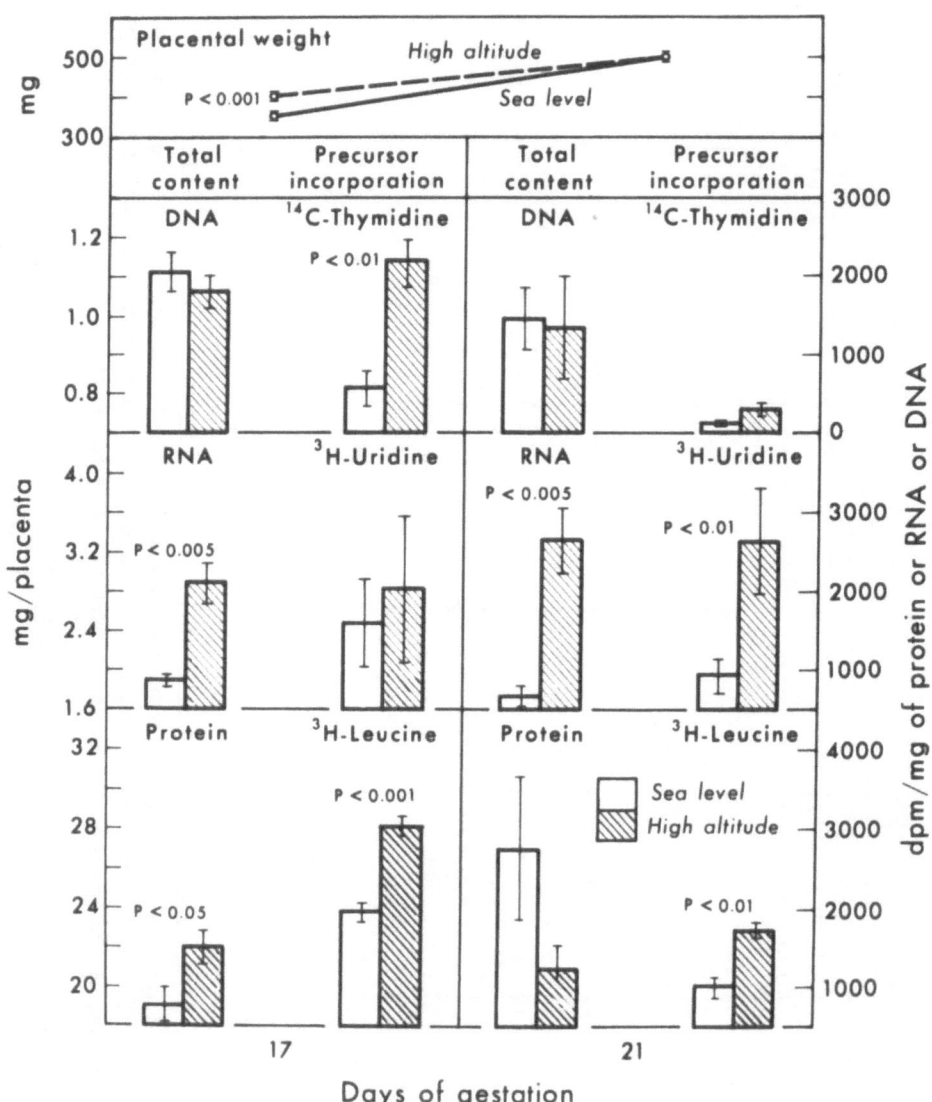

Fig. 2. Placental metabolic changes in pregnant rats at high altitude.

vessels of sheep native to HA was similar to that of SL controls, confirming the assumption that the mother is able to secure adequate oxygen supply for the fetus, these findings have not been duplicated either by Metcalfe or by others, the experimental period was circumscribed to late gestation, and a different animal species was utilized; thus the belief that no significant impairment of oxygen supply to the fetal brain occurs at HA, because of maternal protection, remains questionable. Secondly, even though the present data and those of others (cf. Petropoulos and Timiras, 1973) indicate that the placenta is capable of making necessary adaptations to the oxygen deficiency of HA, it is quite possible that its adjustments are predominantly geared to securing and maintaining proper oxygen levels for the fetus, to the detriment perhaps of other functions, important to fetal welfare, such as procuring nutrients and secreting hormones (Sobrevilla et al., 1968). In this context, both malnutrition and hormonal imbalances during gestation have been clearly related to the incidence, extent and severity of brain damage in fetus and newborn (Abdul-Karim et al., 1970; Wallace and Michie, 1966; Zamenhof et al., 1971b). In addition, the postulated metabolic resistance of the fetuses and newborns to anoxia (Himwich, 1951; Windle, 1943) has been challenged by Racker (1955) and it is now well documented that the neonatal brain does sustain permanent developmental damage (Hicks et al., 1962) under experimental anoxic conditions previously considered to be harmless. Finally, the increased cosmic radiation at HA (Petropoulos and Timiras, 1973) also should be considered in evaluating the mechanisms by which fetal brain development is altered at HA, for irradiation during pregnancy has been amply shown to lead to severe developmental abnormalities in the brain of the progeny (Kirrmann and Wolff, 1964; Maletta et al., 1967; Miller, 1956; Vernadakis et al., 1968).

CONCLUSIONS

In contrast with previous beliefs, the evidence presented here indicates that fetal brain maturation is delayed at HA, and that as with drugs found to affect fetal brain development, the effects of HA depend on the duration of exposure and the maturational stage of the CNS at the time of such exposure. The observations from this study point to hypoxia as the major factor influencing brain development; however, other factors, such as placental insufficiency and increased cosmic radiation, play a role. Evidence reported by others on the adverse effects of HA on fetal development in general has been presented, and, examined in context with the present findings, suggests that the HA environment is not entirely harmless during prenatal life. Accordingly, therapeutic handling of abnormal pregnancies in HA natives must take into consideration the possibility of interaction between drug effects and effects of hypoxia; such an interaction would most likely result in a mutual enhancement of the action of these two factors, leading to a more severe fetal impairment than either of these factors would bring about alone.

ACKNOWLEDGMENTS

This study was supported by USPHS grant NS 08989. The authors express their thanks to Miss Pat Shannon for skillful technical assistance throughout this study, to Dr. K.B. Dalal and Miss J. Csejtey for determination of brain lipids, to Mrs. L. Cook for editorial advice, and to Mrs. Christine Lazootin for typing assistance.

REFERENCES

Abdul-Karim, R.W., Drucker, M., and Rizk, P., 1970, Influence of estrogen on the cholinesterase content of fetal brain, Obst. Gynec. 36: 719.

Baird, B., and Cook, S.F., 1962, Hypoxia and reproduction in swiss mice, Am. J. Physiol. 202: 611.

Baker, P.T., 1969, Human adaptation to high altitude, Science 163: 1149.

Becker, E.J., and Kreuzer, F., 1968, Sympathoadrenal response to hypoxia, Pflügers Arch. 304: 1.

Chabes, A., Pereda, J., Hyams, L., Barrientos, N., Perez, J., Campes, L., Monroe, A., and Mayorga, A., 1968, Comparative morphometry of the human placenta at high altitude and at sea level, Obst. Gynec. 31: 178.

Dalal, K.B., Valcana, T., Timiras, P.S., and Einstein, E.R., 1971, Regulatory role of thyroxine on myelinogenesis in the developing rat, Neurobiology 1: 211.

Dalal, K.B., Petropoulos, E.A., and Timiras, P.S., 1973, The effects of hypoxia on 2',3'-cyclic nucleotide-3'-phosphohydrolase activity in brain myelin of the developing rat, Environ. Physiol., in press.

Delaquerriere-Richardson, L., and Valdivia, E. 1967, Effects of simulated high altitude on pregnancy; placental morphology in albino guinea pigs, Arch. Pathol. 84: 405.

Fisher, R.A., 1950, "Statistical Methods for Research Workers", Hofner, New York.

Frisancho, A.R., 1970, Developmental responses to high altitude hypoxia, Am. J. Phys. Anthropol. 32: 401.

Grahn, D., and Krathcman, J., 1963, Variation in neonatal death rate and birth weight in the United States and possible relations to environmental radiation, geology and altitude, Am. J. Human Genet. 15: 329.

Heim, L.M., 1965, Spinal cord convulsions in the developing rat at high altitude, Nature 207: 299.

Heim, L.M., and Timiras, P.S., 1964, Brain maturation measured by electroshock seizures in rats at high altitude (12,470 ft; 3,800 m), Nature 204: 1157.

Hicks, S.P., Cavanaugh, M.C., and O'Brien, E.D., 1962, Effects of anoxia on the developing cerebral cortex in the rat, Am. J. Pathol. 40: 615.

Himwich, H.E., 1951, Cerebral metabolism during growth of lower mammals. A biochemical basis for neurophylogenesis, in "Brain Metabolism and Cerebral Disorders", Chapter 7, pp. 124-176, Williams and Wilkins, Baltimore.

Jilek, L., Trojan, S., and Trávnickorá, E., 1966, Lactic acid and glycogen changes in the rat brain due to aerogenic (altitude) hypoxia during ontogenesis, Physiol. Bohemoslov. 15: 532.

Kelley, F.C., and Pace, N., 1968, Etiological considerations in neonatal mortality among rats at moderate high altitude (3,800 m), Am. J. Physiol. 214: 1168.

Kirrmann, J., and Wolff, E., 1964, Teratogenic effects of ionizing radiation on the embryonic development of the higher vertebrates, Int. Rev. Exp. Pathol. 3: 365.

Krüger, H., and Arias-Stella, J., 1970, The placenta and the newborn infant at high altitudes, Am. J. Obst. Gynec. 106: 586.

Lichty, J.A., Ting, R.V., Brums, P.D., and Dyar, E., 1957, Studies of babies born at high altitudes: I. Relation of altitude to birth weight; II. Measurement of birth weight, body length and head size; III. Arterial oxygen saturation and hematocrit values at birth, Am. Med. Ass. Dis. Child. 93: 666.

Maletta, G.J., Vernadakis, A., and Timiras, 1967, Acetylcholinesterase activity and protein content of brain and spinal cord in developing rats after prenatal X-irradiation, J. Neurochem. 14: 647.

Metcalfe, J., Meschia, G., Hellegers, A., Prystowsky, H., Huckabee, W., and Barron, D.H., 1962a, Observations on the placental exchange of the respiratory gases in pregnant ewes at high altitude, Quart. J. Exp. Physiol. 47: 74.

Metcalfe, J., Meschia, G., Hellegers, A., Prystowsky, H., Huckabee, W., and Barron, D.H., 1962b, Observations on the growth rate, and organ weights of fetal sheep at altitude and sea level, Quart. J. Exp. Physiol. 47: 305.

Metcalfe, J., Novy, M.J., and Peterson, E.N., 1967, Reproduction at high altitudes, in "Comparative Aspects of Reproductive Failure", (K. Benirschke, ed.), pp. 447-457, Springer-Verlag, New York.

Miller, R.W., 1956, Delayed effects occurring within the first decade after exposure of young individuals to the Hiroshima Atomic Bomb, Pediatrics 18: 1.

Nelson, M.L., and Srebnik, H.H., 1970, Comparison of the reproductive performance of rats at high altitude (3,800 m) and at sea level, Int. J. Biometeor. 14: 187.

Petropoulos, E.A., 1973, Maternal and fetal factors affecting the growth and function of the rat placenta, Acta Endocrinol. (Kbh) 72, Suppl. 176, pp. 1-69.

Petropoulos, E.A., and Timiras, P.S., 1973, Biological effects of high altitude as related to increased radiation, temperature fluctuations, and reduced partial pressure of oxygen, in "Progress in Biometeorology; Progress in Human Biometeorology", (S.W. Tromp, ed.), Sect. A., vol. 1, Swets and Zeitlinger, Amsterdam, in press.

Petropoulos, E.A., Vernadakis, A., and Timiras, P.S., 1969, Nucleic acid content in developing rat brain after prenatal and/or neonatal exposure to high altitude, Federation Proc. 28: 1001.

Petropoulos, E.A., Vernadakis, A., and Timiras, P.S., 1970, Neuro-chemical changes in rats subjected neonatally to high altitude and electroshock, Am. J. Physiol. 218: 1351.

Petropoulos, E.A., Dalal, K.B., and Timiras, P.S., 1972a, Effects of high altitude on myelinogenesis in brain of the developing rat, Am. J. Physiol. 223: 951.

Petropoulos, E.A., Lau, C., and Liao, C.L., 1972b, Neurochemical changes in the offspring of rats subjected to stressful con-ditions during gestation, Exp. Neurol. 37: 86.

Racker, E., 1955, The mechanisms of glycolysis, in "Neurochemistry; the Chemical Dynamics of Brain and Nerve", (K.A.C. Elliott, I.H. Page and J.H. Quastel, eds.), pp. 134-152, Charles C. Thomas, Springfield, Ill.

Shivers, R.R., and Roofe, P.G., 1966, Cerebral cell population under hypoxia, Anat. Rec. 154: 841.

Sobrevilla, L.A., Romero, I., Kruger, F., and Whittembury, J., 1968, Low estrogen excretion during pregnancy at high altitude, Am. J. Obst. Gynec. 102: 828.

Timiras, P.S., 1964, Comparison of growth and development of the rat at high altitude and at sea level, in "The Physiological Effects of High Altitude", (W.H. Weihe, ed.), pp. 21-30, Pergamon Press, Oxford.

Timiras, P.S., and Woolley, D.E., 1966, Functional and morphological development of brain and other organs of rats at high altitude, Federation Proc. 25: 1312.

Vernadakis, A., Casper, R., and Timiras, P.S., 1968, Influence of prenatal X-radiation on brain lipid and cerebroside content in developing rats, Experientia 24: 237.

Wallace, S.J., and Michie, E.A., 1966, A followup study of infants born to mothers with low oestriol excretion during pregnancy, Lancet 2: 560.

Windle, W.F., 1943, Developmental physiology, Ann. Rev. Physiol. 5: 63.

Zamenhof, S., Gravel, L., and van Martens, E., 1971a, Study of possible correlations between prenatal brain development and placental weight, Biol. Neonate. 18: 140.

Zamenhof, S., van Marthens, E., and Gravel, L., 1971b, DNA (cell number) in neonatal brain: second generation (F_2) alteration by maternal (F_0) dietary protein restriction, Science 172: 850.

THYROID HORMONES IN RELATION TO DEVELOPMENT OF THE NERVOUS SYSTEM

Donald H. Ford

Department of Anatomy, State University of New York

Downstate Medical Center, Brooklyn, New York

Modern interest in hormone research may be said to have commenced with the use of aqueous extracts of dog and guinea pig testicles by the French neurologist, Brown-Sequard (1889) to restore male sex drive in man, one may presume by an action on the nervous system. However, since it is to be doubted that an aqueous extract could remove the lipid soluble steroid hormone from the testicular tissue, it would seem that the reported beneficial effect was psychological. Interest in thyroid hormone in relation to its effect on the nervous system undoubtedly is of more ancient origin, based on early observations available in the literature on mental retardation in cretins. Additional evidence for a thyroid hormone effect in development was presented in 1924 by Allen who demonstrated that metamorphosis in amphibians was thyroid hormone dependent and that in the absence of thyroxine the brain failed to attain normal growth. Then, in 1952 investigations conducted by Beach demonstrated that gonadal hormones influence reproductive behavior. However, little direct evidence had accumulated at this time to support a hormonal action on the nervous system. The concept of a critical period in the development of the brain wherein the presence or absence of androgens could determine whether or not the hypothalamus regulated a cyclic or acyclic pituitary-gonad relationship was yet to come. Similarly, we did not comprehend the extent to which thyroid hormone was needed in the early postnatal period to promote growth and differentiation of neurons and the myelinization of their axons.

Although from about 1949 numerous reports began to appear concerning the effect of thyroxine (T_4) or triiodothyronine (T_3) on various aspects of development, growth or function of the nervous system, no systematic studies had been performed to specifically relate the presence of thyroid hormones to discrete responses or functions of

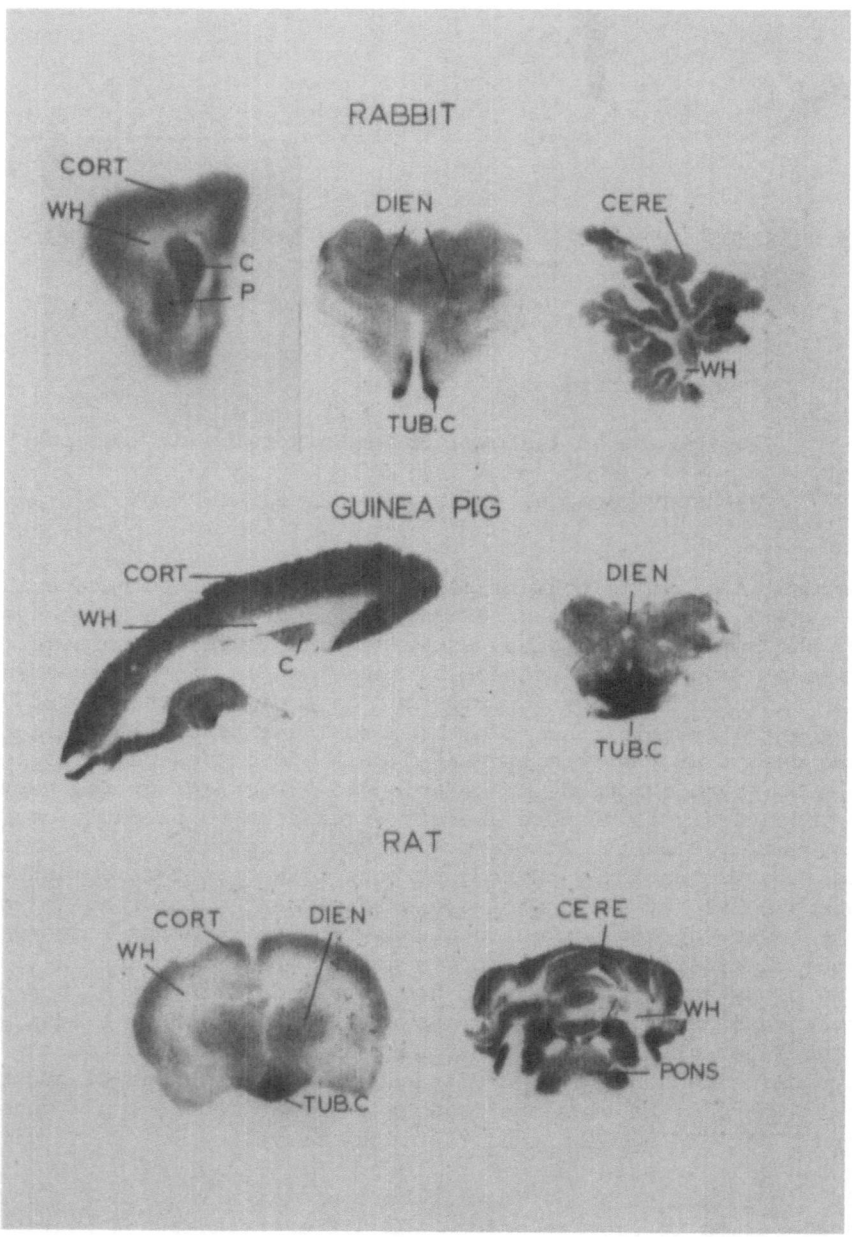

Fig. 1. X-ray radioautographs of sections of the central nervous
system of rat, guinea pig and rabbit demonstrating the sites of accumulation of radioactive material 2 hours after an intravenous injection of ^{131}I-l-triiodothyronine (dose of 0.5 mC/kg in the rabbit and
1.0 mC/kg in the rat and guinea pig). C = caudate nucleus, Cere =
cerebellum, Cort = cerebral cortex, Dien = diencephalon, P = putamen,
Tub.C = tuber cinereum, Wh = white matter.

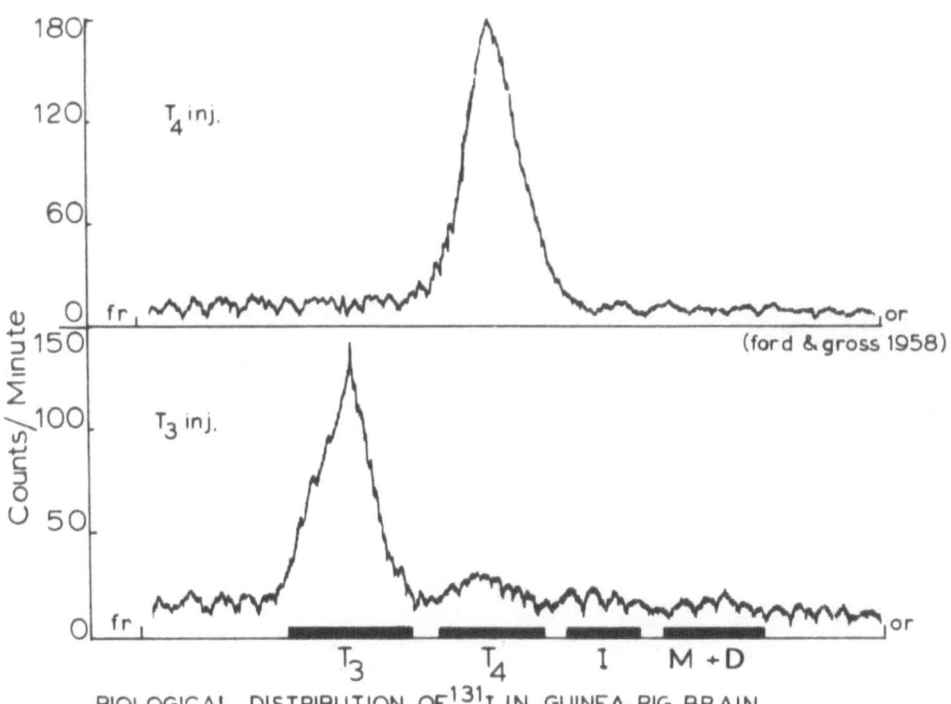

Fig. 2. ^{131}I-activity in the brain of the guinea pig following 4 hr intravenous injection of ^{131}I-labelled triiodothyronine or thyroxine. This is based on scans of radiochromatograms (T$_3$=triiodothyronine, T$_4$=thyroxine, I=iodide, and M+D=the area occupied by mono and diiodothyrosine) (Ford and Gross, 1958b).

the CNS. Experimental proof of its role in brain development awaited quantitative studies of its accumulation in either neurons or the surrounding glia within the neuropil.

Early investigations of Schittenhelm and Eisler (1932) had indicated that the highest concentrations of iodide were to be found in the hypothalamus and midbrain. These observations were later confirmed by the use of radioactive iodide (Courrier et al., 1949; Jensen and Clark, 1951). Subsequent studies demonstrated the accumulation of either T$_4$ or T$_3$ in the brain following intravenous injection of the ^{131}I-labelled hormone in rabbits and guinea pigs (Ford and Gross, 1958a, 1958b). Somewhat later, rats were added to the list of common laboratory animals showing accumulation of T$_3$ (Ford et al., 1959).

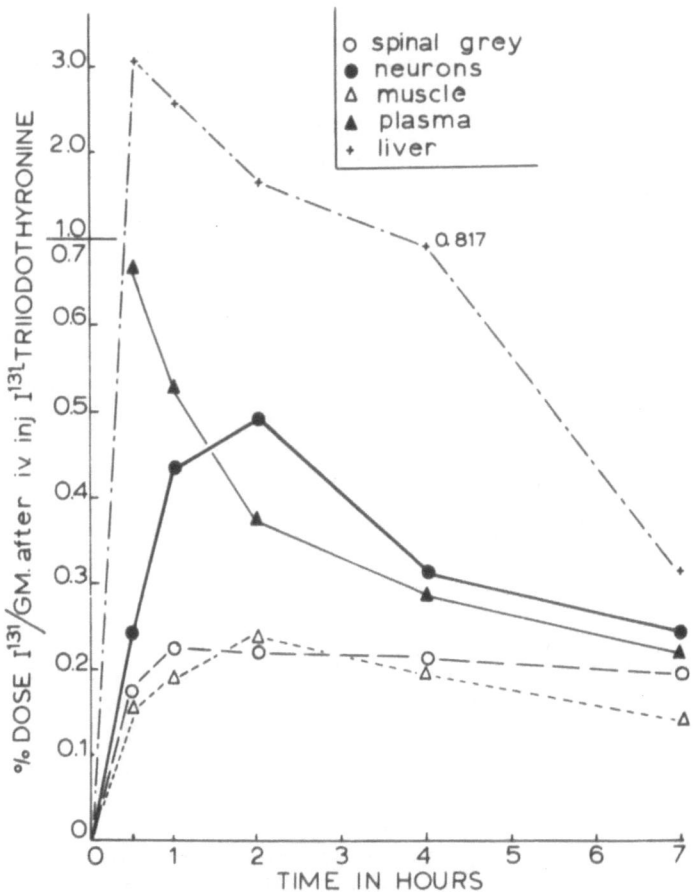

Fig. 3. Levels of accumulation of ^{131}I-triiodothyronine in the spinal grey matter, ventral horn motoneurons, muscle, liver and plasma of the rat at various time intervals after intravenous injection of the labelled hormone (Dose = 19.6 µg/kg, 526.0 µC/kg) (Ford and Rhines, 1967).

X-ray radioautography, by Ford and co-workers, demonstrated that the sites of hormone accumulation were predominantly in the areas most rich in neurons (Fig. 1). Chromatographic analysis of the tissue revealed that most of the radioactivity present was in the form of the injected hormone (Ford and Gross, 1958a, 1958b; Ford, 1961; Bleecker et al., 1971) (Fig. 2). It was also demonstrated that there was a sex difference in T_3 accumulation, the levels of uptake being higher in females (Ford et al., 1962, 1964; Bleecker et al., 1971). Further investigation revealed age differences in T_3 accumulation (Ford and Rhines, 1970; Bleecker et al., 1971). It has also been demonstrated that ^{131}I-T_3 is preferentially accumulated by the neurons

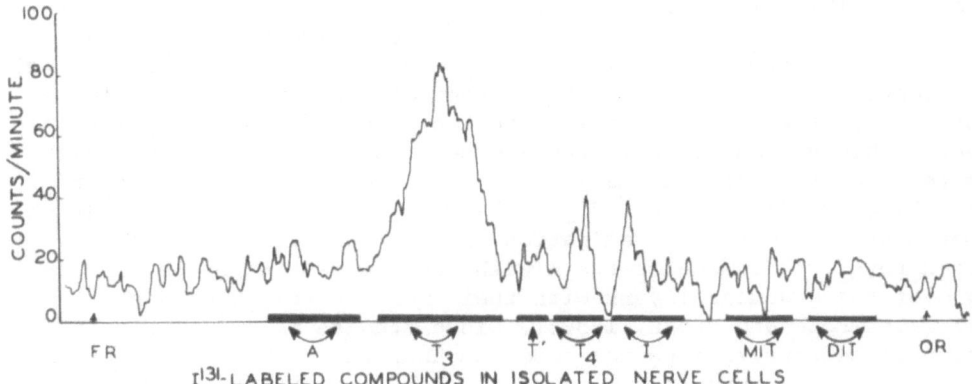

Fig. 4. Distribution of radioactivity on a chromatogram prepared
from an ethanolic extract of 1000 unfixed neurons dissected from the
ventral horn of the spinal cord from an animal injected with ^{131}I-
labelled triiodothyronine. (T_3=triiodothyronine, T_4=thyroxine, I=
iodide, MIT=monoiodotyrosine, DIT=diiodotyrosine, A=probably triio-
dothyroacetic acid, T=unknown, FR-front, OR-origin) (Ford and Rhines,
1967).

(Figs. 3 and 4) in an investigation on the levels of accumulation of
the hormone in ventral horn motoneurons (Ford and Rhines, 1967).
Thus, it seems clear from the foregoing that thyroid hormones do reach
the level of brain tissues and in particular the neurons.

Various studies with amphibians have provided considerable evidence for the role of thyroid hormone in the development of the nervous system commencing in 1924 with the observations of Allen. Investigations by Weiss and Rosetti, Kollros and co-workers, Pesetsky,
Yonazawa and co-workers, to name a few, have provided ample evidence
for the significant role of thyroid hormone in anurans. However, I
wish only at this time to call attention to the important contribu-
tions in this area and to continue on in somewhat more detail considering mammalian data.

In considering the effect of thyroid hormone on the mammalian
brain, one might first examine the results from studies on brain
accumulation of ^{131}I-T_3 following intravenous injection. First,
accumulation of thyroid hormone is greatest in areas containing many
neurons and lowest in white matter. This fact is most clearly evident when comparing accumulation in grey and white matter. Some
degree of species difference has also been noted in the level of
accumulation attained, in that rat and guinea pig have higher levels
of accumulation than rabbit. The difference in accumulation between

grey and white matter is visually well demonstrated by X-ray radioautography (Fig. 1) following i.v. injection of ^{131}I-labelled triiodothyronine. A similar distribution occurs with thyroxine, but
the level of accumulation with essentially equimolar doses is appreciably less. In the cerebellum the extent of exposure of the film is
greater over the granule-Purkinje region than over the molecular
layer. Observations made in the diencephalon and brain stem demonstrated that the areas of maximal accumulation occur in that part of
the film overlying the specific nuclear regions and in particular the
tubercinereum. Careful examination of the autographs of cerebral
cortex reveals a laminar pattern with the greatest exposure occurring over the granular layers with their more densely packed neuronal
cell mass (Ford and Gross, 1958b). Since studies on ^{131}I-T$_3$ accumulation in neurons from spinal cord demonstrated higher levels of hormone than in the surrounding neuropil (Ford and Rhines, 1967), it is
assumed that the higher concentration in layers of cerebral cortex
most packed with neurons is associated with primarily nerve cell
hormone uptake.

   T$_3$ is more readily accumulated in the CNS than T$_4$, presumably
due to the difference in the degree of binding of the two hormones
to the plasma proteins (Robbins and Rall, 1960). T$_3$, which is less
firmly bound to the plasma proteins, is about 3 times more readily
accumulated into neuronal tissue.

   There are other factors which may influence the amount of T$_3$
accumulated in the CNS; for example, levels of accumulation are higher
than normal in hypothyroid and lower than normal in hyperthyroid rats
(Ford et al., 1959; Ford, 1961). Chromatographic analysis of extracts
of brain homogenates suggest that these differences may in part be
due to difference in the rate of degradation through the deiodinative
pathway. This depression of thyroid hormone degradation in the CNS
of hypothyroid rats is associated with a decrease in blood flow (Himwich et al., 1942; Madison et al., 1957; Scheinberg et al., 1950;
Sensenbach et al., 1954; Sokoloff et al., 1953) as well as with a
decrease in glucose and oxygen utilization (Himwich et al., 1942).
The incorporation of ^{3}H-lysine into brain protein is also depressed
in hypothyroid adult rats (Ford et al., 1965), presumably due to a
reduction of the anabolic stimulating activity of thyroid hormone.
The general reduction of protein synthesis could of itself subsequently
lead to a decreased synthesis of those enzymes which degrade the hormone and thus account for the decreased rate of T$_3$ deiodination in
brains of hypothyroid rats. Using similar logic one may associate
the increased ^{131}I-T$_3$ degradation in brains of hyperthyroid adult
male rats with an increased enzyme activity (Ford, 1961), which
we believe is accompanied by an increased turnover of proteins without change in amount.

The gender of the animals has also been observed to influence the levels of accumulation of ^{131}I-T_3 in the nervous system (Bleecker et al., 1971; Ford et al., 1962, 1964; Ford and Rhines, 1970). Higher levels were observed in brains of female than in male rats at ages ranging from 1 week to 24 months. Studies of ^{131}I-T_3 accumulation in castrated male animals suggest that the presence of the male hormone may be in part responsible for these differences between male and female rats (Ford et al., 1964; Bleecker, personal communication).

Finally, age dependent differences have been noted in ^{131}I-T_3 accumulation in the CNS. In an earlier study (Cohan et al., 1967) it was reported that the youngest animals showed higher levels of ^{131}I-T_3 in the brain and that the levels became progressively lower as the animal matured; these findings confirmed the results of Peterson et al. (1966). Our data, however, were reported in terms of the percent of the injected dose present/g of tissue. More recently we have observed that this manner of expression introduces a bias when animals of greatly differing weights are compared. This occurred because the number of counts/min in the injected dose of ^{131}I-T_3 increased proportional to the increase in the weight of the animals. The count/min/g of tissue also showed an increase, but of a lesser magnitude. Since the counts/min/g of tissue were then divided by the counts/min injected, these calculations led to the conclusion that the amount of hormone accumulated became smaller/g of brain tissue as the animals grew larger. However, since the number of counts/min/g of brain tissue was also increasing during early maturation, there was actually an increase in the amount of hormone present/g of tissue. Thus, in more recent studies, we have elected to express the data in terms of the amount of hormone present/g of tissue in a large group of male and female rats two, four, eight and 12-14 weeks of age. The results (Table I) demonstrate that the levels of hormone present in the brain increased during the first eight weeks and then decreased slightly. The lowest level of accumulation occurred during the period of highest accumulation of ^3H-lysine into brain protein (one to three weeks). This same age period is characterized as being the time when ^{14}C-leucine oxidation is greatest (Patel and Balázs, 1971), as is the incorporation of ^{14}C-leucine into the acids of the tricarboxylic acid cycle. This also correlates with the period when the neuronal population density is the greatest (see cell body neuropil coefficient), when nerve cell growth is most rapid in relation to neuron weights and incorporation of ^3H-lysine into neuronal protein (Table I), when gliogenesis is the most active (Schonbach et al., 1968) and when other aspects of morphological and biochemical maturation are most extensive (Eayrs and Goodhead, 1959; Cocks et al., 1970).

In attempting to correlate the observations that the greatest amount of amino acid incorporation into brain protein and neurons occurs during the period when nerve cells are growing the most rapidly (Table I) and undergoing what is actually a dramatic maturation, one is also tempted to consider if the changes in levels of ^{131}I-T_3

TABLE I

ACCUMULATION OF 131I-TRIIODOTHYRONINE IN BRAIN AS COMPARED WITH ^{3}H-LYSINE INCORPORATION INTO PROTEIN IN RELATION TO THE CELL VOLUME NEUROPIL COEFFICIENT IN SPINAL GREY MATTER AND THE WEIGHTS OF VENTRAL HORN MOTONEURONS IN MALE RATS OF VARIOUS AGES

Age in Weeks	ng 131I-T$_3$/ gm in Cerebral Grey	ng ^{3}H-lysine/ gm Brain Protein Fraction[2]	Cell Volume Neuropil Coefficient Spinal Grey[3]	nMole ^{3}H-lysine/gm Spinal Grey Matter[3]	Weight Ventral Horn Motoneuron in ng[4]	nMoles ^{3}H-lysine/gm Ventral Horn Motoneurons[3]
1	–	680	0.256	1.430	11.2	98.2
2	0.050	–	0.165	1.205	15.6	44.1
3	–	820	0.217	1.117	18.2	43.0
4	0.168	–	0.090	0.614	20.0	15.8
5	–	420	–	–	23.5	–
6	–	–	0.098	0.657	25.0	16.9
8	0.175	–	–	–	–	–
12–14	0.115	–	–	0.003	54.0	0.358
24	0.150[5]	–	–	–	–	–

[1]Bleecker et al., In: "Influence of Hormones on the Nervous System", (D.H. Ford, ed.), S. Karger, Basel, 1971, p. 231.

[2]Kartzinel et al., In: "Influence of Hormones on the Nervous System", (D.H. Ford, ed.), S. Karger, Basel, 1971, p. 296.

[3]Ford and Rhines, Acta Neurolog. Scandinav. 45: 529–539, 1969.

[4]Ford and Cohan, Acta Anat. 71: 311–319, 1968.

[5]Ford and Rhines, Brain Res. 21: 265–274, 1970.

accumulation with increasing age may be correlated to these changes. This is because thyroid hormone has been conclusively related to brain protein synthesis in early postnatal development (Sokoloff and Roberts 1971; Garcia Argiz, 1967; Pasquini et al., 1967). Further, levels of T_3 accumulation in brain are inversely related to the general metabolic state of the animal (Ford et al., 1959; Ford, 1961). From this one might infer that T_3 accumulation in the brain might also be low during the neonatal period when protein synthesis is occurring most rapidly and known to have a special relationship to thyroid hormone (Sokoloff and Roberts, 1971). Further, as thyroid hormones must be in the free state to be metabolically effective (Tata, 1964), they are more subject to degradation, which Tata has also shown occurs primarily with the free hormone. Thus, such free hormone, which would be associated with mitochondrial protein synthesis in the neonatal brain would also be more subject to degradation than sequestered (Protein bound) hormone and would be less likely to accumulate. In older animals, when the rate of protein synthesis in whole brain is markedly reduced, as is the rate of accumulation of labelled amino acid into nerve cell protein (Ford and Rhines, 1969) and when brain total protein levels are higher (Fish and Winik, 1969), one might anticipate that more hormone would become bound to cytoplasmic protein, be less rapidly degraded and thus accumulate to higher levels. Further, the fact that neurons, which are the major site of T_3 accumulation, are much larger in adults than in neonates (Ford and Cohan, 1968; Eayrs, 1953, 1955) should contribute to the increasing T_3 uptake in brain during maturation and finally in old age. In neonates, loss of thyroid hormone through degradation, may be further facilitated since thyroid hormone is degraded by an additional pathway which appears to split the molecule at the ether bond (Cohan et al., 1969).

While the above theory may explain the changes in T_3 accumulation in brain between one and eight weeks of age and the final higher level at 24 months, it does not explain the drop in hormone accumulation between eight and twelve weeks of age which is subsequently maintained to at least 17 months of age. We have no answer for this except to note that this is a period of marked stability in the rat CNS in relation to growth. Also, the final elevation of T_3 accumulation at 24 months of age may actually be caused by quite different factors. Furthermore, despite what appear as interesting temporal relationships, data is still lacking to relate conclusively levels of thyroid hormone accumulation in the brain to the rate of growth and protein receptors with age. Nevertheless, the close association between thyroid hormone and protein synthesis and the binding of the hormone to intracellular proteins would suggest such a correlation.

During the period of most active neuronal growth, the morphologic effects of thyroid hormone deficiency has been dramatically demonstrated by Eayrs and his colleagues (1951, 1953, 1955, 1960, 1961, 1964) in experiments wherein neonatal animals were deprived of thyroid

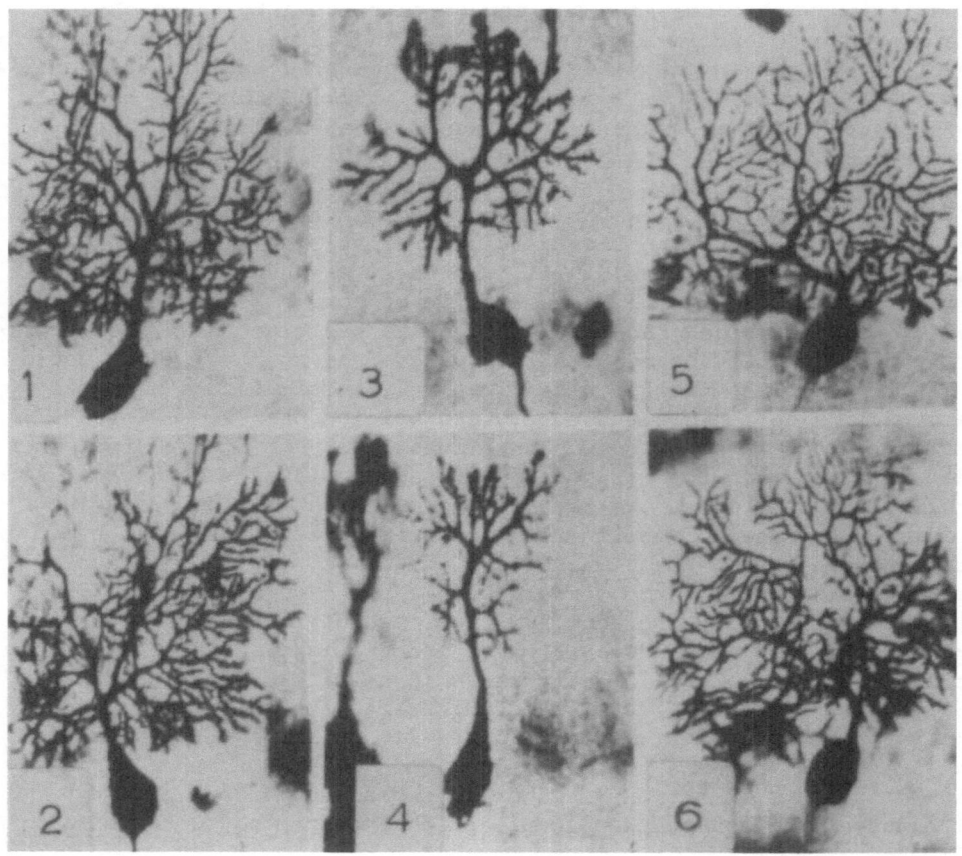

Fig. 5. A montage of illustrations of Golgi-Cox preparations demonstrating Purkinje cells in normal (1 and 2), hypothyroid animals
(3 and 4), and in animals treated with PTU, but which had also received thyroxine during the first postnatal week (5 and 6). All
animals were 14 days old when killed. The Purkinje cells of the PTU-
treated animal receiving the thyroxine supplement are essentially
identical to the cells in the controls (From Legrand, 1967b).

hormone. Cell packing density was increased and the growth of the
cell bodies and their processes severely depressed. Working with
cerebellar tissue, Legrand (1967a, 1967b) noted that the external
granule cell layer in hypothyroid rats persisted longer than in normal rats due to a delay in migration of the cells. He also noted a
severe inhibition in the maturation of Purkinje cells (Fig. 5). The
period of thyroid hormone dependence is most marked during the first
ten days of life and rapidly decreases thereafter. The depression

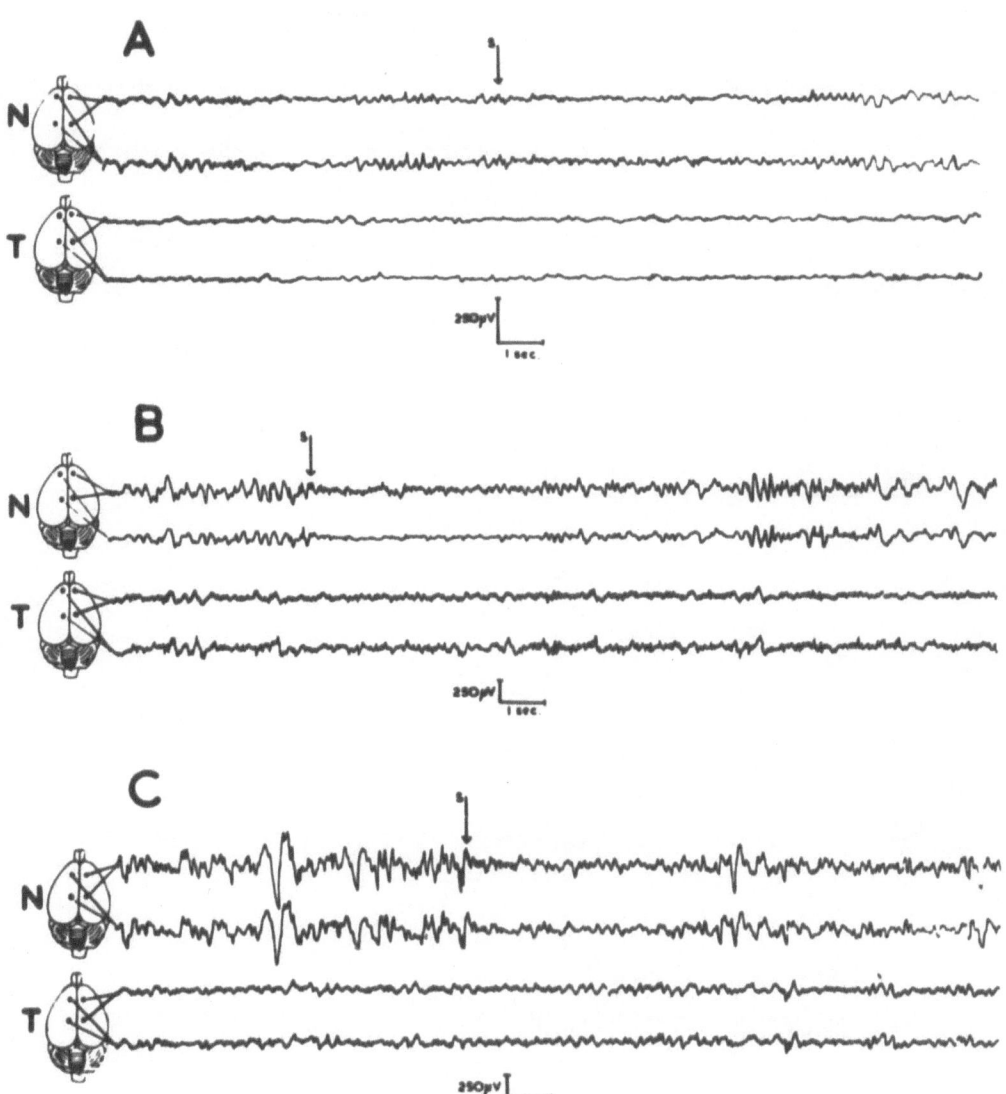

Fig. 6. EEG recordings made from normal (N) and hypothyroid (T) rats
at 15 days (A), 18 days (B) and 24 days (C) of age. S indicated when
an alerting auditory stimulus was applied. The animals were thyroidectomized at birth by radiothyroidectomy with 150-200 μc ^{131}I. Note
the maturation of the EEG during the period between 15 and 24 days
in controls in contrast to the very slight changes occurring in the
hypothyroid animals. (From Bradley et al., 1960, Fig. 2).

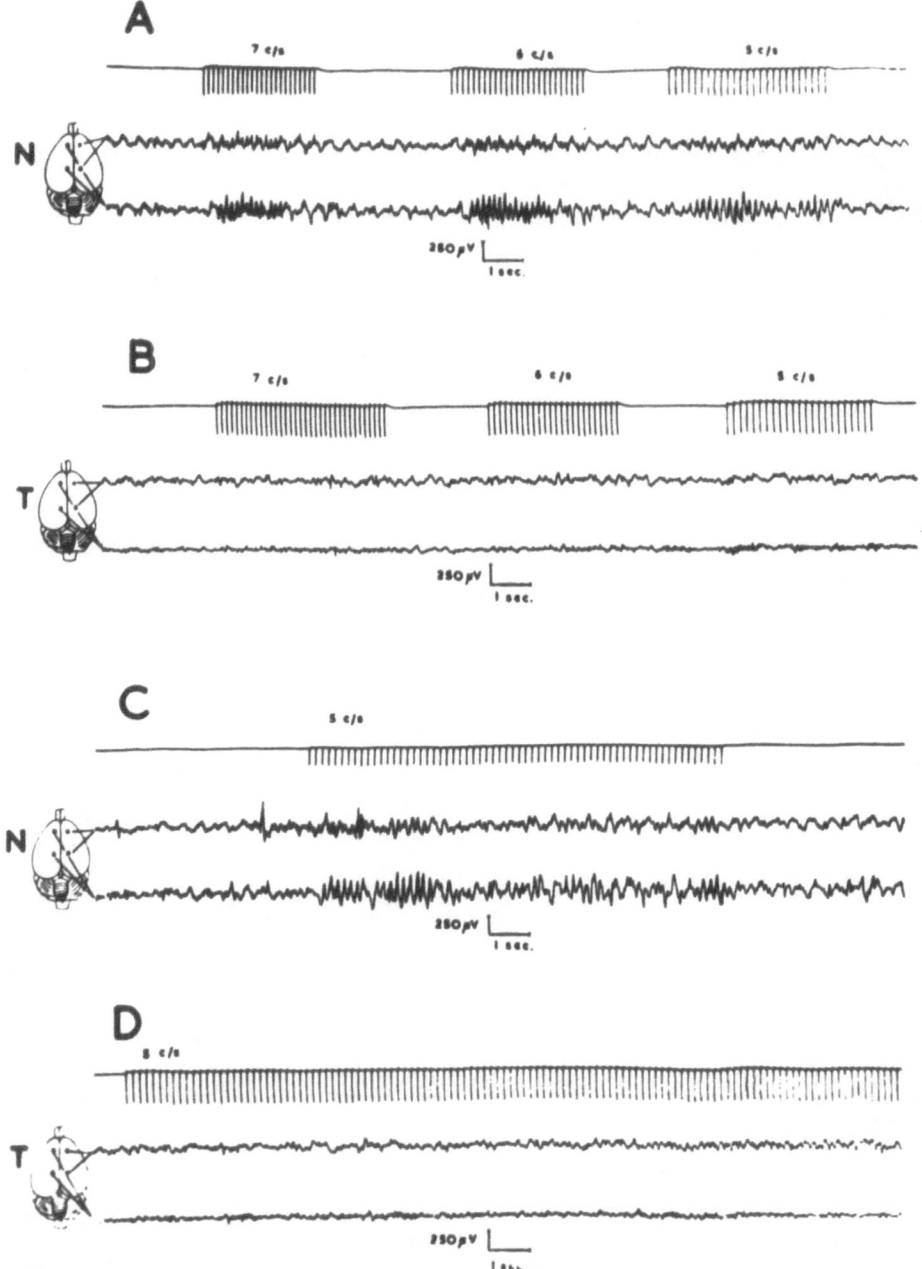

Fig. 7. EEG recordings made from normal (N) and hypothyroid (T) rats
exposed to rhythmic photic stimuli. The top tracing in each record
is that of the photocell recording the times of stimulation. The
record in D shows the appearance of a low amplitude response in the
cretin after prolonged stimulation. Rats were 48 days old and radio-
thyroidectomized at birth (From Bradley et al., 1960, Fig. 4).

in neuronal growth is further associated with a decrease in the activity of the EEG detected in the rat cerebral cortex (Bradley et al.,
1960; Figs. 6 and 7). A defect in the electrical activity has also
been reported by Hatotani and Timiras (1967) for the transcallosal
response in the rat. Hypothyroidism increased the peak latency period,
increased the duration of the wave response, increased the threshold
and decreased the amplitude of the response. Hyperthyroidism had an
essentially opposite though less marked effect. Further, thyroid
hormone treatment of neonates has been observed to accelerate the
development of innately organized behavior and the formation of dendritic spines (Eayrs, 1968) and the electrophysiological activity of
neurons.

The thyroid state of neonatal animals also influences RNA metabolism (Geel and Valcana, 1971) which was clearly depressed in hypothyroidism (Pasquini et al., 1967). Neonatal hypothyroidism decreases
acetylcholinesterase (AChE) and choline acetyltransferase activity
in the cerebral cortex and AChE in the hypothalamus (Geel and Timiras,
1967; Valcana, 1971). Valcana (1971) further notes that the depression
of enzyme activity varies with the subcellular fraction studied and
the maturational state of the animal. Other enzymes, such as aspartate aminotransferase, succinic dehydrogenase, glutamic acid decarboxylase, GABA transaminase and Na^+-K^+ ATPase are also depressed in
hypothyroid animals (Pasquini et al., 1967; Garcia Argiz et al., 1967;
Hamburgh and Flexner, 1957; Balázs et al., 1968; Balázs, 1970). Glutamate dehydrogenase is, however, much less affected, whereas aldo-
lase and cytochrome oxidase are not affected (Hamburgh and Flexner,
1957). These findings suggest that the effect of thyroid hormone on
the synthesis of enzymes in the developing mammalian brain is somewhat selective, not influencing all facets of protein synthesis
equally. Such a conclusion may well be related to the observation of
Patel and Balázs (1971) that even though changes in the thyroid state
have little effect on the developmental changes in brain amino acids,
they may markedly effect metabolic compartmentation, which is advanced by treatment with T_3.

Other aspects of thyroid hormone influence on the developing
brain have been amply reviewed by Hamburgh (1969). Of particular
interest is the observation by his group that thyroid hormone stimulates myelinogenesis of cerebellar explants in culture. In his
review, Hamburgh discusses a role for thyroid hormone which is somewhat different from that of a simple direct stimulus of protein and
RNA synthesis. As a result of his and other studies (Balázs et al.,
1971a, 1971b; Kovacs et al., 1969) the concept emerges that thyroid hormones play a significant role in stimulating the conversion of neurons
from the proliferative phase of development to the differentiative phase.
Excess thyroid hormone (T_3) accelerates this process as well as the
development of innately organized behavior; however, when such animals mature, their performance in adaptive behavior testing situations
is depressed (Eayrs, 1968). While it is not clear as yet how thyroid

hormones produce their effects, to conclude that it is achieved by
stimulating protein synthesis seems an oversimplification. They could
possibly act at the level of the DNA code by repression or derepression
of the genes coding for various types of proteins (i.e. enzymes) which
then themselves would be capable of exerting an effect on the growth
and differentiation of neurons (Villee and Fujii, 1969; Tata, 1965,
1966, 1971). In this context, current ideas relating to cyclic AMP
and adenyl cyclase in mediating hormone-target interaction may also
be relevant (Robinson et al., 1968; Sutherland et al., 1965).

To conclude, a review of the literature clearly illustrates that
in all the animal forms thus far studied, thyroid hormones exert
powerful influences on the proliferation of neurons and glia, and on
their subsequent maturation into functional systems. How this action
is mediated is as yet uncertain, although RNA and protein synthesis
appear to be important endpoints in the process. In view of the data
suggesting that other hormones act at the level of the nucleus, possibly affecting the manner in which the DNA code is interpreted, it
seems possible that thyroid hormone might also utilize a similar path.

ACKNOWLEDGMENTS

The author would like to express his appreciation for the tire-
less assistance of Mr. Ralph K. Rhines, whose dedicated labors have
made possible much of the work emanating from this laboratory.

This work has been supported in part by a U.S. Public Health
Service Research Grant (NB 04568 for 8 years) and by a Research
Contract with the Physiology Branch of the Office of Naval Research
(NONR 4018 (00)).

REFERENCES

Allen, B.M., 1924, Brain development in anuran larvae after thyroid or
    pituitary gland removal, Endocrinology 8: 639.

Garcia Argiz, C.A., Pasquini, J.M., Kaplún, B. and Gómez, C., 1967,
    Hormonal regulation of brain development. II. Effect of neonatal
    thyroidectomy on succinate dehydrogenase and other enzymes in
    developing cerebral cortex and cerebellum of the rat, Brain Res.
    6: 635.

Balázs, R., 1970, Carbohydrate metabolism. In: "Handbook of Neuro-
    chemistry", Vol. 3, (Lajtha, ed.), Plenum Press, New York.

Balázs, R., Kovacs, S., Teichgraber, P., Cocks, P. and Eayrs, J.T.,
    1968, Biochemical effects of thyroid deficiency on the develop-
    ing brain, J. Neurochem. 15: 1335.

Balázs, R., Cocks, W.A., Eayrs, J.T. and Kovacs, S., 1971a, Biochemical effects of thyroid hormones on the developing brain. In: "Hormones in Development", (Hamburgh and Barrington, eds.), Appleton-Century-Crofts, New York.

Balázs, R., Kovacs, S., Cocks, W.A., Johnson, A.L. and Eayrs, J.T., 1971b, Effect of thyroid hormone on the biochemical maturation of rat brain: Postnatal cell formation, Brain Res. 25: 555.

Barron, K.D. and Tuncbay, T.O., 1964, Phosphatase histochemistry of feline cervical spinal cord after brachial plexectomy, J. Neuropathol. Expt. Neurol. 23: 368.

Beach, F.A., 1952, Mechanisms of hormone action upon behavior, Ciba Foundation Colloq. Endocrinol. 3: 209.

Bleeker, M.L., 1971, Accumulation of ^{131}I-1-triiodothyronine in the rat brain: Effect of age, sex and castration, Thesis dissertation, Downstate Medical Center, Brooklyn.

Bleeker, M.L., Ford, D.H. and Rhines, R.K., 1971, Accumulation of ^{131}I-1-triiodothyronine in the rat brain: Effect of age and sex. In: "Influence of Hormones on the Nervous System", (Ford, ed.), S. Karger, Basel.

Bradley, P.B., Eayrs, J.T. and Schmalback, K., 1960, The electroencephalogram of normal and hypothyroid rats, Electroenceph. Clin. Neurophysiol. 12: 467.

Brown-Sequard, de M., 1889, Des effects produits chez l'homme par des injections sous-cutanees d'un liquide retire testicules frais de cobaye et de chien, C.R. Soc. Biol. (Paris) 41: 415.

Cocks, J.A., Balázs, R., Johnson, A.L. and Eayrs, J.T., 1970, Effect of thyroid hormone on the biochemical maturation of rat brain: Conversion of glucose-carbon into amino acids, J. Neurochem. 17: 1275.

Cohan, S., Ford, D.H. and Rhines, R.K., 1967, The effect of age on the uptake and degradation of thyroid hormone by the brain and skeletal muscle, Acta Neurol. Scandinav. 43: 11.

Cohan, S., Ford, D.H., Rhines, R.K. and Thompson, D., 1969, The effect of neonatal X-irradiation in the accumulation and degradation of ^{131}I-1-triiodothyronine in the maturing rat central nervous system, Acta Neurol. Scandinav. 45: 129.

Courrier, R., Horeau, A., Marois, M. and Morel, F., 1949, Etude quantitative de la penetration de la radiothyroxine dans les cellules hypophysaires, Compt. Rend. Soc. Biol. 143: 935.

Eayrs, J.T., 1953, Hormones and the maturation of the central nervous system with special reference to the rat, Brit. J. Animal Behavior 1: 144.

Eayrs, J.T., 1955, The cerebral cortex of normal and hypothyroid rats, Acta Anat. 25: 160.

Eayrs, J.T., 1960, Influence of thyroid hormone on the central nervous system, Brit. Med. Bull. 16: 122.

Eayrs, J.T., 1961, Age as a factor determining the severity and reversibility of the effects of thyroid deprivation in the rats, J. Endocrinol. 22: 409.

Eayrs, J.T., 1964, Endocrine influence on cerebral development, Arch. Biol. 75: 529.

Eayrs, J.T., 1968, Developmental relationships between brain and thyroid. In: "Endocrinology and Human Behaviour", (Michael, ed.), Oxford University Press, London.

Eayrs, J.T. and Goodhead, B., 1959, Postnatal development of the cerebral cortex in the rat, J. Anat. 93: 385.

Eayrs, J.T. and Horn, G., 1955, The development of the cerebral cortex of hypothyroid and starved rats, Anat. Rec. 121: 53.

Eayrs, J.T. and Taylor, S.H., 1951, Effect of thyroid deficiency induced by methyl thiouracil on the maturation of the central nervous system, J. Anat. 85: 350.

Fish, I. and Winick, M., 1969, Cellular growth in various regions of the developing rat brain, Pediat. Res. 3: 407.

Ford, D.H., 1961, The effect of hyperthyroidism on the uptake of I^{131}-labelled triiodothyronine by the brain and pituitary of the male rat, Gen. Comp. Endocr. 1: 59.

Ford, D.H. and Cohan, G., 1968, Changes in weight and volume of the rat spinal cord motor neurons with increasing age, Acta Anat. 7: 311.

Ford, D.H. and Gross, J., 1958a, The metabolism of I^{131}-labelled thyroid hormones in the hypothesis and brain of the rabbit, Endocrinology 62: 416.

Ford, D.H. and Gross, J., 1958b, The localization of I^{131}-labelled triiodothyronine and thyroxine in the pituitary and brain of the male guinea pig, Endocrinology 63: 549.

Ford, D.H. and Rhines, R.K., 1967, Accumulation of ^{131}I-triiodothyro-nine in neurons and other tissues following intravenous inject-ion of the labelled hormone, Brain Res. 6: 481.

Ford, D.H. and Rhines, R.K., 1969, ^{3}H-lysine accumulation in spinal cord grey matter and central horn montoneurons in the rat as related to age and neuronal cytoplasmic volume, Acta Neurol. Scandinav. 45: 529.

Ford, D.H. and Rhines, R.K., 1970, Effect of age on the accumulation of ^{131}I-triiodothyronine in male and female rat brains and other tissues, Brain Res. 21: 265.

Ford, D.H., Kantounis, S. and Lawrence, R., 1959, The localization of I[131]-labelled triiodothyronine in the pituitary and brain of normal and thyroidectomized male rats, Endocrinology, 64: 977.

Ford, D.H., Fishmap, S.K. and Rhines, R.K., 1962, The uptake of I[131]-labelled-1-triiodothyronine by the brain, pituitary and muscle of diestrous and estrous female rats as compared with the uptake in male rats, Gen. Comp. Endocrinol. 2: 480.

Ford, D.H., Hartstein, M. and Rhines, R., 1964, Further studies on differences in the uptake of ^{131}I-triiodothyronine in the brains of male and female rats, Acta Endocrinol. 45: 219.

Ford, D.H., Rhines, R., Hartstein, M. and Rhodes, A., 1965, The up-take of DL-lysine-H[3] into the nervous system as compared with other tissues in euthyroid and dysthroidal male rats, Acta Neurol. Scandinav. 41: 215.

Geel, S.E. and Timiras, P.S., 1967, Influence of neonatal hypothyroid-ism and of thyroxine on the acetylcholinesterase and cholin-esterase activities in the developing central nervous system of the rat, Endocrinology 80: 1069.

Geel, S.E. and Valcana, T., 1971, Cerebral RNA metabolism and thyroid function in early life. In: "Influence of Hormones on the Nervous System", (Ford, ed.), S. Karger, Basel.

Hamburgh, M., 1969, The role of thyroid hormone and growth hormone in neurogenesis, Curr. Top. Dev. Biol. 4: 109.

Hamburgh, M. and Flexner, L.B., 1957, Biochemical and physiological differentiation during morphogenesis. XXI. Effect of hypothyroid-ism and hormone therapy on enzyme activities of the developing cerebral cortex of the rat, J. Neurochem. 1: 279.

Hatotani, N. and Timiras, P.S., 1967, Influence of thyroid function on the postnatal development of the transcallosal response in the rat, Neuroendocrinology 2: 147.

Himwich, H.E., Daly, C., Fazekas, J.F. and Herrlich, H.C., 1942, Effect of thyroid medication on brain metabolism in cretins, Amer. J. Psychiat. 98: 489.

Jensen, J.M. and Clark, D.E., 1951, Location of radioactive 1-thyroxine in the neurohypophysis, J. Lab. and Clin. Med. 38: 663.

Kollros, J.J., 1943, Experimental studies on the development of the corneal reflex in amphibia. II. Localized maturation of the reflex mechanisms effected by thyroxine-agar implants in the hindbrain, Physiol. Zool. 16: 269.

Kollros, J.J., 1957, Influence of thiourea on the growth of cells in the midbrain of frogs, Proc. Soc. Exptl. Biol. & Med. 95: 138.

Kollros, J.J., 1958, Hormonal control of onset of corneal reflex in the frog, Science 128: 1505.

Kollros, J.J. and McMurray, V.M., 1956, The mesencephalic V nucleus in anurans. II. The influence of thyroid hormone on cell size and cell number, J. Exptl. Zool. 131: 1.

Kovacs, S., Cocks, W.A. and Balázs, R., 1969, Incorporation of (2-^{14}C) thyrmidine into deoxyribonucleic acid of rat brain during postnatal development: Effect of thyroid hormone, Biochem. J. 114: 60.

Legrand, J., 1967a, Analyse de l'action morphogenetique des hormones thyroidiennes sur le cervelet du jeune rat, Arch. d'Anat. Morph. Exptl. 56: 205.

Legrand, J., 1967b, Variations en fonction de l'age, de la response du cervalet a l'action morphogenetique de la thyroide chez le rat, Arch. d'Anat. Microscop. 56: 291.

Madison, L., Sensenback, W. and Ochs, L., 1957, Effect of hyperthyroidism and myxedema upon the cerebral blood flow and metabolism, Amer. J. Med. 11: 246.

Pasquini, J.M., Kaplun, B., Garcia, C.A. and Gomez, C.J., 1967, Hormonal regulation of brain development. I. The effect of neonatal thyroidectomy upon nucleic acids, protein and two enzymes in the developing cerebral cortex and cerebellum, Brain Res. 6: 621.

Patel, A.J. and Balázs, R., 1971, Effect of thyroid hormone on metabolic compartmentation in the developing rat brain, Biochem. J. 121: 469.

Paul, E., 1967, Über die Typen der Ependymzellen und ihre regionale Vertielung bei Rana temporaria L. Mit Bemerkungen über die Tanycytenglia, Z. Zellforsch. Mikroskop. Anat. 80: 461.

Pesetsky, I., 1962, The thyroxine stimulated enlargement of Mauthner's neurons in anurans, Gen. Comp. Endocrinol. 2: 229.

Pesetsky, I., 1965, Thyroxine stimulated oxidative enzyme activity associated with precocious brain maturation in anurans. A histochemical study, Gen. Comp. Endocrinol. 5: 411.

Pesetsky, I., 1969, Altered thyroid state and change in nucleoside phosphtase activity in ependymoglial cells of anuran amphibians, Gen. Comp. Endocrinol. 2: 238.

Pesetsky, I., 1971, The role of thyroid hormone in neurogenesis: glial activity following alteration in thyroid state. In: "Influence of Hormones on the Nervous System", (Ford, ed.), S. Karger, Basel.

Pesetsky, I. and Kollros, J.J., 1956, A comparison of the influence of locally applied thyroxine upon Mauthner's cells and adjacent neurons, Exptl. Cell Research 11: 477.

Peterson, N.A., Nataf, B.M., Chaikoff, I.L. and Ragupathy, E., 1966, Uptake of injected ^{131}I-labelled thyroxine, triiodothyronine and iodide by rat brain during various stages of development, J. Neurochem. 13: 933.

Robbins, J. and Rall, J.E., 1960, Proteins associated with the thyroid hormone, Physiol Rev. 40: 415.

Robinson, G.A., Butcher, R.W. and Sutherland, E.W., 1968, Cyclic AMP, Ann. Rev. Biochem. 37: 149.

Scheinberg, P., Stead, F.A.J., Brannan, E.S. and Warren, J.V., 1950, Correlative observations on cerebral metabolism and cardiac output in myxedema, J. Clin. Invest. 29: 1139.

Schittenhelm, A. and Eisler, B., 1932, Thyroxine und Zentral nervensystem, Klin. Wchnschr. 11: 9.

Schonbach, J., Hu, K.H. and Friede, R., 1968, Cellular and chemical changes during myelination: Histologic, autoradiographic, histochemical and biochemical data on myelination in the pyramidal tract and corpus callosum of rat, J. Comp. Neurol. 134: 21.

Sensenbach, W., Madison, L., Eisenberg, S. and Ochs, L., 1954, Cerebral circulation and metabolism in hyperthyroidism and myxedema, J. Clin. Invest. 33: 1434.

Sjöstrand, J., 1966, Changes of nucleoside phosphatase activity in the hypoglossal nucleus during nerve regeneration, Acta Physiol. Scandinav. 67: 219.

Sokoloff, L. and Roberts, P., 1971, Biochemical mechanisms of action of thyroid hormones on nervous and other tissues. In: "Influence of Hormones on the Nervous System", (Ford, ed.), S. Karger, Basel.

Sokoloff, L., Wechsler, R.V., Mangold, R., Balls, K. and Kety, S.S., 1953, Cerebral blood flow and oxygen consumption in hyperthyroidism before and after treatment, J. Clin. Invest. 32: 202.

Sutherland, E.A., Oye, I. and Butcher, R.W., 1965, Action of epinephrine and the role of adenyl cyclase in hormone action, Recent Prog. Hormone Res. 21: 623.

Tata, J.R., 1964, Distribution and metabolism of thyroid hormones. In: "The Thyroid Gland", (Pitts-Rivers, ed.), Butterworth, London.

Tata, J.R., 1965, Turnover of nuclear and cytoplasmic ribonucleic acid at the onset of induced amphibian metamorphosis, Nature 207: 378.

Tata, J.R., 1966, Requirement for RNA and protein synthesis for induced regression of the tadpole tail in organ culture, Develop. Biol. 13: 77.

Tata, J.R., 1971, Cell structure and biosynthesis during hormone-mediated growth and development. In "Hormones in Development", (Hamburgh and Barrington, eds.), Appleton-Century-Crofts, New York.

Torack, R.M. and Barrnett, R.J., 1963, Nucleoside phosphatase activity in membranous fine structures of neurons and glia, J. Histochem. Cytochem. 11: 763.

Valcana, T., 1971, Effect of neonatal hypothyroidism on the development of acetylcholinesterase and choline acetyltransferase activities in the rat brain. In: "Influence of Hormones on the Nervous System", (Ford. ed.), S. Karger, Basel.

Villee, C.A. and Fujii, T, 1971, Growth of seminal vesicle and
    prostrate: Role of RNA following testosterone stimulation.
    In: "Hormones in Development", (Hamburgh and Barrington, eds.),
    Appleton-Century -Crofts, New York.

Weiss, P. and Rossetti, F., 1951, Growth responses of opposite sign
    among different neuron types exposed to thyroid hormones, <u>Proc.
    Natl. Acad. Sci.</u> 37: 540.

Yonezawa, T., Bornstein, M.B., Peterson, M.A. and Murray, M.R., 1962,
    A histochemical study of oxidative enzymes in myelinating cul-
    tures of central and peripheral nervous tissues, <u>J. Neuropath.
    Exptl. Neurol.</u> 21: 479.

THERAPEUTICS
J. Gordon Millichap, Chairman

NEUROPHARMACOLOGY OF HYPERKINETIC BEHAVIOR: RESPONSE TO METHYL-

PHENIDATE CORRELATED WITH DEGREE OF ACTIVITY AND BRAIN DAMAGE

J. Gordon Millichap

Departments of Neurology and Pediatrics, Northwestern

University Medical School, Chicago, Illinois

Neurological mechanisms of hyperkinesia are not completely understood. Diffuse brain lesions are thought to be a major cause of a
large percentage of clinical cases of hyperactive behavior (Strauss
and Lehtinen, 1947). In a recent study (Millichap et al., 1968) on
hyperkinesia in children, fifty-seven per cent of the patients had
a history of brain injury or other cerebral damage, and all but one
patient had neurological signs of minimal brain dysfunction. In certain cases where the diagnosis of brain damage may be uncertain, other
etiological factors such as delayed maturation of the brain and psychogenic disorders have been invoked (Eisenberg, 1964). In many
patients the hyperactivity may be controlled and learning disabilities
benefited by various drugs (Millichap and Fowler, 1967), and central
nervous system stimulants such as methylphenidate (Ritalin) and dextroamphetamine (Dexedrine) are most effective. In contrast, phenobarbital has an excitant effect (Millichap and Millichap, 1966) and is
contraindicated in the treatment of hyperactive behavior. The paradoxical calming effect of stimulants on hyperactive children has not
been fully explained and the present clinical and laboratory studies
were designed to investigate the relation of the degree of activity
and brain damage to the drug response and to develop an experimental
model for the development of new pharmacological therapies for hyperactivity.

Experimental neuroanatomical studies of hyperkinesia have been
concerned with the effects of destruction of different cortical and
subcortical structures on locomotor activity. Bilateral removal of
the prefrontal and frontal areas in the monkey causes the greatest
total increase in activity (Kennard et al., 1941). Lesions in Walker's
area 13 of the orbital surface produce, for any single cortical area,
the most extreme degree of hypermotility (Ruch and Shenkin, 1943;

475

Livingston et al., 1948). Parietal lobe lesions in both the monkey
(Mettler, 1967) and rat (Beach, 1941) can result in hyperactivity,
but this is not as marked as in frontal lobe lesions. Destruction
of subcortical structures, such as the striatum (Davis, 1958), inter-
penduncular nucleus (Bailey and Davis, 1942), and parts of the hypothalamus (Maire and Patton, 1954; Wheatley, 1944) can induce hyperactivity. These experimental findings are of importance in understanding the clinical observation that diffuse brain damage is of
significance in the etiology of hyperkinesis in children.

METHODS AND RESULTS

Clinical Studies

Methods. Twenty-eight children, 5 to 14 years of age, were
evaluated because of hyperactive behavior and associated learning
disabilities. Twenty-four patients were male and four were female.
A history of brain injury or other cerebral damage was obtained in
17 (61%) patients, and the electroencephalogram was abnormal in 14
(50%). The neurological signs of minimal brain dysfunction and their
frequency (shown in parentheses) were as follows: impairment of rapid
alternating movements of forearms (13); impaired finger tapping (11);
dyspraxic tandem gait (9); cortical sensory loss, mainly graphanes-
thesia (9); impaired hopping (7); finger-to-nose incoordination (6);
Babinski signs (6); speech disorder (4); involuntary movements, mainly
choreiform, when arms are held in outstretched posture (4).

The degree of motor restlessness and hypermotility was measured
by an actometer, a method shown to be reliable in studies of drug
effects on motor activity (Schulman and Reisman, 1959; Millichap and
Boldrey, 1967). The instrument consists of an automatically winding
calendar wrist watch with the pendulum attached directly to the hands
of the watch. The pendulum rotates in a plane parallel to the face,
and movements with a component at right angles to this plane are recorded. The actometer was worn on the wrist of the nondominant arm
during the 45-minute test periods, and the activity was measured in
units of hours and minutes. The effect of methylphenidate on motor
activity was evaluated using double-blind technique and random allo-
cation of patients to drug treatment or placebo groups. The tablets
of methylphenidate and the placebo were indistinguishable. The subjects were divided into two groups, one received the placebo, the
other methylphenidate according to a system of random permutations.
After three weeks of the initial medication a cross-over design was
employed and the alternate medication was given for another three-
week period in the same dosage schedule as the first course of treatment. The initial daily dose of each medication was 0.5 mg/kg body
weight given in two equal divided amounts after breakfast and lunch;

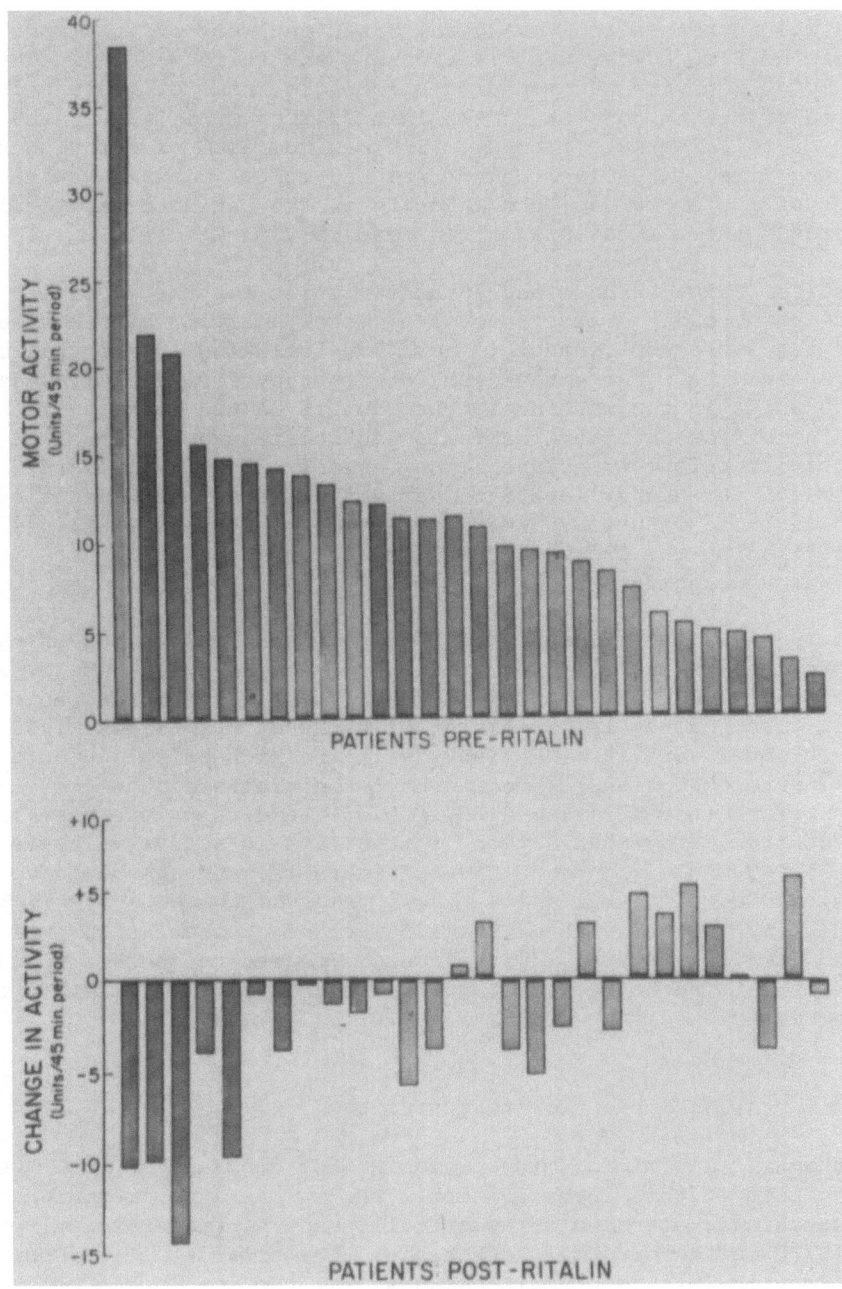

Fig. 1. Motor activity of 28 patients before treatment with methylphenidate correlated with the change in activity after treatment.

the dose was increased to 1 mg/kg/day after one week of treatment
and a dose of 2 mg/kg/day was given during the third week. The degree of motor activity was measured before the trial of medication,
at the end of the third week of the initial treatment, and on the
last day of the alternate therapy. The maximum dose of methylphenidate at the time of testing ranged from 0.3 to 2.0 mg/kg/day with a
mean dose of 1.5 mg/kg/day; the majority of the patients had received
and tolerated the largest prescribed dose of 2 mg/kg daily.

Results. Fig. 1 shows the actometer units for the 28 patients
arranged in the order of their level of motor activity before treatment and the subsequent change in activity following administration
of methylphenidate. The activity before therapy varied from a maximum of 38 units in the most active to 2 units in the least active
child. The effect of methylphenidate was related to the level of
motor activity before treatment; a depressant effect was recorded in
patients with the higher levels of activity whereas a stimulant effect
occurred in those with lower activity levels. Nineteen (68%) patients
were benefited by the drugs; 8 (28%) showed an increase in activity
and one was unchanged.

Fig. 2 shows the frequency of abnormal neurologic signs in patients arranged as in Fig. 1, according to the pre-treatment level
of activity, in decreasing order from left to right; the degree of
neurologic abnormality is correlated with the methylpheidate-induced
changes in motor activity. Patients with the highest incidence of
abnormal neurologic signs tended to have the greatest degree of motor
activity before therapy (r, + 0.38; P<0.05), and they were most likely
to benefit from methylphenidate by a reduction in activity levels
(r, -0.59; P<0.005). In responsive patients the average number of
neurologic abnormalities was 3.4 ± 0.42, whereas in the subjects made
more active by the drug, the average number of abnormal signs was
$1.0 \pm .69$ (t=3.15; P<0.01). The placebo appeared to cause a reduction
in activity but the degree of change was significantly less than that
following methylphenidate (t =5.45; P<.01).

Laboratory Studies

Methods. Male albino mice, weighing 20-38 gm and 10 to 20 weeks
old, were used in this investigation. Thirty-one experimental animals
were successfully operated on aseptically under intraperitoneal pentobarbital (60 mg/kg) or ether anesthesia. The prefrontal lesions were
made by suction through a small cannula. At the conclusion of the
experiments the animals were sacrificed by a lethal dose of pentobarbital; the brains were removed, fixed in formalin and preserved
for macroscopic and microscopic study. The brains were sectioned
and then stained with the Kluver-Barrera combination stain for fibers
and cells of the nervous system. Unilateral prefrontal lestions were

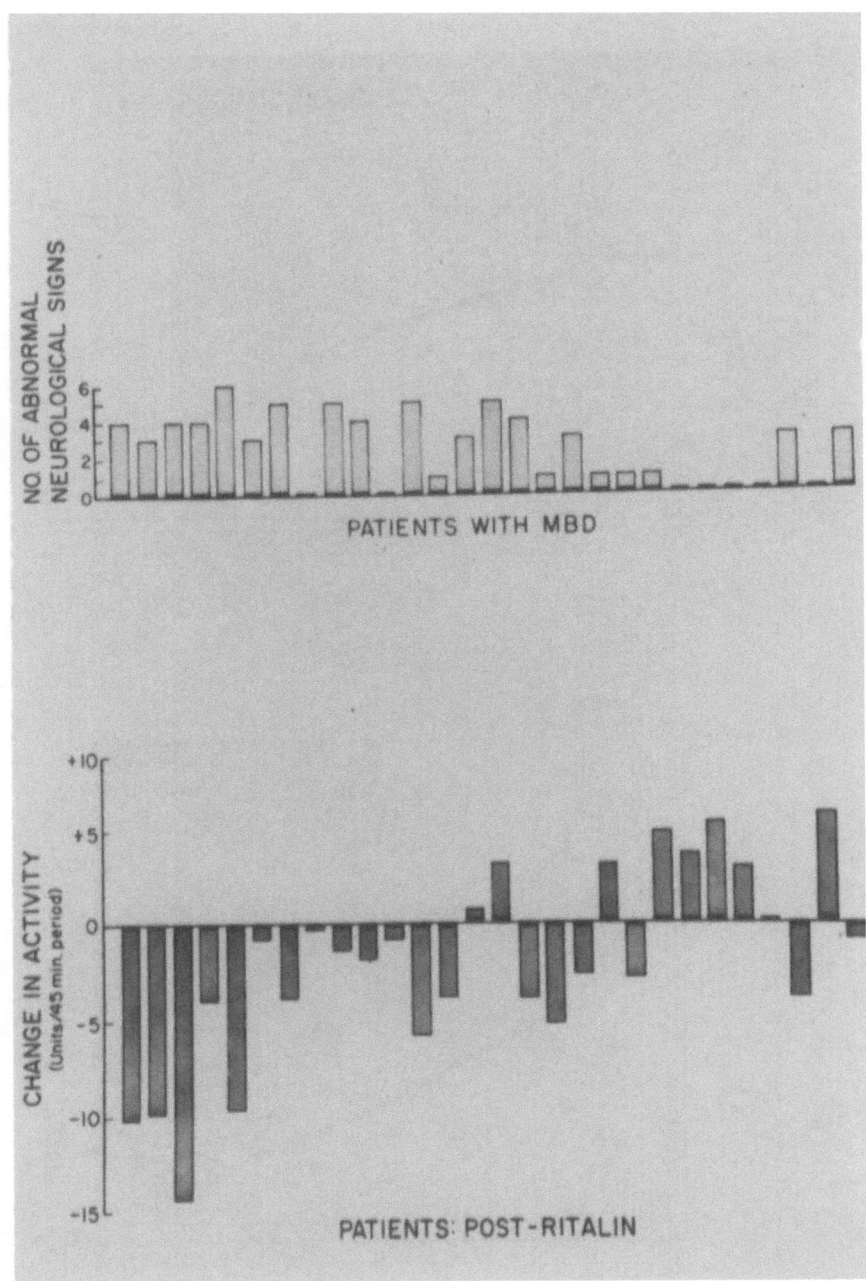

Fig. 2. Number of abnormal neurologic signs in patients arranged in order shown in Fig. 1, and correlated with the change in activity after methylphenidate.

(a)

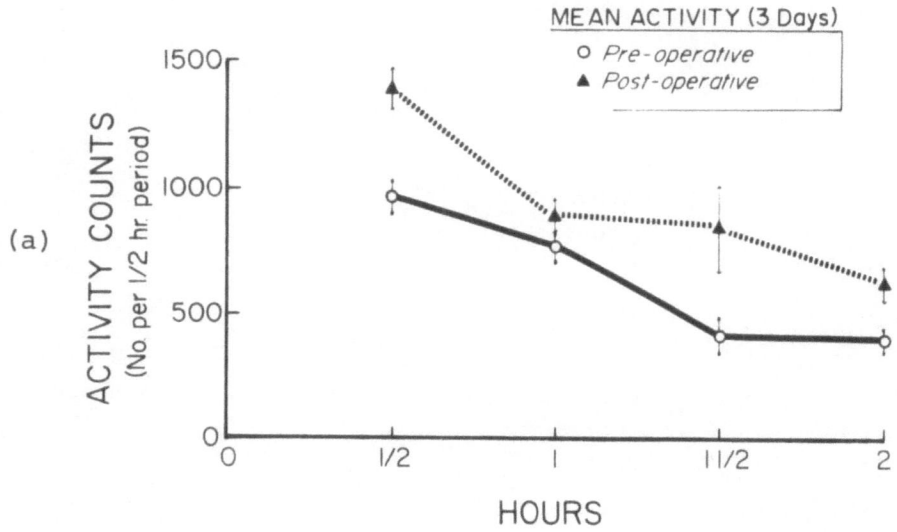

(b)

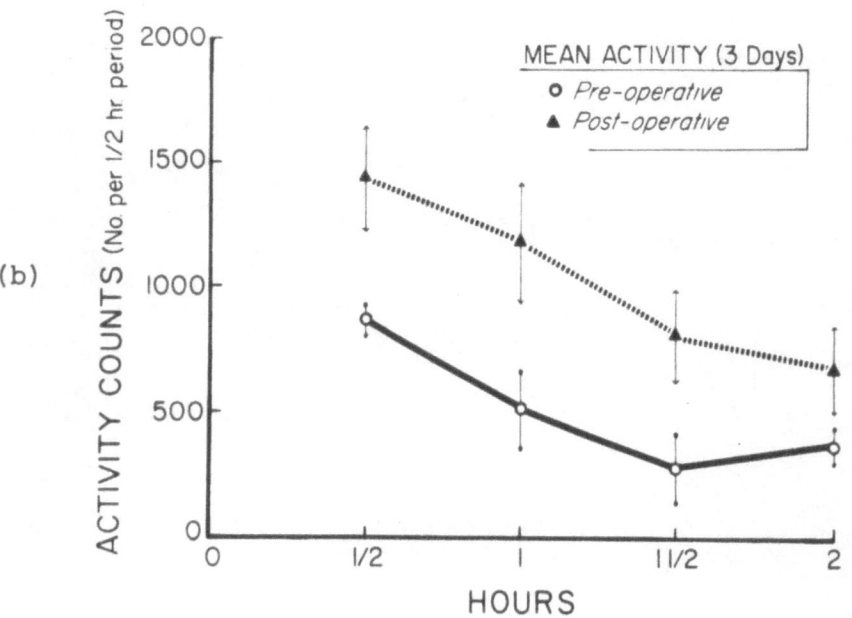

made in twenty-five mice, and bilateral lesions in a one stage operation in six mice. A second operation was carried out on four of the
animals with unilateral lesions at which time the other prefrontal
region was destroyed. Four mice in the unilateral group died after
the pre-operative and post-operative activity levels were determined.

Locomotor activity was measured by means of six activity cages,
the center having a cylinder that serves as the housing for the intra-
red generator which emits beams of light. As the animal moves about
the circular raceway these beams are broken, initiating electrical
impulses which operate the counter automatically. A similar system
of recording has been compared with other methods and has been found
to give an accurate measure of locomotor activity in small animals.
Cumulative readings of total activity were taken during each of four
half-hour periods in the three successive days comprising the pre-
operative, the post-operative, and the post-operative drug period,
for a total of nine days. The mean activity counts and standard
errors of the means were then calculated from the activity measurements on the animals at each half-hour period for the sum of three
day experimental periods and these results were compared. Methylphenidate hydrochloride (Ritalin Hydrochloride) was administered by
the intraperitoneal route to the operated mice in a dose of 25 mg/kg.
The activity counts per half hour for three days at four readings per
day were summed and the means of the animals benefited versus the
animals not benefited by methylphenidate were compared by the Student's
t-test.

Results. Figs. 3a and 3b show the effects of unilateral and bilateral prefrontal cortical lesions, respectively, on the locomotor
activity of mice. An increase in activity was observed following
operation in all except six animals of the unilateral lesion group,
and five of these showed a reduction in activity. Fig. 4 shows (a)
the percentage change in activity following operation and (b) the
effect of methylphenidate on the post-operative activity level in each
animal tested. Six mice with the highest levels of post-operative
activity responded to methylphenidate with a reduction in locomotor
activity, whereas twenty-five mice with lesser degrees of hyperactivity
or hypoactivity following operation were stimulated by methylphenidate.
A somewhat proportional relationship between the degree of post-
operative activity and the effect of methylphenidate was observed.
In animals with greater than 250% increases in activity post-opera-
tively, methylphenidate had a quietening effect, whereas those with

---

Fig. 3. (a) Effect of unilateral prefrontal lesions on locomotor
activity in 25 mice. (b) Effect of bilateral prefrontal lestions
on locomotor activity in 10 mice.

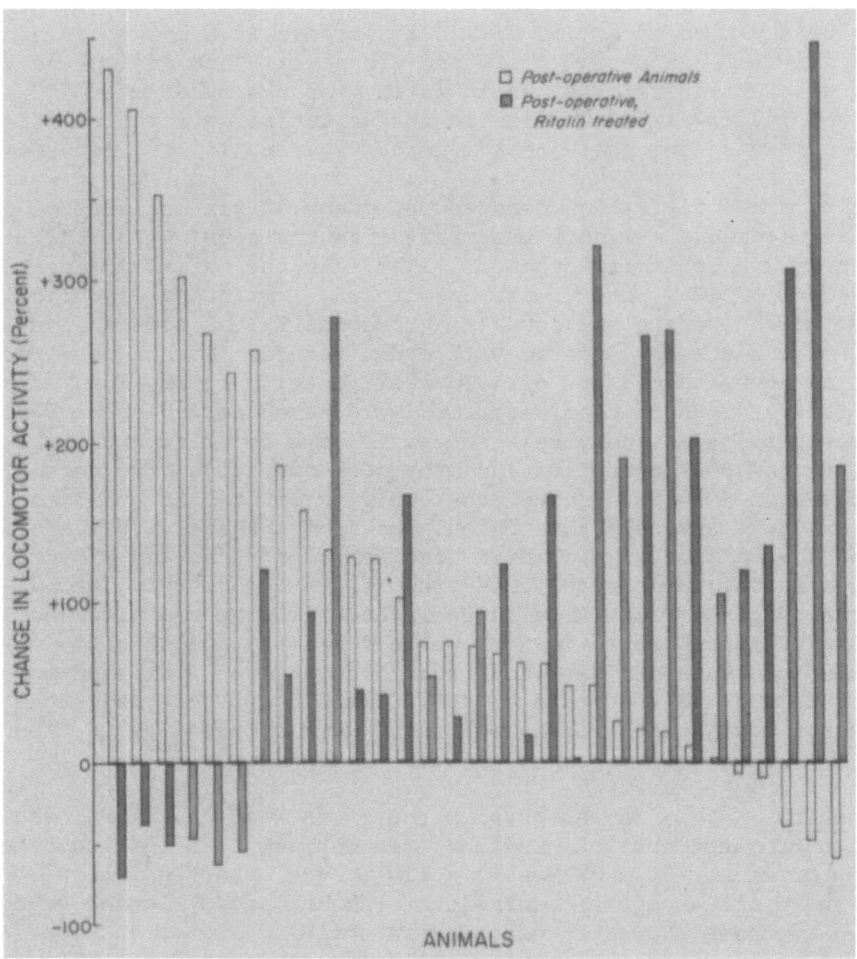

Fig. 4. Change in locomotor activity of 31 mice after prefrontal
lobectomy (unshaded columns) and following treatment with methylphenidate (shaded columns).

activity changes of 75% to 200% and less than 50% showed moderate
and severe degrees of stimulation, respectively, following methylphenidate. Fig. 5a illustrated the reduction in activity following
methylphenidate in the six mice with maximal post-operative activity
levels. Fig. 5b shows the stimulant effect of methylphenidate on
25 mice with low to moderate post-operative activity levels. Table I
compares and contrasts the means of the summed activity counts in
pre-operative, post-operative and post-operative drug treated animals,
grouped according to drug response. There are significant differences
between the activity levels of the two post-operative groups and the
changes following methylphenidate, whereas the activity levels of
the two pre-operative groups of mice were not significantly different.

TABLE I

EFFECTS OF METHYLPHENIDATE (RITALIN) ON HYPERKINETIC BEHAVIOR
INDUCED BY PREFRONTAL LESIONS IN MICE

Response to Ritalin	No. of Animals	Locomotor Activity in Mice[a]		
		Pre-Operative	Post-Operative	Post-Operative Ritalin
Depressant	6	592 ± 52 (<.01)[b]	1932 ± 45 (<.01)[c]	1334 ± 142
		(N.S.)[d]	(<.01)[d]	(<.05)[d]
Stimulant	25	544 ± 29 (<.01)[b]	793 ± 49 (<.01)[c]	1769 ± 69
Total	31	599 ± 28 (<.01)[b]	958 ± 44 (<.01)[c]	1690 ± 61

[a] Mean activity counts ± standard errors per 1/2 hour period.

[b] P values for comparison of pre-operative to post-operative activity.

[c] P values for comparison of post-operative to post-operative drug treated activity.

[d] P values for comparison between same groups.

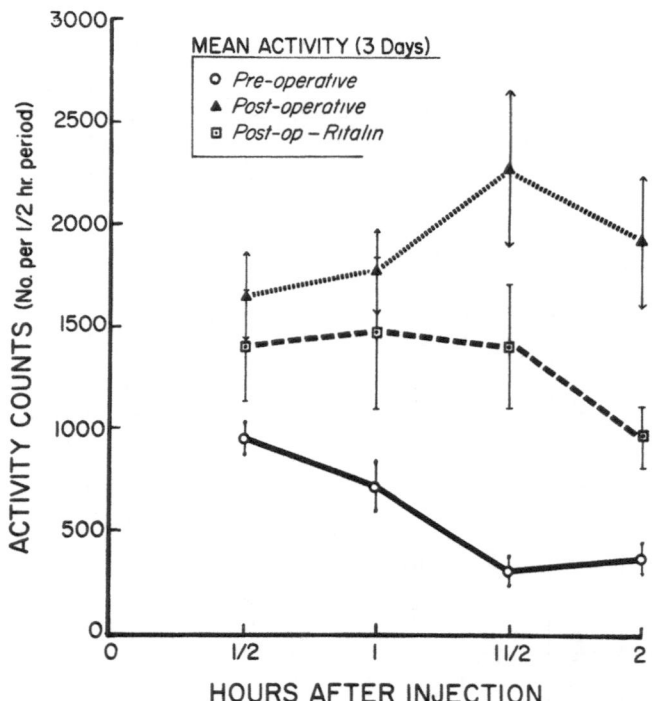

Fig. 5. (a) Effect of methylphenidate in 6 brain-injured mice with maximal post-operative hyperactivity.

DISCUSSION

The central nervous system stimulants, methylphenidate and dextroamphetamine, are the most effective agents presently available for the treatment of children with hyperactivity and minimal brain dysfunction. The results of the present study show a close correlation between the clinical and laboratory evaluations of methylphenidate. The beneficial effect of methylphenidate on hyperactivity is related to the level of motor activity before treatment and the incidence of abnormal neurological signs. Patients with the greatest number of signs of minimal brain dysfunction tend to be the most active and are more likely to benefit from the drug whereas those with lower levels of activity and fewer signs may be unaffected or made worse. The laboratory observations also show that methylphenidate has a depressant effect on the hypermotility of those animals which are the most active following prefrontal brain lesions, and a stimulating action on those with lower activity following operation and in normal

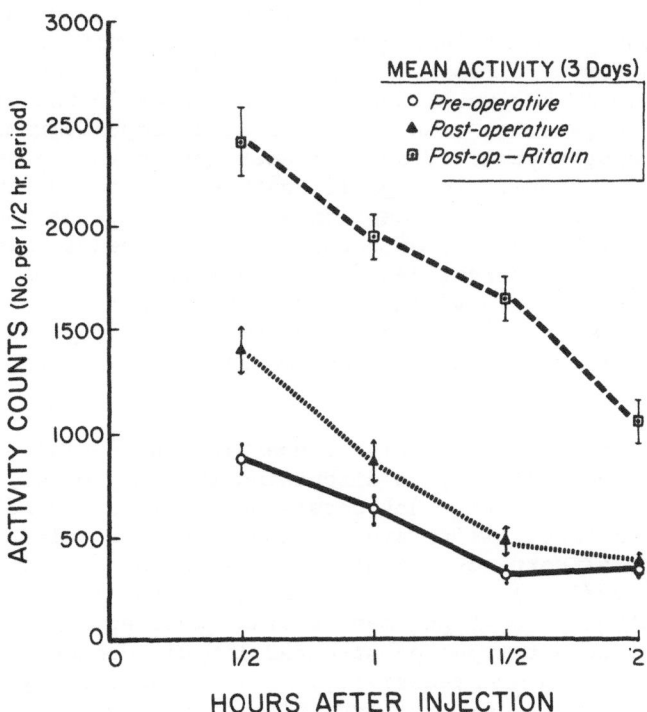

Fig. 5. (b) Effect of methylphenidate in 25 brain-injured mice with minimal post-operative hyperactivity.

---

non-brain-damaged animals. Patients with a relatively high level of motor activity and a high incidence of minimal abnormalities on neurological examination should be selected for treatment with methylphenidate. Animals with prefrontal cerebral lesions are valuable experimental models for the testing of new drugs for potential clinical efficacy against hyperactive behavior.

Drugs with optimal efficacy in the management of minimal brain dysfunction should control hyperactivity, but in addition, learning should be facilitated by effects on attention span, reduction of impulsiveness, and improvements in perception. Drug therapy should be used as an adjunct to remedial education. In a previous clinical study (Millichap et al., 1968), methylphenidate was found to cause a significant improvement in the "Draw-a-Man" test of general intelligence and in the Frostig test of visual perception; auditory perception was not benefited by this central nervous system stimulant. In

a subsequent investigation of the effects of medications on auditory
perception, diphenylhydantoin sodium was found to increase the auditory perception for word memory and recall and this effect was related
to the occurrence of paroxysmal seizure discharges in the electroencephalogram; in patients with normal electroencephalograms or only
mild nonspecific dysrhythmias, auditory perception was unchanged
(Millichap et al., 1969). In a preliminary uncontrolled study of
pemoline (Cylert), auditory perception was improved, but the effect
was unrelated to the presence of paroxysmal electroencephalographic
changes (unpublished observations). The manifestations of minimal
brain dysfunction are diverse and future studies should determine
the specificity of action on visual and auditory perception, reading
ability, coordination, conduct and personality, as well as the effect
on hyperactivity.

There are a number of theories concerning the neural basis of
hyperkinesia. Magoun (1963), in discussing the subject of the inhibition of behavior, states that persistent exploratory behavior
and heightened distractibility are attributable to a release from
frontal or temporal cortico-reticular inhibition of ascending systems.
Mettler's concept (1967) about hyperkinesia is that within the spectrum of hyperactivity two types can be distinguished and correlated
with somewhat different types of structural brain damage. Frontal
lobe injury results in overreactivity, i.e., hyperactivity directly
related to the degree of external stimulation or distractibility.
The other type of hyperkinesia, "essential overactivity", is subdivided into a transient deprivative hyperkinesia which he feels is
due to lesions in the striatum and not to decortication. In this
theory the striatum holds back proprioceptively driven activity by
its outflow to the pallidum, which is the efferent limb of the route
from the thalamus for proprioceptive-associated movement. That the
striatum receives a large system of fiber projections from the frontal
cortex is now a definitive observation and since part of the fronto-
striatal system originates and ends in those areas which, if damaged,
are associated with hyperkinesia, it seems reasonable that both a
structural and functional relationship exists.

One part of the limbic lobe, the orbital frontal region, pro-
jects on the hypothalamus and this system may also be implicated in
the inhibition of behavior since hyperactivity results following its
destruction (Livingston et al., 1948; Maire and Patton, 1954). Primitive motor mechanisms of the visceral brain and olfactory system
have been described, the exploratory or primitive search behavior
being a function of olfaction used for the detection of food. The
experimental work of Bailey and Davis (1942) and Mettler (1967) in
which lesions are placed in the interpeduncular nucleus and habenulo-
peduncular tract resulting in obstinate progression indicates that
the olfacto-habenulo-peduncular system is involved in motility.
Physiological drives have been studied in relationship to activity

as influenced by stimulation by hormones, illumination, temperature
and nutritional requirements, and an internal activity drive, quite
apart from that reaction to any type of stimulation, may also be a
neural basis for abnormal hyperactivity.

One might postulate that the site of action for methylphenidate
is on the inhibitor systems such as the reticular formation, striatum,
cortical regions, or limbic areas and its beneficial effect is produced by stimulation of such inhibitory mechanisms which in turn then
suppress the hyperkinetic behavior. Further studies of experimentally-
induced hyperactivity in animals should be of value both in the elucidation of the mechanism of action and in the development of potential new therapies for hyperactive behavior in children.

ACKNOWLEDGMENT

Dr. F.H. Johnson, Research Associate in the Division of Neurology,
Children's Memorial Hospital, contributed to the laboratory studies.

REFERENCES

Baily, P. and Davis, E.W., 1942, The syndrome of obstinate progression in the cat, Proc. Soc. Exp. Biol. Med. 51: 307.

Beach, F.A., 1941, Effects of Brain lesions upon running activity
in the male rat, J. Comp. Psychol. 31: 145.

Davis, G.D., 1958, Caudate lesions and spontaneous locomotion in
the monkey, Neurology 8: 135.

Eisenberg, L., 1964, Behavioral manifestations of cerebral damage
in childhood, in: "Brain Damage in Children", (Birch, ed.),
Williams & Wilkins, Baltimore.

Kennard, M.A., Spencer, S., and Fountain, G., Jr., 1941, Hyperactivity in monkeys following lesions of the frontal lobes,
J. Neurophysiol. 4: 512.

Livingston, R.B., Fulton, J.F., Delgado, J.M.R., Sachs, E.,
Brendler, S.J. and Davis, G.D., 1948, Stimulation and regional
ablation of orbital surface of frontal lobe, in: "The Frontal
Lobes", Res. Publ. Ass. Nerv. Ment. Dis. 27: 405.

Magoun, H.W., 1963, The Waking Brain, Charles C. Thomas, 2nd ed.

Maire, F.W. and Patton, H.D., 1954, Hyperactivity and pulmonary
edema from rostral hypothalamic lesions in rats, Amer. J.
Physiol. 178: 315.

Millichap, J.G. and Boldrey, E.E., 1967, Studies in hyperkinetic
    behavior. II. Laboratory and clinical evaluations of drug
    treatments, Neurology 17: 467.

Millichap, J.G. and Fowler, G.W.,1967, Treatment of minimal brain
    dysfunction syndromes: Selection of drugs for children with
    hyperactivity and learning disabilities, in: "Pediatric
    Neurology," Ped. Clin. N. Amer. 14: 767.

Millichap, J.G. and Millichap, P.A., 1966, Circadian analysis of
    phenobarbital-induced hyperkinesia in mice and hamsters,
    Proc. Soc. Exp. Biol. Med. 121: 754.

Millichap, J.G., Egan, R.W., Hart, W.H. and Sturgis, L.H., 1969,
    Auditory perceptual deficit correlated with EEG dysrhythmias.
    Response to diphenylhydantoin sodium, Neurology 19: 870.

Millichap, J.G., Aymat, F., Sturgis, L.H., Larsen, K.W. and Egan,
    R.A., 1968, Hyperkinetic behavior and learning disorders. III.
    Battery of neuropsychological tests in controlled trial of
    methlphenidate, Am. J. Dis. Child. 116: 235.

Ruch, T.C. and Shenkin, H.A., 1943, The relation of area 13 on
    orbital surface of frontal lobes to hyperactivity and hyper-
    phagia in monkeys, J. Neurophysiol. 6: 349.

Schulman, J.L. and Reisman, J.M., 1959, An objective measure of
    hyperactivity, Amer. J. Ment. Def. 64: 455.

Strauss, A.A. and Lehtinen, L.E., 1947, Psychopathology and Edu-
    cation of the Brain Injured Child", Grune & Stratton, New
    York.

Wheatley, M.D., 1944, The hypothalamus and affective behavior in
    cats. A study of the effects of experimental lesions, with
    anatomic correlations, Arch. Neurol. Psychiat. 52: 298.

OCCULT MECHANISMS OF BRAIN DYSFUNCTION

John W. Olney

Washington University School of Medicine, Department of

Psychiatry, St. Louis, Missouri

It is clear from Dr. Millichap's presentation that important
advances in the diagnosis and treatment of seizure disorders and minimal brain dysfunction syndromes have been realized in recent years.
Unfortunately, significant progress toward the companion goal of prevention remains seriously hampered by our poor understanding of the
etiology and pathogenesis of these conditions. Genetic factors undoubtedly play at least a predispositional role in many cases, but
the potential contribution of an adverse environment deserves constant emphasis, particularly in that corrective measures are more
easily brought to bear upon the environment than upon the gene.
Dr. Nair, in discussing the toxic effects of drugs upon the developing CNS, touched upon an important theme worth reiterating here;
that, in contrast to the gross malformations which characteristically
result from exposure to toxic agents in early stages of development,
exceedingly subtle forms of brain damage capable of defying current
methods of detection may occur from exposure in later developmental
stages. Dr. Millichap indicated, and I think many would agree, that
the more carefully one examines children with minimal brain dysfunction,
the more convinced one becomes that some sort of subtle brain damage
underlies these conditions. Observations similar to those of Drs.
Nair and Millichap led me to begin studying mechanisms which might
inconspicuously give rise to brain damage in relatively late stages
of development. I shall confine this discussion to certain subtle
types of brain damage which we and others have been able to induce
in experimental animals by exposing infants or late gestation fetuses
to select chemicals which are commonly encountered by the immature
human under ordinary circumstances. Implicit in the title "Occult
Mechanisms of Brain Dysfunction" is the suggestion that the neurotoxic mechanisms we have been examining could underlie human brain
dysfunction syndromes without our being aware of it; whether they

do, in fact, contribute to brain dysfunction in the human is an open
question which has not been adequately explored.

The first compound I shall discuss, glutamic acid (Glu), occurs
in the ordinary diet as a natural constituent of protein. The sodium
salt, monosodium glutamate (MSG) is an extensively used food additive.
Fifteen years ago, Lucas and Newhouse (1957) reported that retinal
ganglion cells rapidly degenerate following subcutaneous administration of MSG to infant mice - a surprising finding in view of the high
concentrations of Glu normally present throughout the mammalian CNS,
including the retina.

From a series of more recent investigations, it is now known
that certain populations of nerve cells in the developing brain are
also destroyed by MSG administration (Olney, 1969; Olney, 1971a;
Burde et al., 1971; Abraham et al., 1971; Everly, 1971; Murakami and
Inouye, 1971; Johnston and Reynolds, 1972); that oral doses in the
range of 0.5 to 1 mg/g body wt are effective in producing such damage
(Olney and Ho, 1970; Olney et al., 1972a; Burde et al., 1971; Abraham
et al., 1971; Johnston and Reynolds, 1972); that lesion formation is
accompanied by selective uptake and accumulation of Glu in the brain
areas where neurons are being destroyed (Perez and Olney, 1972); that
several animal species, including mice (Olney, 1969), rats (Burde
et al., 1971; Everly, 1971), chicks (Snapir, 1971) and rhesus monkeys (Olney and Sharpe, 1969; Olney et al., 1972a) are susceptible
to MSG-induced brain damage and, a point to be emphasized for our
present purposes, that the neurodegenerative reaction to MSG can occur
in the developing brain in the absence of outward signs of distress,
yet give rise later in life to sequelae ranging from obesity and
various neuroendocrine disturbances (Olney, 1969; Knittle and Ginsberg-Feller, 1970; Matsuyan, 1970; Redding et al., 1971) to deficits
in discrimination learning (Pradhan and Lynch, 1972). Further, unless the brain is examined in the acute stages of the degeneration
process it is exceedingly difficult to establish whether brain damage
even occurred (Olney, 1971b). Destroyed neurons are phagocytized and
degeneration products disposed of so efficiently that there are few
traces of the tissue reaction, other than a decreased number of neurons, if examination of the brain is delayed even for a few days
(Olney, 1971a).

One of the very intriguing biological properties of Glu is its
ability to excite neurons when introduced into their surroundings by
the delicate procedure of microelectrophoresis. Curtis and colleagues
(Curtis and Watkins, 1960, 1963) clarified the molecular specificity
of this effect by demonstrating that a select group of acidic amino
acids which are fundamentally similar to Glu in molecular structure,
also excite neurons when administered by microelectrophoresis. These
compounds (glutamic, aspartic, cysteic, cysteine sulfinic, homocysteic
acids and certain of their substituted synthetic congeners) were designated the "neuroexcitatory amino acids". In recent experiments

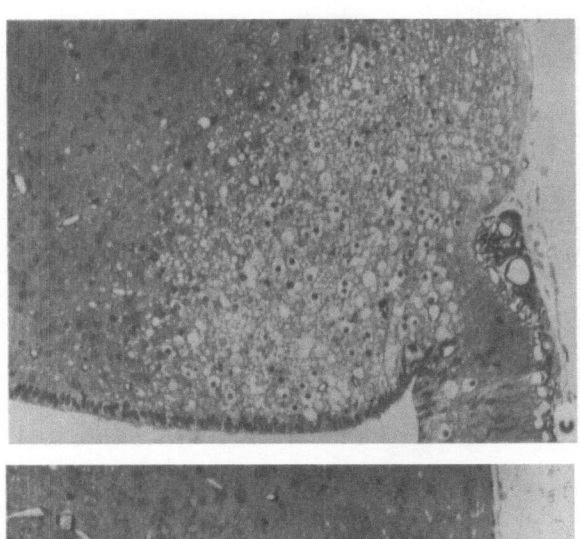

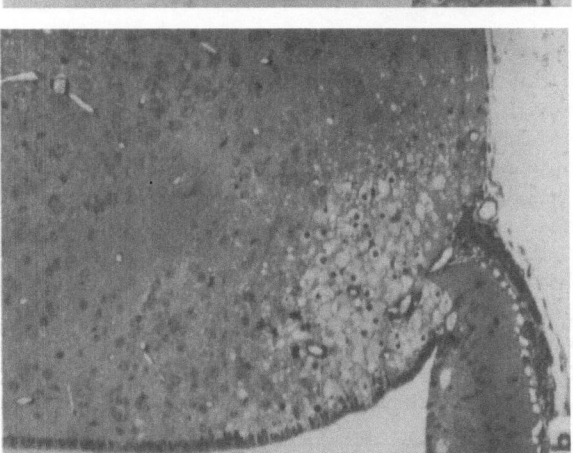

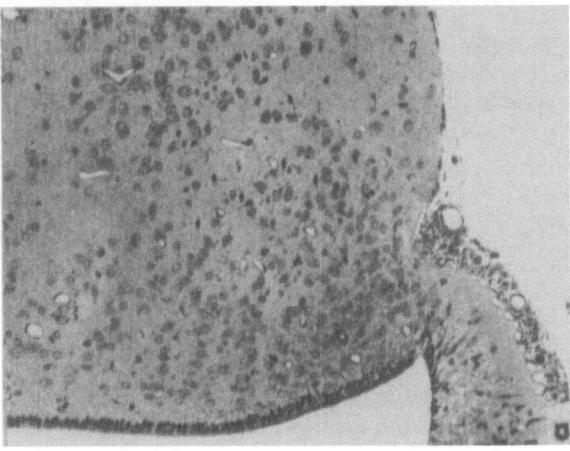

Fig. 1. Sections through the arcuate nucleus of the 10 day old mouse hypothalamus, 3 hours following different treatment regimens, all given subcutaneously. a) L-MSG, 0.75 mmol/kg. The arcuate nucleus appears normal. When the sodium salts of L-aspartic, cysteic or cysteine sulfinic acids are given in the same dosage (0.75 mmol/kg) there is also no reaction in the arcuate nucleus. b) A combination of the above 4 agents, each at a dose of 0.75 mmol/kg (total dose of acidic amino acids = 3.0 mmol/kg). The small lesion in the arcuate nucleus is approximately the same size any of the 4 agents given separately at 3.0 mmol/kg would produce. c) A combination of the above 4 agents each at a dose of 3 mmol/kg (total dose of acidic amino acids = 12 mmol/kg). The large lesion involving essentially the entire arcuate nucleus is similar in size to the lesion which any of the agents would produce if given separately at 12 mmol/kg. Note that doses are expressed in mmol/kg for purposes of the comparisons being made in this experiment rather than mg/g as is used elsewhere in this paper and in the literature. Histology as described elsewhere (Olney, 1971a;). Mag. about 100X.

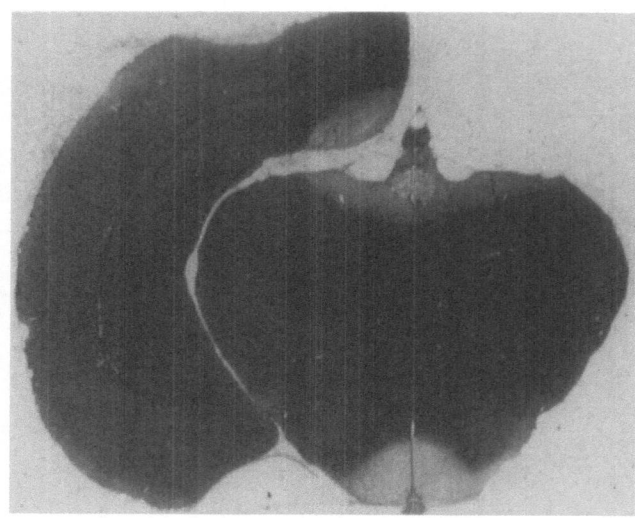

Fig. 2. Coronal section of 10 day old mouse brain 3 hours following
a large subcutaneous dose (4 mg/g) of cysteine sulfinic acid. Areas
surrounding the roof and floor of the third ventricle stain lightly
because of the edematous lesion selectively affecting these regions.
This is the pattern of damage produced by any of the neuroexcitatory
amino acids. When smaller doses are given the lesion tends to affect
only the arcuate nucleus (See Figs. 1b and 1c). This is a maximal
MSG-type lesion. Infant mice often convulse and die when the lesion
begins spreading in this fashion to include all midline areas bordering on the roof of the third ventricle between the psalterium rostrally and the superior colliculus caudally. Histological procedures
as described in Olney (1971a); Mag. about 10X.

---

we have found that the glutamate type of neurotoxic reaction can be
reproduced in the infant mouse hypothalamus by subcutaneous administration of any one of the "neuroexcitatory amino acids" but not by
a variety of other amino acids or non-amino acid compounds (Olney
et al, 1971.) This suggests that a similar mechanism may be responsible for both the neuroexcitatory and neurotoxic properties of Glu.
When neuroexcitatory amino acids are administered in combination with
one another the toxic reaction is augmented in an additive manner
(Fig. 1).

     One of the amino acids tested for neurotoxic potential, L-cys-
teine, requires separate consideration. Doses of L-cysteine in the
range of 1 mg/g do not produce the MSG type lesion; instead, a slightly
delayed and much more widespread neurodegenerative reaction affecting
the thalamus, hippocampus, amygdala and cerebral cortex develops over
the course of 24-48 hrs (Olney et al., 1972b). Rats sustaining this

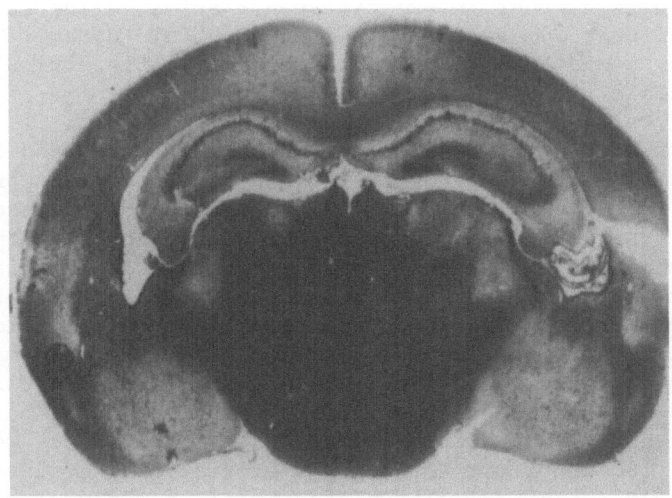

Fig. 3. Coronal section of a 9 day old mouse brain 24 hours following a 1 mg/g dose of L-cysteine. Light areas about the amygdala,
cerebral cortex, hippocampus and thalamus are those typically affected
by L-cysteine. Although the infant survived treatment for 24 hours
while the lesion was developing, this is a severe degree of brain
damage from which death might have ensued later. Some infants treated
with similar doses of L-cysteine, particularly younger infants, sustain milder degrees of brain damage but the pattern is the same.
Neither the habenular nor arcuate nuclei at the roof and floor of
the third ventricle, respectively, is affected, in contrast to the
MSG-type lesion (Fig. 2) which localizes about these regions. Histological procedures as described in Olney (1971a); Mag. about 10X.

---

type of brain damage from a single dose of L-cysteine in infancy
appear grossly normal as adults but perform learning tasks very poorly
(Sharpe, Olney, Olendorf and Zimmerman, unpublished). Both cysteine
(Olney et al., 1972b) and MSG (Murakami and Inouye, 1971) produce
their respective types of brain damage in fetal rodents when the amino
acids are administered to the pregnant dam in late gestation. Susceptibility of the primate fetus to transplacentally-induced brain
damage has not been studied for either compound.

    In brief, available evidence indicates that there are two basic
brain damage syndromes (MSG-type and cysteine-type) which can be induced by administering single amino acid loads to immature animals.
The acidic (excitatory) amino acids such as glutamic, aspartic, cysteine sulfinic, cysteic and homocysteic acids tend to produce a focal
pattern of brain damage (MSG-type) restricted to midline tissue zones
boardering on the roof and floor of the third ventricle (Fig. 2).

Cysteine, which is neither an excitatory nor acidic amino acid, produces a more diffuse and extensive pattern of brain damage (Fig. 3)
which curiously tends to spare the diencephalic periventricular zones
affected by acidic amino acids.

The fact that Glu is found in very high concentrations in brain
under normal circumstances makes it both enigmatic and of considerable
interest that ingestion of this amino acid can rapidly destroy CNS
neurons. An important key to understanding this phenomenon may lie
in distinguishing between intracellular and extracellular brain Glu
concentrations. It has been shown in microelectrophoretic studies
that it is the extracellular and not intracellular application of
Glu which excites neurons (Coombs et al., 1955). The same may be
true for the neurotoxicity of Glu. While a high intracelluar content of Glu is the normal state of health for the central nervous
system, relatively slight extracellular concentrations may be a state
of emergency - leading first to neuronal excitation (depolarization)
and finally, if the extracellular milieu is not rapidly corrected,
to neuronal necrosis. Blood brain barriers and homeostatic mechanisms
within brain are probably geared toward maintaining the extracellular
environment of central neurons relatively free from Glu. Assuming
that these barriers and mechanisms are underdeveloped in the immature
organism, this might explain the greater vulnerability of immature
animals to brain damage from exogenous loads of Glu.

In the absence of regulatory restrictions on the use of MSG in
foods, children in the United States, including those with seizure
disorders and minimal brain dysfunction syndromes, routinely consume
commercially processed foods containing added MSG. Some foods intended specifically for infants are supplemented with free amino
acid mixtures (protein hydrolysates) which include several of the
compounds (glutamic, aspartic and cysteic acids) shown to have additive
brain damaging effects on infant animals. The majority of human
infants raised in the United States over the past twenty years were
weaned on foods containing up to 0.6% added MSG. One small jar (130 g)
of baby food supplemented with 0.6% added MSG would expose a three
month old infant weighing 6 kg to an exogenous load of 0.13 g/kg or
about 1/4 the oral dose (0.5 g/kg) required to destroy hypothalamic
neurons in the infant animal brain. The fact that human infants and
children typically exhibit no signs of distress from MSG intake could
be dangerously misleading in that infant monkeys, while sustaining
brain damage from the ingestion of MSG, also manifest no signs of
acute distress (Olney et al., 1972a). It has also been demonstrated
in infant monkeys that it requires only a transient and moderate elevation of blood Glu to produce brain damage (Olney et al., 1972a)
and in infant mice that vulnerable brain regions rapidly accumulate
Glu within minutes after blood concentrations begin to rise (Perez
and Olney, 1972). Whether the average human infant can metabolize
Glu efficiently enough to prevent dangerous levels from developing
in local brain regions following ingestion of MSG-supplemented foods

is not known nor is it known to what extent the Glu metabolizing capabilities of some infants or children deviate from the average. Blood Glu curves monitored in human adults following an ingested MSG load (Himwich and Peterson, 1954) are characterized by marked individual variation with some individuals reaching much higher peak values than others. Whether similar studies, if conducted on infants and children, would reveal even more extreme variability and a tendency of some individuals to develop very high peak values from a modest MSG load warrants serious consideration.

Menkes et al. (1962) reported on a family in which five male children, although normal at birth, soon developed severe seizures followed by spastic paraplegia and death by 3 years of age with autopsy findings of cerebral and cerebellar degeneration. Blood Glu concentrations, although only investigated in two infants, were repeatedly (moderately) elevated. Yoshida et al. (1964) described a child, apparently normal at birth, who soon developed severe mental retardation, cortical atrophy and, despite only slightly elevated blood Glu concentrations, has CSF levels of Glu 4 times higher than normal. Various relatives died in infancy from a similar syndrome but were not examined for blood or CSF abnormalities. Assuming that these were Glu-mediated neurodegenerative syndromes, (no other plausible mechanism was uncovered), it is of interest that a substantial CSF elevation of Glu, when looked for, was found even though resting blood Glu levels were not markedly elevated. This would be consistent with a genetic error expressed primarily as a disturbance within the CNS, perhaps involving an excessive CNS build-up of extracellular Glu with consequent brain degeneration. Worth contemplating is the possibility that such a pathological process occurs more commonly in mild form - for example, manifesting itself as seizure or minimal brain dysfunction syndromes - but is not identified as a Glu-related process because Glu-tolerance curves and CSF assays for Glu are not obtained on such patients. Adding MSG to the diet, in such cases, might be detrimental.

Years ago Price et al. (1943) reported that oral administration of MSG was beneficial in some cases of epilepsy; however, they described one child who had an increase to approximately three times his ordinary seizure frequency each time he was given MSG. Recently, Dr. M.G. Stemmerman (personal communication) notified me of a young child in his pediatric practice with frequent seizures which respond poorly to ordinary anticonvulsants but can be controlled by avoiding foods containing added MSG. It is instructive that the connection between MSG and seizures in this patient was only discovered because Dr. Stemmerman was persistent in testing the hypothesis that such a connection might exist. The fact that a Glu mediated mechanism has not been implicated more frequently in the pathogenesis of seizure or minimal brain dysfunction syndromes may signify that such a connection is of rare occurence. It would be unwise, however, to ignore the alternative possibility that the connection is a common but subtle

and cryptic one which, unless suspected and looked for, will simply
not be found.

The ability of L-cysteine to produce an extensive pattern of
brain damage is of particular interest in that cysteine is a pivotal
compound in sulphur amino acid metabolism and errors of amino acid
metabolism are frequently associated with neuropsychiatric disturbances. It is not clear whether L-cysteine has neurotoxic properties in its own right or damages brain by intracerebral conversion
to another compound; for example, to one of its acidic analogues.
The acidic analogues of both cysteine and homocysteine have excitatory
and neurotoxic properties (Olney et al., 1972b) so that an accumulation of such analogues in the CNS, particularly in the extracellular
compartment, might be expected to produce neuropsychiatric disturbances. Homocystinuria, the second most common error of amino acid
metabolism known, may be a case in point. In this condition a block
in the enzymatic condensation of homocysteine with serine to form
cystathionine results in a deficiency of brain cystathionine and
probably an accumulation of hymocysteine and related metabolites.
The latter, although poorly studied, may be important in the pathogenesis of the neuropsychiatric disturbances (mental retardation,
seizures and schizophrenia-like syndromes) which are common among
homocystinurics. Wong et al. (1972), postulating that the deficiency
of brain cystathionine gives rise to these disturbances, have advo-
cated treating homocystinurics with massive doses of cysteine (to
stimulate alternate pathways of cystathionine synthesis). We would
suggest, however, that restricting dietary intake of the homocysteine
precursor, methionine, while avoiding massive doses of any sulphur
amino acid, may be more rational therapy since there is a least evidence in experimental animals that exogenous loads of cysteine itself
and acidic metabolites of cysteine and homocysteine induce brain damage but no evidence that cystathionine deficiency is toxic or requires correction. In that the several acidic (excitatory) amino
acids are synergistic in neurotoxic action (Fig. 1), it must also be
kept in mind that an endogenous disturbance giving rise to abnormal
extracellular accumulations of one such compound in the CNS (for
example, an acidic sulphur amino acid accumulating in homocystinuria)
might be aggravated by exogenous loads of another such compound (for
example, MSG being added to foods).

A brief word should be included about an additional compound,
hexachlorophene - an antibacterial soap which is absorbed readily
through the skin and for years has been used routinely in 3% solution
for total body bathing of human infants. It was recently reported
that when mean blood levels of hexachlorophene reach 1.2 µg/ml in
rats it produces cystic degeneration of axon tracts in the CNS (Gaines
and Kimbrough, 1971); that blood concentrations exceeding 1/2 this
level were detected in the human infant after only 5 daily washings
with 3% hexachlorophene (Curley et al., 1971) and that when infant

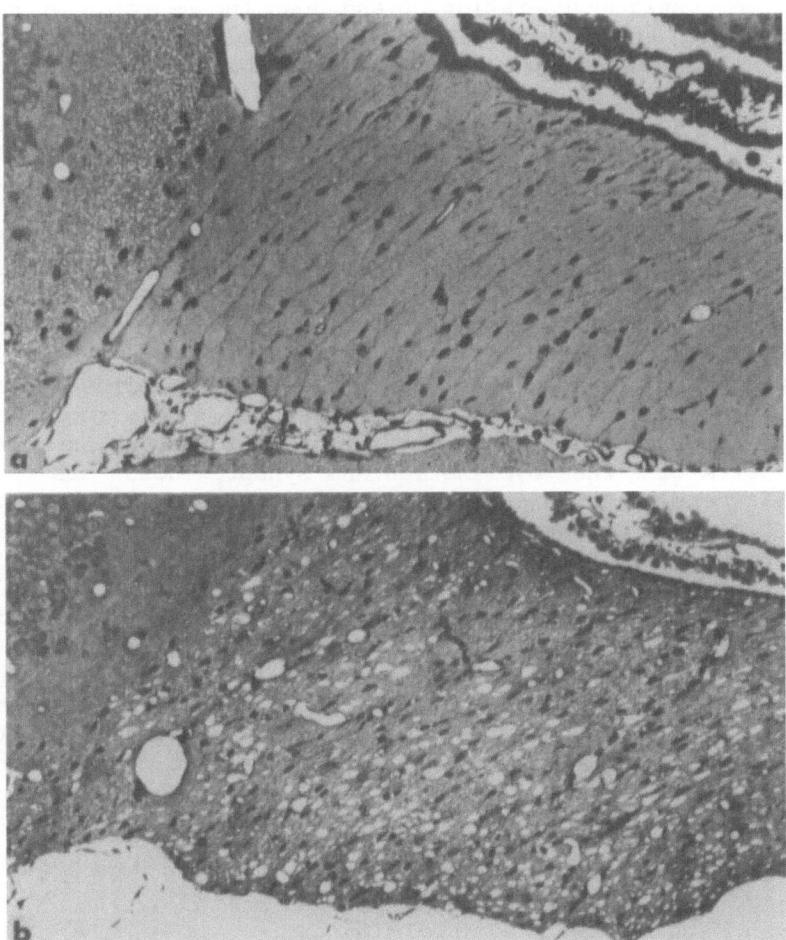

Fig. 4.   a) Fimbria of hippocampus from 19 day old control mouse
following 8 daily subcutaneous injections of olive oil (the vehicle
used to deliver hexachlorophene in Fig. 4b).   There are no pathological changes.   b) Fimbria of hippocampus from 19 day old mouse
following 8 daily subcutaneous injections of hexachlorophene (25 mg/kg).
The animal was asymptomatic despite rather marked edematous changes
in structures of the fimbria which preliminary electron microscopic
examination revealed to be grossly dilated myelin-bound compartments,
the contents of which require further study to determine the extent
of axonal involvement.   Histology as described elsewhere in Olney
1971a; Mag. about 100X.

monkeys were bathed daily for 90 days with 3% hexachlorophene they developed mean blood levels of 2.3 μg/ml and CNS examination revealed well developed cystic degeneration up and down the neuraxis with spinal cord, brain stem,· cerebellar and cerebral white matter areas all being involved (Winthrop Laboratories, unpublished; cited in FDA Drug Bulletin, Dec. 1971). Over the spring and summer months of this year (1972) approximately 40 human infants died in France from skin exposure to a talcum powder which, by accident, contained 6% hexachlorophene.

We have begun studying the effects of hexachlorophene on infant rodents and have encountered rather widespread edematous degeneration of the developing myelin sheath (the degree of axonal involvement is uncertain) in various CNS regions, including the developing optic pathways, corticospinal tracts at various CNS levels and the fimbria of the hippocampus (Fig. 4). The CNS changes are sometimes detectable for days or weeks before clinical symptoms appear. This suggests the need for studies to determine whether hexachlorophene exposure in infancy, at a time when myelination and synaptogenesis are in progress, has detrimental effects on the axon which, although asymtomatic at time of exposure, might become clinically manifest in later years; for example, in the form of a hyperkinetic syndrome.

Occult processes underlie many of the brain dysfunction syndromes encountered in pediatric medicine today. I have drawn attention to several common constituents of the chemical milieu of the developing CNS which have the potential to function as occult neurotoxins in order to emphasize the need for research aimed at clarifying what role, if any, such agents play in the pathogenesis of human brain dysfunction syndromes.

REFERENCES

Abraham, R., Doughtery, W., Goldberg, L. and Coulston, F., 1971, The response of the hypothalamus to high doses of monosodium gluta- mate in mice and monkeys. Cytochemistry and ultrastructural study of lysosomal changes. Exp. Molec. Path. 15: 43.

Burde, R.M., Schainker, B. and Kayes, J., 1971, Monosodium glutamate: Acute effect of oral and subcutaneous administration on the ar- cuate nucleus of the hypothalamus in mice and rats, Nature 233: 58.

Coombs, J.S., Eccles, J.C. and Fatt, P., 1955, The specific ionic conductances and the ionic movements across the motoneuronal membrane that produce the inhibitory postsynaptic potential, J. Physiol. 130: 326.

Curley, A., Hawk, R.E., Kimbrough, R.D., Nathenson, G. and Finberg, L., 1971, Dermal absorption of hexachlorophene in infants, Lancet, 2: 296.

Curtis, D.R. and Watkins, J.C., 1960, The excitation and depression of spinal neurons by structurally related amino acids, J. Neuro- chem. 6: 117.

Curtis, D.R. and Watkins, J.C., 1963, Acidic amino acids with strong excitatory actions on mammalian neurons, J. Physiol. 166: 1.

Everly, J.L., 1971, Light microscopic examination of MSG-induced lesions in brain of fetal and neonatal rats, Anat. Rec. 169: 312.

Gaines, T.B. and Kimbrough, R.D., 1971, The oral and dermal toxicity of hexachlorophene, Paper read at the 10th annual meeting of the Society of Toxicology in Washington, D.C., March 7-11.

Himwich, W.A. and Peterson, I.M., 1954, Ingested sodium glutamate and plasma levels of glutamic acid, J. Appl. Physiol. 7: 196.

Johnston, N. and Reynolds, W.A., 1972, Incidence and extent of brain lesions in mice following ingestion of MSG, Anat. Rec. 172: 354.

Knittle, J.L. and Ginsberg-Feller, F., 1970, Cellular and metabolic alterations in obese rats treated with monosodium glutamate during the neonatal period, Bulletin Am. Peds. Soc. Gen. Meeting, Program Abstracts, p.6.

Lucas, D.R. and Newhouse, J.P., 1957, The toxic effect of sodium L-glutamate on the inner layers of the retina, AMA Arch. Ophth. 58: 193.

Matsuyan, S., 1970, Studies on experimental obesity in mice treated with MSG. Jap. J. Vet. Science 32: 206.

Menkes, J.H., Alter, M., Steigleder, G.K., Weakley, D.R. and Sung, J.H., 1962, A sex-linked recessive disorder with retardation of growth, peculiar hair and focal cerebral and cerebellar degeneration, Pediatrics 29: 764.

Murakami, U. and Inouye, M., 1971, Brain lesions in the mouse fetus caused by maternal administration of monosodium glutamate, Congenital Anomalies 11: 171.

Olney, J.W., 1969, Brain lesions, obesity and other disturbances in mice treated with monosodium glutamate, Science 164: 719.

Olney, J.W., 1971a, Glutamate induced neuronal necrosis in the infant mouse hypothalamus. An electron microscopy study, J. Neuropath. Exp. Neurol. 30: 75.

Olney, J.W., 1971b, Monosodium glutamate effects, Science 172: 294.

Olney, J.W. and Ho, O.L., 1970, Brain damage in infant mice following oral intake of glutamate, aspartate or cysteine, Nature 227: 609.

Olney, J.W. and Sharpe, L.G., 1969, Brain lesions in an infant monkey treated with monosodium glutamate, Science 166: 386.

Olney, J.W., Ho, O.L. and Rhee, V., 1971, Cytotoxic effects of acidic and sulphur containing amino acids on the infant mouse central nervous system, Exp. Brain Res. 14: 61.

Olney, J.W., Sharpe, L.G. and Feigin, R.D., 1972a, Glutamate induced brain damage in infant primates, J. Neuropath. Exp. Neurol. 31: 464.

Olney, J.W., Ho, O.L., Rhee, V. and Schainker, B., 1972b, Cysteine induced brain damage in infant and fetal rodents, Brain Res. 45: 309.

Perez, V.J. and Olney, J.W., 1972, Accumulation of glutamate by arcuate nucleus of infant mouse hypothalamus, J. Neurochem. 19: 1777.

Pradhan, S.N. and Lynch, J.F., 1972, Behavioral changes in adult rats treated with monosodium glutamate in the neonatal stage, Arch. Int. Pharmacodyn. 197: 301.

Price, J.C., Waelsch, H. and Putnam, T.J., 1943, DL-Glutamic acid hydrochloride in treatment of petit mal and psychomotor seizures, JAMA 122: 1153.

Redding, T.W., Shalley, A.V., Arimura, A. and Wakaboyashi, I., 1971,
    Effects of monosodium glutamate on some endocrine functions,
    Neuroendocrin. 8: 245.

Snapir, N., Robinson, B. and Perek, M., 1971, Brain damage in male
    domestic fowl treated with monosodium glutamate, Poultry Science
    50: 5.

Wong, P.W.K. and Fresco, R., 1972, Tissue cystathionine in mice
    treated with cysteine and homoserine, Pediat. Res. 5: 172.

Yoshida, T., Tada, K., Mizuno, T., Wada, Y., Akabane, J., Ogasawara,
    J., Minagawa, A., Morikawa, T. and Okamura, T., 1964, A sex-
    linked disorder with mental and physical retardation characterized
    by cerebrocortical atrophy and increase of glutamic acid in the
    cerebrospinal fluid, Tohoku J. Med. Sci. 83: 26.

MANAGEMENT OF SEIZURE DISORDERS IN INFANCY, CHILDHOOD AND ADOLESCENCE

Gerhard Nellhaus

Department of Pediatrics and Medicine (Neurology)

University of Colorado School of Medicine

Denver, Colorado

The approach of the clinician to the management of seizures remains largely symptomatic and pragmatic. The many publications about the epilepsies and the continuing need to develop modes of anticonvulsant treatment more effective than those available bear witness to the gap between the base provided by experiments such as reported in this Symposium and the exigencies of the clinical situations. Guidelines may be given on how to bridge the gap, but not a set of rules; knowing one's patient and experience with a drug or drugs are among the prime ingredients of good seizure management.

Seizures in the younger age groups present special problems in their pathophysiology, manifestations and prognosis, and in the sheer size of the population involved. In newborns, about one of every 125 full-term (and more among the premature and small-for-date infants) suffer convulsions, and these spell either death or impairment of neurologic and intellectual functions for over half of them (Brown et al., 1972). Febrile convulsions - or initial seizures associated with high fever - occur in at least 2% of children in the first three years of life (Millichap, 1968; van den Berg and Yerushalmy, 1969); in 50-70% seizures may recur, while in about 15% of cases, such convulsions mark the onset of chronic epilepsy (Taylor and Ounstead, 1971). Altogether, anywhere from 5% to over 10% of our population up to 15 years of age is reported to have had one or more seizures (Abernathy, 1966; Graham and Rutter, 1968; Metrakos and Metrakos, 1960).

TYPES OF SEIZURES

The more common types of seizures seen in the differing age groups in children, their manifestations, some of the causative factors, EEG findings, and preferred drugs for therapy have been compiled in Table I, and the drugs commonly employed in the United States at present are indicated in Table II. Notable omissions from Table I are those seizures called by many names, such as autonomic, visceral, or abdominal epilepsy. It is often far more important for a physician to familiarize himself with the effectiveness, limitations and side-effects of certain drugs, and to push these to the limit of toxicity to gain control of seizures, than to switch drugs frequently. Parents and older patients may, in most instances, be trusted to report when drugs fail, or result in undesirable side effects, such as the hyperirritability and undirected constant activity produced paradoxically by phenobarbital in the toddler and pre-school child.

The rather high incidence of neonatal seizures with its attendant morbidity and mortality may well be reduced, not so much by better anticonvulsants as by preventive measures, both social and medical. Preliminary data from Sweden suggests, for example, a decreasing incidence of low birth weight diplegia (Hagberg et al., 1973). Every effort must be made to identify a specific remediable cause of seizures, whether metabolic, infectious or vascular, in the neonates. Metabolic disturbances occur in a high percentage of brain-damaged convulsing newborns and "differentiation" between brain-damage associated and metabolic convulsions in less effective than differentiation based on neurological and behavioral criteria (Brown et al., 1972). Though mannitol administration does not influence seizures once they have occurred, early and proper treatment with this hyperosmolar agent may prevent some of the neurologic sequelae of neonatal brain damage (Marchal et al., 1972). Of great concern are the infants and small children presented clinically with frequent and often massive myoclonic seizures. Those seen usually before the end of their first year of life with infantile spasms, many of whom also have hypsarrhythmic electroencephalograms, are labeled as suffering from the West syndrome, named for Dr. W.J. West who in a letter to Lancet in 1841 described the peculiar seizures and psychomotor regression in his own son. The many approaches to treatment indicate how much is yet to be learned. But the remarkable normalization of the EEG which occurs, almost as rapidly as with the pyridoxine-dependent infant, within hours or a day or so of intravenously administered adrenocorticotropin (preferred by the writer to either corticosteroids or diazepam) is unfortunately not accompanied by improvement in mentation. Reflective of the extensive underlying neuronal damage, from whatever cause, is the fact that, despite control of infantile spasms, about 90% of the infants are doomed to varying degrees of mental retardation.

Etiologically as variable and prognostically as ominous are the seizures, usually having their onset in the second to third year of life or later, characterized by myoclonic jerks, tonic posturing and often sudden dragging of the head or violent propulsion of the body either to one side or forward. But, other seizure forms may occur as well. This severe type of childhood epilepsy, sometimes called the Lennox-Gastant syndrome, is defined for the electroencephalographer by the 1.5-2.5 cps diffuse spike waves, or "petit mal variant", or even by a hypsarrhythmic EEG pattern; indeed a significant number of affected children have a history of infantile spasms. In many instances there is evidence of multifocal or diffuse brain damage, and the outlook for mental normality is limited. Some of the children respond to hormonal therapy; some to a "cocktail" of phenobarbital, methsuximide and acetazolamide, some to diazepam; but these seizures are as notoriously resistant to treatment as they are to classification (Aicardi, 1973).

TREATMENTS

Ketogenic Diet. In such cases of intractable seizures in childhood, particularly of the varieties just described, some of us have fallen back on the ketogenic diet, first introduced by Wilder over half a century ago (Wilder, 1921). It is, as repeatedly reported, neither an easy nor inexpensive form of seizure management, and hence proper selection of the patient and the ability to predict whether the diet might be effective are of primary importance. Recently, the writer reported that the EEG may normalize as ketosis develops during the fast, even before the diet is instituted and EEG monitoring may thus help the physician within a few days to decide whether through this regimen the child's seizures are likely to come under control (Nellhaus, 1971a).

The mechanism by which the diet works is not entirely clear. What has intrigued the writer most is that both short chain fatty acids and ketones act as CNS depressants and anticonvulsants (Harper et al., 1966). There is evidence that there is utilization of ketone bodies in preference to glucose by the brain of very young animals (Spitzer and Weng, 1972). Clinical and experimental studies have shown that the ketosis and its anticonvulsant effect are rapidly negated by the feeding of carbohydrates; likewise in the mouse, as in children, the anticonvulsant effect of the diet diminishes as the brain matures, with essentially no protection afforded to the adult mouse (Uhlemann and Neims, 1972). But children in whom the ketogenic diet controls the seizures, regardless of their etiologies, and in whom the EEG becomes normal, can often after two or three years of this regimen terminate the diet and remain seizure-free (Keith, 1963; Livingston, 1972). More recently, a dietary regimen substituting medium-chain triglycerides, which produce ketone bodies, has been introduced by Huttenlocker and co-workers (Huttenlocker et al., 1971) but experience with this is quite limited and apparently not wholly satisfactory (personal communication).

Depakine. In the search for the ideal anticonvulsant that is highly effective in terminating at least some seizure forms, as well as virtually non-toxic, the past months have afforded the author some familiarity with di-n-propylacetic acid or "Depakine". This drug has been used throughout much of Western Europe since 1964. It is a fatty acid with two unbranched symmetrical side chains, and has been shown to raise the level of gamma-aminobutyric acid in the brain of experimental animals, possibly by inhibiting GABA-transaminase (Godin et al., 1969).

Chemically, di-n-propylacetic acid is most effective against "absences", or, together with phenobarbital whose action it poten-tiates, against "mixed" generalized and absence seizures. In the more problematic cases of the myoclonic forms of epilepsy discussed earlier, a few cases apparently resistant to conventional anticon-vulsants have been reported to have come under control (or to have been better managed) with di-n-propylacetic acid, at least temporarily. Of course, almost any change of drugs - or even better, of the pa-tient's environment - will have a beneficial effect for a while. In focal seizures of the temporal lobe type, di-n-propylacetic acid, despite some reports to the contrary, appears to be less effective, and it is not at all effective against focal motor and Jacksonian epilepsy. The compound by itself is not sedating, is said to have no toxic effects other than mild gastric irritability, and, as a rule, EEG normalization correlates well after weeks or months with clinical improvement (Scollo-Lavizzari and Corbat, 1970; Bergamini et al., 1970; Forester, 1972).

Phenobarbital. The difficulties of management of certain con-vulsive disorders in childhood are matched by the problems of whether and how to treat such common seizures as those considered benign febrile convulsions (Dodge, 1971). The writer has tended to treat children with such seizures, regardless of their duration, family history, or initial EEG findings rather than wait for one or two recurrences, and has usually used phenobarbital, 5-7 mg/kg, maintain-ing a serum level above 1 mg/100 ml, until the child is about 4 years of age and is then less likely - unless there is an underlying chronic seizure disorder - to have further febrile convulsions (Faero et al., 1972). Continuous anticonvulsant therapy to prevent recurrences of febrile seizures has been endorsed more definitely than previously this past year (Aicardi, 1972; Lennox-Buchthal, 1972).

Carbamazepine. A strong impetus toward treatment has been a series of studies suggesting an intimate association between chronic temporal lobe epilepsy and localized hypoxic neuronal damage with severe convulsions associated with fever in early childhood (Taylor

and Ounsted, 1971). Age, sex, genetic factors as well as certain
types of viral illnesses seem to play a part.

Related to this is the problem of early recognition of those
focal seizures with complex symptomatology in early childhood, whether
they are called psychomotor, temporal lobe of limbic seizures. Beginning almost at any time, but usually not recognized until after
the age of three years, the epileptic phenomena observed are mani-
fold and often bizarre. In each child, however, they are repeated
in a rather stereotyped fashion. As a result of the odd behaviors,
sensations of fear or pain, or long vacant and glassy-eyed looks,
the children are often diagnosed initially as either emotionally
disturbed or as having "petit mal", and then are treated, usually
without much success, accordingly. The diagnostic and therapeutic
problems presented by such children are many; among the most difficult are the adolescents who feign their own seizures so that the
physician may no longer know what he is treating. While treatment
with diphenylhydantoin, alone or in combination with, for example,
primidone, is well established, the search continues for a drug or
drugs with fewer side-effects.

Carbamazepine has been used as the drug of choice in such
seizures in children for years by neurologists in Europe (Gamstorp,
1970; Fichsel and Heyer, 1970; Scheffner and Schiefer, 1972) and
received the strongest endorsement recently by Livingston (1972).
Structurally this drug is more nearly related to the tricyclic antidepressants of the imipramine class, which it resembles in toxicity,
including extrapyramidal symptoms and autonomic and behavioral
effects. The usual starting dose is about 10-20 mg/kg. Whether the
oft-cited psychic benefits are due to the drug itself is not clearly
defined; they may be related to other factors.

CONCLUSIONS

With afflicted children and adolescents, the physician should
strive to reduce or abolish seizures employing the least amount of
a medication with the least toxic effects and, above all, he should
assist in developing the support of the child by his family, peers
and school authorities. Success with these latter factors will
facilitate management of seizures. Sometimes the physician must
content himself with less than complete control of the seizures,
either because of the severity of the underlying pathophysiological
mechanisms, or because complete control carries with it too steep a
price in terms of the child's behavior and development. Many aspects
of seizure-management in the maturing human being have not been discussed. Whether to treat only for 3 years of a seizure-free period,
or through adolescence, or perhaps for a lifetime will be dependent
on both the individual patient and the risk of recurrence the patient
and physician are willing to take. The magnitude and complexity of
the clinical problems allow for no ready prescription, but constitute
challenges for clinicians and researchers alike.

TABLE I

SEIZURES BY AGE OF ONSET AND PREFERRED TREATMENT

Age Group and Seizure Type	Neonatal seizures. Birth - 2 weeks.
Clinical Manifestations	Often "atypical" - sudden limpness or tonic posturing with apnea and cyanosis; odd cry; eyes "rolling up" or nystagmus; twitchiness or clonic movements - focal, multifocal, general-ized.
Causative Factors	Neurologic insults (intracranial hemorrhage, hypoxia) tend to present more in first 3 or after 8th day; metabolic disturbances alone between 3rd and 8th day; hypoglycemia, hypocal-cemia, hypophosphatemia, hyper- & hyponatremia often with brain damage. Pyridoxine deficiency & other metabolic errors cause seizures after 1st week. Meningitis unpredictable.
Electroencephalo-graphic (EEG) Pattern	Highly variable - often rhythmic slowing, independent abnormalities of the hemispheres. Focal abnormalities may shift.
Other Diagnostic Studies	<u>Musts:</u> LP; Ca^{++}; PO_4^-; Glucose; Mg^{++}; BUN; amino acid screen; consider NH_4; organic acid screen.
Treatment and Comments	Phenobarbital 5-8 mg/kg and/or 10 mg/kg I.V. diphenylhydantoin. Diazepam, approximately 0.2 mg/kg. Treat underlying disorder. Seizures 2^0 brain damage often very resistant to anticonvulsants.

TABLE I
(cont'd)

SEIZURES BY AGE OF ONSET AND PREFERRED TREATMENT

Age Group and Seizure Type	West Syndrome "Infantile Spasms". 3 mo. - 18 mo.
Clinical Manifestations	Usually sudden symmetric adduction and flexion of limbs with concomitant flexion of head and trunk; also abduction and exterior movements - like Moro reflex.
Causative Factors	Pre- or perinatal damage or malformations in approximately 1/3; biochemical, infectious, degenerative causes in approximately 1/3; unknown in approximately 1/3. With early onset, pyridoxine deficiency, amino- or organic acidurias. Tuberous sclerosis 5-10%. Chronic inflammatory disease and toxoplasmosis.
Electroencephalo-graphic (EEG) Pattern	Hypsarrhythmia - chaotic pattern of high voltage slow waves and random spikes in all leads in 90%; other abnormalities in rest.
Other Diagnostic Studies	Skull X-rays, fundoscopic and skin examination; trial of pyridoxine. Amino- and organic acid screen. Chronic inflammatory disease, Toxo titres.
Treatment and Comments	Corticotropin preferred (4-5 mg/kg/day 1st 10-14 days) then slow withdrawal. Some prefer oral corticosteroids. Diazepam. In resistant cases, ketogenic diet (see text). Retardation in approximately 90% of cases.

TABLE I
(cont'd)

SEIZURES BY AGE OF ONSET AND PREFERRED TREATMENT

Age Group Seizure Type	Febrile convulsions. 6 mo. - 4 years.
Clinical Manifestations	Usually generalized seizures, less than 15 minutes; rarely focal onset. May lead to status epilepticus.
Causative Factors	Non-neurological febrile illness (temperature rise to $40^{\circ}C$ or greater); family history frequently positive for febrile convulsions.
Electroencephalo- graphic (EEG) Pattern	Normal interictal EEG, especially when obtained 8-10 days after seizure.
Other Diagnostic Studies	In infants or whenever suspicion of meningitis exists, LP.
Treatment and Comments	Treat underlying illness, fever. Preferred: phenobarbital 5 mg/kg continuously, keeping blood level 1 mg/100 ml or greater (see text).

TABLE I
(cont'd)

SEIZURES BY AGE OF ONSET AND PREFERRED TREATMENT

Age Group and Seizure Type	Myoclonic and akinetic seizures. 2-7 years, but may have onset any time in childhood.
Clinical Manifestations	Shock-like violent contractions of one or more muscle groups, singly or irregularly repetitive; may fling patient suddenly to side, forward or backward. Usually no or only brief loss of consciousness. 50% or more have generalized seizures.
Causative Factors	Multiple causes, usually resulting in diffuse neuronal damage: History of West syndrome; pre- or perinatal brain damage; vital meningo-encephalitides; subacute sclerosing panencephalitis; CNS degenerative disorders; lead or other encephalopathies; structural abnormalities, e.g. porencephaly.
Electroencephalo-graphic (EEG) Pattern	Atypical slow spike-wave complexes ("petit mal variant") and frequent bursts of high voltage generalized spikes. For Lennox-Gastant Syndrome, see text.
Other Diagnostic Studies	As dictated by index of suspicion. LP with measles antibody titre and CSF Ig G. Nerve conduction studies. Urine for lead, arylsulfatase A, etc. Brain biopsy may be justified.
Treatment and Comments	Phenobarbital; "cocktail" of phenobarbital + methsuximide + acetazolamide. Diazepam. Di-n-propylacetic acid. Ketogenic/or medium chain triglyceride dietary regimen. Occasionally adrenocorticotropin or corticosteroids. Often resistant to drug therapy.

TABLE I
(cont'd)

SEIZURES BY AGE OF ONSET AND PREFERRED TREATMENT

Age Group and Seizure Type	Absences ("Petit Mal"). 3 - 15 years.
Clinical Manifestations	Brief lapses of consciousness or vacant stares, usually in "clusters", often with blinking of eyelids or other movements. Sometimes automatisms.
Causative Factors	Unknown. Genetic component. Rarely may usher in childhood form of CNS lipidoses.
Electroencephalographic (EEG) Pattern	3 c/sec bilaterally synchronous, symmetrical, high voltage spikes and waves.
Other Diagnostic Studies	Hyperventilation when patient not on medication often evokes attacks.
Treatment and Comments	Ethosuximide; since many patients may also have generalized seizures, add phenobarbital if EEG suggests other abnormalities. Acetazolamide-Di-n-propylacetic acid. Rarely "diones".

TABLE I
(cont'd)

SEIZURES BY AGE OF ONSET AND PREFERRED TREATMENT

Age Group and Seizure Type	Psychomotor seizures (temporal lobe seizures). Any age, usually from age 3 on.
Clinical Manifestations	See text. (loss of consciousness, usually with semipurposeful inappropriate activity. Stereotyped symptomatology may combine psychic, motor, sensory or visceral phenomena.)
Causative Factors	Birth injury, inflammatory processes, prolonged febrile convulsions or status epilepticus, trauma, tumors. Genetic component.
Electroencephalographic (EEG) Pattern	Variety of patterns, including focal spike or slow wave activity, limited to or predominant in anterior temporal lobe in 1/3 of cases.
Other Diagnostic Studies	Occasionally EEG with nasopharyngeal leads. Neurodiagnostic studies as indicated by clinical index of suspicion.
Treatment and Comments	Carbamazepine (see text). Diphenylhydantoin or diphenylhydantoin plus primidone. Rarely phenacemide. Frequent need for supportive psychologic care, especially in adolescent. Occasionally anterior temporal lobectomy.

TABLE I
(cont'd)

SEIZURES BY AGE OF ONSET AND PREFERRED TREATMENT

Age Group and Seizure Type	Focal seizures (Motor/Sensory/Jacksonian). Any age.
Clinical Manifestations	Seizure may involve any part of body; may spread in fixed pattern (Jacksonian march), becoming generalized. In children, focus may shift.
Causative Factors	Often 2^O to birth trauma, inflammatory process, vascular accidents, meningoencephalitis, etc. If seizures coupled with new or progressive neurologic defirils, structural lesion, e.g. tumor, likely.
Electroencephalo-graphic (EEG) Pattern	Focal spikes or slow waven in appropriate cortical region; sometimes diffusely abnormal or even normal.
Other Diagnostic Studies	If seizures difficult to control, or progressive deficits, neurodiagnostic studies imperative (see text).
Treatment and Comments	Phenobarbital and/or diphenylhydantoin. Primidone. Carbamazepine. Di-n-propylacetic acid. "Cocktail" of phenobarbital + methsuximide + acetazolamide.

TABLE I
(cont'd)

SEIZURES BY AGE OF ONSET AND PREFERRED TREATMENT

Age Group and Seizure Type	Generalized seizures (Grand Mal). Any age.

Clinical Manifestations	Loss of consciousness; tonic, clonic movements, often preceded by vague aura or cry. Bladder and bowel incontinence in approximately 15%. Post-ictal confusion; sleep. Often mixed with other seizure patterns.

Causative Factors	Often unknown. Genetic component. May be seen with metabolic disturbances, trauma, infections, intoxications, degenerative disorders, etc.

Electroencephalographic (EEG) Pattern	Bilaterally synchronous, symmetrical multiple high voltage spikes, spikes and waves; mixed patterns. Often normal in children under 4 yrs.

Other Diagnostic Studies	Usually skull films, glucose, Ca^{++}, PO_4^-, BUN. Other studies as clinically indicated.

Treatment and Comments	Phenobarbital in 1st 6-12 mo; or after 5-6 years. Diphenylhydantoin. Carbamazepine. Combinations with primidone, methsuximide, acetazolamide. See text.

TABLE II

GUIDE TO ANTICONVULSANT DRUG THERAPY

Seizure Pattern	Drug	Average Total (mg/kg/day)	in	Divided Doses	Toxicity and Precautions	Remarks
All seizures	Phenobarbital	3–5	:	1–3	Irritability and overactivity in many children; sedative effects in others. Mild ataxia, nystagmus, skin rash.	Safest overall drug. Bitter taste.
	Mephobarbital (Mebaral)	4–10	:	1–3	As above.	Tasteless. Twice the quantity of phenobarbital required for comparable effect.
	Primidone (Mysoline)	10–25	:	3–4	Drowsiness, ataxia, vertigo, anorexia, nausea, vomiting, rash.	Start out slowly with 1/4 or 1/3 expected maintenance dose and increase every 2 days until full dose is reached.
	Methsuximide (Celontin)	15–30	:	3–4	Drowsiness, ataxia, headache, diplopia, skin rash.	Effective with phenobarbital in "mixed patterns" where other drugs may be contraindicated.
	Bromides	25–75	:	3–4	Rash, drowsiness, toxic psychosis, mental dullness. Check blood bromide levels regularly.	Rarely used now. Try when usual drugs fail, especially in infantile spasms and "minor motor" seizures.
	Metharbital (Gemonil)	5–15	:	2–3	Drowsiness, irritability, rash.	Not a satisfactory drug. May be useful in seizures due to organic brain damage.
Adjuncts to above	Acetazolamide (Diamox)	5–20	:	3–4	Anorexia; numbness and tingling; increase in urinary frequency.	Supplement to other medications, especially in petit mal and other minor patterns. Also in females 4 days prior to and in the first 2–3 days of menstrual periods.
	Diazepam (Valium)	0.20 ± 0.05	:	3	Somnolence.	Most useful in minor motor seizures and infantile spasms but often ceases to be effective after a few weeks or months.
	Carbamazepine (Tegretol)	Individualize (10–25)	:	2–3 times a day with meals	Bone marrow and liver toxicity.	Experience limited. Useful in psychomotor and generalized seizures. Improved behavior reported.
	Dextroamphetamine (Dexedrine)	0.25–0.75	:	Breakfast and noon	Nervousness, palpitations, anorexia, insomnia.	To counteract sedative effect of other drugs. Narcolepsy. In behavior disorders of younger children.
	Amphetamine (Benzedrine)	0.25–0.75	:	Breakfast and noon	As above.	As above. Less potent, but sometimes better tolerated than Dexedrine.
Any seizures except petit mal absences, akinetic, or myoclonic	Diphenylhydantoin (Dilantin)	5–9	:	1–2	Gum hypertrophy, hirsutism, ataxia, nystagmus, diplopia, rash, anorexia, nausea. Rare: macrocytic anemia, lymph node involvement, exfoliative dermatitis, peripheral neuropathy.	Generally very effective and safe. Will not cause behavior disturbances in children. Good dental hygiene reduces gum hyperplasia. May aggravate petit mal and myoclonic seizures. Severe toxicity may cause pseudodementia and liver damage.

Seizure type	Drug	Dosage		Doses/day	Toxicity / Warning	Remarks
	Ethotoin (Peganone)	15–30	:	2–3	As above.	Not very effective. Worth trying if others fail.
	Mephenytoin (Mesantoin)	4–15	:	2–3	Mild: Rash, drowsiness, ataxia. *Warning:* Aplastic anemia, agranulocytosis. Obtain at least monthly blood counts.	A good anticonvulsant, but fear of bone marrow depression limits use.
Psychomotor Occasionally primarily akinetic and myoclonic attacks	Phenacemide (Phenurone)	25–50	:	2–4	Rash, anorexia, nausea. *Warning:* Hepatitis, psychosis, blood dyscrasias. Monthly blood counts, liver function tests.	Especially effective in temporal lobe seizures when all other drugs fail.
Petit mal absences	Ethosuximide (Zarontin)	10–25	:	3–4	Nausea, gastric discomfort. Take with food. Rare: bone marrow depression.	Drug of choice for petit mal. Occasionally aggravates generalized seizures.
Akinetic and myoclonic attacks	Trimethadione (Tridione)	20–50	:	3–4	Rash, photophobia, irritability. *Warning:* Leukopenia, agranulocytosis, nephrosis, LE phenomenon. Monthly blood counts and urinalysis.	Useful in petit mal absences if Zarontin fails. May aggravate generalized seizures.
	Paramethadione (Paradione)	20–50	:	3–4	As above.	As above.
	Phensuximide (Milontin)	20–40	:	3–4	Drowsiness, headache, slight nephrotoxicity. Monthly urinalysis.	Not very effective, but may be useful when other drugs fail, or in combination.
Status epilepticus, grand mal, focal, psychomotor, and myoclonic	Diazepam (Valium)	0.2 ± 0.05 mg/kg IV initially. Repeat dose 0.1 mg/kg.			Administer slowly IV. Monitor pulse and BP. May cause respiratory depression if given to patient who has already received phenobarbital.	May need to be repeated every 3–4 hours. Follow with phenobarbital or diphenylhydantoin for long-range control.
	Phenobarbital	7–10 mg/kg IV initially. Repeat dose 5 mg/kg IV.			Less if patient has already received barbiturates.	Rule out pyridoxine deficiency, water intoxication.
	Paraldehyde	0.1–0.15 ml/kg IV; 0.2–0.3 ml/kg rectally.			Administer slowly IV mixed in saline; rectal dose in vegetable oil. Avoid in patient with pulmonary disease or in croup.	Avoid IM administration if possible: may cause fat necrosis.
	Lidocaine (Xylocaine)	2 mg/kg IV			Administer slowly.	Useful especially when reluctant to give more barbiturates or paraldehyde. Effect brief.
	General anesthesia if other measures fail.					
Infantile Spasms	Use of corticotropin or corticosteroids and of ketogenic diet discussed in text.					

FROM: Nellhaus, 1972b

REFERENCES

Abernathy, R.S., 1966, A survey of 156 seizure patients in a general
    pediatric clinic, J. Lancet 86: 115.

Aicardi, J., 1973, The problem of the Lennox syndrome, Dev. Med.
    Child Neurol. 15: 77.

Aicardi, J., 1972, Les convulsions hyperpyretiques de l'enfant,
    Arch. Franc. Ped. 29: 5.

Bergamini, L., Mutani, R., Furlan, P.M. and Riccio, A., 1970, Le
    Depakine dans le traitement de l'epilepsie essentielle on
    idiopathique, Arch. Swisse Neurol. Neurochirur. Psychiat. 106: 1.

Brown, J.K., Cockburn, F. and Forfar, J.O., 1972, Clinical and
    chemical correlates in convulsions of the newborn. The Lancet
    I: 135.

Dodge, P.R., 1971, Febrile convulsions, J. Pediat. 78: 1083.

Faero, O., Kastrup, K.W., Lykkegaard, E., Nielsen, J., Melchior, C.
    and Thorn, D., 1972, Successful prophylaxis of febrile con-
    vulsions with phenobarbital, Epilepsia 13: 271.

Fichsel, H. and Heyer, R., 1970, Carbamazepin in der behandlung
    kindlicher epilepsien, Deutsch. Med. Wschr. 47: 2367.

Forster, C., 1972, Antikonvulsive behandling mit dipropylessigsaure
    in kindesalter, Munch. Med. Wschr. 114: 399.

Gamstorp, I., 1970, Long-term follow-up of children with severe epi-
    lepsy treated with carbamazepine (Tegretol^R), Acta Pediat. Scand.
    206: 96.

Godin, J., Heiner, L., Mark, J. and Mandel, P., 1969, Effects of
    di-n-propylacetate, and anticonvulsive compound on GABA meta-
    bolism, J. Neurochem. 16: 869.

Graham, P. and Rutter, M., 1968, Organic brain dysfunction and child
    psychiatric disorders, Brit. Med. J. 3: 695.

Hagberg, B., Olow, I. and Hagberg, G., 1973, Decreasing incidence of
    low birth weight diplegia - an achievement of modern neonatal
    care, Acta. Pediat. Scand. 62: 192.

Harper, N.J., Simmonds, A.B., Wakama, W.T., Hall, G. and Vallance,
    D.K., 1966, Some basic ketones with central nervous system de-
    pressant activity, J. Pharm. Pharmac. 18: 150.

Huttenlocher, P.R., Wilborun, A.J. and Signore, B.S., 1971, Medium-chain triglycerides as a therapy for intractable childhood epilepsy, Neurology 21: 1097.

Keith, H., 1963, "Convulsive Disorders in Children", Little, Brown, Boston.

Lennox-Buchthal, M.A., 1972, Febrile convulsions, aspects of prevention, 8th Int'l Study Group on Child Neurology and Cerebral Palsy, Oxford.

Livingston, S., 1972, "Comprehensive Management of Epilepsy in Infancy, Childhood and Adolescence", Charles C Thomas, Springfield.

Marchal, C., Leveau, M., André, M., Gardia-Lang, M. and Costagliola, P., 1972, Traitment des souffrances cérébrales néo-natales, Pédiatrie 27: 709.

Metrakos, J.D. and Metrakos, K., 1960, Genetics of convulsive disorders I. Introduction, problems, methods and baselines, Neurology 10: 228.

Millichap, J.G., 1968, Definitions and statistics, in "Febrile Convulsions", p.11, The Macmillan Co., New York.

Nellhaus, G., 1971a, The ketogenic diet reconsidered: Correlation with the EEG. Abstract presented to the Am. Acad. of Neurology, New York.

Nellhaus, G., 1971b, Neuromuscular disorders, in "Current Pediatric Diagnosis and Treatment", pp. 496-497, Lange Med. Publications, Los Altos, California.

Scheffner, D. and Schiefer, I., 1972, The treatment of epileptic children with carbamazepine. Follow-up studies of clinical course and EEG. Epilepsia 13: 819.

Scollo-Lavizzari, G. and Corbat, F., 1970, A clinical note on a new anti-epileptic, "Depakine[R]", Europ. Neurol. 4: 312.

Spitzer, J.J. and Weng, J.T., 1972, Removal and Utilization of ketone bodies by the brain of newborn puppies, J. Neurochem. 19: 2169.

Taylor, D.C. and Ounsted, C., 1971, Biological mechanisms influencing the outcome of seizures in response to fever, Epilepsia 12: 33.

Uhlemann, E.R. and Neims, A.H., 1972, Anticonvulsant properties of the ketogenic diet in mice, J. Pharm. Exp. Therap. 180: 231.

van den Berg, B.J. and Yerushalmy, J., 1969, Studies on convulsive
     disorders in young children. I. Incidence of febrile and non-
     febrile convulsions by age and other factors, <u>Pediat. Res.</u> 3:
     298.

Wilder, R.M., 1921, The effect of ketonemia on course of epilepsy,
     <u>Mayo Clin. Bull.</u> 2: 307.

LIST OF INVITED PARTICIPANTS

JOSEPH ALTMAN   Laboratory of Developmental Neurobiology,
                              Department of Biological Sciences, Purdue
                              University, Lafayette, Indiana 47907

SAMUEL BARONDES   Department of Psychiatry, University of
                              California, San Diego, La Jolla, California
                              92037

STANELY M. CRAIN   Department of Physiology, Albert Einstein
                              College of Medicine, Yeshiva University,
                              Bronx, New York 10461

J. FOLCH-PI   McLean Hospital, Belmont, Massachusetts
                              02178

DONALD H. FORD   Department of Anatomy, State University of
                              New York, Downstate Medical Center,
                              Brooklyn, New York 11203

WILLIAMINA A. HIMWICH   Nebraska Psychiatric Institute, University
                              of Nebraska College of Medicine, Omaha,
                              Nebraska 68105

DOHERTY B. HUDSON   Department of Physiology-Anatomy,
                              University of California, Berkeley,
                              California 94720

CONRAD E. JOHANSON   Department of Pharmacology, College of
                              Medicine, University of Utah, Salt Lake
                              City, Utah 84112

ABEL LAJTHA   New York State Research Institute for
                               Neurochemistry and Drug Addiction, Ward's
                               Island, New York, New York 10035

J. GORDON MILLICHAP   720 North Michigan Avenue, Chicago,
                               Illinois 60611

BERNARD L. MIRKIN   Departments of Pediatrics and
                               Pharmacology, Division of Clinical
                               Pharmacology, College of Medicine,
                               University of Minnesota, Minneapolis,
                               Minnesota 55455

VELAYUHAN NAIR   Department of Pharmacology and
                               Therapeutics, The Chicago Medical School,
                               Chicago, Illinois 60612

GERHARD NELLHAUS   Departments of Pediatrics and Medicine,
                               University of Colorado School of Medicine,
                               Denver, Colorado 80220

JOHN W. OLNEY   Department of Psychiatry, Washington
                               University School of Medicine, St. Louis,
                               Missouri 63110

ALAN PETERS   Department of Anatomy, Boston University
                               School of Medicine, Boston, Massachusetts
                               02118

EVANGELOS A. PETROPOULOS Department of Physiology-Anatomy,
                               University of California, Berkeley,
                               California 94720

DOMINICK P. PURPURA   Department of Anatomy, Albert Einstein
                               College of Medicine, Yeshiva University,
                               Bronx, New York 10461

ELIZABETH R. EINSTEIN   Institute of Human Development,
                               University of California, Berkeley,
                               California   94720

C.O. RUTLEDGE   Department of Pharmacology, University of
                            Colorado School of Medicine, Denver,
                            Colorado 80220

SHELDON B. SPARBER   Department of Pharmacology, University of
                            Minnesota Medical School, Minneapolis,
                            Minnesota 55455

PAOLA S. TIMIRAS   Department of Physiology-Anatomy,
                            University of California, Berkeley,
                            California 94720

THEONY VALCANA   Department of Physiology-Anatomy,
                            University of California, Berkeley,
                            California 94720

ANTONIA VERNADAKIS   Department of Psychiatry and Pharmacology,
                            University of Colorado School of Medicine,
                            Denver, Colorado 80220

J.C. WAYMIRE   Department of Psychobiology, University
                            of California, Irvine, California 92664

NORMAN WEINER   Department of Pharmacology, University
                            of Colorado School of Medicine, Denver,
                            Colorado 80220

RICHARD E. WHALEN   Department of Psychobiology, University
                            of California, Irvine, California 92664

C.D. WITHROW   Department of Pharmacology, School of
                            Medicine, University of Utah, Salt Lake
                            City, Utah 84112

DIXON M. WOODBURY   Department of Pharmacology, School of
                            Medicine, University of Utah, Salt Lake
                            City, Utah 84112